AAAP Review of Addiction Psychiatry

Carla Marienfeld • Maryam Soltani
Editors

AAAP Review of Addiction Psychiatry

Clinical Practice and Board Preparation

Second Edition

Springer

American Academy *of* Addiction Psychiatry
Translating Science. Transforming Lives.

Editors
Carla Marienfeld
Department of Psychiatry
University of California San Diego
La Jolla, CA, USA

Maryam Soltani
Department of Psychiatry
University of California San Diego
La Jolla, CA, USA

ISBN 978-3-032-24173-3 ISBN 978-3-032-24174-0 (eBook)
https://doi.org/10.1007/978-3-032-24174-0

This Springer imprint is published by the registered company Springer Nature Switzerland AG
The registered company address is: Gewerbestrasse 11, 6330 Cham, Switzerland

Acknowledgments

The development of *AAAP Review of Addiction Psychiatry: Clinical Practice and Board Preparation* would not have been possible without the time and contributions of the members of American Academy of Addiction Psychiatry (AAAP)'s Board of Directors, Continuing Professional Development Committee, and staff. Thank you to the following individuals for reviewing this manuscript and providing formative feedback to drive its development and ensure the success of this endeavor.

2024–2025 AAAP Board of Directors
- John Mariani, MD
- Larissa Mooney, MD
- Kevin Sevarino, MD, PhD
- Tim Fong, MD
- Rebecca Payne, MD
- Kevin Gray, MD
- Carol Weiss, MD
- Jose Vito, MD
- Frances Levin, MD
- Jennifer Creedon, MD
- Alena Balasanova, MD
- Carla Marienfeld, MD
- Adina Bowe, MD
- Elie Aoun, MD
- Inbal Gafni, MD
- Alexis Ritvo, MD, MPH
- Thomas Kosten, MD
- Joseph Liberto, MD
- Lewei (Allison) Lin, MD
- David Lott, MD
- David Marcovitz, MD
- Sanchit Maruti, MD
- Ismene Petrakis, MD
- John Renner, MD
- Justine Welsh, MD
- Cornelius Stanciu, MD

- Laurence Westreich, MD
- Danae DiRocco, MD, MPH
- Stanley Nkemjika, MD, MPH
- Alfred Tager, MD, MPH

AAAP Continuing Professional Development Committee

- Carla Marienfeld, MD
- Subhadeep Barman, MD
- Nitigna Desai, MD
- William Hinds, MD
- Mary-Anne Kowol, MD
- Sonya Longest, MD
- Vanessa Loukas, MSN, FNP-C
- Nikhil Teja, MD
- Dave Cundiff, MD
- Joseph Bravoco, MD
- Poorvanshi Alag, MD
- Eversley Clarence, MD
- Markos Emmanouel, MD
- Elizabeth Guevara, MD
- Jolomi Ikomi, MD
- Jonathan Lee, MD
- Rebecca Payne, MD
- Kevin Sevarino, MD, PhD
- Shram Shukla, MD
- Cornelius Stanciu, MD
- Douglas Ziedonis, MD, MPH
- Andrew Bartholomew, BS, MD

AAAP Staff

- Kathryn Cates-Wessel, ED
- Michelle Dirst, AED
- Beth Welch

A special thank you to Kevin Sevarino, MD, PhD (Board of Directors, Continuing Professional Development Committee) and Poorvanshi Alag, MD (Continuing Professional Development Committee) for reviewing and providing feedback to several chapters—often at the last minute!

Contents

Contributors

Matthew P. Abrams Department of Psychiatry, University of California San Diego, La Jolla, CA, USA

Bachaar Arnaout Department of Psychiatry, Yale School of Medicine, New Haven, CT, USA

Jonathan Avery New York-Presbyterian Hospital, New York, NY, USA

Weill Cornell Medical College, New York, NY, USA

Leo Beletsky Department of Medicine, University of California San Diego, La Jolla, CA, USA

School of Law & Bouvé College of Health Sciences, Northeastern University, Boston, MA, USA

Katerina Christodoulides New York-Presbyterian Hospital, New York, NY, USA

Weill Cornell Medical College, New York, NY, USA

Hector A. Colon-Rivera Asociación Puertorriqueños en Marcha, Inc (APM), Philadelphia, PA, USA

UPMC Jameson Partial Hospitalization Program | Intensive Outpatient Program, New Castle, PA, USA

Intrinsic Me TM Psychiatry, Bluebell, PA, USA

Natasia S. Courchesne-Krak Department of Psychiatry, University of California San Diego, La Jolla, CA, USA

David Dadiomov University of Southern California Mann School of Pharmacy and Pharmaceutical Sciences, Los Angeles, CA, USA

Peter J. Davidson Department of Medicine, University of California San Diego, La Jolla, CA, USA

Joao P. De Aquino Department of Psychiatry, Yale School of Medicine, New Haven, CT, USA

Department of Psychiatry, West Haven Veteran Affairs, West Haven, CT, USA

Jeffrey J. DeVido Addiction Services, Behavioral Health and Recovery Services, Marin County California, Department of Health and Human Services, San Rafael, CA, USA

Behavioral Health Clinical Director, Partnership HealthPlan of California, Fairfield, CA, USA

Department of Psychiatry and Behavioral Sciences, Weill Institute for Neurosciences, University of California San Francisco, San Francisco, CA, USA

Charles Dike Department of Psychiatry, Yale University School of Medicine, New Haven, CT, USA

Javad J. Fatollahi Department of Psychiatry, University of California San Diego, La Jolla, CA, USA

Nafisa Ferdous San Diego State University, School of Social Work, Joint Doctoral Program in Interdisciplinary Research on Substance Use, San Diego, CA, USA

Thirdhand Smoke Resource Center, San Diego State University, San Diego, CA, USA

Kavita K. Fischer Community Care Behavioral Health, Pittsburgh, PA, USA

University of Pittsburgh School of Medicine, Pittsburgh, PA, USA

Natassia Gaznick Private Practice, Los Angeles, CA, USA

Katia M. Harlé Department of Psychiatry, University of California San Diego, La Jolla, CA, USA

VA San Diego Health System, La Jolla, CA, USA

Stephanie L. Hsia Department of Clinical Pharmacy, University of Southern California Alfred E. Mann School of Pharmacy and Pharmaceutical Sciences, Los Angeles, CA, USA

Theddeus Iheanacho Department of Psychiatry, Yale University School of Medicine, New Haven, CT, USA

Soohyun Joe Department of Psychiatry, University of California San Diego, La Jolla, CA, USA

Ayana Jordan Department of Psychiatry, New York University Grossman School of Medicine, New York, NY, USA

Kristopher A. Kast Vanderbilt University Medical Center, Nashville, TN, USA

Mashal Khan Department of Psychiatry, NewYork-Presbyterian Weill Cornell Medical Center, New York, NY, USA

Edwin Kim Federation of State Physician Health Programs, Mechanicsburg, PA, USA

Christine LaGrotta Department of Psychiatry, James J. Peters Bronx VA Hospital, Bronx, NY, USA

Eve Lasswell Department of Psychiatry, University of California San Diego, La Jolla, CA, USA

Jonathan C. Lee The Farley Center at Williamsburg Place, Williamsburg, VA, USA

Victor Manuel Magaña San Diego State University, School of Social Work, Joint Doctoral Program in Interdisciplinary Research on Substance Use, San Diego, CA, USA

Sanchit Maruti Department of Psychiatry, Larner College of Medicine, University of Vermont, Burlington, VT, USA

Aaron Meyer Department of Psychiatry, University of California San Diego, La Jolla, CA, USA

Stephanie A. Meyers-Pantele Division of Infectious Diseases and Global Public Health, University of California San Diego, La Jolla, CA, USA

María Luisa Mittal Department of Medicine, University of California San Diego, La Jolla, CA, USA

Justin Morales NYU School of Medicine, New York, NY, USA

Howard B. Moss Department of Psychiatry and Neuroscience, University of California at Riverside School of Medicine, Riverside, CA, USA

Julio C. Nunes Department of Psychiatry, Yale School of Medicine, New Haven, CT, USA

Department of Psychiatry, West Haven Veteran Affairs, West Haven, CT, USA

Ismene Petrakis Department of Psychiatry, Yale University School of Medicine, New Haven, CT, USA

VA Connecticut Healthcare System, West Haven, CT, USA

Angela Praecht Addictions Division, Centre for Addiction and Mental Health, Toronto, ON, Canada

Amutha Rajagopal Department of Medicine, Oregon Health and Science University, Portland, OR, USA

Ricardo Restrepo-Guzman Department of Psychiatry, Veterans Health Administration Long Beach, Long Beach, CA, USA

Department of Psychiatry, University of California Riverside, Riverside, CA, USA

Department of Psychiatry, Charles Drew University, Los Angeles, CA, USA

Sarah A. Rojas San Ysidro Health San Diego, San Diego, CA, USA

Roberto D. Sanchez Baylor College of Medicine, Houston, TX, USA

Abdo Semaan Department of Psychiatry, NewYork-Presbyterian Weill Cornell Medical Center, New York, NY, USA

Irshan Shaik BronxCare Health System, New York, NY, USA

Matthew E. Sloan Addictions Division, Centre for Addiction and Mental Health, Toronto, ON, Canada

Department of Psychiatry, Temerty Faculty of Medicine, University of Toronto, Toronto, ON, Canada

Maryam Soltani Department of Psychiatry, Veterans Health Administration San Diego, La Jolla, CA, USA

Department of Psychiatry, University of California San Diego, La Jolla, CA, USA

Kyle Street Department of Psychiatry, University of California San Diego, La Jolla, CA, USA

Anil Thomas Department of Psychiatry, NYU Grossman School of Medicine, New York, NY, USA

Louis Trevisan Yale University School of Medicine, New Haven, CT, USA

Marina Tsoy-Podosenin Catholic Health Services of Long Island, Long Island, NY, USA

Jose Vito NYU School of Medicine, New York, NY, USA

Robert B. Werner Department of Psychiatry, Yale University School of Medicine, New Haven, CT, USA

Stephanie Yarnell-MacGrory Department of Psychiatry, Yale University School of Medicine, New Haven, CT, USA

Penelope P. Ziegler Emerita Florida Professionals Resource Network, Fernandina Beach, FL, USA

María Luisa Zúñiga San Diego State University, School of Social Work, Joint Doctoral Program in Interdisciplinary Research on Substance Use, San Diego, CA, USA

Part I

Diagnosis, Treatment Modalities and Settings, and Recovery

Health Services for Addiction Treatment and Levels of Care

1

Howard B. Moss and Soohyun Joe

High-Yield Review Points

- Health services for substance use disorders are best addressed in a chronic disease model.
- Addiction treatment is provided along a continuum or levels of care treatment settings and intensities.
- The American Society of Addiction Medicine (ASAM) Criteria Level Assessment and the ASAM Criteria Treatment Planning Assessment are fundamental to the clinical matching of persons to the appropriate level of therapeutic services and then making a comprehensive treatment plan.
- Successful addiction treatment should address patient engagement, retention, and patient-centered outcomes.
- Fiscal and resource management is now an essential aspect of addiction treatment delivery.
- Treatment congruence with quality performance measures is likely to influence the future delivery of addiction treatment.

H. B. Moss (✉)
Department of Psychiatry and Neuroscience, University of California at Riverside School of Medicine, Riverside, CA, USA

S. Joe
Department of Psychiatry, University of California San Diego, La Jolla, CA, USA

C. Marienfeld, M. Soltani (eds.), *AAAP Review of Addiction Psychiatry*,
https://doi.org/10.1007/978-3-032-24174-0_1

Introduction

The Complexity of Health Services for Persons with Addictive Disorders

The status of the health services environment is central to the daily work of the addiction psychiatrist. It is about where we work, who people are, how we evaluate people, how people pay for our services, and how we get compensated for the work we do. All of this occurs within our political, technological, and sociocultural environment. Move from your town, city, county, state, or country to another venue, and the health services environment can be radically different. Likewise, moving to and from an academic medical center, a group practice, a community clinic, a veteran's hospital, or a private office will change the parameters of the health services you are providing. The diligent addiction psychiatrist needs to be aware and understand these complexities of care to best provide quality services to our patients.

What Do We Mean by Health Services?

Health services are the multidisciplinary factors such as treatment models, social factors, financing systems, organizational structures and processes, health technologies, and personal behaviors that affect access to healthcare, as well as the quality and cost of healthcare, and a patient's health and well-being. Health services for addictive disorders have changed over the past decades. We have new treatments, emerging public policies, evolving organizational structures, recent technologies, shifting social perceptions of our patients, innovative approaches to the funding of care, and new perspectives on the disorders we treat. It is a dynamic process requiring our ongoing attention and efforts to broaden the implementation of evidence-based practices and then educating and empowering providers to feel more confident in treating substance use disorders.

Health Services Research in Addiction Treatment

Health services research drives many of the policies and procedures in addiction treatment at the federal, state, and local levels. This applied health services research provides data, evidence, and tools to make addiction treatment affordable, safe, effective, equitable, accessible, and patient-centered. For example, products stemming from addiction health services research serve to enable providers and persons with substance use disorders to make better clinical decisions regarding treatment options, as well as informing public policy.

Key Concepts That Influence the Current Best Practices Treatment Models for Addictive Disorders

Addiction

According to the American Society of Addiction Medicine (ASAM), addiction is a treatable, chronic medical disease involving complex interactions among brain circuits, genetics, the environment and an individual's life experiences. People with addiction use substances or engage in behaviors that become compulsive and often continue despite harmful consequences. Prevention efforts and treatment approaches for addiction are generally as successful as those for other chronic diseases.

Addiction as a Chronic Disease

In the past, physicians, policymakers, persons with substance use disorders, and families have supposed or expected that people entering addiction treatment should be "cured" and able to maintain lifelong abstinence or recovery following a single episode of specialized treatment. When a single episode is ineffective, it is not unusual for these same individuals to become discouraged when a relapse occurs. Yet Dennis and others [1] have shown that more than half the people entering publicly funded addiction programs require multiple episodes of treatment over several years to achieve and sustain recovery. The clinical course of many people is marked by cycles of recovery, relapse, and repeated treatments, which may span many years before resulting in the goal of long-term recovery. The presence of co-occurring psychiatric and medical disorders further complicates the trajectory. Persons who have co-occurring psychiatric disorders are more likely to experience difficulties with treatment and medication adherence, and they experience shorter treatment episodes or leave treatment against medical advice. In addition, individuals may be administratively discharged, experience compromised functional status, have difficulties adjusting to their communities, or have reduced quality of life resulting in poorer outcomes [1]. Thus, it has become increasingly clear that addiction should be viewed as a chronic, rather than acute condition, and that the treating addiction psychiatrist, particularly when managing patients with significant psychiatric comorbidity, needs to appreciate the cyclical and chronic nature of the disorder and maintain appropriate expectations and resources. The contemporary perspective is to view substance use disorders more like chronic diseases such as hypertension or diabetes rather than acute conditions like pneumonia [2]. New models of addiction treatment now accommodate the natural history of the disorder, and policymakers are beginning to follow suit, allowing for more appropriate treatment and better outcomes.

The Continuum of Care

- The concept of a continuum of care has been applied as a central concept in the management of a wide variety of disorders and conditions that require caregiving. The World Health Organization (WHO) highlights the following dimensions of a continuum of care:
- *Integrated and coordinated services*: This refers to a "place and approach" dimension that emphasizes a comprehensive system where different levels and types of care work together seamlessly. This includes various settings (community, hospital, specialized clinics) and approaches (prevention, treatment, rehabilitation, palliative care).
- *Continuity of care*: This relates to the dimension of "timing" of care, stressing uninterrupted care over time and across different life stages. It involves smooth transitions between services and ongoing support to meet evolving needs. WHO's focus is on ensuring that health systems provide a range of services that are:
- *Accessible Care*: Available, affordable, and acceptable to everyone.
- *Equitable Care*: Fairly distributed, meeting the needs of the most vulnerable.
- *Comprehensive Care*: Covering all levels of care, from health promotion and prevention to treatment and rehabilitation. Quality: Safe, effective, people-centered.

Clinical Matching of Persons with Substance Use Disorders to Therapeutic Services

For many decades, it has been recognized that persons with addictive disorders, despite similarities in diagnoses, have their own complex pattern of psychiatric, psychological, medical, legal, social, and family problems that can impact their success in treatment. Thus, not all people will respond to the specifics of a single unitary type of treatment program. Consequently, there has been substantial effort directed toward the matching of the patient's clinical presentation and needs to treatment program content or program services within the continuum of care [3].

By determining the specific treatment needs of a patient that are addressed by a given therapeutic program and then assigning a patient with those needs to that program, it is hoped that there will be an improvement in the overall level of treatment success. Importantly, this strategy emphasizes the conduct of a *systematic clinical assessment* to be used for initial treatment placement recommendations or for the determination of continuing care needs. Structured and focused clinical assessments such as the Level of Care Utilization System (LOCUS) [4] and the Addiction Severity Index (ASI) [5] have successfully been used for this purpose, and the multidimensional clinical evaluation system offered by the ASAM Criteria [6] (below) is now widely employed and accepted in the determination of treatment level recommendations along the continuum of care. Thus, much of our current system of addiction treatment services relies upon the quality of the initial multidimensional clinical assessment and the serial clinical assessments during the treatment process.

The ASAM (American Society of Addiction Medicine) Criteria [6] uses six dimensions to assess and determine the appropriate level of care for individuals with substance use disorders. These dimensions are:

1. *Acute intoxication and/or withdrawal potential*: Evaluates the immediate risk of severe withdrawal symptoms or intoxication.
2. *Biomedical conditions and complications*: Assesses medical conditions that may affect treatment.
3. *Emotional, behavioral, or cognitive conditions and complications*: Considers mental health issues and cognitive impairments.
4. *Readiness to change*: Measures the individual's willingness and ability to engage in treatment.
5. *Relapse, continued use, or continued problem potential*: Evaluates the risk of relapse or continued substance use.
6. *Recovery environment*: Looks at the individual's living situation and support network.

These dimensions help create a comprehensive, holistic assessment of the patient's needs, guiding the selection of the most appropriate treatment levels.

Patient Engagement and Retention

One of the most critical tasks for an effective drug and alcohol treatment program, clinic, or office-based practice is to encourage persons with substance use disorders to enter and remain in treatment. Retention in treatment is an important outcome that is linked with other beneficial outcomes for persons with substance use disorders [7]. Unfortunately, evidence has shown that many persons either fail to attend their first treatment session or drop out of treatment after attending only a few sessions. To improve entry and retention, efforts have been directed toward an examination of the process by which persons are referred to treatment, attend their first session, and continue in accordance with the treatment plan. In recognition of this need, SAMHSA's Center for Substance Abuse Treatment (CSAT), in partnership with the Addiction Technology Transfer Center Network (ATTC Network), and the Robert Wood Johnson Foundation and academic partners have developed the Network for Improvement in Addiction Treatment or NIATx program. This program teaches drug and alcohol treatment centers and providers how to use process improvement strategies to improve access to and retention in quality addiction treatment [8]. The specific aims of this program are to reduce waiting times between the first request for service and the first treatment session, reduce the number of persons who do not keep an appointment, increase admissions to treatment, and increase continuation in treatment with a focus on the first through the fourth treatment sessions. Evaluations of this program have been quite positive [9], yet there remain many addiction professionals who are unaware of its existence or its utility.

Health Insurance, Managed Care, Parity, and Federal and State Financing for Addiction Treatment Services

The concept of *health insurance* in the United States began over concerns for payment during the economic downturn of the Great Depression of the 1930s. Thirty-five years later, *Medicare* was introduced as government-sponsored health insurance to provide coverage to older and retired Americans. By the 1980s, spiraling healthcare costs prompted the emergence of what we now think of as *managed care,* which was an effort to employ greater fiscal responsibility in the allocation and payment for healthcare resources. Managed care introduced price competition by encouraging insurance companies to selectively contract for services such as addiction treatment and mental health services, and award contracts to the most economical providers. By the 2000s, efforts began to control costs by encouraging insured individuals to pay more out-of-pocket using high-deductible health plans. This shift in responsibility for the payment of healthcare services to the person disproportionately affected individuals from lower socioeconomic strata and those with limited health insurance benefits, ultimately prompting the passage of the *Patient Protection and Affordable Care Act* (ACA) in 2010.

The early 2000s also showed an organizational shift to *integrated healthcare delivery systems* from hospital-based "vertical" systems of care. In an integrated healthcare delivery system, a single organization, or a closely aligned group of organizations, offers a broad range of patient care and support services in a unified manner. However, many of the early integrated healthcare systems avoided incorporating addiction or mental health treatment in their menu of services. The primary argument against providing addiction and mental health treatment was the fear that the cost to third-party payers would be too high, and the outcomes too variable. Many doubted the practicality of requiring insurance providers to cover the costs of parity of substance use and mental health treatment services with medical and surgical treatment despite the scientific evidence supporting the benefits of doing so. Key studies conducted by the Substance Abuse and Mental Health Services Administration (SAMHSA) and the RAND Corporation showed that the costs of parity for addiction and mental health treatment are relatively small and that the demonstrable benefits to individuals, employers, and society are highly significant. Consequently, Congress enacted the *Mental Health Parity and Addiction Equity Act* (MHPAEA) of 2008, which now requires health insurers and group health plans to provide the same level of benefits for mental health and/or substance use treatment and services as they do for medical/surgical care. The Affordable Care Act (ACA) further expands the MHPAEA's requirements by ensuring that qualified plans offered cover many behavioral health treatments and services. Specifically, it creates an "essential health benefit" or mandated benefit for the coverage of mental health and substance use disorder services in several specific insurance financing arrangements.

States also have a significant role in the financing of addiction treatment. *Medicaid* is a Federal/State partnership with shared authority and financing. It is a health insurance program for low-income individuals and people with disabilities. Participation is optional, although all 50 states participate in the Medicaid program to a greater or lesser extent. However, eligibility for specific Medicaid benefits such as those for addiction and/or mental health treatment varies widely among the states. Currently, the Centers for Medicare and Medicaid Services (CMS) supports a voluntary expansion of *Medicaid* addiction treatment services through a mechanism called Section 1115 demonstration projects that allows states to test innovative policy and treatment delivery for substance use disorders.

Treatment Settings and Levels of Care for Those with Addictive Disorders

The addiction psychiatrist practices in a variety of treatment settings ranging from dedicated addiction treatment programs to general psychiatric and medical/psychiatric specialty venues. The current standardized definitions of the levels of care for addiction treatment cross-cut specialized addiction, psychiatric, medical, and specialty clinical settings. For the practitioner, these defined treatment settings have significant clinical ramifications in terms of appropriateness and availability of treatment type given the individual's clinical needs, established criteria for entry into a given type of treatment, the intensity and duration of treatment, and the financing and reimbursement for the treatments provided. For the program administrator in the managed care environment, these defined treatment settings provide a framework of programmatic standards to assess needs, offer a mechanism to establish and maintain program content, provide a context for program policies and procedures, and compare service coverage with other providers in other venues.

Standardized Levels of Care in Addiction Treatment

The current conceptualization of levels of care for addiction treatment was developed and is best exemplified by the American Society for Addiction Medicine (ASAM) Criteria [6]. The ASAM Criteria provide an integrated crosswalk of individual characteristics with appropriate levels of care and intensity along the continuum of care, matching clinical needs and characteristics with the appropriate treatment services to manage those needs and behaviors. A more detailed explanation of the matching of characteristics to a given level of care is available from ASAM [6]. The ASAM criteria have been examined rigorously in terms of their predictive validity for resource utilization and patient outcomes (e.g., [10]). As a result, commercial health insurers recognized the utility of this system of levels of addiction treatment and criteria for entry into a given level of care and began adopting these criteria for both resource management and placement.

The passage of the ACA's Medicaid Expansion stimulated the creation of the Medicaid Innovation Accelerator Program (IAP) as a demonstration project to ensure that addiction treatment is delivered consistently with industry standards. This program employs the ASAM levels of care and criteria because they have become the industry standard, and Medicaid is utilizing these criteria in hopes that beneficiaries will receive the most appropriate addiction treatment services given their clinical needs [11]. It is important to note that not all localities have all these levels of care available, despite encouragement by Medicaid agencies.

The ASAM/Medicaid Adult Levels of Care The ASAM Criteria outlines a structured approach to addiction treatment, providing two key assessments: the Level of Care assessment and the Treatment Planning assessment. The Level of Care assessment determines the most appropriate care level for a person by considering biomedical, psychological, and sociocultural factors. The Treatment Planning assessment then utilizes this information to develop a comprehensive treatment plan. Both assessments are multidimensional, ensuring a holistic and patient-centered approach to care [6].

Addiction treatment is organized into various levels to address the diverse needs of persons with substance use disorders. The ASAM Criteria categorizes these levels into four main groups, with sublevels defining the intensity and type of care provided. Understanding the services, supervision, and staffing requirements for each level is essential for effective treatment planning and delivery. Persons with substance use disorders are continually reassessed throughout their treatment to ensure they receive the most appropriate level of care recommendation, whether more intensive, less intensive, or consistent with their current needs.

Level 1: Outpatient Services

- *Level 1.0—Long-term remission monitoring:*
  Designed for persons who are in sustained remission from substance use disorders (SUDs), Level 1.0 is based on a chronic care model, which anticipates periods of remission and potential recurrence. This level emphasizes regular check-ins and early interventions to maintain therapeutic relationships, with the primary goal of ensuring quarterly checkups to facilitate rapid reengagement in treatment if necessary. Services are flexible and can be provided in various settings, making them accessible. Recovery management checkups, including biopsychosocial screening and assessment, are crucial at this level to identify current or emerging treatment needs.
- *Level 1.5—Outpatient:*
  This level serves medically managed outpatient care focused on withdrawal management and biomedical services. Offering less than 9 h per week of clinical services, it is designed for persons who require medical oversight but can be treated in an outpatient setting. Key services include vital sign monitoring, glucose monitoring, basic first aid, AED availability, wound care, injectable epinephrine, naloxone, and point-of-care pregnancy testing. Outpatient individual and group therapy treatment can be included at this level, at frequencies commensurate with need and availability, typically ranging from weekly to monthly. A medical director oversees this level, supported by clinical staff, including

nurses, therapists, and advanced practice providers, who are available during clinic hours. This level is ideal for persons needing ongoing medical management while remaining in their communities.

Level 2: Intensive Outpatient and High-intensity Outpatient Services

- *Level 2.1—Intensive outpatient treatment:*
  Level 2.1 supplies 9–19 h per week of direct psychosocial services. It is intended for persons needing more structured support than outpatient therapy but not requiring 24-h supervision. Services typically include counseling, psychoeducation, and group therapy, delivered by a program director and allied health staff. This level helps persons develop skills and strategies to manage their recovery while living in their community.
- *Level 2.5—High-intensity outpatient treatment:*
  Providing 20 or more hours per week of intensive outpatient services, Level 2.5 is designed for persons who require high-intensity services but do not need 24-h residential care. This level often includes a medical director, program director, and allied health staff to provide comprehensive care. The focus is on intensive psychotherapy and psychosocial interventions to address complex treatment needs.
  Level 2.7—Medically managed intensive outpatient treatment:
  Similar to Level 2.5, Level 2.7 includes additional direct withdrawal management and biomedical services, with nursing and medical oversight as integral components. It is suitable for persons stepping down from medically managed care or those needing extended nurse monitoring. Level 2.7 programs are led by a medical director, typically specializing in addiction medicine, with medical staff available during program hours and on-call 24/7. Clinical staff, including a program director, may be on staff or affiliated with the program. These programs provide medical management of intoxication and withdrawal, as well as care for biomedical and psychiatric comorbidities. Additional capabilities include echocardiograms, vaccine administration, and phlebotomy services.

Level 3: Residential Services

- *Level 3.1—Clinically managed low-intensity residential treatment:*
  This level offers 9–19 h per week of direct psychosocial services in a residential setting, providing a therapeutic environment with 24-h structure and support. It is ideal for individuals who need a stable, structured environment to support their recovery.
- *Level 3.5—Clinically managed high-intensity residential treatment:*
  Level 3.5 provides 20 or more hours per week of high-intensity psychosocial services with 24-h supervision by direct staff. It includes comprehensive care

provided by a medical director, physicians, nursing staff, and allied health staff. This level is for persons with significant treatment needs who require constant supervision in a residential setting.

- *Level 3.7—Medically managed residential treatment:*
  This level offers 24-h supervision with comprehensive medical and psychiatric management, including direct withdrawal management and biomedical services. Staffed by board-certified addiction specialists and 24/7 nursing, Level 3.7 is suitable for persons with complex medical and psychiatric needs requiring intensive, round-the-clock care.
  Level 3.7 BIO—Biomedically enhanced residential treatment:
  In addition to the services provided at Level 3.7, Level 3.7 BIO offers intravenous fluids, medications, and advanced wound care, facilitating the transition from acute care to sustained addiction treatment. It is ideal for persons with severe medical conditions needing specialized biomedical interventions alongside addiction treatment.

Level 4: Medically Managed Inpatient Treatment

- *Level 4—Addiction specialty unit:*
  Level 4 provides the highest intensity of care, with 24-h supervision in addiction specialty units within acute care hospitals. It includes comprehensive medical, psychiatric, and psychosocial services, making it suitable for persons with severe addiction and co-occurring conditions.
- *Level 4—General hospitals:*
  These hospital services should collaborate with addiction specialists to manage intoxication, withdrawal, and SUD, ensuring that persons receive appropriate ongoing addiction management.
- *Level 4—Psychiatric care:*
  Designed for persons with co-occurring SUD and severe psychiatric disorders, this level integrates mental health and addiction treatment to provide comprehensive care.

Recovery Residences

The ASAM Criteria may recommend recovery residences in addition to outpatient care based on a comprehensive assessment of the patient's needs. These residences provide a structured, substance-free environment that supports long-term recovery, complementing outpatient treatment services.

Program Management and Integration

- *Clinically managed programs:*
  Levels x.1 and x.5 programs are led by clinical staff and focus on counseling and psychoeducation, with varying levels of intensity.
- *Medically managed programs:*
  Levels x.7 programs are overseen by medical staff, focusing on withdrawal management and biomedical services, including medications for addiction treatment, with integrated psychosocial support.
- *Mental health integration:*
  Mental health care is integrated across all levels of care, with specialized programs for persons with severe psychiatric concerns.
- *Withdrawal management and biomedical services:*
  Integrated into medically managed levels, these services provide comprehensive treatment for intoxication, withdrawal, medications for addiction treatment, and co-occurring medical conditions.
- *Medical oversight and coordination of care:*
  Medical directors are essential at every level, with specific responsibilities that vary according to the care's intensity. Effective care coordination involves blending medical, psychiatric, and psychosocial services to provide well-rounded treatment. This approach includes specialized services such as referral systems for medical, psychiatric, cognitive care, and laboratory testing, ensuring persons receive all the necessary care.

Transitions and Continued Service

Persons are regularly reassessed throughout treatment, ensuring that their care level is adjusted as needed based on their progress. This continuous reassessment informs the treatment plan and helps ensure that individuals receive the appropriate level of care throughout their recovery journey.

Levels of Care for Adolescent Treatment

It is well-recognized that the manifestations of addictive disorders and the treatment needs of adolescents may not be congruent with those for adults. The biopsychosocial environment for adolescents is quite different from that of adults, and the factors that bring adolescents into treatment and their responses to treatment are frequently quite different from adults. In recognition of these differences, the most recent version of the ASAM criteria [6], and the ASAM/Medicaid criteria, has incorporated specific matching criteria for the level of care, the appropriateness of treatment venues (e.g., school-based clinics, after-school and weekend treatment programming), and the intensity of treatments based upon the best evidence of the needs of the adolescent patient.

Quality Performance Measures and Health Services for Addictive Disorders

Providers, persons, and payers are increasingly emphasizing the measurement of value and performance in the delivery of health services. Consequently, the treatment of addictive disorders is the focus of quality and performance scrutiny, and the development of suitable measures of quality performance is underway. The most advanced of these measures is derived from ASAM's Standards of Care for the Addiction Specialist Physician [11]. Currently, nine specific performance measures have been developed by ASAM for the treatment of alcohol use disorders and opioid use disorders [12]. These measures are:

- *MEASURE #1*: Percent of patients prescribed a medication for alcohol use disorder (AUD)
- *MEASURE #2*: Percent of patients prescribed a medication for opioid use disorder (OUD)
- *MEASURE #3*: Number of patients receiving a 7-day follow-up visit after withdrawal management
- *MEASURE #4*: Presence of screening for psychiatric disorder
- *MEASURE #5:* Presence of screening for tobacco use disorder
- *MEASURE #6:* Number of patients receiving primary care visit follow-ups within 6 months of treatment initiation
- *MEASURE #7:* All cause inpatient, residential re-admission following initial treatment episode
- *MEASURE #8*: The presence of SUD diagnosis documentation in addiction treatment regardless of setting
- *MEASURE #9*: Number of psychiatric disorder diagnoses present

Medicaid and several commercial health insurers are testing the utility of these ASAM quality performance measures to determine their acceptability, feasibility, and informativeness. While these and other quality performance indicators are not yet a part of our current practice requirements, such measures are soon likely to have a significant role in the practice of addiction psychiatry.

Chapter Review Questions

Part I: JB, a 39-year-old salesman, has a longstanding history of heavy alcohol use that began during his teenage years. Following the recent loss of his job, his drinking escalated to daily heavy consumption, which he struggled to control. During a routine physical exam, lab results revealed significantly elevated AST and ALT levels, prompting his primary care physician (PCP) to assess him for alcohol use disorder using the Michigan Alcoholism Screening Test (MAST). JB tested positive for alcohol use disorder, leading his PCP to discuss his drinking habits and recommend reducing his alcohol intake.

Initially resistant to the idea of change, JB denied any issue with alcohol. However, after multiple motivational interviewing sessions with his PCP, he recognized the need to address his drinking. When JB attempted to quit alcohol entirely, he experienced severe withdrawal symptoms, including intense anxiety, tremors, and profuse sweating. Feeling overwhelmed, he went to the emergency department but left before being seen due to discomfort in the waiting area. His symptoms subsided only after consuming three shots of alcohol. Eventually, JB reached out to his PCP to describe the incident. Although he expressed doubts about the effectiveness of treatment, he agreed to be referred for an intake evaluation at a local substance use treatment facility.

1. What is the purpose of the intake evaluation?

   A. To verify if JB has any outstanding legal issues
   B. To establish the most suitable level of care for JB's treatment
   C. To introduce JB to the treatment program's team
   D. To alleviate the primary care physician's workload
   E. To determine whether JB has healthcare insurance

   Best Answer: B. To establish the most suitable level of care for JB's treatment
   Explanation: The intake evaluation involves a comprehensive multidimensional assessment to determine the level of care that best aligns with JB's clinical needs.

2. Which of the following was most influential in determining JB's initial level of care?

   A. His choice of alcoholic beverages
   B. His problematic work performance
   C. His acute alcohol withdrawal symptoms
   D. His transaminitis
   E. His denial of drinking problems.

   Best Answer: C. His experiences with alcohol withdrawal symptoms
   Explanation: According to the ASAM/Medicaid criteria, the risk of withdrawal symptoms is a key factor in deciding whether a patient needs more intensive medical monitoring or inpatient care.

   Part II. JB was admitted to a medically supervised residential treatment program at ASAM Level 3.7. Over the first 5 days, his moderate alcohol withdrawal symptoms were successfully managed by the medical team. After a week, JB started participating in group discussions and therapy sessions. Despite his abstinence from alcohol, his mood remained persistently low, and he was diagnosed with major depressive disorder. The program physician initiated a trial of antidepressant medication, and the treatment team continued to monitor JB for other potential clinical concerns. Alongside these evaluations, the team began planning his discharge, recommending that he transition to an Intensive Outpatient Program within the same community addiction treatment network upon completing his residential stay.

3. ASAM Standards of Good Clinical Practice in addiction treatment suggest that persons should be evaluated for which of the following?

   A. Tobacco use disorder
   B. Pharmacogenetic metabolic status
   C. Needs for transportation and housing
   D. Need for marital or couple's therapy
   E. Employment and financial situation

   Best Answer: A. Tobacco use disorder

   Explanation: The ASAM's Standards of Care for Addiction Specialist Physicians highlight the importance of screening for tobacco use disorder as a key quality performance measure in addiction treatment.

4. What does JB's transition from a residential treatment program to an Intensive Outpatient Program reflect?

   A. His inadequate response to the initial treatment
   B. The availability of an appropriate step-down level of care in the continuum of care
   C. Concerns about the affordability of the residential program
   D. Potential for conflicts with other persons
   E. Persistent depressive symptoms

   Best Answer: B. The availability of an appropriate step-down level of care in the continuum of care

   Explanation: The "continuum of care" in addiction treatment refers to a flexible treatment approach where persons start at the level of care appropriate to their needs and then progress to more or less intensive treatment, as necessary. JB's move to an Intensive Outpatient Program indicates a step to a less intensive level of care, reflecting this continuum.

References

1. Dennis M, Scott CK. Managing addiction as a chronic condition. Addict Sci Clin Pract. 2007;4(1):45–55.
2. McLellan AT, Lewis DC, O'Brien CP, Kleber HD. Drug dependence, a chronic medical illness: implications for treatment, insurance, and outcomes evaluation. JAMA. 2000;284(13):1689–95.
3. McLellan AT, Woody GE, Luborsky L, O'Brien CP, Druley KA. Increased effectiveness of substance abuse treatment. A prospective study of patient-treatment "matching". J Nerv Ment Dis. 1983;171(10):597–605.
4. Sowers W, Pumariega A, Huffine C, Fallon T. Level-of-care decision making in behavioral health services: the LOCUS and the CALOCUS. Psychiatr Serv. 2003;54(11):1461–3.
5. McLellan AT, Kushner H, Metzger D, Peters R, Smith I, Grissom G, et al. The fifth edition of the addiction severity index. J Subst Abus Treat. 1992;9(3):199–213.
6. Waller RC, Boyle MP, Daviss SR, et al., editors. The ASAM criteria: treatment criteria for addictive, substance-related, and co-occurring conditions, volume 1: adults. 4th ed. Hazelden Publishing; 2023.

7. Hser YI, et al. Relationship between drug treatment services, retention, and outcomes. Psychiatr Serv. 2004;55(7):767–74.
8. Hoffman KA, Green CA, Ford JH II, Wisdom JP, Gustafson DH, McCarty D. Improving quality of care in substance abuse treatment using five key process improvement principles. J Behav Health Serv Res. 2012;39(3):234–44.
9. Rutkowski BA, Gallon S, Rawson RA, Freese TE, Bruehl A, Crèvecoeur-MacPhail D, et al. Improving client engagement and retention in treatment: the Los Angeles County experience. J Subst Abus Treat. 2010;39(1):78–86.
10. Sharon E, Krebs C, Turner W, Desai N, Binus G, Penk W, et al. Predictive validity of the ASAM patient placement criteria for hospital utilization. J Addict Dis. 2003;22(Suppl 1):79–93.
11. C.M.S. Overview of substance use disorder (SUD) care clinical guidelines: a resource for states developing SUD delivery system reforms [PDF]. Washington, DC: U.S. Department of Health and Human Services; 2017. [updated 04/2017; cited 2018]. Available from: https://www.medicaid.gov/state-resource-center/innovation-accelerator-program/iap-downloads/reducing-substance-use-disorders/asam-resource-guide.pdf.
12. (ASAM) ASAM. Standards of care for the addiction specialist physician. 2014. Available from: https://www.asam.org/docs/default-source/publications/standards-of-care-final-design-document.pdf.

Laboratory Testing for Substance Use Disorders

2

David Dadiomov and Kyle Street

High-Yield Review Points

- Drug screening interpretation can be highly affected by patient-specific factors such as time since last use, metabolism, genetics, age, and weight.
- Knowledge of drug-specific factors such as half-life, tissue binding, and metabolism can help the clinician properly interpret a drug screening result.
- A thorough and accurate patient history is necessary prior to drug screening to interpret possible false-positives or negatives.
- Certain medications require baseline medical laboratory testing, which should be conducted and followed to ensure safe use.

Introduction

Laboratory drug testing is an important tool utilized by clinicians for the comprehensive assessment of patients with substance use disorders. Drug screening, typically using immunoassay tests on urine samples, gives a clinician objective evidence regarding the presence of various substances or metabolites with which inferences can be made about consumption of substances. Drug screens may be commonly utilized in nonmedical settings (such as for employment or legal purposes);

D. Dadiomov (✉)
University of Southern California Mann School of Pharmacy and Pharmaceutical Sciences, Los Angeles, CA, USA
e-mail: dadiomov@usc.edu

K. Street
Department of Psychiatry, University of California San Diego, La Jolla, CA, USA
e-mail: kyle.street@va.gov

C. Marienfeld, M. Soltani (eds.), *AAAP Review of Addiction Psychiatry*,
https://doi.org/10.1007/978-3-032-24174-0_2

however, it is important to discern these tests from those utilized in clinical practice. In the employment setting, false positives may carry severe implications, and thus, detection limits for these are often higher. When drug testing is done for legal purposes, there are often significant consequences with results, and there are specific cutoff points that are defined. These samples should follow clear chain-of-custody processes. In the clinical setting, many factors may impact the result of a drug screen and knowledge and understanding of the nuance is warranted when ordering and interpreting laboratory drug screen results.

Due in part to the societal stigma associated with drug screening, patients may have concerns that should be addressed. The reason for laboratory testing should be communicated, and both the patient and provider should have an agreement or understanding about how and why drug screens are conducted. Broadly speaking, they are commonly used for external accountability for substance use, as well as for providing the clinician with medical information for use in safety and treatment considerations. For example, understanding what substances may be in a person's system can inform acute management for intoxication or withdrawal states, as well as considerations for longer-term treatment and medication management. In general, testing should be conducted in accordance with the patient's pattern of use, their stage in the recovery process, the substances used, and any practical considerations (such as transportation and schedule). This chapter will discuss the fundamentals of testing across different clinical scenarios.

Prior to interpreting drug screens, it is imperative that the clinician attempt to obtain a thorough history of all products a patient has used and the time of last use. This medication history should include all licit, illicit, over-the-counter, and herbal products the patient may be using. Effective interviewing techniques (such as utilizing open-ended questions and a non-judgmental stance) should be employed to elicit an accurate history. Many substances have the potential to be detected as false positives; these instances can be excluded if known. In addition, substances can vary significantly in their pharmacokinetic properties, and the timing of last use can help a clinician properly interpret results.

Principles of Laboratory Testing

Laboratory screening in substance use disorders (SUD) can be conducted for two major purposes: either to assess the safety of a given medication and conduct general medical testing or to assess the presence of substances or their metabolites. When conducting general medical testing, typically clinicians may obtain baseline labs to ensure a patient doesn't have a contraindication to a particular therapy (e.g., renal or hepatic impairment), as well as monitoring for laboratory abnormalities potentially caused by the medication or other substances. In contrast, when conducting drug screening, the primary goal may be to assess that the patient is adherent to their prescribed regimen. It may also serve to assess whether a patient is diverting the medication or utilizing other substances. This chapter will focus primarily on drug screening; however, other elements of laboratory testing will be discussed when relevant.

A variety of drug screening tools are currently available to clinicians. Likely the most familiar of these tests will be immunoassay tests. These are commonly "dip-stick" or cup-based urine tests, sometimes called point-of-care tests, which can be used for initial screening; however, they have lower sensitivity and specificity than confirmatory or laboratory tests via liquid chromatography/mass spectrometry (LC/Dual MS). Immunoassays, often called a screening test, are biochemical test that measures the presence or concentration of a molecule in a solution using an antibody or antigen. Alternatively, liquid chromatography/mass spectrometry (LC/Dual MS), often called confirmatory or definitive testing, combines liquid chromatography with mass spectrometry to analyze volatile compounds. This works by chromatography, first separating components in a liquid phase, followed by mass spectrometry, identifying them by mass-charge ratio. Immunoassays are limited by their qualitative nature and higher proportion of false-positive and false-negative test results compared to the quantitative LC/Dual MS tests. Urine immunoassays typically have a threshold, above which a specimen is positive. In many settings, an immunoassay is used as a preliminary tool. If the test returns positive, it can be sent for further confirmatory testing [1]. Despite several disadvantages, urine immunoassays are typically quick and easy to conduct and are inexpensive. Often immunoassays may be employed as a cost-saving tool when a high level of precision is not needed.

It is important for clinicians in addiction psychiatry to be aware of the detection limits of any test they are employing for clinical decision-making. The average detection limit for urine immunoassays tends to be relatively high to minimize the occurrence of false positives. There are a set of mandatory federal guidelines for workplace urine drug screening, which includes both initial cutoff levels used for screening and definitive cutoff levels used for confirmatory testing (Table 2.1) [2]. The Department of Health and Human Services (HHS) previously provided a

Table 2.1 Federal urine drug screening cutoffs [2, 3]

Substance	Initial cutoff value	Definitive cutoff value	Typical urine detection window
Marijuana (Δ9THC)	50 ng/mL	15 ng/mL	Single use—2–3 days Moderate use—5–7 days Chronic use—>30 days
Cocaine (benzoylecgonine)	150 ng/mL	100 ng/mL	3 days
Codeine/morphine	2000 ng/mL	2000 ng/mL	2 days
Hydrocodone/hydromorphone	300 ng/mL	100 ng/mL	3 days
Oxycodone/oxymorphone	100 ng/mL	100 ng/mL	3 days
6-Acetylmorphine (heroin metabolite)	10 ng/mL	10 ng/mL	2 days
Phencyclidine	25 ng/mL	25 ng/mL	8 days
Fentanyl/norfentanyl[a]	1 ng/mL (fentanyl)	1 ng/mL (norfentanyl)	3 days
Amphetamine/methamphetamine	500 ng/mL	250 ng/mL	2 days
MDMA/MDA	500 ng/mL	250 ng/mL	2 days

[a]A fentanyl immunoassay must have at least 5% cross reactivity to norfentanyl

standard guideline for workplace drug screening known as the "standard 5-panel drug test." However, after the HHS issued a rule in January 2025 adding fentanyl and its metabolite norfentanyl to the mandatory drug testing panels, federal workplaces began testing for fentanyl in 07/07/2025. The current panel includes screening for marijuana, cocaine, phencyclidine (PCP), amphetamines, hydrocodone/hydromorphone, oxycodone/oxymorphone and fentanyl/norfentanyl. As discussed further in this chapter, there are limitations to specific substances that can be detected on the standard drug screen [2, 3].

Within addiction psychiatry, however, obtaining quantitative tests may be of greater clinical utility. With standard immunoassays, a patient's sample may be falsely negative for a variety of reasons including genotypic metabolism differences, a subthreshold positive result, or the particular substance or metabolite is not detected [1]. Furthermore, urine immunoassays may have false positives and false negatives that limit their utility in addiction settings. A false-positive test may be the result of a substance used that has a similar chemical structure to the assayed chemical and thus shows up as a positive result. Agents that can cross-react for a false-positive test include prescribed medications, herbal supplements, and food products.

Clinicians also have a variety of sampling methods for drug screenings (Table 2.2). The most utilized are urine, blood, hair, nail, and breath tests. Urine tests are the most employed due to their relative ease of collection and good detection window for most substances or their metabolites. Blood sampling may be more useful for detecting acute intoxication as it has a shorter detection window and can be more sensitive. Conducting hair and nail testing leads to the longest detection window; however, there is also a delay for the substance to appear in the sample after use, and there are specific guidelines about how to collect hair and nail samples to improve the yield. Breath testing is also typically used primarily to detect acute intoxication of volatile substances such as ethanol and is fairly easy to administer in most environments [3].

In addition to ordering the best test for the setting and need, it is imperative that an addiction psychiatrist can interpret tests correctly. As mentioned previously, knowledge of a full medication history is important as many substances may cause

Table 2.2 Benefits and drawbacks of different drug screening methods

Sampling method	Benefits	Drawbacks
Urine	Relatively inexpensive, readily available, quick results, noninvasive sample collection	Limited accuracy for certain compounds, adulteration risk if unsupervised
Blood	May determine acute intoxication, relatively inexpensive	Invasive, will not determine past drug use
Hair	Long period (3–6 months) of detecting past use, noninvasive sample collection	Will not detect recent drug use, expensive
Nail	Long period of drug detection in hair test, noninvasive collection	Will not detect recent drug use, expensive
Breath	Readily available, inexpensive, determines acute intoxication	Primarily only for volatile drugs (ethanol)

Table 2.3 Potential cross-reactive substances by misused substance type [1]

Substance	Potential positive result
Amphetamines	Aripiprazole, atomoxetine, bupropion, ephedrine, labetalol, MDMA, phentermine, pseudoephedrine, ranitidine, selegiline, trazodone, Vicks inhaler
Benzodiazepines	Efavirenz, sertraline
THC	Dronabinol, efavirenz, nabilone
Opioids	Dextromethorphan, diphenhydramine, poppy seeds, quinolone antibiotics
Phencyclidine	Dextromethorphan, doxylamine, ketamine, tramadol, venlafaxine

Table 2.4 Homeostatic urinalysis ranges

Criteria	Range
Urine creatinine	18–200 mg/dL
pH	4.5–8.0
Specific gravity	1.002–1.030
Temperature	90–100 °F

false positives in immunoassays. The clinician should consider the false-positive and false-negative rates of many available immunoassays (Table 2.3), though this can vary by manufacturer for each test. Knowledge of the physical properties of various substances is important to being able to predict the results of a given drug screen. For instance, the metabolic pathway of a given substance may produce analytes that could incorrectly be interpreted as the use of a different substance if the interpreter doesn't recognize the full pathway. This is important for opioids. Information on specific substances will be discussed in this chapter. Other pharmacokinetic considerations should be noted, such as the half-life and tissue binding of a substance and/or its metabolites, which would dictate the time frame that a test may be valid. Finally, individual pharmacogenomics may alter the analytes in a specimen as well. This may occur when individuals are poor or ultrarapid metabolizers of a substance.

Clinicians should also consider potential manipulation of the sample if there is an incentive to do so. While some samples are less likely to demonstrate interference (such as blood or breath tests), unobserved urine samples may lend themselves to adulteration. A urinalysis can provide additional information to guide urine drug screen interpretation. The sample would be expected to have a temperature close to normal body temperature. The color of the sample, urine creatinine, specific gravity, and pH should be within normal homeostatic ranges (Table 2.4) [4].

Drug-Specific Information

Opioids

Opioids broadly describe the substances that have agonist activity at the mu opioid receptors, as well as other opioid receptors. Naturally occurring opioids can be further classified as opiates, whereas semisynthetic and fully synthetic opioids require

Fig. 2.1 Opioid metabolism [5]

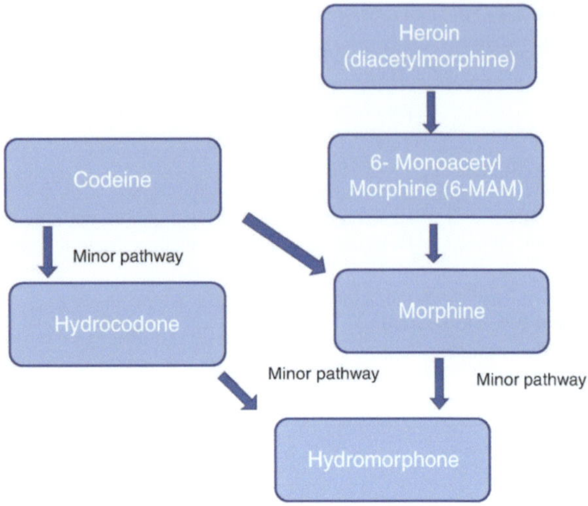

some manipulation for their manufacture and are chemically distinct from opiates. Opioids are a class containing many distinct substances with potentially differing pharmacokinetic properties that can vary depending on their specific biologic properties or formulations (e.g., extended-release tablets). These different properties carry implications for detection in drug screens. For instance, opioids that are formulated in a long-acting or extended-release formulation may be detectable in specimens for a longer period. Additionally, many urine drug screens were designed to detect opiates and are not as sensitive for semisynthetic opioids such as oxycodone and hydrocodone nor synthetic opioids such as fentanyl. In instances where the clinician wishes to test for those opioids, a specific immunoassay test is usually used unless specifically included in the test panel.

Another important consideration for those caring for patients with opioid use disorders is the metabolism of the different opioids. Figure 2.1 demonstrates a general pathway for opioid metabolism. Of note, the opioid metabolism pathway of many opioids may converge at several common metabolites. For instance, a patient taking either codeine, morphine, or heroin may produce a urine specimen that contains morphine. Therefore, a person that is prescribed acetaminophen and codeine tablets and takes a urine drug screen (UDS) that shows a positive result for morphine should not necessarily be understood to have used other substances. Similarly, utilizing various analytes and their concentrations may help discern the use of one substance from another. A patient that is using heroin (aka diacetyl morphine) would show morphine in their UDS, just as a person taking prescribed or illicit morphine or codeine would. A test for the analyte 6-monoacetyl morphine is specific to the heroin metabolite and would indicate heroin use. However, 6-monoacetyl morphine has a short detection window in the urine of as few as 8 h with limited use [1].

Clinicians should be aware that many synthetic opioids (such as fentanyl, methadone, or buprenorphine) are not detected by the traditional standard SAMHSA

5-drug panel and have typically required a specific lab test for these agents [1]. Though fentanyl may not be a "standard" test in many health systems, it's prevalence in laboratory orders as either an immunoassay or the more specific GCMS or LCMS is increasing. As noted above, HHS issued a rule in January 2025 adding fentanyl and its metabolite norfentanyl to the mandatory drug testing panels and federal workplaces began testing for fentanyl in 07/07/2025. Though fentanyl continues to be the largest cause of drug overdoses in the United States, a published data tracker showed that the fentanyl testing rate in emergency department overdose encounters was approximately 27% in Q4 of 2024 in a sample of hospitals that utilize the Epic electronic medical record (EMR) software [6]. As of early 2023, Epic was the most common EMR utilized in acute care hospitals in the United States [7]. This will likely begin to improve as health systems include fentanyl in their drug testing panels.

Starting approximately in 2013, the emergence of an illegal market in new synthetic opioids (largely fentanyls) has become a major global public health issue, associated with a substantial increase in unintentional overdoses and drug-related deaths. Synthetic opioids can include fentanyl, its analogues and emerging non-fentanyl-derived synthetic opioids such as U-compounds (benzamides and 2-phenylacetamides), MT-45, xylazine, metotomidine and related compounds, benzimidazole opioids (such as nitazenes) and brorphine. Although many states are funding efforts to improve specialized or enhanced toxicology testing for these novel compounds in cases of overdose deaths, they are not yet commonly available to most clinicians [8].

Fentanyl is highly lipophilic, allowing for fast diffusion between blood plasma and the central nervous system [9, 10]. In those who use fentanyl regularly, this high lipophilicity can allow fentanyl to be stored in adipocytes or other tissues, like the effect seen with THC in marijuana use. Although pharmacokinetic studies of single-dose fentanyl administration show renal clearance to be 1.5–7 h, some studies in daily users show a mean clearance of 2 weeks (range of 4–26 days) which is thought to be due to lipophilic sequestration. Oftentimes those with opioid use disorder are exposed to fentanyl daily which may lead to protracted withdrawal during treatment, or precipitated withdrawal with buprenorphine induction [11].

Buprenorphine is a synthetic opioid commonly used in both the treatment of pain and the treatment of opioid use disorder. Clinicians may wish to order buprenorphine urine testing for several reasons. Since it is a mu-opioid partial agonist, there is a potential for buprenorphine misuse. Patients may be acquiring illicit buprenorphine, and the provider wishes to assess the use pattern. Another reason for buprenorphine drug screening is to ensure adherence to the prescription regimen for opioid use disorder. This serves as a marker of medication ingestion and to minimize diversion of buprenorphine. Urine testing of buprenorphine/naloxone products should include buprenorphine and norbuprenorphine (major metabolite) [12]. Providers should carefully consider the pattern of detection that would be expected with adherence as compared to adulterated samples. A patient taking buprenorphine/naloxone formulation would be expected to produce a sample containing buprenorphine and norbuprenorphine. Buprenorphine is primarily metabolized by hepatic cytochrome P450 3A4 (CYP3A4) to its active metabolite norbuprenorphine. Buprenorphine and norbuprenorphine are eliminated primarily by the biliary system, with 10–30% excreted into the urine. Drugs or conditions that inhibit or induce CYP3A4 and genetic polymorphisms affecting CYP3A4 decrease or increase buprenorphine metabolism [13].

Both buprenorphine and norbuprenorphine can be detected in urine for 2–4 days in people who are taking buprenorphine regularly [14]. The buprenorphine level, norbuprenorphine level, and the norbuprenorphine-to-buprenorphine ratio are useful when interpreting results. The presence of the metabolite norbuprenorphine can be used to show adherence to the medication. However, a very high buprenorphine level with a negative norbuprenorphine level indicates likely buprenorphine "spiking" (adding buprenorphine to the urine sample directly) with no recent dosing. Some studies suggest using an N:B ratio of 0.02 as a threshold for identifying urine spiked with unconsumed buprenorphine [15].

Additionally, some laboratories may report naloxone concentrations; a proportion of the naloxone may be absorbed sublingually and thus be detectable in the urine. Some laboratories may report naloxone concentrations as either free naloxone, naloxone-3-glucuronide, or total naloxone concentrations [16, 17]. Analysis of free naloxone in urine may indicate adulteration, whereas naloxone-3-glucuronide is the expected analyte from first-pass metabolism of oral or sublingual naloxone.

Methadone is another synthetic opioid that is commonly used for both the treatment of pain and opioid use disorder. Typically, confirmatory testing is required to detect methadone in the urine, as it is less commonly included in urine immunoassay drug screening panels. Methadone testing is prone to adulteration of urine with the drug for persons who have diverted methadone. To determine if methadone was added to urine (as opposed to being present via excretion of the drug into urine), clinicians may choose to order a test for methadone's metabolite 2-ehtylidene-1,5-dimethyl-3,3-diphenylpyrollidine (EDDP). The presence of EDDP would indicate that the patient has ingested and metabolized methadone [1].

Alcohol

Alcohol is one of the most commonly used substances and may often co-occur with other substance use or mental health disorders. Alcohol has slightly different pharmacokinetics from many other substances. In general, ethanol undergoes metabolism that is termed "zero-order" kinetics, or saturable pharmacokinetics. This implies that the metabolism of alcohol occurs at a given metabolic rate (20 mg/dL/h) regardless of the concentration of alcohol in the body; thus, the metabolism is "saturable." Several factors may affect this metabolic rate such as sex (women eliminate alcohol faster, though they have higher blood alcohol concentrations because of a smaller volume of distribution), race, whether someone is in the fed nutritional state, and body mass [18].

The usual laboratory measurement for alcohol in clinical settings is the blood alcohol content (BAC) expressed as mg of ethanol per dL of blood. BAC may be recognized as its expression of a percentage, as in the legal limit to operate a motor vehicle that is 0.08%. A BAC of 0.1% corresponds to 100 mg ethanol/dL blood. A "standard drink" in the United States is defined as 14 g of ethanol, or 0.6 fluid ounces of pure ethanol. Similarly, this corresponds to a 12 oz beer (5% Alcohol By Volume (ABV)), a 5 oz glass of wine (12% ABV), or 1.5 oz of spirit (40% ABV).

BAC is easily estimated using a Breathalyzer machine, which can give clinicians a quick reading of estimated BAC. Due to the ease and affordability of testing, the comorbid presence of alcohol use disorders with other substance use disorders, and the negative implications of alcohol intoxication to recovery, many clinicians will utilize a Breathalyzer in routine outpatient follow-up. In addition, inpatient units or emergency departments may obtain a blood draw for newly presenting patients to determine their blood alcohol level (BAL) and guide further treatment considerations.

In addition to labs to detect acute intoxication, several other forms of laboratory testing may be utilized to assess patients with alcohol use disorders. While ethanol has a short half-life, it is metabolized to ethyl glucuronide and ethyl sulfate, which are excreted in the urine. Ethyl glucuronide may be detected for up to 3–4 days after alcohol consumption. Ethyl sulfate may be used concurrently to increase the specificity of the ethyl glucuronide test [19]. Another test for recent ethanol consumption utilized is phosphatidyl ethanol, which is a biomarker only formed in the presence of ethanol via phospholipase D [20]. Phosphatidyl ethanol is elevated in the presence of approximately 4–5 standard drinks per day for at least 3 weeks. It remains elevated for up to 14 days after discontinuing alcohol [19]. Gamma glutamyl transferase (GGT) is a liver enzyme that is increased in individuals with chronic heavy alcohol use. In patients without chronic heavy alcohol use, GGT levels are expected to be below 54 IU/L. It should be noted that certain anticonvulsant medications may increase GGT even without alcohol use. GGT may also be increased in certain hepatic conditions, and so it is not specific for alcohol use. Carbohydrate-deficient transferrin (CDT) is a protein that exists in blood and is increased with heavy alcohol use. Elevations in carbohydrate-deficient transferrin may be noted sooner than elevations in GGT. A value greater than 1.6% indicates heavy alcohol consumption. Finally, standard liver function test (LFT) panel labs may be assessed in alcohol use disorder. Liver enzymes such as aspartate aminotransferase (AST) and alanine aminotransferase (ALT) (measured in LFT panels) and mean corpuscular volume (MCV) (measured in complete blood count (CBC) panels) may be increased with repeated alcohol use, with AST being more specific for alcohol-induced liver damage than ALT. An AST/ALT ratio >2 is considered suggestive of alcohol as the cause of liver dysfunction [21]. Elevations in LFTs have been associated with hepatic cellular damage due to toxins, and MCV elevations are more likely a result of direct hematologic toxicity of ethanol, rather than vitamin deficiencies. These tests are not as sensitive or specific as those previously listed [19].

Benzodiazepines

Benzodiazepines are commonly used agents for anxiety and related disorders that are often misused. As with other substances, it is important to consider the pharmacokinetics of the specific agent that is being detected. Benzodiazepines vary in their duration of action and half-lives (that can also vary from person to person based on individual characteristics and metabolism), with some having a half-life as short as 10 h (alprazolam), and others lasting 3 days or longer (diazepam). Diazepam has a half-life of 72 h; however, its active metabolite, desmethyldiazepam, has a half-life of 160 h. Due to the drug lingering in the body for so long, diazepam may be detected from 10 days up to 30 days with moderate to heavy use [1, 3].

Benzodiazepines undergo phase I (hepatic oxidation and reduction by cytochrome P450) and phase II (glucuronide conjugation) metabolic pathways. Alprazolam, triazolam, midazolam, and diazepam undergo hydroxylation while clonazepam undergoes nitro-reduction. CYP2C19 and CYP3A4 are the enzymes most involved in the metabolism of benzodiazepines that undergo phase I metabolism. Phase I metabolism tends to be reduced in the elderly, along with polypharmacy, predisposing elderly patients to CYP450-related interactions. However, phase II metabolism remains relatively preserved in the elderly. Benzodiazepines that undergo phase II glucuronidation, but not cytochrome phase I p450 metabolism, include lorazepam, oxazepam, temazepam (LOT) and are the recommended benzodiazepines in the elderly for this reason [22, 23].

Urine immunoassays for benzodiazepines, unfortunately, have a high rate of false negatives. Most assays are designed to detect diazepam or its metabolites such as nordiazepam or oxazepam. Benzodiazepine metabolites because of glucuronidation in liver metabolism (such as metabolites of alprazolam or lorazepam) are often not detected on standard immunoassays. Similarly, clonazepam is metabolized by nitroreduction, and its metabolite is not often detected unless the clonazepam dose is sufficiently high (Fig. 2.2). For this reason, false negatives are common with benzodiazepine immunoassay screening, particularly with detecting lorazepam and clonazepam and may require definitive or confirmatory testing [24].

A small proportion of the benzodiazepines alprazolam, lorazepam, and clonazepam are partially excreted in the urine unchanged and may therefore be detected by urine drug screens. Careful consideration is warranted for the assay's cutoff value for detection. Potent agents requiring lower doses (such as alprazolam or lorazepam) may not show up on an assay if the cutoff for detection is 300 ng/mL. Agents that undergo metabolism that is not readily detectable on an immunoassay further decrease the likelihood of detection as only a small proportion of the original dose is available to be detected.

Tests that are specific to these compounds can be helpful in detecting an individual's use of benzodiazepines. In some instances, lower detection cutoffs may be available and useful for detecting potent or glucuronidated benzodiazepines. Finally, some laboratories can enzymatically alter the benzodiazepine metabolites to the parent drug via hydrolysis of the urine sample [1].

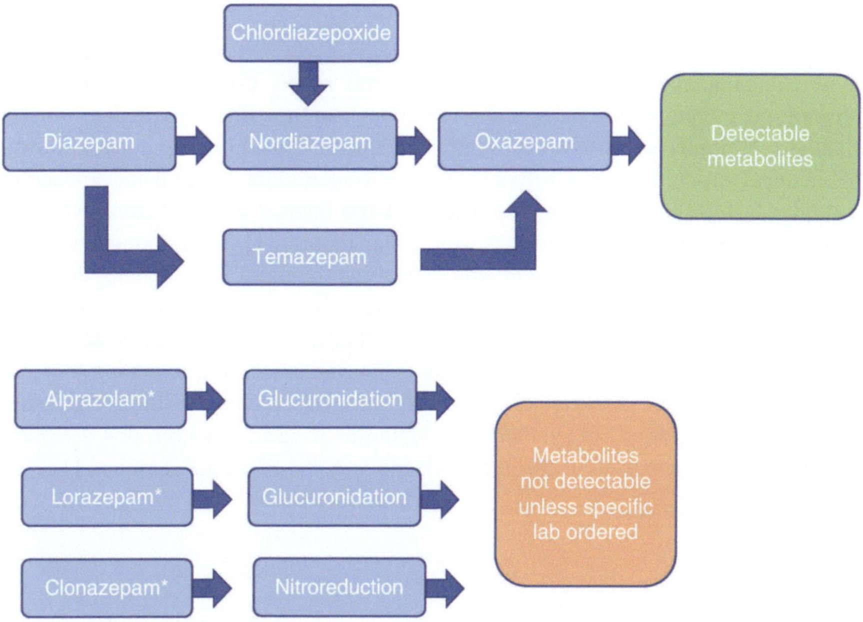

*A small minority of these benzodiazepines are excreted unchanged in the urine. Even without specific lab testing, they may be detected but usually with less sensitivity and at high concentrations.

Fig. 2.2 Benzodiazepine metabolites

Marijuana

Urine drug screens focus on detecting a metabolite of the main psychoactive component of marijuana, delta-9 tetrahydrocannabinol (THC). Typically, the federal cutoff limit for detection is 50 ng/mL, with a confirmatory test cutoff of 15 ng/mL [2]. Several factors may affect how long THC may be detectable in an individual. The first consideration should be whether the use is consistent or not. With infrequent use, THC may be detectable for only 3 days. However, chronic heavy use may be detectable for 30 days or longer due to elution of THC that is stored in body tissues. A positive immunoassay will not be able to distinguish acute intoxication from consistent use that may have ceased several days or weeks ago.

A commonly held misconception about marijuana is that passive inhalation (such as from a concert) may produce a positive result. This has been tested in a controlled environment, and while high potency THC exposure in an enclosed environment had some THC metabolites detectable on GCMS (mean ranging from 7.5 to 28.3 ng/mL depending on THC concentration in marijuana and whether ventilation was in the room), the results demonstrated that only 1 of the 6 subjects had a positive result above the federal threshold of 50 ng/mL. The result was only positive at the single time point 4–6 h post exposure, and subsequent specimens fell below 50 ng/mL. Therefore, it is highly unlikely to test positive with passive inhalation in an instance where exposure is not obvious [25].

Synthetic Cannabinoids

Synthetic cannabinoids have been developed and widely used due to their similar physiologic effects, action on cannabis receptors, and their difficulty in detection on standard immunoassay drug tests. Synthetic cannabinoids represent a diverse array of chemical structures that are often sprayed onto inert plant material and smoked in a similar fashion to marijuana [26]. The DEA has banned many of these synthetic compounds because of numerous poison center reports [1]. Even though standard federal panels do not test for synthetic cannabinoids, there is increasing development of urine immunoassays to detect the most common of these substances. Several validated immunoassays are available, but it is important for clinicians to recognize that not all synthetic cannabinoids have an associated screening tool and further development of novel cannabinoids may occur in the future. The usual detection time reported for synthetic cannabinoids is 72 h; however, this detection window may be increased in chronic users and vary based on the chemical [1].

Stimulants

The stimulant class includes drugs such as amphetamine(s), methylphenidate, methamphetamine, and cocaine, as well as nicotine. Stimulant medications are commonly prescribed for disorders such as ADHD, though they can be misused as well. UDS for stimulants can be challenging for clinicians due to the poor selectivity of these assays, specifically those screening for amphetamines. Due to chemical similarities, the distinction between amphetamine and methamphetamine is difficult to make without a more definitive laboratory analysis [1]. Clinicians should be aware that many prescribed and over-the-counter medications may cause false positives (and even some "true" positives) on UDS. For instance, the MAOI selegiline is metabolized to methamphetamine in the body and may trigger a positive UDS. Oxymetazoline (Vicks) nasal spray has also been shown to produce a positive urine screen after following manufacturer-recommended dosing [1]. False positives for amphetamine screens may include aripiprazole, atomoxetine, bupropion, chlorpromazine, ephedrine, metformin, MDMA, phentermine, pseudoephedrine, ranitidine, and trazodone, among others. The standard federal 5-panel drug screen includes confirmatory testing for MDMA (methalenedioxymethamphetamine or "ecstasy") as well as MDA (methylenedioxyamphetamine). If a urine screen is positive for amphetamines, it is recommended to utilize quantitative confirmatory testing (e.g., GCMS testing) to verify the result. Amphetamines or methamphetamines are typically detected in the urine for about 48–72 h after use [1, 3]. It should be noted that to detect methylphenidate accurately, a specific laboratory test for it should be ordered, as it does not cross-react with the amphetamine immunoassay since it is chemically different, though still acting as a stimulant.

Cocaine is detected on a urine immunoassay drug screen via its metabolite benzoylecgonine, which has a high level of specificity, and no false positives have been identified for this assay [1, 3]. Benzoylecgonine is detectable in the urine for approximately 2–5 days after use [1, 3]. Cocaine is a Schedule II substance by the FDA and is used licitly as an eye drop in ophthalmic procedures. It is reasonable that use under these circumstances may produce a positive test result; however, other aminoester or aminoamide local anesthetics (such as benzocaine and lidocaine) do not produce false-positive results [1].

Nicotine is the legal stimulant present in tobacco leaves and sold over the counter in gums, patches, and lozenges. It is present in many "vapes" as a heated and inhaled liquid. When assessed, providers can order a urine screen for nicotine's major metabolite, cotinine. Cotinine can be detected in the urine of heavy smokers for up to 2 weeks [28].

Dissociatives

Dissociative drugs include phencyclidine (PCP), ketamine, and dextromethorphan. These agents produce perceptual disturbances, hallucinations, and characteristic out-of-body (dissociative) experiences. PCP is included in the standard federal 5-panel drug test. While PCP is a Schedule I controlled substance, ketamine (Schedule III) and dextromethorphan (not scheduled) are commonly used in medical care. These agents have the potential to show up as a false positive for PCP on immunoassay screening. The use of these agents should be excluded prior to interpreting a positive UDS. PCP is typically detected in the urine for up to 8 days following its use [3].

Hallucinogens and Other Drugs

Hallucinogens include substances such as psilocybin (active ingredient in psychedelic mushrooms), lysergic acid diethylamide (LSD), and mescaline (found in peyote cactus), which have not historically been detected on standard urine drug screens. In many instances, these substances have short half-lives or are sufficiently potent that only a small amount of drug is needed for recreational use. While specialized laboratory testing is available, it is fairly uncommon in clinical practice. Other substances besides hallucinogens that may be difficult to detect on a urine screen include gamma-hydroxybutyrate (GHB), inhalants, synthetic cathinones ("bath salts"), and non-fentanyl-derived synthetic opioids as described above [3].

Chapter Review Questions

1. A patient presents to your clinic seeking a buprenorphine prescription for opioid use disorder. The patient states that they have recently taken prescribed oral pain medications, which belong to a family member. The patient submits a urine drug screen, which results positive for morphine but negative for 6-monoacetyl morphine. There is also a small amount of hydromorphone detected. Which of the following substances did the person most likely take?

A. Oxycodone
B. Fentanyl
C. Heroin
D. Codeine
E. Methadone

Correct answer: D. Codeine

Explanation: Codeine is an opiate and prodrug of morphine, mainly used to treat pain, coughing, or diarrhea. As seen in Fig. 2.1 above, Codeine's major pathway is conversion into morphine which could then potentially be converted into hydromorphone via a minor pathway. Codeine also has another minor pathway where it could be converted into hydrocodone.

2. A patient is prescribed buprenorphine/naloxone for opioid use disorder. The patient has also struggled with cocaine in the past and was previously admitted to selling buprenorphine to get money to buy cocaine and then regretted it because of buprenorphine withdrawal symptoms. Which of the following urine drug screen results would most likely indicate medication adherence to the prescribed buprenorphine/naloxone?

A. High levels of buprenorphine only
B. High levels of naloxone only
C. High levels of buprenorphine and norbuprenorphine
D. High levels of buprenorphine and EDDP
E. High levels of norbuprenorphine and EDDP

Correct answer: C. High levels of buprenorphine and norbuprenorphine

Explanation: When a patient is taking buprenorphine/naloxone as prescribed, both buprenorphine and its major metabolite norbuprenorphine, should be present in the urine. The presence of both indicates that the medication has been ingested and metabolized. High levels of buprenorphine alone might suggest sample adulteration, while naloxone or EDDP are not relevant for buprenorphine adherence testing. Occasionally patients who metabolize buprenorphine rapidly may have just norbuprenorphine in their urine.

3. A patient with a known history of attention deficit hyperactivity disorder (ADHD) who takes methylphenidate for ADHD is taking over-the-counter medications for cold symptoms. The patient's urine screen is positive for amphetamines, but they deny any non-prescribed stimulant use. Which medication could explain the positive test result?

A. Lorazepam
B. Methylphenidate
C. Pseudoephedrine
D. Gabapentin
E. Naloxone

Correct answer: C. Pseudoephedrine

Explanation: Pseudoephedrine can cause a false positive for amphetamines on urine immunoassays due to its chemical similarity. Confirmatory testing, such as GC-MS, is recommended to differentiate between pseudoephedrine and amphetamine use. Methylphenidate is a stimulant that is chemically distinct from amphetamines and does not cross-react with the amphetamine immunoassay.

4. A patient with a history of alcohol use disorder reports being abstinent for the past 2 weeks after completing a medically supervised detoxification followed by an intensive outpatient program. The clinician wants to objectively verify this claim. Which of the following laboratory tests would be most appropriate to detect heavy alcohol use over the past several weeks?

   A. Blood alcohol content (BAC)
   B. Ethyl glucuronide
   C. Gamma glutamyl transferase (GGT)
   D. Phosphatidyl ethanol
   E. Carbohydrate-deficient transferrin (CDT)

   Correct answer: D. Phosphatidyl ethanol

   Explanation: Phosphatidyl ethanol is the most appropriate test for detecting heavy alcohol use over the past several weeks. It is a biomarker only formed in the presence of ethanol via phospholipase D. Phosphatidyl ethanol is elevated in the presence of 4–5 standard drinks per day for at least 3 weeks and remains elevated for around 14 days after discontinuing alcohol. Blood alcohol content (BAC) only detects very recent alcohol consumption. Ethyl glucuronide can be detected for up to 3–4 days after alcohol consumption. Gamma glutamyl transferase (GGT) can indicate chronic heavy alcohol use but is less specific and may not accurately reflect use over the past month as well as phosphatidyl ethanol.

5. A patient presents to the emergency room exhibiting signs including lethargy, slowed breathing, pupil constriction and cold/clammy skin. They are quickly provided with intranasal naloxone, and a urine drug screen immunoassay is obtained by the nursing staff. Which of the following substances is least likely to be detectable by an initial standard 5-panel urine immunoassay?

   A. Diazepam
   B. Fentanyl
   C. Morphine
   D. Heroin
   E. Codeine

   Correct answer: B. Fentanyl

   Explanation: Fentanyl is not part of the standard 5-panel immunoassay and would need to be specifically ordered or detected in confirmatory testing, depending on the facility/lab. The Department of Health and Human Services (DHHS) has established a standard guideline for workplace drug screening, typically known as the "standard 5-panel drug test." This panel includes screening for marijuana (THC), cocaine (benzoylecgonine), phencyclidine (PCP), amphetamines, and certain opioids (codeine/morphine, 6-Monoacetyl Morphine, hydrocodone/hydromorphone, oxycodone/oxymorphone).

References

1. Moeller KE, Kissack JC, Atayee RS, Lee KC. Clinical interpretation of urine drug tests: what clinicians need to know about urine drug screens. Mayo Clin Proc. 2017;92(5):774–96.
2. Mandatory Guidelines for Federal Workplace Drug Testing Programs-Authorized Testing Panels. 2025. Federal Register. https://www.federalregister.gov/documents/2025/01/16/2025-00425/mandatory-guidelines-for-federal-workplace-drug-testing-programs-authorized-testing-panels.
3. Nelson ZJ, Stellpflug SJ, Engebretsen KM. What can a urine drug screening immunoassay really tell us? J Pharm Pract. 2016;29(5):516–26.
4. Verstraete AG. Detection times of drugs of abuse in blood, urine, and oral fluid. Ther Drug Monit. 2004;26(2):200–5.
5. Cook JD, Caplan YH, Lodico CP, Bush DM. The characterization of human urine for specimen validity determination in workplace drug testing: a review. J Anal Toxicol. 2000;24(7):579–88.
6. Pesce A, West C, Egan city K, Strickland J. Interpretation of urine drug testing in pain patients. Pain Med. 2012;13(7):868–85.
7. Chishtie J, Sapiro N, Wiebe N, Rabatach L, Lorenzetti D, Leung AA, Rabi D, Quan H, Eastwood CA. Use of epic electronic health record system for health care research: scoping review. J Med Internet Res. 2023;25:e51003.
8. EHRN. Epic research [Internet]. Epic Research. 2025. Available from: https://www.epicresearch.org/data-tracker/fentanyl-and-opiate-toxicology.
9. Shafi A, Berry AJ, Sumnall H, Wood DM, Tracy DK. Synthetic opioids: a review and clinical update. Ther Adv Psychopharmacol. 2022;12:20451253221139б.
10. Lötsch J, Walter C, Parnham MJ, Oertel BG, Geisslinger G. Pharmacokinetics of non-intravenous formulations of fentanyl. Clin Pharmacokinet. 2012;52(1):23–36.
11. Henthorn TK, Liu Y, Mahapatro M, Ng K. Active transport of fentanyl by the blood-brain barrier. J Pharmacol Exp Ther. 1999;289(2):1084–9.
12. Huhn AS, Dunn KE. Challenges for women entering treatment for opioid use disorder. Curr Psychiatry Rep. 2020;22:1.
13. Hull MJ, Bierer MF, Griggs DA, Long WH, Nixon AL, Flood JG. Urinary buprenorphine concentrations in patients treated with suboxone as determined by liquid chromatography-mass spectrometry and CEDIA immunoassay. J Anal Toxicol. 2008;32(7):516–21.
14. Elkader A, Sproule B. Buprenorphine. Clin Pharmacokinet. 2005;44(7):661–80.
15. Tzatzarakis MN, Vakonaki E, Kovatsi L, Belivanis S, Mantsi M, Alegakis A, et al. Determination of buprenorphine, norbuprenorphine and naloxone in fingernail clippings and urine of patients under opioid substitution therapy. J Anal Toxicol. 2015;39(4):313–20.
16. Warrington JS, Warrington GS, Francis-Fath S, Brooklyn J. Urinary buprenorphine, norbuprenorphine and naloxone concentrations and ratios. J Addict Med. 2020;14(6):e344–9.
17. Danso D, Langman LJ, Jannetto PJ. Targeted opioid screening assay for pain management using high-resolution mass spectrometry. Methods Mol Biol. 1872;2019:41–50.
18. Fang WB, Chang Y, Mccance-katz EF, Moody DE. Determination of naloxone and nornaloxone (noroxymorphone) by high-performance liquid chromatography-electrospray ionization-tandem mass spectrometry. J Anal Toxicol. 2009;33(8):409–17.
19. Jones AW. Pharmacokinetics of ethanol - issues of forensic importance. Forensic Sci Rev. 2011;23(2):91–136.
20. Tavakoli HR, Hull M, Michael OL. Review of current clinical biomarkers for the detection of alcohol dependence. Innov Clin Neurosci. 2011;8(3):26–33.
21. Perilli M, Toselli F, Franceschetto L, Alessandro Cinquetti, Ceretta A, Cecchetto G, et al. Phosphatidylethanol (PEth) in blood as a marker of unhealthy alcohol use: a systematic review with novel molecular insights. Int J Mol Sci [Internet] 2023 [cited 2024 Mar 1];24(15):12175–5. Available from: https://www.ncbi.nlm.nih.gov/pmc/articles/PMC10418704/.
22. Oh RC, Hustead TR, Ali SM, Pantsari MW. Mildly elevated liver transaminase levels: causes and evaluation. Am Fam Physician. 2017;96(11):709–15.

23. Mihic SJ, Harris RA. Hypnotics and sedatives. Goodman and Gilman's pharmacological basis of therapeutics. 12th ed. New York: McGraw-Hill; 2011. p. 457–80.
24. Melton ST, Kirkwood CK. Anxiety disorders: generalized anxiety, panic, and social anxiety disorders. In: DiPiro JT, Talbert RL, Yee GC, Matzke GR, et al., editors. Pharmacotherapy: a pathophysiologic approach. 10th ed. New York, NY: McGraw-Hill; 2017.
25. Mullins GR, Reeves A, Yu M, Goldberger BA, Bazydlo LAL. Improved clinical sensitivity of a reflexive algorithm to minimize false-negative test results by a urine benzodiazepine immunoassay screen. J Appl Lab Med. 2018;2(4):555–63.
26. Cone EJ, Bigelow GE, Herrmann ES, et al. Non-smoker exposure to secondhand cannabis smoke. I. Urine screening and confirmation results. J Anal Toxicol. 2015;39(1):1–12.
27. Arntson A, Ofsa B, Lancaster D, Simon JR, Mcmullin M, Logan B. Validation of a novel immunoassay for the detection of synthetic cannabinoids and metabolites in urine specimens. J Anal Toxicol. 2013;37(5):284–90.
28. Vine MF, Hulka BS, Margolin BH, et al. Cotinine concentrations in semen, urine, and blood of smokers and nonsmokers. Am J Public Health. 1993;83(9):1335–8.

Epidemiology, Genetics, and Neurobiology of Substance Use and Disorders

3

Katerina Christodoulides, Kristopher A. Kast, and Jonathan Avery

High-Yield Review Points

- The 12-month prevalence of any SUD in the United States has remained relatively stable across time, representing 10–15% of the general population, with tobacco, alcohol, cannabis, and opioid use disorder being the most common.
- Tobacco and underage alcohol use have declined over the past two decades, but cannabis use and use disorder have risen, alongside a rise in heavy alcohol use among women aged 12–20 years (closing the historical gender gap).
- Only a minority of individuals with SUD (23.6% in 2023) received any addiction treatment, marking a significant treatment gap.
- Addiction is a highly heritable (40–70% in family and twin studies), polygenic disorder with multiple risky genes of small effect size that interact with environmental influences (gene-by-environment interactions) and epigenetic mechanisms (including histone modification, DNA methylation, and microRNA regulation) to produce the syndrome of a substance use disorder.
- The three-stage addiction cycle of binge intoxication, withdrawal/negative affect, and craving corresponds to specific neuroanatomical substrates (the

K. Christodoulides · J. Avery
New York-Presbyterian Hospital, New York, NY, USA

Weill Cornell Medical College, New York, NY, USA
e-mail: apc9022@nyp.org; joa9070@med.cornell.edu

K. A. Kast (✉)
Vanderbilt University Medical Center, Nashville, TN, USA
e-mail: kristopher.a.kast@vumc.org

C. Marienfeld, M. Soltani (eds.), *AAAP Review of Addiction Psychiatry*,
https://doi.org/10.1007/978-3-032-24174-0_3

striatum, extended amygdala, and prefrontal cortex, respectively). Each of these involves complex neurocircuitry that governs:

- Compulsive behavior (cortico-striatal-pallidal-thalamic-cortical feedback loops)
- Hedonic reward (mesolimbic dopaminergic system)
- Homeostatic antireward (allostatic change of the mesolimbic dopaminergic firing rate and activation of the stress-response neurotransmitter systems, including CRF, dynorphin, and norepinephrine)
- Prefrontal Go/Stop systems (cholinergic projections from the anterior cingulate and dorsolateral prefrontal cortex, and orbitofrontal and ventrolateral prefrontal cortex)

Introduction

Addiction is a complex, chronic, relapsing neuropsychiatric disorder with genetic and epigenetic risk, conserved common neuropathology, significant prevalence across populations, severe medical and psychiatric comorbidity, and social and occupational impairment with resulting large individual and societal cost. This chapter will focus on (1) the epidemiology of substance use, unhealthy use, and use disorder; (2) genetic and epigenetic risk and resilience for addiction; and (3) the common neuropathology of the three stages of the addiction cycle. This chapter offers a number of perspectives that translate the historically moralized and stigmatized clinical syndrome of addiction into the language of medicine and psychiatry. In addition, it reviews clinically useful data that argues against culturally prevalent stigma toward patients with these life-threatening disorders.

Epidemiology of Substance Use, Unhealthy Use, and Use Disorder

Substance Use Disorders

The prevalence of alcohol and illicit substance use disorders among Americans aged >12 years was 17.1% in 2023 (exclusive of the 22.7% prevalence of past-month tobacco product or nicotine vaping use) [1]. For reference, this exceeds the prevalence of major depression among adult Americans over the same period (8.5% in 2023) [1]. The majority of those with any SUD have a tobacco or alcohol use disorder (1), while 9.6% have an illicit or cannabis drug use disorder. The most common illicit drug use disorder is cannabis use disorder (6.8% of the general population), with opioid use disorder second most prevalent (1.9% using prescription opioids; 0.2% using heroin; illicitly manufactured fentanyl (IMF) tracked differently (details later in chapter)), and CNS stimulant use disorder the third most prevalent (1.5%).

The remaining substance categories occur at <1% prevalence. These numbers are based on the 2023 National Survey on Drug Use and Health, which utilized multimode data collection through both in-person and web-based surveys. As a result, comparisons with NSDUH data from years prior to 2021, which did not use this methodology, may be challenging.

Substance use disorder prevalence has been relatively stable over time, with consistent reports of 10–15% over the past two decades, though differences in samples, diagnostic instruments, and data collection across different national surveys contribute to some variability in findings [2, 3]. For example, the 2012–2013 National Epidemiologic Survey on Alcohol and Related Conditions (NESARC) found a 13.9% 12-month prevalence of alcohol use disorder, though this sample includes only those individuals >18 years old (compared to the finding of 10.2% in the 2023 National Survey of Drug Use and Health, which collects data for those aged >12 years) [1, 4]. Table 3.1 reviews the four major national surveys of SUD and related conditions, comparing their data collection periods, sample sizes, differences in inclusion criteria, and diagnostic instruments.

Substance Use and Recent Trends

Substance use (without the addiction syndrome) is far more common than substance use *disorder*. Alcohol is the most used substance in the United States, with 134.7 million current (i.e., "past month") users in 2023 (47.5% of the general population aged >12 years) [1]. Tobacco products or nicotine vaping are second, with 64.4 million current users (22.7%). Cannabis is third, with 43.6 million current users (15.4%). Opioids are fourth, with 8.9 million current past-year users (8.6 million using prescription opioids; 0.66 million using heroin), accounting for 3.1% of the general population; this does not account for fentanyl, including illegally made fentanyl (IMF), misuse. Data on the IMF is tracked separately and shows 0.2% of IMF misuse [1]. The remaining substance categories (cocaine, hallucinogens, inhalants, and other prescription psychotropics) each have <1% of the general population as current past month users.

Noteworthy epidemiological trends in substance use over the past two decades include (1) a decline in tobacco users from 26% in 2002 to 21.4% in 2023, (2) a decline in underage alcohol use from 28.8% of 12- to 20-year-olds in 2002 to 14.6% in 2023, and (3) a rise in cannabis use from 6.2% in 2002 to 15.4% in 2023 (driven by increased use among >18-year-olds). The substances with the most new users in 2023 are nicotine vaping (5.9 million), alcohol (4.2 million), tobacco (3.5 million), cannabis (3.5 million), and hallucinogens (1.5 million).

Unhealthy Substance Use

Addiction (or substance use disorder) is more clearly defined than *unhealthy* use, the latter being an umbrella term for any substance use above *low or lower risk* use

Table 3.1 Major cross-sectional surveys studying the prevalence of substance use disorders in the United States

Survey name	Dates of data collection	Population size surveyed	Representativeness of the sample	Diagnostic instrument used	Data reported	Notable findings
NIMH Epidemiologic Catchment Area (ECA)	1980–1984	$n = 20{,}000$	Five metropolitan catchment areas in the United States	Diagnostic interview schedule (DSM-III criteria)	Incidence and service-use data for all psychiatric disorders, including SUD	First attempt at a nationally representative sample
National Comorbidity Survey	1990–1992; 2001–2002	$n = 9000$	Nationally representative sample (though smaller than later surveys); ages 15–54 (younger sample than other surveys)	Composite international diagnostic interview (modified; DSM-III-R criteria)	Lifetime and 12-month prevalence data for SUD and psychiatric disorders	Lifetime prevalence of any SUD was 35% (tobacco 29%; alcohol 13%; illicit drug 8%); 12-month prevalence of any SUD was 13% (tobacco 11%; alcohol 3%; illicit drug 1.4%)
National Epidemiologic Survey on Alcohol and Related Conditions (NESARC)	2001–2002; 2004–2005; 2012–2013	$n = 43{,}000$ in 2004–2005 survey; $n = 36{,}000$ in 2012–2013	Nationally representative sample; ages 18 and older	Alcohol use disorder and associated disabilities interview schedule (DSM-IV criteria)	Lifetime and 12-month prevalence data for SUD and psychiatric comorbidity; also collected saliva DNA samples from participants in the most recent sample	Closing gender gap between men and women for alcohol use disorders; significant comorbidity of SUD and mood, anxiety, and personality disorders; significant treatment gap (only 19.8% of those with lifetime alcohol use disorder were ever treated)
National Survey on Drug Use and Health (NSDUH)	Conducted annually since 1971; at the time of publication most recent data from 2023	$n = 70{,}000$ in most recent survey	Randomly selected national sample; ages 12 and older	In-person interview; NSDUH-specific instrument	Prior year prevalence of substance use and use disorder, as well as psychiatric comorbidity	Most recent data are summarized in the chapter text

This table presents the four nationally representative epidemiological surveys conducted in the United States since 1980. The dates of data collection, sample size, unique features of the sample, diagnostic instruments, data reported, and important findings are reviewed

[5]. Unhealthy use includes the entire spectrum of substance use associated with any health consequences, including substance use disorder (or addiction), harmful use (or use that has led to specific health consequences for an individual; e.g., alcohol intoxication that has resulted in a fall with bone fracture), and hazardous or at-risk use (or an amount of use known to increase the risk of adverse health consequences, such as *heavy* alcohol use). The concept of *unhealthy* use captures all conditions related to substance use that warrant targeted interventions (whether preventive or therapeutic), including those states that do not (yet) meet diagnostic criteria for substance use disorder.

For most substances, no amount of use is known to be completely safe, and single episodes of intoxication may risk sequelae (e.g., myocardial infarction with first cocaine use); thus, any amount of use may be hazardous or at-risk. Alcohol is a notable exception, where *heavy use* known to increase risk of adverse health outcomes has been defined using epidemiological data; these are 5 or more standard 14-gram drinks in a day or >14 drinks per week for men; these amounts are adjusted to 4 or more drinks per day or 7 per week for women or men aged >65 years [5]. In 2023, 21.7% of the general population aged >12 years endorsed drinking 5 or more drinks in a day (4 or more drinks in a day for females), with a notable peak among 18- to 25-year-olds (28.7% of this age group) [1]. Notably, alcohol use under these levels may still be hazardous or harmful, as intoxication may occur with less intake and result in impaired functioning and injury.

Transition from Substance Use to SUD

Of individuals who have ever used certain substance categories, relatively few develop addiction. The highest rates of conversion from "ever used" to SUD occur for tobacco (14%), heroin (10%), alcohol (7.8%), prescription opioids (5.2%), cannabis (3.8%), and cocaine (2%) [2]. The proportion of current past-year users who have a SUD differs across substance categories; some, like heroin, prescription opioids, and tobacco, have >50% of current users with an associated SUD, whereas current cannabis and alcohol users are less likely (15% and 10%, respectively) to have a current SUD. Risk of developing SUD is elevated in individuals who initiate use in adolescence, with subsequent development of SUD in 34% of those whose first use occurred in <14-year-olds (vs. 14% with first use >21 years old) [2].

The Closing Gender Gap

Historically, women in the US and most cultures around the globe have been less likely to use alcohol and illicit substances, leading to greater SUD rates among men (rates of use and SUD among men have been consistently twice that found among women in the US) [3]. However, this gender gap has not been static in the United States; in more recent studies, women aged 12–20 years have greater rates of heavy alcohol use than age-matched men. Further, the likelihood of transitioning from substance use to addiction is equal for men and women, leading to the increasing concern that the historical gender gap, likely related to cultural norms, is closing [6]. This is especially important given the increased risk for negative health and reproductive or perinatal outcomes for women with smaller amounts of alcohol, compared to men.

Culture, Race, Ethnicity, Immigration, and SUD

Differences in rates of SUD exist across racial and ethnic groups in the United States [7]. American Indian or Alaska Native have elevated rates of SUD compared with the general population (25.3% vs. 17.1% in 2023); Asian Americans have lower rates (9.2%). Black Americans (17.6%), Latino Americans (15.6%), and White Americans (17.8%) have rates comparable to national averages [7]. However, even for populations with relatively similar rates of SUD, there are disparities in medical and psychiatric sequelae; as an example, Black Americans experience higher mortality from alcohol use disorder than white Americans despite similar prevalence, though socioeconomic status may be a confounding variable [3]. Additionally, increasing attention has been paid to disparities in criminal justice system involvement for racial minorities with SUD [3].

Populations immigrating to the United States generally have a lower risk of SUD than native-born Americans, though risk normalized with duration of residence >10 years [8]. Among more disadvantaged immigrant populations (undocumented Mexican groups being most frequently studied), alcohol, tobacco, and illicit drug use are elevated compared with both American and control populations in the home country; in one sample, 42.3% of Mexican migrants report at-risk alcohol use, 31.4% smoke tobacco, and 17.7% use illicit substances [9].

Further, cultural norms for low-risk alcohol use (and perhaps for other substances) differ markedly internationally, leading to large geographical differences in reported prevalence of alcohol use disorder despite using standardized SUD diagnostic criteria. Among European countries, estimated prevalence of alcohol use disorder in 2010 ranged between <1% (in Italy and Spain) and >12% (in Latvia)—though the per capita consumption only varied threefold; further, reported use in countries with religious prohibition against alcohol consumption leads to markedly elevated per capita consumption rates, most likely representing underreporting of individual use [10].

The Treatment Gap for SUD

Of individuals with SUD in the United States, only 23.6% received any treatment (this includes treatment via the inpatient, outpatient, telehealth, or prison/jail setting, as well as people receiving medications for addiction treatment); this marks a significant treatment gap. Of those 18+ who do not receive needed treatment, only 5.3% perceive a need for treatment, highlighting an important attitudinal barrier to accessing care. Of those who do not believe they need treatment,74.1% believe they can handle their use on their own; 65.6% are not ready to start treatment; 60.1% are not ready to stop using [1].

Comorbidity

SUDs are highly comorbid with psychiatric disorders, often complicating treatment and prognosis. The 2023 prevalence of any mental illness was 22.8% of Americans >18 years old (5.7% of all adults having serious mental illness or SMI) [1]. One third of all Americans >18 years old with mental illness had co-occurring SUD, while one half of Americans >18 years old with SMI had co-occurring SUD. Affective, anxiety, personality, and psychotic disorders, as well as attention-deficit hyperactivity disorder (ADHD), are the most common comorbid psychiatric disorders in patients with SUD; 15–25% of individuals with SUD have comorbid ADHD (and 10–45% of those with ADHD have a SUD), 20–29% have comorbid mood or anxiety disorders, and 30–40% have comorbid personality disorders (most commonly antisocial, histrionic, or dependent) [2, 11]. Comorbid SUD among individuals with schizophrenia is markedly elevated, reaching 50% lifetime prevalence; 60–90% use tobacco, with 28% having a nicotine use disorder, and rates of other SUD range from 20% to 65% [12].

Among adolescents aged 12–17 years, 18.1% experienced a major depressive episode in 2023; these depressed adolescents experienced elevated rates of substance use as compared to adolescents who did not experience a major depressive episode (28.4% vs. 11.6%). For adolescents with a past year major depressive episode rates of past month substance use were higher than rates experienced by adolescents without a major depressive episode: past month tobacco or nicotine use were 14.9% vs. 5.7%; past month binge alcohol use were 7.1% vs. 3.1%; past month marijuana use were 21.9% vs. 8.7%; and past month opioid misuse were 3.5% vs. 1.9% [1].

Consequences of Use

SUD has adverse effects on nearly every organ system. Infectious disease transmission, particularly for viral hepatitis and HIV, is a serious consequence of intravenous drug use (IVDU), with 6–9% of new HIV cases in 2016 associated with IVDU [13]. Further, the incidence of new hepatitis C viral infections doubled between 2004 and 2014 in the United States, mirroring an associated rise in admissions for injection opioid use over the same period [14].

Despite increased rates of SUD remission during pregnancy (ranging from 70% to 90% for illicit drugs and alcohol; around 30% for tobacco), 5–15% of pregnant women continue to use substances in the United States (5.9% use illicit drugs, 8.5% drink alcohol, and 15.9% smoke tobacco) [15]. Adverse obstetrical and neonatal outcomes associated with substance use include fetal mortality, congenital anomalies, preterm delivery, low birthweight, neonatal opioid withdrawal syndrome

(NOWS) (for opioid-exposed newborns), and neurodevelopmental disorders (including fetal alcohol syndrome). As of 2018, six neonates have NOWS, and nine have fetal alcohol spectrum disorders for every 1000 live births in the United States [16]. Additionally, high rates of postpartum SUD relapse for mothers lead to deficits in the caregiving environment for infants, risking neglect and sudden infant death syndrome.

Overall, SUD-related deaths have substantially increased since 2000 [17]. Specifically, deaths from drug overdose in the United States have risen dramatically since 2000, at greater than 100,000 from 2021 onward (compared to less than 20,000 deaths in 2000) [18]. These overdoses have largely been driven by increasing rates of fentanyl contamination of the nonprescription drug supply and "prescription" nonsynthetic opioids (excluding methadone), with 22.7 overdose deaths involving these drugs per 100,000 standard population in 2022 [18]. For every opioid overdose death, there are >20 emergency department visits related to opioid use disorder [16]. Emergency department (ED) visits related to substance use have increased in parallel with the opioid epidemic (doubling between 2004 and 2011, reaching 1626 ED visits per 100,000 population in 2011) [19].

Genetics and Epigenetics of SUD

Genetic Risk for SUD

Family and twin studies demonstrate that substance use disorders (SUDs) have significant heritability, with complex genetic influence accounting for 40–70% of the variation in the phenotypic expression of addictive behavior [20, 21]. Addiction is a polygenic disorder, with the relatively large cumulative genetic risk being a sum of multiple "risky" genetic alleles, each with a small individual effect size. This means that the genetics of addiction are non-Mendelian (i.e., there are no dominant, recessive, or X-linked patterns of intergenerational transmission) and that no single gene fully determines whether an individual will develop an SUD. Genetic influences appear to be most important for progressing to (and maintaining) substance use disorder, though there is some evidence for limited effects on initiation and early use [22].

Exemplar Genes

Hundreds of specific genetic loci associated with the risk of SUD have been identified using candidate gene and genome-wide linkage and association studies [22]. Not all have been replicated. Heuristically, we can categorize these genes by their function in (1) substance-specific metabolism, (2) addiction-related neurocircuits, and (3) those requiring further study to understand their relationship to SUD pathogenesis.

Genes Implicated in Substance Metabolism

Genes encoding proteins involved in substance metabolism may affect the amount of a psychoactive substance available to the central nervous system (CNS) or may be involved in the clearance of toxic metabolites. The alcohol dehydrogenases (including ADH1A, 1B, and 1C, ADH4, ADH5, and ADH7) have been identified across genetic studies as affecting risk of developing alcohol use disorder [20, 21]. ADH converts alcohol into acetaldehyde, a toxic intermediate that leads to an aversive "flushing" response. Increased ADH function or decreased acetaldehyde dehydrogenase (ALDH2) function (the latter a phenotype commonly found in Asian populations), both lead to accumulation of acetaldehyde and the aversive reaction, which appears to reduce the risk of developing alcohol use disorder.

Genes Implicated in Addiction-Related Neurocircuits

Genes involved in neurotransmitter systems known to be associated with the neurobiology of addiction have also been implicated. The GABAA receptor gene cluster (specifically, GABRA2) modulates risk of developing alcohol use disorder via anxiety-related phenotypes and sensitivity to the hedonic effects of alcohol consumption [20]. Glutamatergic pathways (specifically CNIH3, involved in ionotropic AMPA-receptor conductance) have been associated with opioid use disorder in genome-wide association studies, or GWAS (a study design that uses markers of genetic variation across the genome to compare cases and controls, identifying specific genetic loci associated with a specific diagnosis) [21, 22]. Nicotinic cholinergic receptors (including alpha-5 and beta-3, CHRNA5 and B3) are associated with nicotine use disorder, amount of daily cigarette consumption, vulnerability to tobacco smoking in schizophrenia, and development of lung cancer [16, 20, 21]. The mu opioid receptor (specifically OPRM1) has been implicated in the pathogenesis of multiple SUDs, with an A118G polymorphism (encoding Asn40Asp amino acid substitution) leading to functional differences in the opioid receptor that appear to confer risk of progressing to SUD, especially in Asian populations where the allele is most common [20]. Single-nucleotide polymorphisms, or SNPs (a single DNA base pair at a specific chromosomal locus that is polymorphic across a population, serving as an easily identifiable surrogate marker to compare large quantities of genetic material between cases and controls in a study), associated with the kappa opioid receptor (responsible for aversive effects; encoded by OPRK1) and its ligand prodynorphin (encoded by PDYN) have also been associated with alcohol use disorder.

The dopamine D2 receptor (DRD2), given its function in the reward system circuit, has been intensively studied, but significant controversy exists around the findings [20, 21]. DRD2 has been associated with multiple SUD phenotypes, but it is unclear if the association is due to this locus or nearby cytoskeletal genes.

Finally, voltage-gated potassium channel (KCNC1, G2, A4) and calcium-dependent signaling (phosphatidylinositol transport gene PITPNM3) genes important for long-term potentiation have been associated with opioid use disorder, linking neural correlates of learning to SUD development.

Genes with Unknown SUD-Related Function

GWAS have identified several genetic loci linked to SUD with unclear function in the pathogenesis of addiction, though these offer promising leads for novel pathways in SUD neurobiology. The family with sequence similarity 53, member B (FAM53B) and cyclin-dependent kinase 1 (CDK1) are associated with cocaine use disorder; autism susceptibility candidate 2 (AUTS2), serine incorporator 2 (SERINC2), and chromosome 15 open reading frame 53 (C15orf53) are associated with alcohol use disorder [20, 21].

Gene-by-Environment Interaction

Known additive genetic influences alone, like those loci reviewed above, account for only a small proportion of the total variance in SUD. Thus, the interaction between genetic influence and environmental exposures has been studied to account for further risk affecting the development of SUD.

Early studies of gene-by-environment interactions focused on the hypothalamic-pituitary-adrenal (HPA) axis, given the role of activation of this system and its corticosteroid mediators in response to environmental stress. The serotonin transporter polymorphic region, or 5-HTTLPR short allele, known to mediate risk of depression in relation to stressful life events, also affects risk of SUD. The short allele possesses a glucocorticoid response element in its promoter region (allowing for HPA-axis-mediated stress response) and has been found to mediate risk of heavy drinking and unprescribed drug use in homozygous individuals with multiple negative life events [22].

Additionally, the genetic risk of tobacco smoking attributable to CHRNA5 (nicotinic cholinergic receptor, alpha-5 subunit) has been shown to be modulated by parental monitoring and exposure to peer tobacco use, again demonstrating a gene-by-environment interaction [22].

Epigenetic Influences

Epigenetic mechanisms are influences on DNA transcription and protein expression that are not encoded in the genetic sequence. These include (1) reduction in gene expression via methylation of specific genetic loci; (2) histone modification via acetylation, impacting availability of genetic loci for transcription; and (3) microRNA regulation of protein translation. Given the significant proportion of risk for SUD not accounted for by genetic variance, epigenetic mechanisms may play an additional role.

Candidate gene methylation studies have demonstrated differential methylation of genes associated with major and minor neurotransmitter systems (monoamines including dopamine and serotonin, cannabinoid, and opioid systems) as well as drug metabolism (CYP2D6 involved in nicotine metabolism; COMT for catecholamines) for alcohol- and nicotine-dependent individuals [22].

Histone modifications via acetylation (making genetic loci available for transcription) and deacetylation (preventing transcription) lead to brain region and cell-type-specific changes that are longer-lasting and may play roles in neuroadaptations that lead to alcohol withdrawal effects [22].

MicroRNA expression in the brain affects synapse development and neuronal plasticity in response to substance exposure. These effects are mediated by adaptation responses in neurotransmitter systems, cytoskeletal organization, and regulation of transcription. For example, the mRNA of neuronal voltage-gated potassium channel BK decreases rapidly following exposure to alcohol, an effect mediated by the microRNA miR-9 [22]. Further microRNAs have been identified that regulate dopamine receptor (miR-382 and D1 receptor) and brain-derived neurotrophic factor (miR-206 and BDNF) expression [22].

Relevance to Treatment

Individual genetic differences are important in understanding differential treatment response in SUD. Response to naltrexone for alcohol use disorder may be modulated by the OPRM1 Asp40 allele (though this difference appears to be overcome by additional treatment modalities) [23]. Response to interventions for nicotine use disorders is highly heritable (40–60% heritability in twin studies), and GWAS have identified multiple genes associated with successful smoking cessation, with the further finding that those who respond to bupropion and nicotine replacement appear to differ genetically [24].

Of relevance to opioid use disorder treatment, the half-life of methadone ranges from 5 to 130 h (mean of 22 h) between individuals; this pharmacokinetic variability is mediated by differences in hepatic CYP enzyme function. Methadone's metabolism is complex, involving multiple CYP enzyme subtypes with different effects on the S- and R-enantiomers present in racemic methadone and multiple active and inactive methadone metabolites produced. CYP2B6 is responsible for a great proportion of methadone clearance, and there are 38 CYP2B6 protein variants with different catalytic activity and expression across studied populations (with a 300-fold inter-individual variability) [25]. CYP2D6 also participates in methadone metabolism and exhibits phenotypic variability in methadone clearance across ultra-rapid and poor metabolizers [25]. Although the pharmacogenomics have yet to be fully characterized, we can expect that some individuals (e.g., those with the CYP2B6*4 SNP) may require higher doses of methadone to overcome rapid hepatic clearance of methadone, while others with slower clearance may require lower methadone doses to avoid respiratory depression (from R-methadone's agonism of the mu opioid receptor) or cardiac arrhythmia (due to the blockade effect of S-methadone on voltage-gated potassium channels in cardiac tissue).

Neurobiology of SUDs

Tripartite Addiction Cycle and Associated Neuroanatomy and Circuitry

The dominant contemporary neurobiological model of addiction consists of three stages: (1) binge/intoxication, with associated classical conditioning to drug-related cues; (2) withdrawal/negative affect; and (3) craving (preoccupation/anticipation) [2, 16, 26]. Three major neuroanatomical regions are known to be important in each stage of the addiction cycle: (1) the striatum (binge/intoxication stage), (2) the extended amygdala (withdrawal/negative affect stage), and (3) the prefrontal cortex (craving stage).

Binge/Intoxication Stage and the Striatum

Habitual or compulsive behavior is encoded in extrapyramidal motor circuits involving the basal ganglia. These are looped feedback motor systems linking cortical to striatal to pallidal to thalamic, then back to cortical neurons [2]. The role of the striatum in this circuit is important in the binge/intoxication stage of the addiction cycle.

The striatum is anatomically composed of the caudate and putamen; it can be divided into dorsolateral (with predominantly motor input) and ventromedial (largely limbic input) areas; the ventromedial striatum includes the nucleus accumbens (NAc), which mediates the hedonic/rewarding effects of psychoactive substance intoxication in addiction.

The classical mesolimbic reward system requires activation of midbrain dopaminergic neurons in the ventral tegmental area (VTA) that project to the NAc; cocaine and other stimulants lead to increased dopamine release from VTA axon terminals in the NAc [2]. Nicotine activation of a4b2 acetylcholine receptors also modulates dopaminergic activity in the mesolimbic circuit [2, 26]. Opioids, agonizing mu opioid receptors, disinhibit firing of VTA dopaminergic neurons in the NAc (by inhibiting inhibitory GABAergic interneurons) and act independently of the mesolimbic system, directly agonizing mu opioid receptors in the NAc. Alcohol's reinforcing effect is complex but appears to, in part, involve enhancement of GABAA receptor function, which also disinhibits mesolimbic dopaminergic firing. Phencyclidine may inhibit postsynaptic glutamatergic NMDA receptors in the NAc. Cannabinoids agonize CB1 receptors, which modulate both dopamine and opioid activity in the NAc [2, 26]. Figure 3.1 illustrates these sites of action for each substance class.

NAc activation initially reinforces substance use (bingeing) and strengthens classically conditioned associations between substance-induced reward and previously

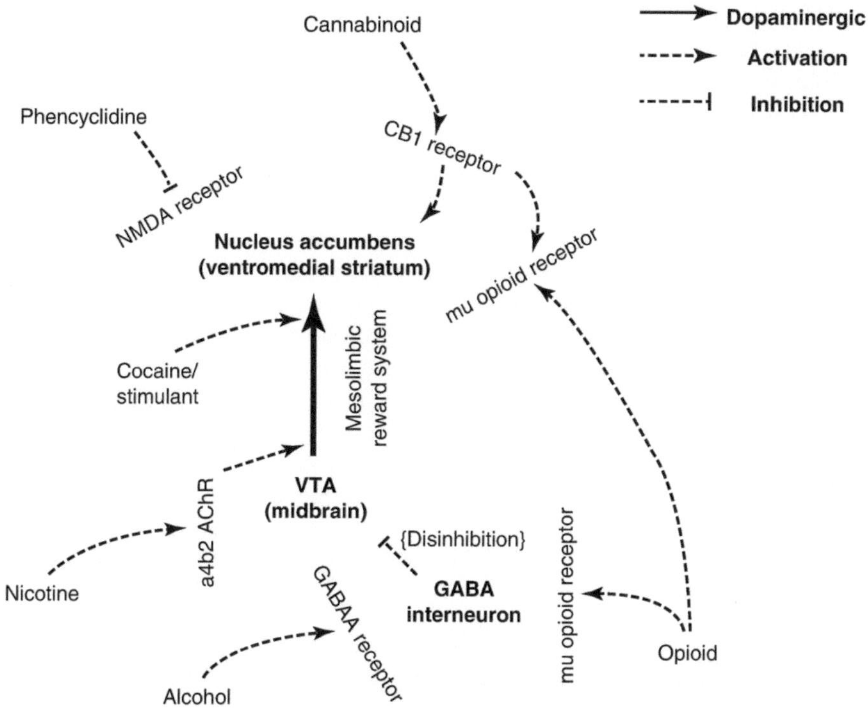

Fig. 3.1 Substance-specific effects on the classical mesolimbic reward system. Dopaminergic projections from the ventral tegmental area (VTA) to the nucleus accumbens (NAc) in the ventromedial striatum compose the mesolimbic reward system, important for the rewarding effects of substance intoxication. Cocaine and other stimulants increase dopamine release from VTA axon terminals in the NAc; nicotine activation of a4b2 acetylcholine receptors in the VTA modulates its dopaminergic activity; opioids agonize mu opioid receptors and disinhibit firing of VTA dopaminergic neurons in the NAc by inhibiting inhibitory GABAergic interneurons and also directly agonize mu opioid receptors in the NAc; alcohol's reinforcing effect involves enhancement of GABAA receptor function, which disinhibits VTA dopaminergic firing; phencyclidine inhibits postsynaptic glutamatergic NMDA receptors in the NAc; cannabinoids agonize CB1 receptors, which modulate both dopamine and opioid activity in the NAc

neutral stimuli (paraphernalia, location of use, etc.) paired with the substance. The conditioned stimuli then can independently induce dopaminergic firing in the NAc, resulting in "incentive salience" and motivation to repeat use (as occurs in the craving characterizing the third preoccupation/anticipation stage) [2, 16, 26].

Withdrawal/Negative Affect Stage and the Extended Amygdala

With repeated substance-induced NAc activation, dopamine release and response in the NAc is attenuated; dopamine D2 receptor density and basal firing rate of mesolimbic dopaminergic neurons decrease with repeated substance exposure [23]. This is thought to be mediated by an opponent-process counter-adaptation in the "anti-reward" system that is in homeostatic balance with the reward system. The introduction of NAc activation by substance intoxication leads to an allostatic shift, where the basal dopaminergic firing rate becomes stably lower than before repeated substance exposure, establishing a new homeostatic equilibrium. This shift is thought to be driven by neuroplastic adaptation involving glutamatergic projections from the amygdala and prefrontal cortex to NMDA and AMPA receptors in the mesolimbic system [23]. This reduction in mesolimbic dopaminergic activity secondarily decreases sensitivity to reward from natural reinforcers (food, sex, etc.), as well.

The homeostatic anti-reward system drives the withdrawal/negative affect stage of the addiction cycle, consisting of a state of dysphoria, anhedonia, stress sensitivity, and anxiety. It involves the central division of the extended amygdala, a circuit composed of the amygdala's central nucleus, bed nucleus of the stria terminalis, and a transition zone in the NAc shell [2]; the habenula has also been implicated more recently [16]. The withdrawal/negative affect stage signals a shift from positive to negative reinforcement as the dominant motivator of addictive behavior; in this stage, seeking relief from the aversive negative emotional state is most salient. The extended amygdala activates stress-response neurotransmitter systems, including corticotropin-releasing factor (CRF), norepinephrine, and dynorphin, which drive the aversive withdrawal state.

Craving (Preoccupation/Anticipation) and the Prefrontal Cortex

As noted above, the craving stage is marked by conditioned stimulus-induced release of dopamine in the NAc, motivating compulsive drug-seeking behavior. The prefrontal cortex's executive function manages this cue-induced impulse using two opposing systems, termed the Go system (which engages automatic habitual behavior) and the Stop system (which inhibits these habitual behaviors) [2]. The Go system is composed of the anterior cingulate and dorsolateral prefrontal cortex, both of which are involved in attention, planning, and self-initiation. The Stop system involves the orbitofrontal cortex and ventrolateral prefrontal cortex, which participate in response inhibition, rule generation, set-shifting, and salience attribution, integrating anticipated reward or punishment [2].

Prefrontal glutamatergic projections from these systems to the VTA and striatum modulate the response to craving, whether it is cue-induced anticipation of reward or withdrawal-induced desire for relief [16, 25]. In the addiction syndrome, the Stop system is hypofunctional, and the Go system is hyperactive alongside a sensitized anti-reward system [2, 16]. This imbalance leads to a great disadvantage for individuals with SUD working to oppose impulses toward relapse.

Neurodevelopment During Adolescence

Ongoing neurodevelopment in adolescence (extending into the third decade of life) implies greater neuroplasticity in this age group than is present in adulthood; this allows for more rapid neuroadaptation to psychotropic substance exposure, and thus faster development of an addiction syndrome [16, 26]. The rate of neurodevelopment is uneven across different circuits, with maturity achieved in the reward-mediating (striatal) and emotional (limbic) systems earlier than the top-down cognitive control circuits of the prefrontal cortex [16]. This leads to greater affective reactivity and reward-seeking behaviors without the (later-to-develop) self-regulation of impulses or exciting risk.

Increased risk-taking and impulsivity, coupled with greater neuroplasticity, are thought to create a uniquely vulnerable period for the development of SUD in adolescence and emerging adulthood.

Summary of Relevant Neurotransmitter Systems

Monoamines play an important role in addiction. Dopamine is predominant, acting on D1 and D2 receptors in the mesolimbic and mesocortical dopaminergic circuits mediating reward and motivation (as discussed above); the nigrostriatal dopaminergic circuit is part of the extrapyramidal motor system, which may also become dysregulated by substance exposure (e.g., emergent stereotypy in stimulant use disorder). Serotonin modulates the dopaminergic system in addiction. Norepinephrine, acting on a1, a2, and b-adrenergic receptors from noradrenergic projections out of the locus coeruleus in the dorsal pons, is involved in the stress response, as well as attention/vigilance and arousal.

The opioid system has three well-known receptors, most importantly mu (mediating euphoria, analgesia, and respiratory drive) and kappa (mediating dysphoria and neuroendocrine stress response); both mu and kappa are implicated in the addictive syndrome. The endocannabinoid receptor, CB1, modulates both the opioid and dopamine systems.

Excitatory glutamatergic input from the cortex and inhibitory GABAergic interneurons also feed into addiction-related circuits, with some substances acting directly on these systems (e.g., phencyclidine blocking NMDA glutamate receptors; alcohol enhancing GABAA receptor activity).

Additional neurotransmitters have been implicated in the stress response system, including corticotropin-releasing factor (CRF acting at CRF1 and CRF2 receptors), vasopressin (V1b receptors), neuropeptide Y (Y1 and Y2 receptors), and nociceptin/orphanin FQ (opioid receptor-like 1, or ORL-1 receptors).

Chapter Review Questions

1. You are evaluating a new patient who endorses alcohol and tobacco use on a screening questionnaire; given the frequent co-occurrence of illicit substance use, you begin to formulate additional questions for the patient, informed by current epidemiological data.

   Tobacco and alcohol are the most common substances associated with a use disorder. What illicit substances have the greatest and second-greatest 12-month prevalence of use disorder?

   A. Cannabis, Opioids
   B. Opioids, Cannabis
   C. Stimulants (including cocaine), Opioids
   D. Hallucinogens, Stimulants
   E. Benzodiazepines, Cannabis

   Answer: A

   Explanation: In 2023, cannabis use disorder saw a 12-month prevalence of 6.8%, with opioid use disorder being the second most prevalent use disorder of the illicit substances at 1.9%.
2. In 2017, after alcohol (with 4.9 million new users), cannabis and prescription opioids had the most new users, with three million and two million new users, respectively. In 2023, which substance has now surpassed these substances for the most new users?

   A. Tobacco
   B. Stimulants (including cocaine)
   C. Nicotine vaping
   D. Benzodiazepines
   E. Nonprescription Opioids

   Answer: C

   Explanation: The substances with the most new users in 2023 are nicotine vaping (5.9 million), alcohol (4.2 million), tobacco (6.2 million), cannabis (3.5 million), and hallucinogens (1.5 million).
3. You are working at a university clinic, and a new patient comes in endorsing drinking "only occasionally," but reports at times having 4 or 5 12-ounce beers in an evening. You are considering how to effectively approach discussing this amount of alcohol use with the patient, using your understanding of the known health risks associated with specific amounts of alcohol exposure.

   While most substances do not have a "safe" amount of use, alcohol has a specific amount of use that has been defined as *hazardous* or at-risk for adverse health outcomes. How many standard 14-gram drinks are considered "heavy" use for women and men aged >65 years?

   A. 4 or more drinks/day or >7 drinks/week
   B. 5 or more drinks/day or >14 drinks/week

C. 7 or more drinks/day or >21 drinks/week
D. 2 or more drinks/day or >7 drinks/week
E. 2 or more drinks/day or >5 drinks/week.

Answer: A

Explanation: 4 or more drinks/day or >7 drinks/week are considered *heavy use* for women or men >65 years. For men younger than 65 years, heavy use is 5 or more drinks/day or >14 drinks/week. Though these amounts are hazardous, drinking less quantities may still be unhealthy and lead to adverse health outcomes (such as injury during acute intoxication).

4. What age group saw the most notable peak in endorsing drinking 5 or more drinks in a day (4 or more drinks in a day for females) in 2023?

A. 12- to 17-year-olds
B. 18- to 25-year-olds
C. 25- to 40-year-olds
D. 41- to 65-year-olds
E. Over 65-year-olds

Answer: B

Explanation: In 2023, 21.7% of the general population aged >12 years endorsed drinking 5 or more drinks in a day (4 or more drinks in a day for females). The age group with a notable peak in such habits was seen among 18- to 25-year-olds (28.7% of this age group).

5. You are treating a patient admitted to your general hospital's inpatient psychiatric unit for major depressive disorder and alcohol use disorder. The patient reports that they have never discussed their drinking with a medical provider before and asks you if there is a connection between alcohol use and mood.

SUD is highly comorbid with other psychiatric disorders, complicating treatment and prognosis. What percentage of individuals with a psychiatric illness have co-occurring SUD? And what percentage of individuals with a mood disorder have co-occurring SUD?

A. 65% and 33%
B. 45% and 20%
C. 50% and 50%
D. 20% and 45%
E. 33% and 25%

Answer: E

Explanation: One-third of all Americans >18 years old with any mental illness had co-occurring SUD, while one half of all Americans >18 years old with SMI had co-occurring SUD. Affective, anxiety, personality, and psychotic disorders, as well as attention-deficit hyperactivity disorder (ADHD), are the most common comorbid psychiatric disorders in patients with SUD, and 20–29% have comorbid mood or anxiety disorders.

6. What percentage of individuals in the general population with a SUD received any treatment in 2023, according to NSDUH data?

   A. 45%
   B. 35%
   C. 25%
   D. 15%
   E. 5%

   Answer: C
   Explanation: 25% (actual number is 23.6%) of individuals with SUD received treatment in 2023. This includes receiving treatment in any of the following settings: inpatient, outpatient, telehealth, or prison/jail setting, as well as people receiving medication-assisted treatment.

7. Your patient has an extensive family history of substance use disorders. The patient reports concerns because he is undergoing a surgical procedure next week and wonders about the risk of developing an SUD if prescribed opioid medication. How is addiction understood to be genetically passed from generation to generation?

   A. Autosomal dominant disorder
   B. Autosomal recessive disorder
   C. Polygenic disorder
   D. Genetic anticipation
   E. Still unknown

   Answer: C
   Explanation: Addiction is a polygenic disorder. 40–70% heritability of SUD has been repeatedly demonstrated by family and twin studies. The genetics are non-Mendelian (without dominant, recessive, or X-linked patterns of transmission) and no single gene determines the development of SUD. The genetic risk appears most important for the progression from use to use disorder.

8. The interaction between genetic risk and environmental exposures influences individuals' risk of progressing to SUD. The genetic risk of tobacco smoking attributable to which gene has been shown to be modulated by factors such as parental monitoring and exposure to peer tobacco use, demonstrating a gene-by-environment interaction?

   A. DRD2
   B. CHRNA5
   C. COMT
   D. SLC6A3
   E. MAOA

   Answer: B
   Explanation: The genetic risk of tobacco smoking attributable to CHRNA5 (nicotinic cholinergic receptor, alpha-5 subunit) has been shown to be

modulated by parental monitoring and exposure to peer tobacco use, again demonstrating a gene-by-environment interaction

9. Your patient, a first-year college student, has found the biological disease model helpful in conceptualizing their newly diagnosed cannabis use disorder, increasing their engagement in multiple treatment modalities and reducing stigma-based shame. They bring their visiting parent to a joint visit and ask that you review this model with them.

   What neuroanatomical regions are associated with each stage of the addiction cycle?

   A. Binge intoxication, striatum; withdrawal, prefrontal cortex; craving, extended amygdala
   B. Binge intoxication, prefrontal cortex; withdrawal, extended amygdala; craving, habenula
   C. Binge intoxication, striatum; withdrawal, extended amygdala; craving, prefrontal cortex
   D. Binge intoxication, extended amygdala; withdrawal, prefrontal cortex; craving, striatum
   E. Binge intoxication, striatum; withdrawal, extended amygdala; craving, habenula

   Answer: C

   Explanation: Binge intoxication, striatum; withdrawal, extended amygdala; craving, prefrontal cortex. The striatum is composed of the caudate and putamen; the ventromedial striatum includes the nucleus accumbens (NAc), which mediates the rewarding effects of intoxication in addiction. The homeostatic anti-reward system drives the withdrawal/negative affect stage of the addiction cycle; it involves the central division of the extended amygdala, a circuit composed of the amygdala's central nucleus, bed nucleus of the stria terminalis, and a transition zone in the NAc shell, as well as the habenula. The craving stage is marked by conditioned stimulus-induced release of dopamine in the NAc, motivating compulsive drug-seeking behavior; the prefrontal cortex's executive function manages this cue-induced impulse using two opposing systems, termed the Go system (which engages automatic habitual behavior) and the Stop system (which inhibits these habitual behaviors). Prefrontal glutamatergic projections from these systems to the VTA and striatum modulate the response to craving. In addition, the Stop system is hypofunctional, and the Go system is hyperactive alongside a sensitized anti-reward system.

10. Increased risk-taking and impulsivity, along with greater neuroplasticity, are believed to make adolescence and emerging adulthood a particularly vulnerable period for developing SUD. Which of the following factors contributes most to this vulnerability during this developmental phase?

    A. Decreased dopamine receptor sensitivity
    B. Reduced neuroplasticity in the prefrontal cortex

C. Underdeveloped prefrontal cognitive control systems
D. Fully matured limbic affective system
E. Heightened cognitive control over impulsive behaviors

Answer: C

Explanation: The Prefrontal (top-down) cognitive control system is underdeveloped relative to the striatal and limbic systems, the latter two motivating impulsive, reward-seeking behavior and greater affective reactivity. This imbalance increases the risk of substance use during a sensitive period of neurodevelopment.

References

1. Substance Abuse and Mental Health Services Administration (SAMHSA). Key substance use and mental health indicators in the United States: results from the 2023 National Survey on Drug Use and Health (HHS Publication No. PEP24-07-021, NSDUH Series H-59). Rockville: Center for Behavioral Health Statistics and Quality, Substance Abuse and Mental Health Services Administration; 2023. Retrieved from https://www.samhsa.gov/data/.
2. Koob GF, Arends MA, Le Moal M. Drugs, addiction, and the brain. Waltham: Academic Press (Elsevier); 2014.
3. Miller SC, Rosenthal RN, Levy S, Saxon AJ, Tetrault JM, Wakeman SE. The ASAM principles of addiction medicine. 7th ed. Wolters Kluwer; 2024.
4. Grant BF, Goldstein RB, Saha TD, et al. Epidemiology of *DSM-5* alcohol use disorder: results from the National Epidemiologic Survey on Alcohol and Related Conditions III. JAMA Psychiat. 2015;72(8):757–66. https://doi.org/10.1001/jamapsychiatry.2015.0584.
5. National Institute on Alcohol Abuse and Alcoholism. What is a standard drink? National Institutes of Health; December 2024. Available at: https://www.niaaa.nih.gov/alcohols-effects-health/what-standard-drink.
6. National Institute on Drug Abuse. Substance use in women: sex and gender differences in substance use. National Institutes of Health; April 2020. Retrieved from https://www.drugabuse.gov/publications/research-reports/substance-use-in-women/sex-gender-differences-in-substance-use.
7. Substance Abuse and Mental Health Services Administration (SAMHSA). 2023 NSDUH: highlights by race/ethnicity for the 2023 National Survey on Drug Use; 2023. Retrieved from https://www.samhsa.gov/data/sites/default/files/NSDUH%202023%20Annual%20Release/2023-nsduh-race-eth-highlights.pdf.
8. Breslau J, Aguilar-Gaxiola S, Borges G, Kendler KS, Su M, Kessler RC. Risk for psychiatric disorder among immigrants and their US-born descendants: evidence from the National Comorbidity Survey Replication. J Nerv Ment Dis. 2007;195(3):189–95.
9. Zhang X, Martinez-Donate AP, Nobles J, Hovell MF, Gudelia Rangel M, Rhoads NM. Substance use across different phases of the migration process: a survey of Mexican migrants flows. J Immigr Minor Health. 2015;17(6):1746–57.
10. Rehm J, Room R. The cultural aspect how to measure and interpret epidemiological data on alcohol-use disorders across cultures. Nordic Stud Alcohol Drugs. 2017;34(4):330–41.
11. Wilens TE. Attention deficit hyperactivity disorder and substance use disorders. Am J Psychiatry. 2006;163:2059–63.
12. Volkow ND. Substance use disorders in schizophrenia–clinical implications of comorbidity. Schizophr Bull. 2009;35(3):469–72.

13. Centers for Disease Control and Prevention. HIV Surveillance Report, 2016; vol. 28. http://www.cdc.gov/hiv/library/reports/hiv-surveillance.html. Published November 2017. Accessed 27 Oct 2018.
14. Zibbell JE, Asher AK, Patel RC, Kupronis B, Iqbal K, Ward JW, Holtzman D. Increases in acute hepatitis C virus infection related to a growing opioid epidemic and associated injection drug use, United States, 2004 to 2014. Am J Public Health. 2018;108(2):175–81.
15. Forray A. Substance use during pregnancy. F1000Res. 2016;5:F1000 Faculty Rev-887.
16. Volkow ND, Boyle M. Neuroscience of addiction: relevance to prevention and treatment. Am J Psychiatry. 2018;175(8):729–40.
17. National Institute on Drug Abuse. Overdose death rates. National Institutes of Health; 2018. Retrieved from https://www.drugabuse.gov/related-topics/trends-statistics/overdose-death-rates.
18. Spencer MR, Garnett MF, Miniño AM. Drug overdose deaths in the United States, 2002–2022. NCHS data brief, no 491. Hyattsville: National Center for Health Statistics; 2024. https://doi.org/10.15620/cdc:135849.
19. Substance Abuse and Mental Health Services Administration. Drug Abuse Warning Network (DAWN), 2011: National estimates of erug-related emergency department visits. HHS Publication No. (SMA) 13-4760, DAWN Series D-39. Rockville; 2013.
20. Gelernter J, Kranzler HR. Genetics of addiction. In: Galanter M, Kleber HD, Brady KT, editors. The American psychiatric publishing textbook of substance abuse treatment. 5th ed; 2015. Accessed 27 Oct 2018 via https://psychiatryonline-org.ezproxy.med.cornell.edu/doi/full/10.1176/appi.books.9781615370030.mg02.
21. Deak JD, Johnson EC. Genetics of substance use disorders: a review. Psychol Med. 2021;51(13):2189–200. https://doi.org/10.1017/S0033291721000969.
22. Prom-Wormleya EC, Ebejerb J, Dickc DM, Bowers MS. The genetic epidemiology of substance use disorder: a review. Drug Alcohol Depend. 2017;180:241–59.
23. Anton RF, Oroszi G, O'Malley S, et al. An evaluation of μ-opioid receptor (OPRM1) as a predictor of naltrexone response in the treatment of alcohol dependence results from the combined pharmacotherapies and Behavioral interventions for alcohol dependence (COMBINE) study. Arch Gen Psychiatry. 2008;65(2):135–44.
24. Uhl GR, Liu Q, Drgon T, et al. Molecular genetics of successful smoking cessation convergent genome-wide association study results. Arch Gen Psychiatry. 2008;65(6):683–93.
25. Ahmad T, Valentovic MA, Rankin GO. Effects of cytochrome P450 single nucleotide polymorphisms on methadone metabolism and pharmacodynamics. Biochem Pharmacol. 2018;153:196–204.
26. Uhl GR, Koob GF, Cable J. The neurobiology of addiction. Ann N Y Acad Sci. 2019;1451(1):5–28.

Screening, Evaluation, and Diagnosis of Substance Use Disorder

4

Eve Lasswell and Katia M. Harlé

High-Yield Review Points

- Positive screenings for SUD should facilitate a more comprehensive assessment that contributes to diagnostic impressions and yields clinically useful information for treatment planning.
- Based on the DSM-5-TR, an SUD is diagnosed when the person meets at least 2 of 11 criteria within the same 12-month period [1].
- A comprehensive clinical diagnostic evaluation for SUD should start with a thorough history of presenting illness followed by a systematic assessment of past and present substance use history, other psychiatric history, family history, social and developmental history, and a psychiatric/mental status exam.
- Most individuals will experience recovery of cognitive and motor functions after an extended period of sobriety, but recovery of specific cognitive functions occurs at different rates and is impacted by many factors including age, polysubstance use, duration, and severity of substance use [2].

E. Lasswell
Department of Psychiatry, University of California San Diego, La Jolla, CA, USA
e-mail: elasswell@health.ucsd.edu

K. M. Harlé (✉)
Department of Psychiatry, University of California San Diego, La Jolla, CA, USA

VA San Diego Health System, La Jolla, CA, USA
e-mail: kharle@health.ucsd.edu

C. Marienfeld, M. Soltani (eds.), *AAAP Review of Addiction Psychiatry*,
https://doi.org/10.1007/978-3-032-24174-0_4

Screening

Screening tests for SUDs are relatively brief measures that are designed to identify someone who may be at risk for alcohol- or substance-related disorders, and who may be offered or referred for further evaluation and treatment. Screening measures are not intended to yield a diagnosis or provide a comprehensive account of alcohol or other substance use history. Positive screenings for SUD should facilitate a more comprehensive assessment that contributes to diagnostic impressions and yields clinically useful information for treatment.

In general, structured or semi-structured interviews can collect more comprehensive, detailed information relative to informal interviews while reducing variability from interviewer differences [3]. Structured interviews are fully scripted, requiring strict adherence to questions and allowing a limited range of responses with no individualized follow-up. Semi-structured interviews also utilize a scripted format but allow for clinical judgment in the use of queries to elicit more detailed information from the respondent. Both interview types deserve consideration because of their standardized administration and rigorous approach to identifying specific diagnostic criteria (typically DSM or ICD elements).

Screening measures can be selected according to how well they perform in specific target populations (e.g., adults versus adolescents, psychiatric inpatients, Veterans, etc.) or particular environments (e.g., primary care clinics, counseling centers, online computerized screening). Many screening measures are self-administered (paper/pencil or computer-based) and require a minimum expenditure of time. Optimal brief screening has been investigated using only a few specific questions derived from larger screening measures. Statistically, screening measures are evaluated in terms of their ability to correctly identify true positives (sensitivity) or true negatives (specificity). The selection of a test based on sensitivity or specificity values usually depends on the significance (in terms of cost or severity of an outcome) of an incorrect result in either condition.

Self-reported information about substance use is typically "pre-screened" using brief, focused questions, such as the National Institute on Alcohol Abuse and Alcoholism's (NIAAA) 3 Question Screen or the National Institute on Drug Abuse's (NIDA) Quick Screen. Adequate screening properties have been achieved with only 2 questions culled from longer screening tools (87.2% sensitivity, 79.8% specificity) in screening tools such as the CRAFFT, discussed below [4]. Generally, a positive response from a 2- or 3-question screen would be followed by a more comprehensive screening test.

Here is a summary of brief, initial screens for substance use:

AlcoholScreening.org**,** managed by Join Together, is a free self-assessment tool that helps identify if a person is endorsing alcohol consumption that may be harmful to their health.

*The CAGE Questionnaire***,** developed by Bowles Center for Alcohol Studies Founding Director Dr. John Ewing, is a 4-item questionnaire that can indicate potential problems with alcohol [5]. Of note, the CAGE AID measure was adapted to include drugs. The CAGE Questionnaire usually takes 5 minutes to administer and was designed to be used in any medical clinic. "CAGE" is an acronym formed from the italicized letters in the questionnaire (cut down-annoyed-guilty-eye opener):

- Have you ever felt you should *C*ut down on your drinking?
- Have people *A*nnoyed you by criticizing your drinking?
- Have you ever felt bad or *G*uilty about your drinking?
- Have you ever had a drink first thing in the morning to steady your nerves or to get rid of a hangover (*E*ye opener)?

Item responses on the CAGE are scored 0 or 1, with a higher score indicating alcohol problems. A total score of 2 or greater is considered clinically significant and warrants further assessment for an alcohol use disorder and possible clinical intervention and/or treatment recommendations.

The CRAFFT screening interview is a 6-question screening instrument designed for individuals under the age of 21 to identify if they have potential problems with alcohol and other drug use. The acronym "CRAFFT" refers to the different situations and consequences assessed by the measure. The measure asks about riding in the Car with someone under the influence, using substances to Relax or try to fit in, using Alone, whether use leads someone to Forget what has happened, whether Friends or family have expressed concern about use, and whether use has led the person completing the measure to get into Trouble.

Part A includes questions about the use of alcohol, marijuana or hashish, and other substances used to get high (illegal drugs, over-the-counter and prescription drugs, or anything used as an inhalant) during the past 12 months. Part B assesses the context of use (drinking with others or alone, reason for use), hazardous conditions (driving or being driven by someone that is high, having gotten in trouble while using, or forgetting actions one did while using), and interpersonal functioning (family or friends asking you to cut down).

The CRAFFT is a 2-part questionnaire—if the person answers yes to any of the first 3 questions, the person will be asked a set of 6 questions. Each "yes" answer earns a score of 1 and after all of the questions have been answered, a total cumulative score is given. The higher the score, the greater the predictive value of future drug misuse and therefore the need to refer the person for a full assessment by a SUD-treating provider. Two or more "yes" answers indicate a need for further assessment.

The NIDA Single Question Screen Test [17] was developed by NIDA to quickly screen for substance use issues. The single question is:

How many times in the past year have you used an illegal drug or used a prescription medication for non-medical reasons (for example, because of the experience or feeling it caused)?

Any substance use indicates a need for more in-depth screening to determine whether a referral for further care is appropriate.

The NIAAA 3 Question Screen was developed by NIAAA to assess problematic alcohol use [6].

1. How many days per week do you drink alcohol?
2. On a typical day when you drink, how many drinks do you have?
3. What is the maximum number of drinks you had on any given day in the past month?

The NIAAA 3-question screen is not scored, per se. Rather, the answers to the questions are used to determine if the person is drinking at levels above or below NIAAA levels for heavy drinking. The NIAAA defines heavy drinking for healthy men up to age 65 as more than 4 drinks in a day and more than 14 drinks in a week. For healthy women (and healthy men over age 65), the definition is more than 3 drinks in a day and more than 7 drinks in a week.

The ASSIST is the **A**lcohol, **S**moking, and **S**ubstance **I**nvolvement **S**creening **T**est [7]. It is a brief screening questionnaire initially developed by the World Health Organization (WHO). It collects information about lifetime and past 3-month use, associated problems, risk of current or future harms, and injection drug use. This screener contains 7 questions about each of 10 substances and 1 question about IV drug use.

This measure provides feedback about each level of risk to the person with continued use (low = 0–3, moderate = 4–26, or high = 27+) with a cumulative score for each substance. The only exception is for alcohol use, where low = 0–10, moderate = 11–26, and high = 27+.

The AUDIT is the **A**lcohol **U**se **D**isorders **I**dentification **T**est (AUDIT), a 10-item screening instrument initially developed by the World Health Organization (WHO) to identify excessive and harmful patterns of alcohol use [8].

The 10 AUDIT questions are scored with responses scaled 0–4, where 0 indicates "never" to 4, "daily or almost daily." A score of 8 or more is associated with harmful or hazardous drinking; a score of 13 or more in women and 15 or more in men is likely to indicate the presence of alcohol use disorder.

The Michigan Alcoholism Screening Test (MAST) is a 28-item screen designed to assess problems with alcohol use [9].

To score this instrument, add up the points for every question answered "yes"; for questions 23 and 24 multiply the number of times by points. A score of 0–3 indicates no apparent problem; a score of 4 indicates that the person is an early or middle problem drinker; and a score of 5 or more indicates that the person taking the measure is a problem drinker.

The Michigan Alcoholism Screening Test—Geriatric Version (MAST-G) [18] is a 24-item screen designed to assess problems in older adults with alcohol use. It differs from the MAST in that the questions highlight the potentially different employment and social situations of someone who is retired, and how this can relate to problematic alcohol use.

To score this instrument, add up the points for every question. A score of 5 or more "yes" responses is indicative of a potential alcohol problem and suggests the need for further assessment.

The Short Michigan Alcohol Screening Test (SMAST) [19, 20] is a 10-item screening tool designed to assess problems with alcohol use. It is easier to use in clinical settings where there are time constraints.

Add up the points for every question. Scores of zero or one do not indicate problems with alcohol use and its consequences; two points indicates possible Alcohol Use Disorder, and three or more points indicates that the person completing the measure should be referred for further assessment and they are likely to meet criteria for a diagnosis of Alcohol Use Disorder.

The Drug Abuse Screening Test (DAST) [21] is a 28-item self-reported scale developed by Harvey Skinner of the Toronto Center for Mental Health [10], which consists of items similar to the Michigan Alcoholism Screening Test (MAST). This scale does not screen for alcohol/tobacco. DAST assesses a pattern of use for the 12 months prior to administration.

All questions are answered on a yes or no basis with a score of 1 point for every yes answer. The cumulative score of all answers is used to rate the degree of intensity of the drug use problem and is used to direct the recommended type of intervention. Scoring is as follows: score of 1–2, possible low level of drug use (it is recommended that the person be reassessed in the future for worsening of drug problems); score of 3–5, possible moderate drug use problem; score of 6–8, possible substantial drug use problem; and score of 9–10, significant drug use problem.

The shorter *Drug Abuse Screening Test—10-item measure (DAST-10)* is a shortened, 10-item version of the DAST. Like the SMAST, it is easier to use in clinical situations where there are time constraints.

Score 1 point for each item answered "yes" except for item #3 where a "no" receives 1 point. Then add up the points for the total DAST-10 score. A "low" score is indicated by 1–2 points, an "intermediate" score is indicated by 3–5 points and means that the respondent likely meets diagnostic criteria for a substance use disorder, a "substantial" score is indicated by 6–8 points and a "severe" score is indicated by 9–10 points out of ten possible points. Intermediate, substantial, and severe scoring categories indicate that the respondent should be referred for further substance use disorder care.

The OWLS [22] is a 4-item self-report scale to screen for likely opioid use disorder, targeting Overuse of the substance, Worrying about use of opioid medicines, Losing interest in usual activities due to opioid medicines, and feeling Slowed down/Sedated, due to opioid medicine (i.e., "OWLS").

Response options are "not at all," "a little," "quite a lot," and "a great deal". All questions are answered "yes" or "no" with a score of 1 point for every "yes" answer. "Not at all" responses are coded 0 and any response greater than or equal to "a little bit" has a positive response of 1. Positive responses are summed with a total cutoff 3, indicating a positive screen.

Standardized Psychometric Tests for Substance Use Disorders (SUD)

An array of evidence-based psychometric tests are available for screening and assessment of SUD. The primary rationale for adding psychometric tests to clinical interviews is to increase the overall diagnostic accuracy and predictive validity of the assessment process. Informal, unstructured clinical interviews are ubiquitous in SUD assessment processes. In addition to basic information gathering, the unstructured interview can foster rapport building, allow a clinician to provide psychoeducation about treatment options, and afford flexibility in dealing with clinical emergencies. However, clinicians using unstructured interviews typically overestimate their diagnostic accuracy wherein increased error variance from interviewer effects (e.g., sociodemographic variables) is more likely to occur when assessing sensitive information like substance use. A multi-method assessment approach that combines a clinical interview with psychometric tests and additional sources of information (i.e., medical records, collateral information, biological tests) can improve the accuracy of the diagnosis, augment clinical characterization, and enhance prediction of treatment outcomes [11].

Psychometric tests and interviews for SUD can be broadly classified according to the purpose and phase (timing) of the assessment. Brief screening measures are used to identify those who may be at risk for these disorders from a larger cohort; structured interviews or self-report instruments provide information for a formal diagnosis based on specific SUD criteria; and comprehensive mental health assessments identify comorbid disorders and help to provide additional diagnostic information for treatment planning. Within these categories, considerations for test selection include choices about (a) clinician-administered measure versus self-report, (b) manual scoring versus computer-assisted scoring, (c) current or recent alcohol/drug use versus lifetime/chronic use, (d) clinical versus research application, and (e) target populations such as non-specific groups versus subgroups with characteristics of interest (age, gender, ethnicity, or race).

Statistical and Psychometric Information for Test Selection

The selection of an appropriate evidence-based test involves both theoretical and pragmatic considerations.

Reliability refers to the accuracy of measurement and sources of error when a test is administered across time, over different settings, and by different administrators. Estimates of test-retest reliability indicate how consistently the test evaluates a given person or group over multiple occasions (i.e., temporal stability). This measure can vary according to how stable or transient a given trait or characteristic might be over a given length of time. Estimates of inter-rater reliability indicate the degree of measurement error attributable to differences between examiners or styles of administration. Internal consistency measures how well the items within a given scale or test correlate with each other. The uniformity of the test content can also be assessed with split-half reliability measures (comparing half of the test items with the remaining half) to determine the extent to which individual test items accurately measure the construct of interest.

Validity is an indicator of how well a test actually samples or measures the characteristic of interest, determining if the test is accurately assessing the condition or trait that it proposes to measure. Within this category, test validity can be evaluated by comparing results to outside performance measure(s). Criterion validity can indicate how well a test measures a specific outcome at the present time (concurrent validity) or at some point in the future (predictive validity). Content validity refers to how well items within a test accurately sample the characteristic, disorder, or domain of interest. Construct validity is established over time as the test is compared with both related and dissimilar characteristics and tests. Construct validity evolves with accrued research on the test, comparing and contrasting it with other constructs. Finally, incremental validity reflects the extent to which the test results yield information over and above what is to be gained through other methods.

Psychometric Assessment

Classification through structured interviews is considered the "gold standard" when comparing predictive validity of other tests. Disadvantages can include lengthy administration time and training time required for correct administration. Frequently used structured and semi-structured interviews include Addiction Severity Index (ASI), Composite International Diagnostic Interview (CIDI), Structured Clinical Interview for DSM-5 (SCID), Alcohol Use Disorders and Associated Disabilities Interview Schedule (AUDADIS-5), Psychiatric Research Interview for Substance and Mental Disorders (PRISM), and Semi-Structured Assessment for Drug Dependence and Alcoholism (SSADDA). It should be noted that the transition to DSM-5 signaled a shift from a largely categorical diagnostic approach to a combination categorical and dimensional approach (e.g., including specifiers for severity and remission status). Additionally, there has been a shift in the substance use disorder treatment field toward detecting and treating co-occurring substance use disorders and other mental health concerns.

Psychiatric comorbidity with substance use is associated with worse health outcomes, more complex clinical management, and increased health care costs [2]. When a co-occurring disorder has been detected, a comprehensive assessment can help distinguish the relative severity of each disorder and identify the functional consequences of comorbidity. Psychiatric comorbidity can complicate substance use disorder treatment and have an adverse effect on the outcome of substance use disorders. Psychodiagnostic inventories can be a useful addition to the SUD assessment process, clarifying diagnoses with similar symptoms and identifying associated risk factors. However, such testing is time-intensive for both administration and interpretation, with high levels of training and expertise required. These inventories can provide information about acute clinical syndromes, personality styles/disorders, interpersonal relationships, and specific potentially dangerous behaviors that are relevant for both diagnosis and treatment of SUD.

Comorbidity can also extend to cognitive dysfunction in SUD. The neurotoxic effects of alcohol and many recreational drugs can have both acute and long-term effects on brain functioning, contributing to mild or major neurocognitive disorders over time. It is not uncommon for an assessment of functional status in SUD to suggest evidence of possible cognitive dysfunction. There are brief cognitive screening measures available that are sensitive (but not specific) for cognitive impairment, and these can prove useful for initial assessments. These include Mini Mental State Exam (MMSE), Montreal Cognitive Assessment (MoCA), and St. Louis University Mental Status Exam (SLUMS). However, these cognitive screening tests should not be administered during acute intoxication, nor should they be used until an individual is medically stable after withdrawal from alcohol or drugs. Cognitive impairment is usually the most severe in the first few weeks of abstinence [2]. If subsequent cognitive screening suggests ongoing impairment, a full neuropsychological assessment is recommended to evaluate all cognitive domains. This comprehensive test battery is not administered in the first few weeks of abstinence from substance(s) because variable attention and information processing deficits can negatively impact overall performance. Most individuals will experience recovery of cognitive and motor functions after an extended period of abstinence, but recovery of specific cognitive functions occurs at different rates and is impacted by many factors including age, polysubstance use, duration, and severity of substance use [2].

The most frequently used psychometric instruments are discussed below.

MMPI2/MMPI2RF

The Minnesota Multiphasic Personality Inventory (version 2, or Revised Format) [3] is a 567-item true/false response inventory that yields dozens of variables pertaining to current mental health disorders, and a host of variables describing specific behaviors and clinical syndromes. A wealth of prior research has yielded specific indices pertaining to individuals with alcohol or substance use disorders. The MMPI2 includes 4 specific scales that assess alcohol/drug use. The Addiction Admission Scale and Substance Abuse Scale are direct measures of substance use and its consequences. The MacAndrew Alcoholism (rev) Scale and the Addiction Potential Scale evaluate use indirectly through endorsement of behaviors or situations highly correlated with substance use disorders. There are also 2 sets of specific "critical items" that are flagged by the MMPI2 to identify potential alcohol/drug use.

MCMI3/4

The Millon Clinical Multiaxial Inventory (versions 3, 4) is a 195-item true/false inventory that emphasizes long-standing characterological traits and identifies possible maladaptive personality styles and disorders [4]. This test may be useful in that it provides scales for specific personality disorders that have often been associated with increased risk for alcohol or drug use. It also measures acute clinical syndromes (Alcohol and Drug Use Scales) in terms of base rates to identify the presence or prominence of key behaviors and symptoms.

PAI

The Personality Assessment Inventory [5] is a 344-item inventory using a 4-point Likert response scale to identify psychopathology and personality styles and the associated treatment variables. This inventory offers 2 individual scales that quantify alcohol problems based on problems with excessive intake and a second scale of drug problems indicating probable excessive recreational drug use. These personality inventories can help to identify additional areas of clinical concern in individuals with SUD and add valuable information for treatment planning.

Evaluation and Diagnosis

What Is a SUD and What It Is Not?

While substance use refers broadly to using a particular substance in any amount, this base-level conception generally excludes excessive levels of use, let alone use that indicates a substance use disorder is present. "At-risk" use refers to a level of use that may be higher than typical use rates in the population and may place someone in a category of individuals at a higher risk of developing a SUD. For instance, "heavy use" involves taking a substance routinely, typically most days or every day (e.g., 7 drinks or more per week for alcohol use). Similarly, "problem use" or "hazardous use" typically refers to a level of use that may put someone's health at risk (e.g., consuming the substance in a context that makes it dangerous, such as driving or operating heavy machinery) or interfere with their financial or social functioning. However, neither type of use may necessarily qualify for an SUD, particularly if this type of use has happened on an occasional or specific basis (e.g., in response to a stressor) and does not happen chronically.

In contrast, the DSM-5 defines a SUD as when a person meets at least 2 of 11 criteria within the same 12-month period. The DSM-5 incorporates some aspects of the old DSM-IV categories of "abuse" and "dependence" (except legal problems), as well as a new one (experience of substance cravings), into a single disorder with three levels of severity –mild, moderate, and severe. This set of criteria provides an overarching structure of 11 general criteria applicable to any substance being considered, with the possibility to diagnose a separate substance-specific SUD (e.g., alcohol use disorder, opioid use disorder). These criteria (paraphrased) include:

1. The drug is often taken in a larger amount or over a longer period than intended.
2. Persistent desire or unsuccessful attempts to cut down.
3. A great deal of time is spent on activities to acquire, use, or recover from the drug.
4. Experience of cravings/urges.
5. Recurrent drug use resulting in failure to fulfill major role obligations (e.g., work, home).
6. Continued drug use despite persistent interpersonal problems caused by the drug.
7. Important social, occupational, or recreational activities are given up/reduced because of drug use.
8. Recurrent drug use in situations in which it is physically hazardous.
9. Continued use of the substance despite knowledge of persistent medical or mental health problems caused by it.
10. Tolerance (i.e., need for markedly increased amounts of drug to achieve intoxication/desired effect, or markedly diminished effect with continued use of the same amount).
11. Withdrawal (i.e., drug-specific symptoms, or the substance, or a closely similar substance, is taken to relieve or avoid withdrawal symptoms).

In terms of severity, individuals who meet 2 to 3 of these criteria qualify for a mild SUD, meeting 4 to 6 criteria indicates a moderate SUD, and meeting 7 or more criteria indicates a severe SUD diagnosis.

Not a SUD

Firstly, legal problems related to substance use, a previously recognized "abuse" and "dependence" criteria from DSM-IV, have been removed from consideration in an SUD diagnosis as this criterion was found to be culturally biased and not reliable across cultures and settings [6]. Having current or past problems with the law may reflect a pattern of substance dealing or criminal activity rather than a personal addictive profile. That being said, parts of a history such as a charge for driving under the influence (DUI) are still critically relevant to a potential SUD diagnosis as they may pertain to several SUD criteria, including tolerance and underestimation of substances' impact on cognition, recurrent use in hazardous conditions, and problems fulfilling major role obligations. Secondly, recent ingestion of a substance resulting in a diagnosis of intoxication does not necessarily reflect a pattern of addictive behavior or necessitate a diagnosis of SUD. Intoxication could relate to a one-time experimentation with a particular substance, or even exposure to a prescribed substance (e.g., opioid medication), and an individual with such presentation should not be diagnosed with an SUD unless they meet at least 2 of the SUD criteria in the same 12-month period. Finally, substance-induced withdrawal, which presents with drug-specific physiological and psychiatric symptoms resulting from recent cessation or reduction of a substance, does not in and of itself constitute an SUD diagnosis unless a more prevalent pattern of use and associated SUD criterion would also be met. That is, while withdrawal symptoms may result from stopping use that was previously heavy or prolonged, such pattern of use should be specially assessed for SUD criteria to determine whether a SUD diagnosis is warranted.

Substance Use Evaluation

To accurately and effectively assess for substance use pathology in a clinical setting, several broad assessment areas should be considered in order to not only make an accurate SUD diagnosis, but to determine potential co-occurring mental and physical illness, the individual's protective and risk factors, and the individual's goals and specific situation. This information will ultimately help to develop an individualized treatment plan. The goal is to obtain a broader picture of the context and long-term behavioral history in which present symptoms are occurring, including potential past SUD diagnoses, recovery and relapse history, co-occurring disorders, personality features, as well as socio-economic, developmental, and interpersonal factors. The American Society of Addiction Medicine (ASAM) provides a useful guideline of features to consider when assessing symptom severity and the person's needs. These six dimensions include: 1) Intoxication, Withdrawal and Addiction Medications, 2) Biomedical Conditions, 3) Psychiatric and Cognitive Conditions, 4) Substance Use-Related Risks, 5) Recovery Environment Interactions, and 6) Person-Centered Considerations [12].

History of Presenting Illness (HPI)

This part of the assessment gathers information on current symptoms and precipitating factors, including substance use and other psychiatric and medical pathology. This is the most open-ended component of the assessment and seeks to collect both factual details on the current clinical symptoms and the subjective perspective and experience of those symptoms as described by the person. Thus, while it is not necessary at this stage to systematically check for use of all substances, a thorough assessment of the level of use and review of SUD criteria should be conducted for each substance mentioned by the interviewee as currently being used.

People may not provide an accurate self-assessment of how much of a substance they consume; evaluators should provide specific, concrete cues to gauge how much is used and how often. Evaluating quantity with objective units (e.g., grams of alcohol, number of cigarettes, grams of THC) is ideal, but not necessarily feasible if the interviewee is not familiar with those standards. Many people will report opioid use in terms of the number of bags or bundles (10 bags) used, but determining the potency or composition (i.e., heroin, fentanyl, morphine) is difficult and varies considerably. Cocaine is sometimes reported in terms of grams or the cost (e.g., $20 per day). Cannabis is often reported in ounces, but newer waxes, edibles, and other forms are often reported based on (often unverified) percentage or grams of Tetrahydrocannabinol (THC) or cannabidiol (CBD). In regard to alcohol, "one drink" is a relatively vague and subjective measure that is unlikely to align with current serving size recommendations. A drink is defined as 14g of ethanol, which corresponds to about 12 ounces of regular 5% alcohol by volume (ABV) beer, 5 ounces of 12% ABV wine, or 1.5 ounces of 40% ABV distilled spirits [13]. Typically, one drink as perceived and endorsed by an interviewee will represent a larger quantity (e.g., a regular bottle of craft beer containing 8% ABV, or large-ounce containers of 5% ABV beer). The speed of drinking within a particular day and the frequency of such drinking sessions will also be critical to estimate, as it could reveal a binging tendency even within seemingly normal daily amounts [13].

Once the level of use has been evaluated, the presence of potential SUD symptoms still needs to be assessed even if the person is not drinking with heavy use patterns. A person may experience significant cravings and related ruminations and functional impairment even if objectively using within what is considered low to moderate use. Similarly, psychological dependence and SUD criteria may be met for substances that may not generally be considered physically addictive. This is illustrated in emerging cases of substance misuse with ketamine (dissociative anesthetic) and xylazine (non-opioid sedative), the latter being most typically combined with fentanyl or ketamine. To understand the context of use, consider potential precipitating events that may have triggered the current illness. Did the person experience a recent loss or breakup? Are there any interpersonal conflict(s) with those close to them? Have there been any recent failures or significant delays at school or work, or a recent loss of employment?

It is important to evaluate common co-occurring conditions like mood and anxiety disorders (see other psychiatric history section below). Determining the timeline of these symptoms with respect to the substance use (i.e., whether one of the symptoms was a triggering factor for the substance use or vice versa) will help with the diagnosis of a primary substance use disorder versus a substance-induced psychiatric disorder. For instance, has depression, anxiety, and/or manic symptoms onset occurred first, leading to substance use? Or did substance use onset/relapse precede the development of the affective symptoms? Do they always or only co-occur together? If available, results from screening questionnaires and mood scales may help to guide the person to identify and verbalize the most salient struggle and maladaptive pattern (i.e., chief complaint), but also to consider all potential ongoing symptoms and difficulties. These can also help refocus the interview while minimizing the risk of omission of important data. With consent from the person being treated, it will be particularly useful to talk to collateral informants (e.g., spouse, close relatives, friends), who may provide more objective or complementary data on the history, current symptoms, and level of functioning. Be aware of potential bias on the part of the informant.

Substance Use and Treatment History

The goal for this section of the assessment is to obtain a thorough, long-term picture of the pattern of use for all main substance types, thus reviewing some substances that may not have been reviewed thoroughly during the HPI. Substances that should be systematically considered are the most used based on the geography, availability of drugs, demographics of the person, and other factors. Common substances needing evaluation include alcohol, cannabis, tobacco, caffeine, methamphetamine/amphetamine, cocaine, benzodiazepines, opioids, and other substances such as hallucinogens like lysergic acid diethylamide (LSD), mushrooms containing psilocybin, 3,4-methylenedioxy-methamphetamine (MDMA; ecstasy), phencyclidine (PCP; angel dust), inhalants, and more. Importantly, use of both prescription and illicit forms of the substance should be queried. For example, maladaptive use of stimulants could involve prescription methylphenidate or mixed amphetamine salts (prescribed or obtained elsewhere) or the illicit methamphetamine. Prescription opioid and benzodiazepine medications used to treat pain, sleep, and anxiety are associated with significant addictive potential and may be more commonly encountered than illicit drugs in certain regions or among certain populations.

For each substance endorsed by the person, the first step should be to determine the general chronology and level of maladaptive use over time. The provider should inquire about the following: name of substance used, when use first started, length of time used, frequency and pattern of use with special emphasis on use during the past week, date and time of last use, route(s) of administration, amount, cost, and purpose (e.g., to get high, to avoid withdrawal, to relieve depression, to sleep, or to relieve side effects of other drugs). Focus on key periods of use with relapse-triggering event(s) and subsequent typical pattern of use (i.e., how much, how often), and phases of recovery. Questions about the impact of the substance on a person and their life should be included in the assessment, as well as assessing for the presence of specific DSM-5 SUD criteria. Substance-specific questions are also helpful. For example, one may ask about overdoses with opioids or benzodiazepines; about blackouts, seizures, or delirium tremens with alcohol; and about cardiac side effects with stimulants. For drugs previously used, ask the following: age at which drug use started, length of time used, typical pattern of use (i.e., how much and how often) and adverse effects. For previous treatment experiences inquire about where, what kind, and the outcome. For prescription drugs currently used inquire about the following: name, reason for use, amount, frequency, duration of use, and last dose. State prescription drug monitoring programs (PDMPs) should be searched when available.

To accurately estimate overall severity, maladaptive use, and relapse cycle, it is important to identify and prioritize a detailed assessment of the period of heaviest use in terms of level and pattern of use and specific physiological and psychosocial SUD criteria. It is also important to remember that substances may be consumed in one or multiple forms (ingested, chewed, smoked, snorted/inhaled, injected into the bloodstream, etc.). In addition, the presence of medical or other physiological consequences of use (e.g., withdrawal, intoxication symptoms, blackouts) will be key factors in determining the severity of use and whether some criteria are (e.g., withdrawal, tolerance). One should assess all criteria for every endorsed substance (or confirm any previously-revealed criterion symptom during the HPI) and get a sense of how many of these criteria were met at different periods of use in the person's past history, starting at the age of first use to present (see Table below).

Key elements of a good substance use history	
Thorough survey of substance categories	Alcohol, cannabis, tobacco, caffeine, stimulants (methamphetamine/amphetamine, cocaine), benzodiazepines, opioids, hallucinogens, 3,4-methylenedioxy-methamphetamine (MDMA; ecstasy), inhalants, etc.
Detailed chronology of use	Date of fist use, age when started, length of use, dates for periods of abstinence
Amount of use	Frequency, doses used, route of administration
Purpose of use	e.g., to cope with stressor/pain, to get high, to help with sleep, etc.
Resources/effort Invested in obtaining substance	Cost/money spent on the substance, behaviors to obtain the substance (e.g., risky behaviors)
Psychosocial impact	Impact of use on relationships, work, finances, etc.
Adverse effects	Medical and physiological consequences of use
Attention to relapse periods	Factors that triggered relapse, resulting use/frequency, behavioral patterns
Attention to heavy use periods	Typical and worse pattern of use during heavy use

Substance use history also includes periods of recovery and remission. According to the Substance Abuse and Mental Health Services Administration (SAMHSA) [14], this is a multi-domain *process of change* which should be assessed in terms of health, home/shelter, purpose (e.g., professional endeavors), and community (i.e., relationships, social networks). Thus, when assessing substance use and treatment history, it is important to recognize that recovery may not necessarily include full abstinence from the problem substance(s) and that recovery happens on a continuum, which may involve non-problematic use. According to the DSM-5, a period of remission is defined as not meeting any of the SUD diagnostic criteria aside from cravings (the person being assessed may experience cravings) and can be classified into "early remission" if this is met for at least 3 months, or "sustained remission" if met for at least 1 year [6]. Inquiring about the person's past ability to initiate and sustain recovery will provide a way to understand the specific protective and risk factors that may foster the individual's successful recovery or impede it.

Other Psychiatric History

Given the high rate of co-occurring disorders among individuals with substance use problems, it is particularly important to get a full psychiatric history and gauge the potential relationship between comorbid disorders and substance use to better inform treatment planning. Anxiety and mood disorders including depression and bipolar disorder are the most common psychiatric comorbidities among individuals with SUD [15]. A comprehensive psychiatric history will thus be essential in disentangling potential comorbidities that may warrant a more integrated intensive treatment plan after assessment. Such assessment should include any history of self-injurious behavior and/or suicide attempt(s) (including the extent to which those potential attempts were planned and to what extent the person struggling sought help), tendency for violence, any known past diagnosis of mental illness, any history of traumatic events (including sexual, verbal, physical abuse), any prior hospitalizations and/or inpatient treatment for psychiatric reasons, any prior experience with psychotherapy and/or other behavioral treatment (and if so how often, for how long, and with what results), and any prior use of psychotropic medications (including dosage and observed effectiveness).

Family History

A family history of psychiatric illness, particularly SUD, is a well-recognized risk factor for developing a SUD [16]. Gathering information on family history may help to corroborate an interviewee's diagnosis and shed light on their potential disposition for recovery and treatment response. In addition, such background can shed light and help focus on the assessment of social and developmental history, e.g., if parents or close relatives were abusive, neglectful, or absent while in treatment. Note which relative exhibited which disorder to provide information on how closely related they are/were to the interviewee and to evaluate potential exposure to emotionally taxing and/or abusive behavior.

Social/Developmental History

Collecting social history can not only provide the assessor with a sense of the interviewee's socio-economic background, education, and financial stability; it can be a critical aspect of assessing for trauma history within their family of origin and the development of early psychiatric pathology in this context. More recent social history can also provide important information about current risk factors for problematic substance use and maintenance of addiction, e.g., having a romantic partner or close friend who is using, being in a living environment that facilitates access to substance(s), and being exposed to violence or abuse. Importantly, it can shed light on how substance use is affecting the person's current level of functioning from a social, professional, and financial perspective, which may not have been fully captured during the HPI. Likewise, this portion of the assessment can help identify activities, hobbies, and types of relationships and friendships that are or have been fulfilling and that can act protectively against maladaptive use to the interviewee. This information can be helpfully incorporated into treatment planning.

Medical History

A medical history assessment should survey for any allergies, current medications and their indications, and any relevant medical conditions that may be related to or commonly co-occur with substance use, could be relevant for medication treatment, or could affect the person's health, functioning, and treatment. Common assessments include the presence of any head injury, seizures, neurocognitive impairment, coronary artery disease and/or arrhythmias, pulmonary problems, thyroid problems, anemia, serious abdominal problems (e.g., pancreatitis, liver disease, kidney failure, hepatitis C), and sexually transmitted or other infections (e.g., HIV, Hepatitis C). Such conditions and the current medication regimen will be particularly relevant to plan recovery and substance use discontinuation in a safe manner. Diseases commonly associated with drug use, particularly among users of opioids by injection, are viral (e.g., HIV, Hepatitis C) and bacterial infections. Other diseases such as sexually transmitted diseases, syphilis, and tuberculosis also have a higher prevalence among people with substance use.

Psychiatric/Mental Status Exam

A mental status exam should include the interviewee's attitude and behavior (e.g., cooperative versus guarded), speech quality, presence of psychomotor retardation or agitation, mood and affect, thought process and content (e.g., linear; goal-directed; associations, psychotic content), perceptual disturbances, suicidal ideation, homicidal ideation, orientation to person/place/time, and attention and concentration. In addition, make note of appearance and grooming, gait and station, presence of tremors, or abnormal movements.

Chapter Review Questions

1. Henry just finished his workday and poured himself a glass of wine. His partner arrives and asks him if he would like to join him for another drink. Henry responds, "I think I should really just have one tonight." They go to a restaurant for dinner and when dessert arrives, he thinks it may not do any harm to have his usual glass of Pinot Grigio, though he feels conflicted about it. He eventually gives in, thinking, "It won't make much difference if I have a glass or two." What does Henry's initial response exhibit based on the screening criteria in the CAGE screener?

   A. The individual has felt he/she should **C**ut down on their drinking.
   B. The individual feels a loss of **C**ontrol on their drinking.
   C. The individual has noticed increased **C**riticism from close ones for their drinking.
   D. The individual has been **C**aught drinking on the job.

E. The individual has **C**onsumed an alcoholic drink first thing in the morning to steady their nerves or to get rid of a hangover.

Correct Answer: A.

Explanation: Henry's behavior is indicative of the criteria of feeling he should "**C**ut down" on his consumption of alcohol, corresponding to the "C" in the CAGE questionnaire. The other "C" responses are not a criterion in the CAGE screener.

2. Betty is a 65-year-old divorced Caucasian female with a past medical history of high blood pressure, gout, diabetes, and complaints of depression since age 40 after her divorce. She started drinking alcohol at age 40 after her divorce, about 3 bottles of wine per week at its peak. She currently has up to 2 drinks per day, but less than 5 total drinks in a week. What standard is Betty currently following that is in accordance with NIAAA Guidelines?

A. Betty is following the guideline that for healthy women no more than 3 drinks in a day.
B. Betty is following the guideline that for healthy women under age 65 no more than 10 drinks in a week.
C. Betty is following the guideline that for healthy women no more than 4 drinks in a day.
D. Betty is following the guideline that for healthy women no more than 8 drinks in a week.
E. For all individuals, the guideline is that you can have more than 4 drinks in a day if they consume only beer, but only 3 drinks per day if they consume only hard liquor.

Correct Answer: A.

Explanation: The NIAAA guidelines for moderated drinking in healthy men up to age 65 are: no more than 4 drinks in a day and no more than 14 drinks in a week. For healthy women (and healthy men over age 65), the guideline is no more than 3 drinks in a day AND no more than 7 drinks in a week.

3. If Betty from the question above begins to drink more than the NIAAA guidelines suggest, which questionnaire would be appropriate to administer?

A. The Michigan Alcoholism Screening Test (MAST)
B. The OWLS
C. The Michigan Alcoholism Screening Test—Geriatric Version (MAST-G)
D. The Drug Abuse Screening Test (DAST)

Correct Answer: C.

Explanation: Betty is likely at a time in her life where she is not working and the MAST-G includes questions that are more relevant to this period of life. The OWLS is designed to assess opioid use and the DAST asks only about drug use, not alcohol or tobacco.

4. Jordan is 20 years old and working on his bachelor's degree in computer science. While he is on track in terms of his grades, he is enjoying the "college life" and regularly goes to parties where he has more than a few drinks. He has also been developing a taste for smoking cannabis, which he feels helps him focus during the day and decrease anxiety at night. Which of the following is a diagnostic criterion for a substance use disorder according to the DSM-5?

   A. Repeated drug use both alone and in interpersonal settings
   B. Experiencing cravings or urges to use the substance
   C. Having been legally prosecuted or arrested in possession of the substance
   D. Significant interpersonal problems (e.g., verbal or physical fights with friends or in intimate relationships)
   E. The substance has been taken at least once at the level of intoxication

   Correct Answer: B.

   Explanation: Continued use alone is not a criterion and does not necessarily indicate problem use unless the use results in interpersonal problems (A). Similarly having significant interpersonal problems, including fights, is not a criterion itself unless it is tied to substance use (i.e., the person was under the influence when fighting, the fight resulted from wanting to acquire substance, etc.) (D). Unless the legal problem or arrest is associated with documented intoxication, this would not constitute a diagnostic criterion based on DSM-5. The DSM-IV diagnosis of substance abuse included the language in answer choice C above. A high level of use, including intoxication, does not constitute a criterion for SUD unless it is persistent or there is evidence of tolerance (E).

5. Hannah is a 32-year-old software salesperson who has been enjoying a blossoming career for the past 3 years since she joined her current company. She has been enjoying going out for a drink or two after work with her colleagues. It helps her to wind down. Based on these descriptions, which cluster of symptoms that Hannah endorses would indicate that she meets the criteria for a SUD?

   A. Hannah endorses mild to moderate use of the substance. Her girlfriend has recently broken up with her because she would not stop drinking, which has been a recurrent problem in their relationship.
   B. Hannah has recently been seen in the emergency deparment (ED) with severe alcohol intoxication and withdrawal symptoms. She stated that she is going through a rough time at work because her sales quota was recently raised, which led her to want to "let loose" and binge drink with her friends during the weekend.
   C. Hannah is experiencing frequent cravings for the substance. She is anxious and depressed because she has alienated a lot of her friends and family members because of her alcohol use.
   D. Hannah has been taking substance in increasingly larger amounts. Despite having successfully stopped drinking during the month of January, she is worried she may have a problem with alcohol. She denies any psychological or physical effects of the substance he is consuming.

E. Hannah had a recent documented DUI after she was driving while intoxicated. She also has a recent history of verbal altercations at work with some of her senior colleagues, who have been commenting on her performance behind her back.

Correct Answer: C.

Explanation: There is both evidence of persistent craving/urges and interpersonal problems resulting from the drug use (meets 2 criteria, which would qualify for mild SUD). Other options include one diagnostic criterion at the most, including potential relationship/interpersonal related to drug use (A), taking substance in increasing amounts (D). Intoxication alone (B), DUI, or interpersonal conflicts which occur independently of using (E) are not criteria and may not necessarily point to an SUD diagnosis.

References

1. American Psychiatric Association. Title of chapter. In Diagnostic and statistical manual of mental disorders (5th ed., text rev.). 2022. https://doi.org/10.1176/appi.books.9780890425787.
2. Sullivan E, Rosenbloom MJ, Pfefferbaum A. Pattern of motor and cognitive deficits in detoxified alcoholic men. Alcohol Clin Exp Res. 2000;24(5):611–21.
3. Samet S, Waxman R, Hatzenbuehler M, Hasin DS. Assessing addiction: Concepts and instruments. Addict Sci Clin Pract. 2007;4(1):19.
4. Mitchell SG, Kelly SM, Gryczynski J, Myers CP, O'Grady KE, Kirk AS, et al. The CRAFFT cut-points and DSM-5 criteria for alcohol and other drugs: a reevaluation and reexamination. Subst Abus. 2014;35(4):376–80.
5. Ewing JA. Detecting alcoholism: the CAGE questionnaire. JAMA. 1984;252(14):1905–7.
6. Alcoholism NIoAAa. Recommended alcohol questions. 2003. Available from: http://www.niaaa.nih.gov/research/guidelines-and-resources/recommendedalcohol-questions
7. Group WAW. The alcohol, smoking and substance involvement screening test (ASSIST): Development, reliability and feasibility. Addiction. 2002;97(9):1183–94.
8. Saunders JB, Aasland OG, Babor TF, De la Fuente JR, Grant M. Development of the alcohol use disorders identification test (AUDIT): WHO collaborative project on early detection of persons with harmful alcohol consumption-II. Addiction. 1993;88(6):791–804.
9. Selzer ML. The Michigan alcoholism screening test: The quest for a new diagnostic instrument. Am J Psychiatr. 1971;127(12):1653–8.
10. Skinner H. The drug abuse screening test (DAST): Guidelines for administration and scoring. Toronto: Addiction Research Foundation; 1982.
11. Swartz MS, Perkins DO, Stroup TS, McEvoy JP, Nieri JM, Haak DC. Assessing clinical and functional outcomes in the Clinical Antipsychotic Trials of Intervention Effectiveness (CATIE) schizophrenia trial. Schizophr Bull. 2003;29(1):33–43.
12. American Society of Addiction Medicine (ASAM). The ASAM Criteria Fourth Edition 2024. https://www.asam.org/asam-criteria
13. Staff CRE. Drinking patterns and their definitions. Alcohol Res. 2018;39(1):17.
14. Del Vecchio P. SAMHSA's working definition of recovery updated. 23–30 Mar 2012. Available from: http://blog.samhsa.gov/2012/03/23/samhsas-working-definition-of-recovery-updated
15. Quello SB, Brady KT, Sonne SC. Mood disorders and substance use disorder: a complex comorbidity. Sci Pract Perspect. 2005;3(1):13.

16. Kendler KS, Davis CG, Kessler RC. The familial aggregation of common psychiatric and substance use disorders in the National Comorbidity Survey: a family history study. Br J Psychiatry. 1997;170(6):541–8.
17. Smith PC, Schmidt SM, Allensworth-Davies D, Saitz R. A single-question screening test for drug use in primary care. Arch Intern Med. 2010;170(13):1155–60. https://doi.org/10.1001/archinternmed.2010.140.
18. Center for Substance Abuse Treatment. A Guide to Substance Abuse Services for Primary Care Clinicians. Rockville (MD): Substance Abuse and Mental Health Services Administration (US); 1997. (Treatment Improvement Protocol (TIP) Series, No. 24.) Appendix C—Screening and Assessment Instruments. Available from: https://www.ncbi.nlm.nih.gov/books/NBK64829/
19. Minnich A, et al. Systematic evaluation of psychometric characteristics of the michigan alcoholism screening Test 13-Item Short (SMAST) and 10-Item Brief (BMAST) Versions. J Counsel Develop. 2019;97(1):15–24. https://doi.org/10.1002/jcad.12231.
20. Selzer ML, Vinokur A, van Rooijen L. A self-administered Short Michigan Alcoholism Screening Test (SMAST). J Stud Alcohol. 1975;36(1):117–26.
21. Skinner, H. Guide for using the drug abuse screening test (DAST). Guide for Using the Drug Abuse Screening Test (DAST). 1982. https://socwel.ku.edu/sites/socwel/files/documents/Research%20Projects/Family%20First/Survey%20Measures/DAST%20Guide%202019%20-%20Remediated.pdf
22. Picco L, Middleton M, Bruno R, Kowalski M, Nielsen S. Validation of the OWLS, a screening tool for measuring prescription opioid use disorder in primary care. Pain Med. 2020;21(11):2757–64.

Psychosocial Treatment of Substance Use Disorders

5

Natassia Gaznick and Eve Lasswell

High-Yield Review Points

- First-wave behavioral therapies operate on the assumption that if behavior is not rewarded or is punished, this target behavior will decrease.
- Second-wave cognitive behavioral therapies assume that thoughts, feelings, and behaviors are interdependent, and as such, altering one will influence the other.
- Third wave therapies incorporate mindfulness into the cognitive-behavioral framework with an emphasis on enhancing one's attention to self and environment in a nonjudgmental manner.
- Psychodynamic approaches can be integrated with cognitive, behavioral, mutual support, and pharmacological approaches to enhance treatment.
- Mutual support therapies encourage reliance on fellow members and accepting responsibility for substance use and addictive behaviors through informational, emotional, and social support.
- Systems-based therapies encourage not only the evaluation of the transactions between the person and his/her support system but also the involvement of that support system in the reinforcement of positive changes.

N. Gaznick (✉)
Private Practice, Los Angeles, CA, USA
e-mail: dr.gaznick@drgaznick.com

E. Lasswell
Department of Psychiatry, University of California San Diego, La Jolla, CA, USA
e-mail: elasswell@health.ucsd.edu

C. Marienfeld, M. Soltani (eds.), *AAAP Review of Addiction Psychiatry*,
https://doi.org/10.1007/978-3-032-24174-0_5

Introduction

Psychotherapeutic treatment for substance use disorders (SUDs) and behavioral addictions has been studied and applied in numerous treatment settings to a wide variety of patient populations. Each treatment described here has been shown to be efficacious in either the reduction of or abstinence from the addictive behavior. Many interventions are aimed at accepting the addictive behavior and making steps toward the reduction of response or exposure to triggers, whether internal or external. While each aims to have a unique element, these treatments can be roughly grouped based on their underlying psychological theories. These include cognitive, behavioral, mindfulness, motivation, mutual support, psychodynamic, and systems theory. This chapter will describe the basics of each intervention, the evidence for its use in various disorders, and the characteristics of persons who would likely benefit from the intervention.

Based on cognitive and/or behavioral theories, contingency management (CM), cognitive behavioral therapy (CBT), and mindfulness-based therapies are well studied in addiction literature. Originating in the behavioral theories of Pavlov, Watson, Skinner, and Bandura, behavioral approaches aim to uncouple the stimulus–response patterns evoked by substance use or other maladaptive behaviors. Cognitive approaches, highly based on the work of Ellis and Beck, aim to maximize one's appreciation of how thoughts, feelings, and behaviors impact addictive behavior. Mindfulness aims to bring attention to the present moment without judgment. Placed on a spectrum, CM relies mostly on behavior (the "first wave" of behavioral therapies), CBT on behavior and cognition (the "second wave"), and mindfulness-based therapies on behavior, cognition, and mindfulness ("the third wave").

Motivational, psychodynamic, mutual help, and systems-based therapies aim to decrease addictive behaviors through understanding one's inner life and interpersonal relationships. The psychodynamic perspective involves the therapist developing an understanding of the person and, in turn, helping the person to understand the self to actualize change. Motivation has been shown to be a critical part of engagement and participation in treatment. Through examining biological, psychological, and social dimensions in motivation-based interventions, the practitioner guides the person to identify personal motivations for change. Miller and Rollnick developed the most well-known techniques and style aimed to help an individual move through the stages of change. Mutual help groups, led either by a clinician or group member, are highly accessible and emphasize personal growth and fellowship as steps to develop self-efficacy and more effective coping behaviors. Systems-based therapies operate on the principle that change in one part of the system can produce change in another and whether these system changes contribute to or help solve the problem. Systems-based therapies identify who is important to and involved in the person's life and work to help change maladaptive patterns in the relationships that perpetuate addictive behavior.

Contingency Management

Contingency management (CM) is based on operant learning and aims to increase the positive consequences of abstinence through timely extrinsic motivators for behavior change and represents the "first wave" of psychological theory translated into treatment. CM uses monetary-based and other reinforcements as reward behaviors including demonstration of abstinence, treatment attendance, and medication adherence. Three key principles in the implementation of CM strategies include (1) frequent behavior monitoring, (2) immediate disbursement of tangible positive reinforcements, and (3) denial of positive reinforcements without the target behavior [1]. Monitoring involves objective assessments, and when reward is based on drug use, it should be tailored to the frequency of drug use and the ability of the test to detect the target drug. Positive reinforcements are commonly prizes or vouchers for goods/services rather than actual monetary rewards due to treatment programs' financial limitations. Rewards can use escalating reinforcement, which involves increasing the prize/voucher amount with an increasing number of desired behaviors, as this promotes longer durations of abstinence and long-term success. Importantly, the positive reinforcements are withheld and reset back to the starting value when the target behavior is not met.

Empiric Evidence

CM is well studied for multiple substances and treatment outcomes. Clinical trials and meta-analyses have demonstrated effectiveness in treating individuals with stimulant (cocaine and methamphetamine), nicotine, alcohol, opioid, cannabis, and sedative (benzodiazepine) use disorders [2, 3]. Evidence has shown the superiority of CM to standard treatment conditions for short-term abstinence, treatment retention, and attendance in therapy [4, 5]. Historically, data have been mixed on the utility of CM in long-term abstinence, as there is contention regarding the ability of extrinsic motivators to improve intrinsic motivation for long-term change [6]. A recent meta-analysis indicates that people who receive CM are significantly more likely to be abstinent from substances at a median of 24 weeks after reinforcers have been discontinued, challenging the long-held belief that the benefit of CM is limited to the active treatment context [4].

For Whom

The persons and treatment settings that may benefit from CM are quite broad. Studies support use in broad socioeconomic, demographic, and mental health populations. There are, however, some instances in which CM may not be optimal. Those that may benefit less from CM include persons with extrinsic motivators elsewhere (e.g., those in the criminal justice system). Clinics or payers with limited funding or no mechanism to provide reinforcements may have limited systems-level support to provide rewards. Additionally, reliance on qualitative drug screens would make the use of CM problematic in harm reduction models, as it would require a quantitative test to measure a decrease in use rather than complete abstinence, although other harm reduction behaviors could be reinforced with CM.

Cognitive Behavioral Therapy

Cognitive behavioral therapy (CBT) is a structured and time-limited intervention that draws on both behavioral and cognitive theories with the aim of understanding and disrupting learned patterns associated with drug and alcohol craving and use. Known as "second wave" therapy (after the "first wave" of behavioral therapy), CBT assumes that psychological distress arises from maladaptive thought processes (cognitions) and behaviors. Thoughts, feelings, and behaviors are interdependent, and as such, altering thought patterns can influence feelings and behaviors. There are several common maladaptive thought processes and beliefs in people with SUDs, including all-or-nothing thinking, denial, and the belief that change is too difficult [7]. CBT for substance use disorders aims to reduce drug use by identifying and altering behaviors and thought processes leading to substance use and finding ways to manage unhelpful thoughts and feelings associated with high-risk behaviors. The therapist functions as an educator and guide who leads the person in a functional analysis of substance use and individualized cognitive and behavioral skills training.

Empiric Evidence

Evidence supports the use of CBT for the treatment of multiple types of substance use disorders including alcohol, cannabis, cocaine, nicotine, opioids, and polysubstance use, as well as behavioral addictions such as gambling disorder, compulsive sexual behavior, and internet addiction [8–12]. Commonly studied and implemented CBT includes 12–16 sessions conducted over about 12 weeks. It has been shown to be effective as a standalone treatment and in combination with medication and other therapeutic modalities. Studies have shown the superiority of CBT in the reduction of substance use at long-term follow-up, likely due to the durability of the skills learned, as those who complete homework during the course of CBT are more likely to stay in treatment longer, have more consecutive days of abstinence, and fewer positive drug screens [13].

For Whom

Adaptations of CBT are applicable to many types of persons and in a variety of treatment settings. While originally conceptualized as an outpatient treatment, this intervention may also be used in the inpatient setting or in group-based treatment. CBT is also helpful for the treatment of SUDs with co-occurring disorders, as seen with Seeking Safety, a CBT-based manualized treatment that has shown efficacy in individuals with posttraumatic stress disorder and SUDs [14]. Despite the wide audience and settings for CBT, there are some clients who may be inappropriate for a standardized outpatient CBT, including those with cognitive deficits, medical or social stressors, and a lack of social resources [15].

Mindfulness-Based Therapies

Mindfulness-based therapies (MBT) integrate traditional Buddhist practices with current psychological practice as part of the "third wave" of cognitive and behavioral therapies. The cognitive aspect of mindfulness aims to enhance one's attention to self and environment in a nonjudgmental manner and includes noticing thoughts and feelings without challenging the content. The behavior aspect aims to strengthen one's ability to experience triggers without defaulting to unhelpful habits. Although initially utilized in treating depression, mindfulness-based treatments have grown in popularity and are accepted as a treatment for substance use disorders and behavioral addictions.

Mindfulness-based relapse prevention (MBRP) is an 8-week manualized outpatient program designed to decrease relapse through increasing awareness of and flexibility to triggers for substance use. The therapy begins with two sessions to introduce the rationale of the therapy and the goal of increasing awareness of external triggers and individual thoughts, feelings, and behaviors that may contribute to relapse. Clients then engage in exercises to strengthen mindfulness in daily life and in high-risk situations, to accept current situations, to see thoughts apart from actions, to improve self-care, and to improve social support [16].

Mindfulness-oriented recovery enhancement (MORE), which is like MBRP, has its roots in mindfulness and CBT; however, it also draws from positive psychology. It is a strength-based intervention with foundations in cognitive control of (1) attention through mindfulness (as described above), (2) negative emotion through reappraisal (reinterpreting stress), and (3) reward processing through savoring (focusing on positive present events). MORE was originally designed as a 10-session protocol that addresses mindfulness, automatic habits, reappraisal, savoring, craving, coping with stress, attachment versus aversion, body impermanence, relationships, meaning, and future orientation.

Empiric Evidence

Mindfulness-based treatment has been shown to be effective in the treatment of alcohol, tobacco, cocaine, amphetamines, cannabis, opiates, and behavioral addictions [17]. MBTs show small to large effect sizes in reducing the frequency and severity of substance use, craving, and stress in those with substance use disorders [18]. A main hypothesis for the effectiveness of MBT is that these therapies improve reactivity to craving cues, possibly through improvement in emotion regulation, decrease in perceived stress, and decrease in stress reactivity [17]. Studies have shown that individuals most frequently rated the "stop observe breathe expand respond (SOBER) breathing space" exercise, which improves proactive rather than reactive behaviors in MBRP, as one of the key elements in helping to maintain sobriety [16].

For Whom

MBTs have been shown to be beneficial in diverse treatment settings and to a diverse population of adults. MBTs may be carried out in either the inpatient or outpatient setting. While many manualized MBTs are closed-group, MBTs may be carried out in individual therapy. Of note, MBT for substances has been beneficial in incarcerated populations and adolescents, but more research is needed [18]. It may be especially helpful in female populations, as women are more likely to relapse due to negative emotions, and those with comorbid depression, as MBTs can improve self-esteem and mood in the setting of difficult experiences [16].

Acceptance and Commitment Therapy

Acceptance and commitment therapy (ACT) is a third-wave cognitive-behavioral therapeutic framework rooted in relational frame theory (RFT). ACT looks at how we as humans use language to assign meaning to our cognition, and the ways in which this can keep us "stuck." Its goal is to increase cognitive flexibility so that a person can see themself as a stable, consistent presence in each situation and move away from using language that exacerbates their pain. ACT does this through the use of six core processes: acceptance, defusion, contact with the present moment, self as context (as opposed to self as content), committed action, and clarification of values [19].

Empiric Evidence

Evidence supports the use of ACT for mental health conditions such as anxiety, depression, and others, as well as for substance use disorders [20]. ACT has demonstrated effectiveness in helping persons with substance use disorders to accept urges related to substance use and other problem-causing behaviors and uses values-congruent action to build a life worth living for them [21]. In studies conducted on its efficacy, ACT has been found to increase abstinence from alcohol and other drugs (AOD) [22], decrease the number of drinks and heavy drinking days amongst drinkers [23], and decrease use of multiple substances over timeframes up to three months [24]. It also shows promise in the treatment of compulsive sexual behavior [10].

For Whom

ACT has been adapted to several presenting concerns and can be used in a variety of treatment settings. In terms of treating substance use disorders, ACT has demonstrated effectiveness for use with Veterans, incarcerated men and women, persons with chronic pain, and persons who use single and multiple substances [22]. It can be adapted in group or individual therapy format across levels of care, including outpatient, intensive outpatient, partial hospitalization, and residential levels of care [25].

Dialectical Behavior Therapy

Dialectical behavior therapy (DBT) is another third-wave cognitive behavioral treatment modality. It uses the Biosocial Model to conceptualize patient distress and was developed to address the unique treatment needs of persons with borderline personality disorder (BPD). Skill development focuses on four areas: mindfulness, emotion regulation, interpersonal effectiveness, and distress tolerance (which contains a small section of content devoted to conceptualizing and skills training for substance use disorders) [26]. With full treatment fidelity, DBT is an intensive, multi-component intervention that includes individual psychotherapy, group-based skills training, phone coaching, and consultation for the therapists administering DBT. Therefore, access to this modality can be limited. However, there are many ways to incorporate components of DBT into psychological treatment.

Empiric Evidence

Studies on DBT often consider persons who have co-occurring BPD and SUD. In this population, DBT has demonstrated effectiveness in increasing days abstinent from alcohol and other drugs (AOD) and gains in global and social adjustment at 16-month follow-up [27]. Researchers have also found efficacy in using standard and SUD-tailored DBT as a standalone treatment for persons with only substance use disorder [28, 29].

For Whom

DBT can be used in group or individual therapy formats at any level of care. Skills training can be done individually or in group settings.

Motivation-Based Therapies

Motivation for change is a critical component for the successful treatment of addictive behaviors. The process of change involves addressing the biopsychosocial dimensions that maintain substance use and addictive behaviors, and as such, motivation-based treatments aim to facilitate change by identifying an individual's personal values and reasons for change. Motivation-based interventions were developed to foster provider-patient relationships that stimulate the individual's process of change and growth over time.

Motivational interviewing (MI) is an interactive style of communication that encourages persons to talk themselves into change based on their own values. The spirit of MI includes partnership, acceptance, compassion, and empowerment between the provider and the person they are treating in a guiding rather than directing style [30]. The core micro-skills for the practitioner include open-ended questions, affirmations, reflections, summaries, and informing/advising. MI has been adapted to brief interventions, use in primary care, and structured motivational enhancement therapy (MET).

MET is a structured therapy, initially developed for research studies, which combines MI and normative feedback, which compares the person's behaviors with population norms. MET is a manualized version of MI that consists of an assessment battery and additional sessions designed to elicit change in a short timeframe. As described for Project MATCH, a 5-year NIAAA study for the treatment of alcohol use disorder, MET was initially developed as four-session intervention. The first two sessions focused on providing structured feedback from the assessment, exploring future plans, and enhancing motivation for change. The final two sessions reinforced progress, encouraged reassessment of goals and strategies, and provided an objective perspective on the change process [31].

Empiric Evidence

Meta-analyses on MI have found that efficacy was related to the amount of "change talk" used by the person being treated, and a greater proportion of change talk was associated with risk behavior reduction [32]. Studies evaluating MET in alcohol use have demonstrated that despite its less intensive nature, MET has equivalent effects on frequency and intensity of alcohol consumption compared to more intensive treatments at 1- and 3-year follow-up [31]. MET in combination with CBT has been successful in treating cannabis-dependent adults, and results are mixed for the use of MET with other drugs of abuse. MI also shows promise in engagement of those with gambling disorder [8, 9]. Other studies, however, suggest MI/MET may be more effective at short-term follow-up with diminishing strength over time in the absence of other modalities [33].

For Whom

Persons who may benefit from MI include those without explicit reasons for change and those with difficulty resolving their ambivalence about the addictive behavior. While studies have demonstrated efficacy in pregnant women, adolescents, and those with co-occurring disorders, MI/MET appears most effective in engaging persons in treatment rather than in providing skills to elicit large-scale behavioral changes. Additionally, MET may be more effective than CBT or 12-step facilitation in persons with a high degree of anger who are undergoing treatment for alcohol use disorder [34].

Psychodynamic Psychotherapy

Individual psychodynamic therapy can be useful in the treatment of substance use disorders in combination with medications for addiction treatment, group and family therapy, and mutual support groups. Its goal is enhanced self-understanding and improved self-reflective capacity in the service of improving substance use. It can also assist persons in accepting that they suffer from addiction and can be used to maintain progress. However, understanding alone does not result in sobriety. Psychodynamic perspectives view addiction as (1) a special adaptation to developmental challenges, (2) an attempt to regulate painful emotions, (3) a primary problem in self-regulation, and (4) a reflection of disorder in personality organization [35, 36]. Modern psychodynamic approaches help persons to identify how their past relationships influence current behaviors and may drive substance use as a coping strategy. It helps to build a stronger sense of self, improve affect regulation, and promote personality integration.

Sessions are generally held 1 to 3 times per week for 45 minutes, and the treatment usually spans several years. Therapists monitor the patient-therapist relationship and use it as a means for understanding the self, and as a vehicle through which to discuss and understand disjunctions and misalliances.

Empiric Evidence

To date there are no controlled studies of traditional long-term psychodynamic treatment of substance use disorders. There are several brief psychodynamic therapies, and of these, supportive-expressive (SE) and interpersonal (IPT) have been studied with success for use with substance use disorders [37]. Additionally, more modern psychodynamic interpretations of the underlying reasons for substance use have yielded discussion about how alcohol and other drugs can help persons in the short term with states of anhedonia, dysphoria, and painful emotional states. Substances are then used to deal with the suffering associated with their self-regulation deficits [36].

For Whom

This approach is indicated for patients who struggle to benefit from other interventions, individuals with comorbid personality disorders, and those who wish for privacy and/or have difficulty with mutual support groups. Persons with high intelligence, a capacity for intimacy, motivation to find meaning in their behavior, and/or a beginning capacity for self-reflection may do well with psychodynamic approaches [38].

Mutual Aid Groups

Mutual aid (also called mutual support, mutual help) approaches are based on individuals changing addictive behavior without the use of health professionals. Mutual support groups are recovery-oriented, nonprofessional groups that rely on their members to support one another by encouraging responsibility for substance use through informational, emotional, and social support for persons with a substance use disorder and their families. There are several mutual aid approaches, including 12-step Groups, Women for Sobriety (WFS), Moderation Management (MM) and SMART Recovery® (Self-Management and Recovery Training).

Twelve-step groups, as initially outlined by Alcoholics Anonymous (AA), have been developed for several substance and behavioral addictions with the goal of abstinence through a series of 12 "steps." These focus on admitting powerlessness of the user over drugs and alcohol and/or particular behavior (not over everything in their life, that is, saying that even a small amount of use or a behavior becomes out of control), exploring past wrongs and the causal character traits, seeking forgiveness for past wrongs, seeking connection to a higher power, and carrying forward these strategies to others who suffer. Twelve-step groups nurture self-worth through prosocial behavior norms (helping others, engaging in service work), connecting with spirituality, and celebrating sobriety milestones. The participants are encouraged to develop a relationship with a sponsor, who is generally a senior member with long-term abstinence who is willing to lead the participant through ("work") the steps. Groups exist for individuals with substance use disorders (e.g., alcohol, nicotine, narcotics, cocaine, marijuana, methamphetamine), behavioral disorders (e.g., gambling, sex, love, internet/technology), and dual diagnosis disorders, as well as for family members (e.g., Families Anonymous, Al-Anon/Alateen, Nar-Anon, and Codependents-Anon). In addition, there are groups such as Refuge Recovery that incorporate Buddhist principles into meetings and literature.

While not a mutual aid group itself, 12-step facilitation (TSF) is a manualized therapy led by a clinician to help a person begin and/or attend 12-step meetings through integration of principles offered in 12-step meetings with medication and psychotherapy for substance use disorders. The three main ideas in TSF include acceptance of addiction as chronic and progressive, surrender to a higher power, and involvement in 12-step meetings.

Women for Sobriety (WFS) is one of the oldest mutual aid programs and was founded as an alternative to traditional 12-step therapy based on the idea that women require a different approach to achieve and maintain sobriety. It focuses on nurturing self-worth through its "New Life" Program. WFS utilizes 13 acceptance statements and 6 levels of recovery to promote behavioral change through a cognitive, behavioral, mindful, and group approach to addictive behaviors.

SMART Recovery® (Self-Management and Recovery Training) utilizes CBT-based rational emotive behavior therapy (REBT) to reverse self-destructive behavior through managing thoughts and feelings that are associated with substance use or behavioral addictions. Through their "4-point Program," SMART aims to enhance motivation and assist the participant in refusing to act on urges, using coping skills, and developing a balanced lifestyle. Like CBT, SMART emphasizes skills training and discussion in the group. Unlike 12-step, SMART does not encourage reliance on a higher power or the notion of "powerlessness," supports graduation from the program, accepts harmful behavior reduction as a goal, and can be led by a facilitator not in recovery.

There are also groups that do not focus on abstinence, but rather encourage moderation in drinking, using, or other behavior that interferes with functioning. Moderation Management (MM) is one such group and offers face-to-face and online meetings, a listserv, a forum, online drinking limit guidelines, a self-help book, and an online calendar to record drinking.

Empiric Evidence

Numerous studies have shown that involvement in 12-step groups is associated with greater rates of abstinence and other recovery outcomes in the treatment of alcohol use disorder and other substances. Studies involving TSF support its utility in increasing membership in 12-step groups and odds of abstinence [39]. WFS and SMART have been shown to be as effective as 12-step groups for those with AUD as the traditional 12-step approach when considering abstinence goals [40]. Researchers have found that MM generally attracts heavy drinkers who are well-educated and middle-class, and who have fewer symptoms of dependence or alcohol-related problems than treatment seekers [41].

For Whom

Mutual aid is a group-based treatment utilized in both inpatient and outpatient recovery. Due to the element of the "higher power," traditional 12-step groups may not be ideal for those with an opposition to its focus on spirituality. TSF has been shown to be helpful in the treatment of alcohol use disorder and may be especially helpful for those with dual diagnoses, as TSF encourages the practitioner to incorporate integrative care that is low-cost and high-frequency. This may facilitate treating the underlying psychiatric illness contributing to substance use. Importantly, those with comorbid psychiatric disorders may have a more difficult time in traditional 12-step groups without formal support due to challenges associated with their psychiatric diagnosis or resistance from some groups to supporting the use of psychotropic medications. Demographically, mutual support functions for adults of both sexes and youth have a high dropout rate (this is true in youth across modalities).

Systems-Based Therapy

Systems-based therapies aim to influence substance use through acknowledging, examining, and utilizing the relationships between an individual and their membership in various groups (systems).

Family- and Couples-Based Treatments

Substance use disorders result from a transaction among multiple individual, genetic, family, and community factors. Factors such as parent psychopathology, relational distance, family conflict, and inadequate parenting are predictors of substance use initiation and maintenance [42]. In turn, substance use seriously impacts family functioning and relationships. Because of these transactions, family therapy has been found to be an important intervention that can facilitate engagement and maintenance in treatment and prevent or minimize relapse.

The focus of family therapy is to intervene in complex relational patterns and to alter them in ways that bring about productive change for the entire family. Family therapy rests on systems theory, which proposes that changes in one part of the system can and do produce changes in other parts of the system, and these changes can improve functioning.

Family-based approaches include separate treatments, each with its own conceptual framework and evidence base. The approaches with the strongest empirical support include (1) brief strategic family therapy (BSFT) [43], based in family systems theory that targets adolescents' substance use and other challenging behaviors by facilitating changes in the family's patterns of interaction; (2) multisystemic therapy (MST) [44], rooted in a social ecology perspective that addresses the risk/protective factors (e.g., family, peer group, school, and neighborhood) that influence substance use behavior among adolescents; (3) multidimensional family therapy (MDFT) [45] that addresses substance use and problematic behaviors in adolescents by intervening on a number of levels similar to MST and integrates family therapy, the social ecology perspective, and developmental psychology; and (4) functional family therapy (FFT) [46] that evolved from both behavioral and systems-oriented theoretical approaches and whose goal is to enhance communication and support within the family while altering maladaptive familial patterns.

The most well-developed and studied couples approach is behavioral couples therapy [47]. It involves an initial agreement for the person misusing substances to commit to sobriety and the partner to reinforce this commitment daily. It also teaches strategies to cope with cravings, manage relapse, communicate, and engage in pleasurable activities together.

Empiric Evidence

Family and couples therapies have been shown to be efficacious in multiple SUDs [48, 49]. While there is some evidence for these therapies in gambling disorder and internet addiction, there is a need for more rigorous investigation into the efficacy of family and couples-based therapies in the behavioral addictions [8, 10, 11].

For Whom

Family involvement in treatment is strongly recommended when the client is living within a family system, for example, as a couple or single parent or both parents and children. Modifying harmful family patterns can facilitate change in behavior and prevent relapse. Family members need support and education as to how to cope with the behaviors of their loved one and how to communicate effectively so that even if therapy is not available, the family can be brought in for education and support sessions. The challenge lies in finding staff who are trained in general family and/or couples therapy since many of the approaches have been manualized and require specific training. Family approaches appear to be the most effective for adolescents compared to treatment as usual [50]. Evidence also supports the use of BSFT, MDFT, and MST family approaches with ethnic minority youth and their families [51].

Matrix Model

The Matrix model combines elements of family approaches, 12-step facilitation, and relapse prevention and was originally designed to treat methamphetamine addiction within an intensive outpatient program. The current model includes three individual or conjoint family sessions and 52 group sessions over 16 weeks. Clients are asked to participate in social support groups weekly during the aftercare phase [52].

Empiric Evidence

A multisite study comparing the Matrix model to treatment as usual was conducted in eight community treatment programs for those struggling with methamphetamine misuse [53]. There were no differences in substance use or psychosocial functioning at discharge or at 6-month follow-up. However, Matrix model participants had better retention and completion rates.

For Whom

This treatment was designed for those suffering from methamphetamine misuse but has been expanded to those with substance use disorders who can benefit from an intensive outpatient program (IOP). Staff must be fully trained in the methodology, and clients must be able to access IOP-level treatment.

Community Reinforcement Approach and Community Reinforcement and Family Training

The community reinforcement approach (CRA) is a CBT-based intervention focused on helping a substance-using individual to identify what they deem rewarding outside of substances and to use new skills to adopt a sober lifestyle that is more rewarding than substance use. Community Reinforcement and Family Training (CRAFT) is an outgrowth of the CRA. It is a skills-based program that impacts families in multiple areas of their lives, including self-care, pleasurable activities, domestic violence precautions, problem-solving, and goal setting. CRAFT addresses the loved one's resistance to change by operating indirectly through the family members rather than the substance user. It teaches families behavioral and motivational strategies for interacting with their loved ones. Participants learn the power of positive reinforcement for positive behavior and of withdrawing it for unwanted behavior, as well as how to use positive communication skills to improve interactions and maximize their influence [54].

Empiric Evidence

CRA originally showed efficacy in the treatment of alcohol use [55]. CRAFT was found to be superior in engaging treatment-resistant individuals compared to traditional programs, demonstrating three times more person engagement than Al-Anon [56, 57].

For Whom

CRA has a strong history of use in individuals with alcohol use disorder, and CRA plus contingency management (CM) is used in those with stimulant use disorders. CRAFT is for family members who are interested in helping themselves and their family member who is using substances.

Digital Interventions

Over the past decade, there has been a rise in digital interventions in medicine. This includes but is not limited to the use of electronic health records, telehealth, digital-based therapy modules, mobile applications, and wearable devices. A subset of digital medicine is "digital therapeutics (DTx)." DTx may be defined as "health software intended to treat or alleviate a disease, disorder, condition, or injury by generating and delivering a medical intervention that has a demonstrable positive therapeutic impact on a person's health [58]." They require clinical evidence, real-world outcomes, and are subject to regulatory oversight. DTx can integrate with other digital medicine and digital health applications and devices. DTx that are prescription-only are classified as prescription DTx (PDTx). Some apps do have FDA approval for the treatment of SUDs and are described below.

Empiric Evidence

Multiple reviews and meta-analyses investigating the efficacy of digital interventions suggest that these platforms show promise for the screening and treatment of behavioral health, including SUDs [59]. Telehealth, which includes video or audio-based delivery of medical and/or psychotherapeutic services, has grown significantly since the COVID-19 pandemic. Two review articles specifically investigating SUD treatment suggest that telemedicine and teletherapy are at least as effective as in-person services, though long-term data and more randomized controlled trials are needed [60, 61].

A well-studied digital-based therapy program for SUDs modelled closely on a CBT manual from the National Institute on Drug Abuse, computer-based training for cognitive behavioral therapy (CBT4CBT), is designed to work in concert with oversight from a healthcare provider and has shown efficacy in a number of treatment outcomes compared to treatment as usual in outpatient care [62]. Evidence for other digital-based therapies and mobile applications is mixed due to the heterogeneous nature of the interventions being studied and the lack of a standardized approach to evaluation. However, they warrant further study due to the potential benefits and minimal risk of adverse events.

Of the thousands of digital health products on the market, only two DTx have received FDA clearance as PDTx for SUDs: reSET (a 90-day program for alcohol, cocaine, cannabis, and stimulant use disorders to increase abstinence) and reSET-O (an 84-day program for opioid use disorder in conjunction with oral buprenorphine to increase treatment retention) [63–66]. Both are internet-delivered interventions that use the Community Reinforcement Approach with a clinician interface to deliver cognitive behavioral therapy as an adjunct to contingency management on an outpatient basis under the supervision of a clinician.

For Whom

Persons who may benefit the most from digital interventions include those with limited access to in-person services due to mobility or rural locations, as well as typically hard-to-reach populations such as youth and those with stigmatized diseases (e.g., SUDs). Importantly, digital interventions may be limited by sociodemographic, economic, and political factors, such as access to technology and digital literacy.

Chapter Review Questions

1. Beth presents to your practice and endorses struggling most recently with Alcohol Use Disorder, Severe. She also notes that she was diagnosed with borderline personality disorder at age 18 and has struggled to maintain healthy relationships in her adult years. Which of the following modalities would be the best fit for co-occurring symptoms of both disorders?

   A. Dialectical behavior therapy
   B. Acceptance and commitment therapy
   C. Cognitive behavioral therapy
   D. Mutual aid groups
   E. Moderation Management

   Correct Answer: A.

   Explanation: DBT is an evidence-based treatment for borderline personality disorder (BPD). It also has applications for the treatment of substance use disorders (SUD). There are some key differences in how Dialectical Behavior Therapy (DBT) is applied when treating BPD alone versus when it's combined with Alcohol or SUD. The following is a breakdown based on current research.

   DBT for BPD alone: (1) Focus: Primarily addresses the core features of BPD, such as emotional dysregulation, interpersonal difficulties, impulsivity, and identity disturbance. (2) Skills Training: Emphasizes mindfulness, distress tolerance, emotion regulation, and interpersonal effectiveness skills. (3) Therapy Structure: Typically includes individual therapy, group skills training, and phone coaching. *DBT for BPD with SUD*: (1) Additional Focus: Integrates strategies to address substance use, including: Dialectical Abstinence, which helps clients navigate the tension between the desire to use substances and the commitment to abstinence; "Clear Mind, " which encourages awareness of the impact of substances on thoughts, feelings, and behaviors; and Relapse Prevention, which develops coping skills to manage cravings and avoid high-risk situations. (2) Modified Skills Training: May include adaptations to standard DBT skills to address substance-related challenges. For example, distress tolerance skills might focus on managing cravings and withdrawal symptoms. (3) Increased Emphasis on Attachment: Recognizes that individuals with BPD and SUD may have difficulties with attachment and commitment to treatment. Therapists may use strategies to strengthen the therapeutic relationship and increase treatment engagement.

Reference: Maffei C, Cavicchioli M, Movalli M, Cavallaro R, Fossati A. Dialectical behavior therapy skills training in alcohol dependence treatment: findings based on an open trial. Subst Use Misuse. 2018;53(14):2368–85. https://doi.org/10.1080/10826084.2018.1480035.

2. You have been seeing John for six months. In your sessions, you explore the language they use to describe unwanted emotions and thoughts and how these impact their experience of distress; their values and how these translate into action; and their willingness to connect to the world around them mindfully. Which intervention are you using with them?

   A. Mindfulness-oriented recovery enhancement (MORE)
   B. Contingency management (CM)
   C. Dialectical behavior therapy (DBT)
   D. Acceptance and commitment therapy (ACT)
   E. Cognitive behavioral therapy (CBT)

   Correct Answer: D.

   Explanation: Acceptance and commitment therapy (ACT) works with the language we use to describe the internal and external events in our lives to increase psychological flexibility. This is facilitated through focus on values, committed action, and connection to the present moment, among other core processes.

3. Kate presents, stating her husband has a problem with the amount of money being lost and the time she is spending on gambling, and that he would leave her if she didn't get help. In the interview you find that she does meet the criteria for a gambling disorder with no other mental health diagnoses. Despite this, she doesn't seem to understand that her gambling is a problem. What is the first type of intervention you might try to engage her in, to continue the discussion of her gambling and to have her vocalize other reasons why it may be a problem?

   A. Dialectical behavior therapy
   B. Cognitive behavioral therapy
   C. Family-based therapy
   D. Mutual aid groups
   E. Motivational interviewing

   Correct Answer: E.

   Explanation: Given that Kate is presenting with limited insight into the problem, it is important to first develop rapport while evoking reasons for change through motivational interviewing. Once she is more engaged, she may benefit from other interventions.

   Reference: Ribeiro EO, Afonso NH, Morgado P. Non-pharmacological treatment of gambling disorder: a systematic review of randomized controlled trials. BMC Psychiatry. 2021;21(1):1–5. https://doi.org/10.1186/s12888-021-03097-2.

4. Alexis has been using substances and this is impacting her relationships with her family members, who would like to learn how to reward the behavior in which they wish to see her engage. Which systems-based therapy is a skills-based

therapy that teaches participants how to utilize positive reinforcement for positive behavior and withdraw it for negative behavior to engage treatment-resistant family members?

A. Mindfulness-based relapse prevention
B. Community reinforcement and family training
C. Motivational enhancement therapy
D. Cognitive behavioral therapy
E. Twelve-step facilitation

Correct Answer: B.

Explanation: CRAFT is a systems-based treatment that teaches families behavioral and motivational strategies for interacting with their loved one. While CRAFT draws on elements of cognitive behavioral therapy and uses motivational strategies, its strength lies in utilizing the family system rather than the person alone.

5. Maria, a 34-year-old single female with multiple substance use disorders whom you have been treating with medication, is now open to starting psychotherapy. She has voiced several intrinsic and extrinsic motivators to remain abstinent. She has been sober for 3 months and is willing to give short-term therapy a try to help with how her negative thoughts and feelings may impact her use. She thinks mindfulness is unhelpful for her and does not want in-depth discussions about her past relationships. Which of the following interventions would be best suited for her at this point?

A. Motivational enhancement therapy
B. Acceptance and commitment therapy
C. Contingency management
D. Cognitive behavioral therapy
E. Psychodynamic therapy

Correct Answer: D.

Explanation: The person has already identified numerous intrinsic reasons for continued change and wants to work on long-term sobriety, so motivational enhancement therapy or traditional contingency management would not be best for her at this time. Cognitive behavioral therapy is a time-limited intervention that is helpful for a number of substance use disorders. It focuses on changing maladaptive thoughts and behaviors. It does not utilize mindfulness-based practices (like acceptance and commitment therapy) and is not based on longer-term treatment and a deeper understanding of the person's personality schema (psychodynamic).

References

1. Walter KN, Petry NM. Motivation and contingency management treatments for substance use disorders. Simpson E, Balsam P, editors. Curr Top Behav Neurosci [Internet]. 2016 [cited 2025 May 18];27:569–81. Available from: http://link.springer.com/10.1007/7854_2015_374

2. Bolívar HA, Klemperer EM, Coleman SRM, DeSarno M, Skelly JM, Higgins ST. Contingency management for patients receiving medication for opioid use disorder: a systematic review and meta-analysis. JAMA Psychiatry. 2021;78(10):1092–102. https://doi.org/10.1001/jamapsychiatry.2021.1969.
3. Bentzley BS, Han SS, Neuner S, Humphreys K, Kampman KM, Halpern CH. Comparison of treatments for cocaine use disorder among adults: a systematic review and meta-analysis. JAMA Netw Open. 2021;4(5):e218049. https://doi.org/10.1001/jamanetworkopen.2021.8049.
4. Ginley MK, Pfund RA, Rash CJ, Zajac K. Long-term efficacy of contingency management treatment based on objective indicators of abstinence from illicit substance use up to 1 year following treatment: a meta-analysis. J Consult Clin Psychol. 2021;89(1):58. https://doi.org/10.1037/ccp0000552.
5. Pfund RA, Ginley MK, Rash CJ, Zajac K. Contingency management for treatment attendance: a meta-analysis. J Subst Abuse Treat. 2022;133:108556. https://doi.org/10.1016/j.jsat.2021.108556.
6. Petry NM. Contingency management treatments: controversies and challenges. Addiction. 2010;105(9):1507–1509. Accessed 18 May 2025. Available from: http://www.ncbi.nlm.nih.gov/pubmed/20707772
7. Beck JS. Cognitive behavior therapy: basics and beyond. 3rd ed. New York: Guilford Publications; 2021.
8. Ribeiro EO, Afonso NH, Morgado P. Non-pharmacological treatment of gambling disorder: a systematic review of randomized controlled trials. BMC Psychiatry. 2021;21(1):1–5. https://doi.org/10.1186/s12888-021-03097-2.
9. Di Nicola M, De Crescenzo F, D'alò GL, Remondi C, Panaccione I, Moccia L, et al. Pharmacological and psychosocial treatment of adults with gambling disorder: a meta-review. J Addict Med. 2020;14(4):e15–23. https://doi.org/10.1097/ADM.0000000000000574.
10. Borgogna NC, Garos S, Meyer CL, Trussell MR, Kraus SW. A review of behavioral interventions for compulsive sexual behavior disorder. Curr Addict Reports. 2022;9(3):99–108. https://doi.org/10.1007/s40429-022-00422-x.
11. Zhang X, Zhang J, Zhang K, Ren J, Lu X, Wang T, et al. Effects of different interventions on internet addiction: a meta-analysis of random controlled trials. J Affect Disord. 2022;313:56–71. https://doi.org/10.1016/j.jad.2022.06.013.
12. Hofmann SG, Asnaani A, Vonk IJJ, Sawyer AT, Fang A. The efficacy of cognitive behavioral therapy: a review of meta-analyses. Cognit Ther Res. 2012;36(5):427–40. https://doi.org/10.1007/s10608-012-9476-1.
13. Decker SE, Kiluk BD, Frankforter T, Babuscio T, Nich C, Carroll KM. Just showing up is not enough: homework adherence and outcome in cognitive-behavioral therapy for cocaine dependence. J Consult Clin Psychol. 2016;84(10):907. https://doi.org/10.1037/ccp0000126.
14. Najavits L. Seeking safety: a treatment manual for PTSD and substance abuse. Guilford Publications; 2002.
15. McHugh RK, Hearon BA, Otto MW. Cognitive behavioral therapy for substance use disorders. Psychiatr Clin North Am. 2010;33(3):511–525. Accessed 18 May 2025. Available from: http://www.ncbi.nlm.nih.gov/pubmed/20599130
16. Witkiewitz K, Bowen S, Harrop EN, Douglas H, Enkema M, Sedgwick C. Mindfulness-based treatment to prevent addictive behavior relapse: theoretical models and hypothesized mechanisms of change. Subst Use Misuse [Internet]. 2014;49(5):513–524. Accessed 18 May 2025. https://doi.org/10.3109/10826084.2014.891845.
17. Garland EL, Howard MO. Mindfulness-based treatment of addiction: current state of the field and envisioning the next wave of research. Addict Sci Clin Pract [Internet]. 2018;13(1):14. Accessed 18 May 2025. Available from: https://ascpjournal.biomedcentral.com/articles/10.1186/s13722-018-0115-3
18. Li W, Howard MO, Garland EL, McGovern P, Lazar M. Mindfulness treatment for substance misuse: a systematic review and meta-analysis. J Subst Abuse Treat [Internet].

2017;1(75):62–96. Accessed 19 May 2025. Available from: http://www.ncbi.nlm.nih.gov/pubmed/28153483
19. Hayes SC, Strosahl KD, Wilson KG. Acceptance and commitment therapy: the process and practice of mindful change. Guilford Press: The Guılford Press; 2011.
20. Lanza PV, García PF, Lamelas FR, González-Menéndez A. Acceptance and commitment therapy versus cognitive behavioral therapy in the treatment of substance use disorder with incarcerated women. J Clin Psychol. 2014;70(7):644–57. https://doi.org/10.1002/jclp.22060.
21. Hayes SC, Pistorello J, Levin ME. Acceptance and commitment therapy as a unified model of behavior change. Couns Psychol. 2012;40(7):976–1002. https://doi.org/10.1177/0011000012460836.
22. Osaji J, Ojimba C, Ahmed S. The use of acceptance and commitment therapy in substance use disorders: a review of literature. J Clin Med Res. 2020;12(10):629–33. https://doi.org/10.14740/jocmr4311.
23. Meyer EC, Walser R, Hermann B, La Bash H, DeBeer BB, Morissette SB, et al. Acceptance and commitment therapy for co-occurring posttraumatic stress disorder and alcohol use disorders in veterans: pilot treatment outcomes. J Trauma Stress. 2018;31(5):781–9. https://doi.org/10.1002/jts.22322.
24. Luoma JB, Kohlenberg BS, Hayes SC, Fletcher L. Slow and steady wins the race: a randomized clinical trial of acceptance and commitment therapy targeting shame in substance use disorders. J Consult Clin Psychol. 2012;80(1):43. https://doi.org/10.1037/a0026070.
25. Morgan TA, Dalrymple K, D'Avanzato C, Zimage S, Balling C, Ward M, et al. Conducting outcomes research in a clinical practice setting: the effectiveness and acceptability of acceptance and commitment therapy (ACT) in a partial hospital program. Behav Ther. 2021;52(2):272–85. https://doi.org/10.1016/j.beth.2020.08.004.
26. Linehan MM. DBT skills training manual. 2nd ed. Guilford Press; 2014.
27. Lee NK, Cameron J, Jenner L. A systematic review of interventions for co-occurring substance use and borderline personality disorders. Drug Alcohol Rev. 2015;34(6):663–72. https://doi.org/10.1111/dar.12267.
28. Warner N, Murphy M. Dialectical behaviour therapy skills training for individuals with substance use disorder: a systematic review. Drug Alcohol Rev. 2022;41(2):501–16. https://doi.org/10.1111/dar.13362.
29. Maffei C, Cavicchioli M, Movalli M, Cavallaro R, Fossati A. Dialectical behavior therapy skills training in alcohol dependence treatment: findings based on an open trial. Subst Use Misuse. 2018;53(14):2368–85. https://doi.org/10.1080/10826084.2018.1480035.
30. Miller WR, Rollnick S. Motivational interviewing: helping people change and grow. 4th ed. Guilford Press; 2023.
31. Miller WR, Zweben A, DiClemente CC, Rychtarik RG. Motivational enhancement therapy manual: a clinical research guide for therapists treating individuals with alcohol abuse and dependence. Rockville: US Department of Health and Human Services; 1995.
32. Magill M, Apodaca TR, Borsari B, Gaume J, Hoadley A, Gordon REF, et al. A meta-analysis of motivational interviewing process: technical, relational, and conditional process models of change. J Consult Clin Psychol. 2018;86(2):140. https://doi.org/10.1037/ccp0000250.
33. DiClemente C, Greene P, Petersen A, Thrash S, Crouch T. Motivational enhancement. In: Galanter M, Kleber HD, Brady KT, editors. The American Psychiatric Publishing textbook of substance abuse treatment. 5th ed. Arlington: American Psychiatric Publishing; 2015. p. 397–409. Accessed 18 May 2025. Available from: http://psychiatryonline.org/doi/10.1176/appi.books.9781615370030.mg27
34. Project MATCH Research Group. Matching alcoholism treatments to client heterogeneity: project MATCH three-year drinking outcomes. Alcohol Clin Exp Res. 1998;22(6):1300–1311. Accessed 19 May 2025. Available from: http://doi.wiley.com/10.1111/j.1530-0277.1998.tb03912.x
35. Khantzian EJ. Understanding addictive vulnerability: an evolving psychodynamic perspective. Neuropsychoanalysis. 2003;5(1):5–21. Accessed 18 May 2025. Available from: http://www.tandfonline.com/doi/abs/10.1080/15294145.2003.10773403

36. Khantzian EJ. Psychodynamic psychotherapy for the treatment of substance use disorders. In: El-Guebaly N, Carra G, Galanter M, Baldacchino A, editors. Textbook of addiction treatment: international perspectives. 2nd ed. Springer; 2021. https://doi.org/10.1007/978-3-030-36391-8_26.
37. Center for Substance Abuse Treatment. Brief interventions and brief therapies for substance abuse. Treatment Improvement Protocol (TIP) series 34. 2012.
38. Lightdale HA, Mack AH, Frances RJ. Psychodynamic psychotherapy. In: Galanter M, Kleber HD, Brady K, editors. Textbook of substance abuse treatment. 5th ed. Washington, DC: American Psychiatric Publishing Co; 2015. p. 365–84.
39. Zemore SE, Kaskutas LA, Mericle A, Hemberg J. Comparison of 12-step groups to mutual help alternatives for AUD in a large, national study: differences in membership characteristics and group participation, cohesion, and satisfaction. J Subst Abuse Treat [Internet]. 2017;73:16–26. Accessed 18 May 2025. Available from: http://www.ncbi.nlm.nih.gov/pubmed/28017180
40. Zemore SE, Lui C, Mericle A, Hemberg J, Kaskutas LA. A longitudinal study of the comparative efficacy of Women for Sobriety, LifeRing, SMART Recovery, and 12-step groups for those with AUD. J Subst Abuse Treat [Internet]. 2018;88:18–26. Accessed 18 May 2025. Available from: https://linkinghub.elsevier.com/retrieve/pii/S0740547217304907
41. Kosok A. The Moderation Management programme in 2004: what type of drinker seeks controlled drinking? Int J Drug Policy. 2006;17(4):295–303. https://doi.org/10.1016/j.drugpo.2006.03.003.
42. Tobler AL, Komro KA. Trajectories or parental monitoring and communication and effects on drug use among urban young adolescents. J Adolesc Heal [Internet]. 2010;46(6):560–568. Accessed 18 May 2025. Available from: https://www.sciencedirect.com/science/article/pii/S1054139X09006764?via%3Dihub
43. Szapocznik J, Hervies O, Schwartz S. Brief strategic family therapy for adolescent drug abuse. NIDA Therapy Manuals for Drug Addiction. Bethesda: National Institute on Drug Abuse; 2003. NIH Publication No. 03-4751
44. Henggeler SSW, Borduin CM. Family therapy and beyond: a multisystemic approach to treating the behavior problems of children and adolescents. Pacific Grove: Brooks/Cole Publishing Company; 1990. Accessed 18 May 2025. Available from: https://catalogue.nla.gov.au/Record/1732491
45. Liddle HA. Multidimensional family therapy for adolescent cannabis users, Cannabis Youth Treatment Series, Volume 5. Rockville (MD): Center for Substance Abuse Treatment, Substance Abuse and Mental Health Services Administration; 2002. DHHS Publication No. (SMA) 02–3660.
46. Sexton TL, Van Dam A, Anderson M. Functional family therapy: a comprehensive, evidence-based treatment for diverse communities. American Psychological Association; 2025.
47. O'Farrell TJ, Fals-Stewart W. Behavioral couples therapy for alcoholism and drug abuse. New York: Guildford Press; 2006.
48. Powers MB, Vedel E, Emmelkamp PMG. Behavioral couples therapy (BCT) for alcohol and drug use disorders: a meta-analysis. Clin Psychol Rev. 2008;28(6):952–962. Accessed 18 May 2025. Available from: https://www.sciencedirect.com/science/article/pii/S0272735808000275?via%3Dihub
49. Hogue A, Schumm JA, MacLean A, Bobek M. Couple and family therapy for substance use disorders: Evidence-based update 2010–2019. J Marital Fam Ther. 2022;48(1):178–203. https://doi.org/10.1111/jmft.12546.
50. Rowe CL. Family therapy for drug abuse: Review and updates 2003–2010. J Marital Fam Ther. 2012;38(1):59–81. Accessed 18 May 2025. Available from: http://www.ncbi.nlm.nih.gov/pubmed/22283381
51. Pina AA, Polo AJ, Huey SJ. Evidence-based psychosocial interventions for ethnic minority youth: the 10-year update. J Clin Child Adolesc Psychol. 2019;48(2):179–202.
52. Center for Substance Abuse Treatment. Counselor's treatment manual: matrix intensive outpatient treatment for people with stimulant use disorders. Rockville; 2006. HHS Publication No. (SMA) 13-4152.

53. Rawson RA, Marinelli-Casey P, Anglin MD, Dickow A, Frazier Y, Gallagher C, et al. A multisite comparison of psychosocial approaches for the treatment of methamphetamine dependence. Addiction. 2004;99(6):708–717. Accessed 18 May 2025. Available from: http://www.ncbi.nlm.nih.gov/pubmed/15139869
54. Meyers RJ, Miller WR, Hill DE, Tonigan JSS. Community reinforcement and family training (CRAFT): engaging unmotivated drug users in treatment. J Subst Abuse. 1998;10(3):291–308. Accessed 18 May 2025. Available from: https://www.sciencedirect.com/science/article/pii/S0899328999000036
55. Hunt GM, Azrin NH. A community-reinforcement approach to alcoholism. Behav Res Ther. 1973;11(1):91–104. https://doi.org/10.1016/0005-7967(73)90072-7.
56. Archer M, Harwood H, Stevelink S, Rafferty L, Greenberg N. Community reinforcement and family training and rates of treatment entry: a systematic review. Addiction. 2020;115(6):1024–37. https://doi.org/10.1111/add.14901.
57. Roozen HG, de Waart R, van der Kroft P. Community reinforcement and family training: an effective option to engage treatment-resistant substance-abusing individuals in treatment [corrected] [published erratum appears in Addiction 2010 Nov;105(11):2040]. Addiction. 2010;105(10):1729–38. https://doi.org/10.1111/j.1360-0443.2010.03016.x.
58. International Organization for Standardization. Health informatics – personalized digital health - digital therapeutics health software systems (Publication number ISO/TR 11147:2023). 2023. Available from: https://www.iso.org/standard/83767.html
59. Philippe TJ, Sikder N, Jackson A, Koblanski ME, Liow E, Pilarinos A, et al. Digital health interventions for delivery of mental health care: systematic and comprehensive meta-review. JMIR Ment Heal. 2022;9(5):e35159. https://doi.org/10.2196/35159.
60. Lin L (Allison), Casteel D, Shigekawa E, Weyrich MS, Roby DH, McMenamin SB. Telemedicine-delivered treatment interventions for substance use disorders: a systematic review. J Subst Abuse Treat. 2019;101:38–49. https://doi.org/10.1016/j.jsat.2019.03.007.
61. Pham H, Lin C, Zhu Y, Clingan SE, Lin L, Mooney LJ, et al. Telemedicine-delivered treatment for substance use disorder: a scoping review. J Telemed Telecare. 2025;31(3):359–75. https://doi.org/10.1177/1357633X231190945.
62. Carroll KM, Ball SA, Martino S, Nich C, Babuscio TA, Nuro KF, et al. Computer-assisted delivery of cognitive-behavioral therapy for addiction: a randomized trial of CBT4CBT. Am J Psychiatry. 2008;165(7):881–8. https://doi.org/10.1176/appi.ajp.2008.07111835.
63. Campbell ANC, Nunes EV, Matthews AG, Stitzer M, Miele GM, Polsky D, et al. Internet-delivered treatment for substance abuse: a multisite randomized controlled trial. Am J Psychiatry. 2014;171(6):683–90. https://doi.org/10.1176/appi.ajp.2014.13081055.
64. US Food and Drug Administration. FDA clears mobile medical app to help those with opioid use disorder stay in recovery programs. FDA News Release. 2018. Accessed 19 May 2025. Available from: https://www.fda.gov/news-events/press-announcements/fda-clears-mobile-medical-app-help-those-opioid-use-disorder-stay-recovery-programs
65. US Food and Drug Administration. FDA permits marketing of mobile medical application for substance use disorder. FDA News Release. 2017. Accessed 19 May 2025. Available from: https://www.fda.gov/news-events/press-announcements/fda-permits-marketing-mobile-medical-application-substance-use-disorder
66. Christensen DR, Landes RD, Jackson L, Marsch LA, Mancino MJ, Chopra MP, Bickel WK. Adding an Internet-delivered treatment to an efficacious treatment package for opioid dependence. J Consult Clin Psychol. 2014;82(6):964.

Recovery from Addiction: Maintenance and Preventing Relapse

6

Ricardo Restrepo-Guzman and Maryam Soltani

High-Yield Review Points

- Recovery is a process of change, not a static event, characterized by voluntarily maintained control over substance use, leading toward health and well-being.
- Components of recovery aside from remission from SUD include physical recovery, emotional and psychological recovery, social recovery, spiritual and personal growth, as well as recovery capital.
- Recovery capital refers to the concept that overcoming addiction entails not only the process of healing but also the development and utilization of various forms of capital—such as personal, social, cultural, and community resources—that contribute to sustained wellness and long-term sobriety.
- Abstinence is often a main goal of treatment, but it does not mean that it is the only measure of progress.
- Psychosocial interventions for SUDs target physical, behavioral, cognitive, emotional, interpersonal, and environmental factors to improve the overall functioning of the individual.

R. Restrepo-Guzman (✉)
Department of Psychiatry, Veterans Health Administration Long Beach, Long Beach, CA, USA

Department of Psychiatry, University of California Riverside, Riverside, CA, USA

Department of Psychiatry, Charles Drew University, Los Angeles, CA, USA
e-mail: ricardo.restrepo-guzman@va.gov

M. Soltani
Department of Psychiatry, Veterans Health Administration San Diego, La Jolla, CA, USA

Department of Psychiatry, University of California San Diego, La Jolla, CA, USA

C. Marienfeld, M. Soltani (eds.), *AAAP Review of Addiction Psychiatry*,
https://doi.org/10.1007/978-3-032-24174-0_6

- Therapeutic intervention can facilitate the identification of triggers and cravings and how to address them.
- Understanding the process of relapse is vital to developing an effective relapse prevention plan.
- Relapse prevention is a treatment approach with the goal of preventing lapses or relapses by providing coping skills and alternatives to repeating previous unwanted behaviors.

Overview from Addiction to Recovery

Engaging in behavioral change requires individuals to confront a range of feelings, thoughts, and actions regarding the maladaptive behaviors they are attempting to modify. In the case of substance use disorders (SUDs), the processes of learning and memory are heavily influenced by neurotransmitters like dopamine. These neurotransmitters, which increase activity in brain circuits, lead to biochemical changes that shape thoughts and memories. This neurochemical activity imprints people, situations, and places on the brain, which are later experienced as cues—stimuli such as friends who use substances, emotions, sounds, places, or objects associated with substance use. Over time, these cues become strongly tied to the effects of the substance [1]. Cues often manifest as triggers, which are external or internal events that evoke thoughts or emotions related to substance use [2]. When individuals encounter triggers, they may experience an urge—an impulsive intention to use. This progression can culminate in a craving, a powerful learned response rooted in specific memories of substance use. Cravings, mediated by brain activity in the amygdala, are particularly common in the early weeks or months of abstinence. Fortunately, as individuals adopt relapse prevention strategies, the intensity and frequency of cravings typically diminish.

The development of SUDs is influenced by a complex interplay of biological, genetic, psychological, social, and cognitive factors. Effective treatment addresses these multiple dimensions, aiming to reduce relapse rates and enhance recovery. Research has categorized the risk factors for SUDs into three groups: fixed factors (e.g., gender, ethnicity, family history, socioeconomic status), contextual factors (e.g., social norms, price controls, access laws), and individual or interpersonal factors (e.g., psychiatric comorbidities, trauma history, family and peer dynamics, housing, education, and employment [3].

Family and twin studies indicate that genetics accounts for approximately 50% of the risk for developing an SUD. Across cultures, males generally exhibit higher rates of substance use than females. Certain ethnic minority groups in the United States, including American Indians, African Americans, and Hispanics, experience disproportionately higher rates of substance use. These disparities often intersect with socioeconomic and geographical factors, such as poverty, high substance availability, and low community cohesion. Additionally, chronic stress or trauma significantly heightens vulnerability to SUDs, as do family and social influences, including observing or modelling substance use behaviors within one's environment [4].

Childhood and adolescence are critical periods for personality development and brain maturation, making early intervention particularly effective. Family-based interventions have been successful in reducing substance use among adolescents by addressing substance use in parents, fostering parental social support, and building strong alliances with healthcare providers. Broader public policy measures, such as increasing taxes on substances, raising the legal drinking or smoking age, and implementing stricter regulations, further contribute to prevention efforts. On an individual or group level, interventions may focus on psychological, pharmacological, or social aspects, delivered by a range of care providers. [5].

Psychosocial interventions play a vital role in addressing the physical, behavioral, cognitive, emotional, interpersonal, and environmental factors underlying SUDs. These interventions improve overall functioning and include approaches like cognitive-behavioral therapy (CBT), contingency management, motivational interviewing, and brief interventions for alcohol and tobacco use. Other strategies include community-based treatment, vocational rehabilitation, supportive housing, psychoeducation for families, peer support services, and integrated care for individuals with co-occurring conditions. By promoting behavioral change, psychosocial interventions serve as an essential component of any comprehensive SUD treatment program, complementing medications for addiction treatment to optimize recovery outcomes [6].

Stages of Change

There are several ways of thinking about the recovery process. A common one, originally developed for smoking cessation, is divided into five non-linear stages of change involved in seeking recovery. This is titled the transtheoretical model of change (TTM) [7] (Fig. 6.1).

Pre-contemplation Stage: This stage is typically characterized by denial of addiction, with limited or no recognition of the negative consequences of substance use. The perceived cons of quitting far outweigh the pros of quitting. There is no intention of taking action in the foreseeable future.

Contemplation Stage: There is intent to make a healthy behavioral change in the foreseeable future. The person recognizes the negative consequences of substance use and adopts a more balanced view of the pros vs. cons of pursuing sobriety. However, some ambivalence may remain.

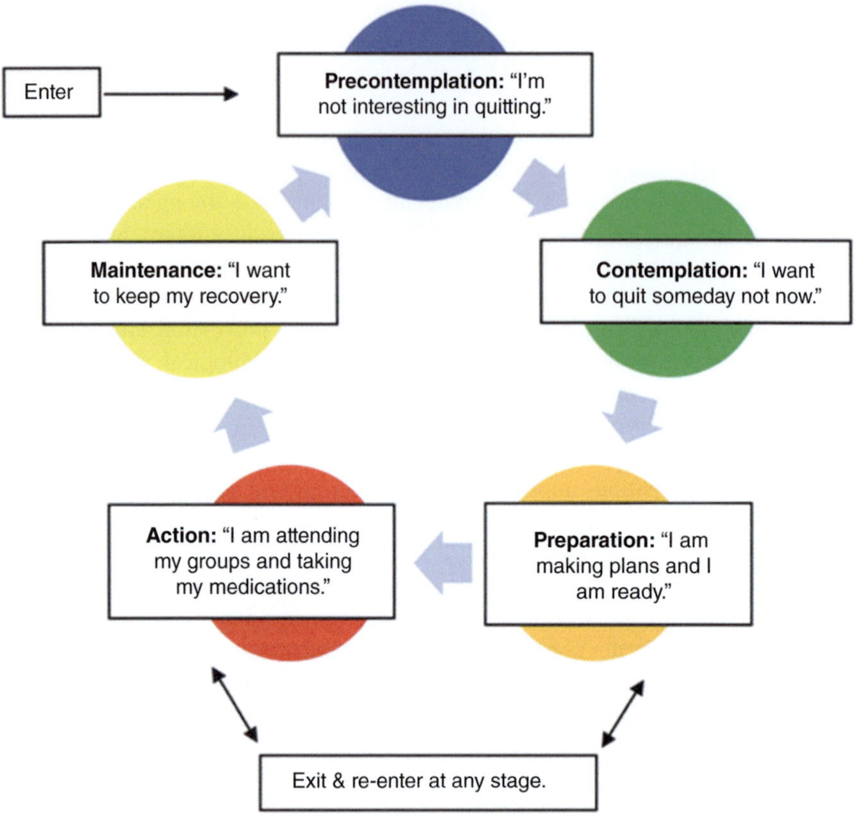

Fig. 6.1 Transtheoretical model of change (TTM)

Preparation Stage: Readiness to take action within the next 30 days. The person is already beginning to take small steps toward sobriety and has fully embraced the belief that sobriety can lead to a healthier and happier life.

Action Stage: The behavior change has been implemented within the last 6 months, and the person intends to continue in this trajectory.

Maintenance and Relapse Prevention: The person has sustained the behavioral change for more than 6 months, intends to maintain this, and is actively practicing RP techniques to avoid falling back to an earlier stage.

Recovery

In the context of addiction treatment, recovery from substance use disorders (SUDs) is recognized as a dynamic and individualized process requiring a comprehensive and long-term approach. A recovery-oriented perspective views SUDs as chronic rather than acute conditions, emphasizing the need for long-term support and focusing on recovery management rather than solely on managing the disease. The Betty Ford Institute Consensus Panel defines *recovery* as "a voluntarily maintained lifestyle composed by sobriety, personal health, and citizenship," focusing on abstinence from substance use, improvements in health and wellness, and the development of personal relationships [8]. The Substance Abuse and Mental Health Services Administration (SAMHSA) defines recovery as "A process of change through which individuals improve their health and wellness, live a self-directed life, and strive to reach their full potential [9]." Other definitions broaden this understanding, highlighting recovery as a progression toward a state of living without the impairments or negative consequences of substance use, whether abstinence is fully achieved.

Recovery is multifaceted and involves various factors beyond cessation of substance use. It includes overcoming physical and psychological dependence on substances, as well as integration into society. The process of recovery is highly individualized, and this is likely the reason why there is no standardized measurement to determine successful treatment [10]. Abstinence can be an end goal but need not be the sole measure of progress. Most people with substance use disorders (SUDs) do not receive treatment. In 2023, an estimated 54.2 million people aged 12 and older needed treatment for a substance use disorder in the past year. Only 23% of those received the treatment they needed. Only 1.6 million of the people classified as needing substance use disorder treatment but who did not receive it felt they needed treatment [11]. For those who do not receive treatment, approximately 30% of all psychosocial SUD treatment episodes are terminated prematurely. When individuals with SUDs are surveyed about why they are not in treatment, "not being ready to stop using substances" is consistently the top reason cited, even among those who acknowledge the need for treatment [12, 13]. Studies aimed at increasing treatment utilization in high-risk SUD populations have found that, even when treatment is offered for free, without waiting lists, and with professional support to help individuals enroll, many (34–92%) still do not enter treatment [14]. While there is a clear need to engage people earlier in treatment, this goal may be more achievable if we allow non-abstinence-based treatments as an initial step toward positive changes for individuals with SUDs. The motivation for change is "action-specific," meaning people are motivated to take specific actions or pursue goals [15]. Aligning the goals of the clinician and patient is key to developing a strong therapeutic alliance and achieving greater treatment outcomes.

Given this, harm reduction plays a crucial role in the recovery process by offering practical and compassionate strategies to support individuals wherever they are in their journey. This approach emphasizes collaboration, aiming to reduce the harmful effects of substance use—such as overdose, disease transmission, or social instability—while promoting incremental steps toward improved health and wellness. By integrating harm reduction into recovery-oriented care, individuals are empowered to make safer choices, address immediate risks, and build a foundation for long-term stability and personal growth. This inclusive perspective recognizes that recovery is not solely defined by abstinence but also by meaningful improvements in quality of life, health, and social connections, aligning with the diverse and individualized pathways that recovery may take.

Progress in Recovery: Should be realistic and measured according to the individual's goals, as there can be a mismatch in clinician expectations for progress and the person's own goals for his or her substance use recovery. The individual may first be encouraged to identify small changes and how these can start to impact his or her well-being. Any positive change can be valued and reinforced by the clinician, such as through motivational interviewing skills. In the same vein, setbacks can be normalized without being minimized while continuing to work toward recovery and identifying positive changes. Reviewing progress in recovery goals at regular intervals is an integral part of a treatment plan. Treatment is dynamic, and changes can lead the team—comprised of the individual with SUD, clinicians and family members—to identify new goals and recovery strategies. As part of an effective approach, progress is not assessed in absolutes, but rather is discussed in an atmosphere where values, trust, and a humanitarian approach are practiced instead of authoritarianism, judgment, fear, and criticism.

Pathways to Recovery

There are different pathways to recovery to choose from based on cultural values, socioeconomic status, psychological and behavioral needs, and the nature of the individual's SUD. Recovery can be achieved by combining various frameworks, including secular, spiritual/religious, natural recovery, peer-assisted, treatment including medications, abstinence-based, moderation-based, and harm reduction-based, among others. The recovery experience is a constant process that needs to be individualized and not generalized. The combination of physical, cognitive, emotional, relational, and spiritual health across the stages of life is fundamental when considering pathways to recovery. Sustained recovery is self-directed and involves personal choices, the support of peers and allies, and community reinforcement, as well as a strength-based approach and the use of research-based interventions [16]. In sum, the pathway to recovery will often include:

1. Physical recovery: Restoring physical health and well-being through detoxification, rehabilitation treatment, and long-term health practices.
2. Emotional and psychological recovery: Addressing the mental and emotional factors that contribute to addiction, such as trauma, stress, and underlying mental health conditions. This may involve therapy, counseling, or other forms of emotional support.

3. Social recovery: Rebuilding relationships, improving social skills, and restoring trust with family, friends, and community. Social support plays a crucial role in maintaining recovery.
4. Spiritual and personal growth: Finding a sense of purpose or meaning in life through spirituality, personal development, or aligning with values that promote a fulfilling and sober life.
5. Recovery capital (RC): Building an ecological model directed to find all internal and external resources a person can access to initiate and maintain recovery [17].

Recovery Capital

The concept of *Recovery Capital (RC)* (Fig. 6.2) emphasizes that recovery from addiction is not just about overcoming substance use but also about building or accessing various forms of capital that can support long-term wellness and sobriety. There are several types of categories encompassed by recovery capital that can pave the pathway to recovery [18, 19]; these are outlined and described below.

RC is seen as a dynamic and evolving resource. As individuals progress in their recovery, their levels of recovery capital can increase or decrease. Successful

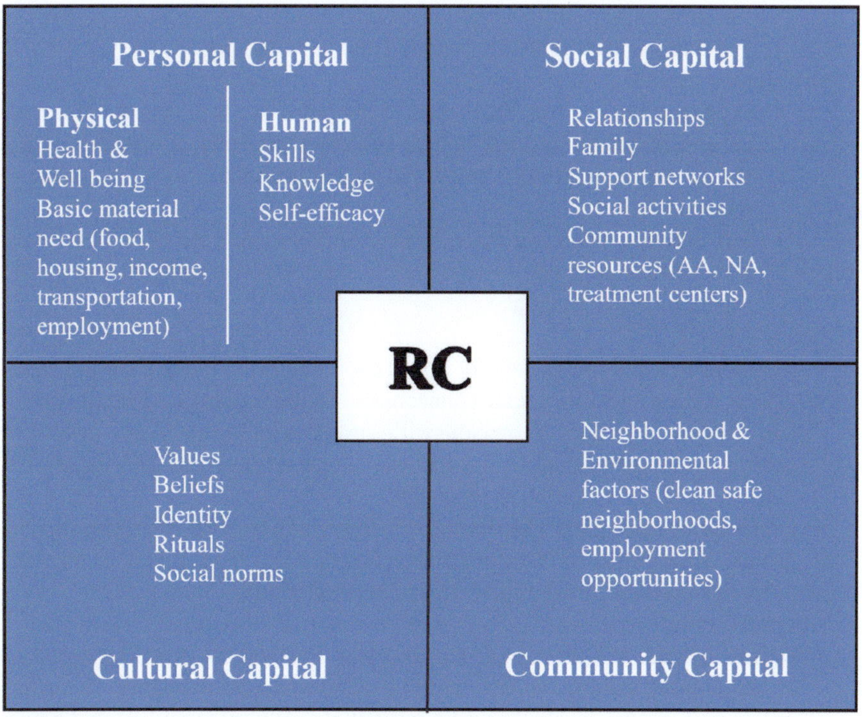

Fig. 6.2 Components of recovery capital (RC)

recovery is often tied to an individual's ability to leverage and build these forms of capital. Central to the theory of RC is the idea that greater RC, fewer barriers, and fewer unmet needs lead to improved recovery outcomes, whereas lower RC, more barriers, and more unmet needs result in poorer outcomes. For example, someone who has strong social and community support but lacks physical or human capital (e.g., education, job or stable health) may face challenges, while someone with a well-rounded portfolio of recovery capital may have more resources to cope with stressors and setbacks.

The concept of RC emphasizes that recovery is not a linear process but rather a complex interaction of multiple factors that can change over time. By focusing on building recovery capital, individuals and treatment professionals can take a more holistic, strengths-based approach to recovery.

1. Personal Capital
   (a) Physical capital:
      - Health & well-being: This includes an individual's physical health, such as being free from the effects of substance use, engaging in regular exercise, having access to medical care, and managing any chronic conditions. Physical capital also encompasses the resources to help with physical healing (e.g., food security, rehabilitation, nutrition, etc.).
      - Basic material needs: Access to housing, food, employment, and financial stability are key components of physical capital. Secure living conditions and financial resources are fundamental to sustaining recovery.

   (b) Human capital:
      - Skills and knowledge: This refers to the individual's personal and practical abilities that contribute to their success in recovery. It includes coping skills, problem-solving, emotional regulation, education, and employment skills.
      - Self-efficacy: The confidence in one's ability to manage life without substances. Building self-esteem and a sense of personal agency is a vital aspect of human capital.
2. Social Capital
   - Relationships and social support: Social capital refers to the quality and quantity of the individual's social connections, including family, friends, peers, and support networks. A person with strong social capital has access to healthy, supportive relationships that encourage sobriety and offer emotional support, which is essential to recovery.
   - Community resources: This includes connections to local recovery support groups (such as AA or NA), treatment centers, recovery coaches, or any network that provides encouragement and accountability.
3. Cultural Capital
   - Values, beliefs, and identity: Cultural capital involves the broader context of an individual's culture, values, traditions, and sense of belonging. It encompasses factors like spiritual or religious beliefs, cultural practices, and how a person relates to their community and society.

  - Social norms: A person's ability to navigate or align with social and cultural norms around recovery. This could also include personal resilience and the ability to find meaning or purpose through their recovery process.
4. Community Capital
  - Neighborhood and environmental factors: Community capital refers to the social and material resources available in the broader community that can support recovery. This includes access to recovery-friendly communities, clean and safe living environments, employment opportunities, and the general support from the community for those in recovery.

Applying Recovery Capital to Treatment

- Assessment: Professionals might assess a person's recovery capital when planning treatment, identifying areas of strength (e.g., strong family support) and areas for growth (e.g., vocational rehab, job readiness or physical health).
- Interventions: Treatment plans might aim to enhance specific aspects of recovery capital. For instance, a person with limited social capital might be encouraged to attend support groups or family therapy, while someone lacking in human capital might benefit from educational programs or vocational training.

In sum, the recovery capital framework encourages a more comprehensive view of recovery that goes beyond just abstaining from substance use and looks at building a resilient, sustainable life that supports ongoing recovery.

Monitoring for Treatment Adherence

The clinician regularly assesses the patient's clinical status throughout treatment. The use of quantitative assessments also can be a valuable tool for monitoring SUD recovery by: providing a common language and clear indicators of progress or deterioration; promoting effective communication between the person with SUD and the clinicians involved in their care, regardless of their area of expertise or level of care; and identifying the need for specific interventions before a lapse or relapse occurs.

Prescription Drug Monitoring Programs

Prescription drug monitoring programs (PDMPs) in the United States are state-level databases that track prescriptions of controlled substances, and their role in the management of SUDs has become increasingly prominent with the rise of opioid use disorders. While the programs themselves may differ from state to state, in general they can serve a key role in clinical decision-making and prescribing. In the context of substance use treatment, PDMPs provide information about a person's past and current prescribed controlled substances, allow for collaboration with the person's other identified prescribers, and may identify concerning activity—for example, undisclosed benzodiazepine use while concurrently receiving buprenorphine treatment—that may not be detected in the snapshot of recent use that a urine drug test provides. Whether PDMP data is accessed as part of an initial intake assessment or a periodic check, a concerning finding is important to discuss with the person for clarification and to arrive at a mutually agreed treatment plan that takes this information into account.

Toxicology

Notwithstanding the abovementioned caveat that urine drug tests are only a detector of recent use, both baseline and unscheduled drug testing are a key component of monitoring treatment adherence in relapse prevention, alongside risk stratification, behavioral assessment, and the PDMPs described in the previous section [20]. Periodic random urine drug tests can test for opioids, though a provider interpreting the results should have an understanding of the test's cut-off thresholds (consider false negatives), each drug of interest and its possible metabolites. Urine testing is also useful for benzodiazepines, particularly for persons on chronic opioid therapy, given their high risk of adverse effects in combination. For alcohol use, a breathalyzer test is a common, affordable option, and urinary testing is also frequently used. Assaying alcohol metabolites EtG and EtS allows for an extended window of detection for recent alcohol use, up to about 4 days after complete elimination of alcohol from the body, depending on the person's use.

With all the above tests, it is important for the provider to keep in mind that drug tests provide information about recent use of drugs, but do not, in themselves, identify SUDs or physical dependence. An unexpected positive drug test result or, in some cases, an unexpected negative drug test result, necessitates careful evaluation and frank, nonjudgmental discussion with the individual. This can rule out false positives from a cross-reacting substance and foster open communication with the individual regarding adjustments to the treatment plan if needed. Similarly, communication and collaboration with the individual's other providers are important, particularly other prescribing providers. Talking with a person who has tested positive, rather than reflexively acting, can prevent inappropriate reactions to a positive test result and begin a collaborative effort to solve a problem.

Relapse

Early onset of SUDs can significantly disrupt the development of essential life skills and lead to chronic deficits in psychosocial functioning. Even individuals who achieve abstinence after prolonged use may struggle to develop effective coping mechanisms that allow them to lead fulfilling lives. These coping mechanisms are crucial for providing a buffer against relapse, especially after structural and functional changes have occurred in the brain.

Relapse is a gradual process closely linked to both intrapersonal and interpersonal factors. At each of the three stages of relapse, there are warning signs and strategies to prevent progression to the next stage. The primary goal of treatment is to prevent physical relapse.

Stages of Relapse

1. *Emotional Relapse*: During this stage, the individual has not started thinking about using substances and has not resumed use. However, the individual may be in denial or experiencing many negative emotions, which leads to strong cravings to use. Warning signs in this stage include negative emotions (anxiety, depression, anger, guilt, shame, embarrassment) and dysfunctional behaviors (isolation or social withdrawal, difficulties attending or engaging in therapy/support groups, poor self-care, refusal of others' support or efforts). It is important for the individual to identify specific triggers and avoid certain people, locations, situations, and emotions. This is a good time to learn coping/relaxation strategies, start positive lifestyle changes, and identify a reliable support network.
2. *Mental Relapse*: During this stage, there are conflicting desires between "wanting to use" and "not wanting to use." At this time, the individual's mind starts to rationalize any negative emotions from the previous stage that have not been resolved. Warning signs include increased cravings to use, romanticizing past use, minimizing consequences of use, reaching out to friends or acquaintances who are still using substances, lying behaviors, and planning to relapse. Consider reviewing the negative consequences that the individual has identified previously and encourage the individual to share his/her thoughts without feeling embarrassed.
3. *Physical Relapse*: During this stage, the individual actively returns to substance use or other dysfunctional behaviors. This stage can be further divided into a *lapse*, that is, an initial use that is a slip or setback in abstinence, versus a full *relapse*, signifying a complete return to previous maladaptive behavior patterns that re-perpetuate the substance use. During this stage, the role of the clinician is to encourage the individual to return to RP plans developed from early stages and practice exit strategies. It is important to reflect on sequences of events preceding physical relapse, as this can be an opportunity to identify issues to process and correct in therapy. It is possible for an individual who has had a brief lapse to return to recovery practices and abstinence with proper support [21].

The Cognitive-Behavioral Framework of Relapse

The CBT framework, which is discussed in a separate chapter, posits that maladaptive cognitive distortions or beliefs are formed from previous experiences, and in turn influence a person's thoughts, feelings, and behaviors in future experiences. In individuals with SUDs, these cognitive distortions end up reinforcing the substance use as the only "solution" to a situation, precluding any consideration of other

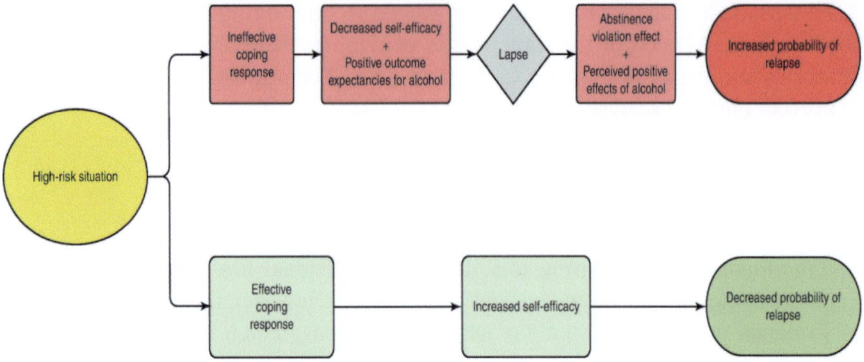

Fig. 6.3 Cognitive-behavioral model of relapse [22]

choices that could be made. Thus, when such an individual is faced with a trigger, the risk of developing cravings and returning to substance use is high. The cognitive-behavioral model of relapse was first conceptualized by G. Alan Marlatt and colleagues in 1985 and has remained one of the most influential models of relapse (Fig. 6.3). Marlatt's work was notable for first making the key distinction between lapse and relapse, as previous behavioral research had strictly defined a relapse as any return of the problem behavior, regardless of its duration or nature. Marlatt's original cognitive-behavioral model of relapse is shown in the figure below.

However, the interplay of the components of the model (including self-efficacy, expectations, and perceptions of the substance) and the intensity of the abstinence violation effect are affected by psychosocial context and are not necessarily sequential as depicted. This led Marlatt and Witkiewitz to propose a revised, more dynamic CBT model of relapse, which accounts for more static risk factors called distal risks such as family history, comorbid psychiatric conditions, and social support or lack thereof, alongside contextual cues and the proximal or immediate risks presented by the specific high-risk situation [22]. The revised model also serves to highlight more points of intervention for RP techniques, including identifying warning signs and high-risk situations, building a social network for recovery, challenging personal cognitive distortions, appropriate transitioning through levels of care, and developing strategies to improve treatment adherence. The top three precipitants of relapse, as identified in a study by Cummings, Gordon, and Marlatt, were negative emotional states, interpersonal conflict, and social pressure. RP is based on the biopsychosocial model of addiction. According to this model, addictive behaviors are conceptualized as acquired, overlearned habits with biological, psychological, and social determinants and consequences (Marlatt & Gordon, 1985). RP consists of a collection of strategies intended to strengthen self-control and self- awareness [23].

In recent years, the concept of "mindfulness"—which entails an active attentiveness to experiencing the present moment and accepting it as it is—is included in substance use treatment. Mindfulness-based relapse prevention, or MBRP, integrates mindfulness-based meditation practices into traditional psychotherapy for

RP. The goal of mindfulness-based meditation in this context includes meditation, self-care and compassion to help persons better tolerate psychological discomforts, such as those accompanying cravings or withdrawal symptoms, that might otherwise lead to a relapse [24].

Other additional interventions used in RP include medication for addiction treatment, contingency management (CM), social reinforcement, mutual help groups, network support, continuing care, recovery management check-ups, and technological innovations.

Conclusion

In this chapter, we have provided key definitions and approaches for relapse and recovery, but it is important to emphasize that these processes are multifaceted and individualized. We have identified the biopsychosocial factors that affect the risk of relapse as well as the trajectory of recovery and have described means of monitoring and measuring progress in SUD treatment. As our understanding of SUDs has expanded over time, more treatment modalities have become available in the realms of medical management, psychotherapeutic interventions, and interdisciplinary collaboration.

Chapter Review Questions

1. A 37-year-old transgender female patient you see in your outpatient practice who was smoking opioids (fentanyl) and methamphetamines (crystal) had been able to stop their use for 2 months while trying to return to work. For the past 3 weekends in a row prior to the holidays, the patient reports use of opioids and methamphetamines on Friday and Saturday. You sit down with your patient to discuss a recent relapse. You start by identifying both internal and external "triggers," which include?

   A. Feelings, thoughts, and emotions
   B. Ideals, psychologies, and therapies
   C. People, places, and things
   D. Coping strategies
   E. People, places, activities, feelings, thoughts, and emotions

   Correct Answer: E.

   Explanation: Triggers are internal and external cues that cause a person in recovery to crave drugs and eventually relapse. External triggers are people, places, activities, and objects that elicit thoughts or cravings associated with substance use. Individuals in recovery can stay away from the dangers of external triggers by developing action plans to avoid triggers that remind them of past drug use. Internal triggers are more challenging to manage than external triggers. They involve feelings, thoughts, and emotions formerly associated with substance abuse.

A. Feelings, thoughts and emotions are internal triggers.
B. Ideals, psychologies, and therapies are not triggers. Humanistic and existential approaches (including empathy, encouragement of affect, reflective listening, and acceptance of the individual's subjective experience) are useful in any type of brief therapy session, whether it involves psychodynamic, strategic, or cognitive-behavioral therapy. They help establish rapport and provide grounds for meaningful engagement with all aspects of the treatment process.
C. People, places and things are examples of external triggers.
D. Coping strategies provide a substitute or alternative that leads to healthier ways of dealing with triggers.

Reference: Daley DC, Marlatt GA. Overcoming your alcohol or drug problem: effective recovery strategies: therapist guide. 2nd ed. Oxford: Oxford University Press; 2006.

2. Which of the following best describes the concept of Recovery Capital?

A. The financial resources needed to undergo treatment
B. The network of people in one's life who can offer support
C. The combination of internal and external resources that help individuals in recovery
D. A program that provides medication-assisted treatment
E. Access to transportation and employment

Correct Answer: C.

Explanation: Recovery Capital refers to the combination of internal and external resources that individuals can draw upon to support their recovery journey. Internal resources include personal strengths, such as resilience, coping skills, and motivation, while external resources encompass social support networks, access to healthcare, stable housing, and community services. Together, these resources provide the foundation for an individual's recovery, helping them navigate challenges, maintain long-term sobriety, and improve their overall well-being.

A. The financial resources required for treatment are just one component of Recovery Capital (RC), specifically under Personal Capital. This category includes not only financial resources but also access to health care, well-being, and the basic material needs necessary for an individual to successfully undergo treatment.
B. The network of people in one's life who can offer support is an important component of Recovery Capital (RC), specifically under Social Capital. This category includes supportive relationships with family, friends, peers, and others who play a key role in fostering recovery and providing emotional, social, and practical support.
C. A program that provides medication-assisted treatment (MAT) would be considered a part of Recovery Capital under Physical Capital. This is because Physical Capital encompasses resources related to health, well-being, and basic material needs, which include access to medical treatments and interventions like MAT.

D. Access to transportation and employment are components of recovery capital that fall under the basic material needs portion of physical capital. Other key components are access to housing, food, and financial stability. Secure living conditions and financial resources are fundamental to sustaining recovery.

Reference: Best D, Hennessy EA. The science of recovery capital: where do we go from here? Addiction. 2022;117(4):1139–1145. https://doi.org/10.1111/add.15732. Epub 2021 Dec 1. PMID: 34729852; PMCID: PMC9209877

3. Luca (they/them) has been in recovery for six months after completing a medically supervised detox, attending a residential treatment program and starting IM naltrexone. While they have been abstinent from opioids and alcohol, they continue to struggle with managing stress and difficult emotions, which sometimes leads them to feel overwhelmed and anxious. Luca reports experiencing frequent feelings of frustration, anger, and sadness, especially when dealing with personal or professional challenges. They have a history of using opioids and alcohol to cope with these negative emotions but are now seeking healthier alternatives. Based on their current needs, which of the following groups would be most appropriate for referring Luca to?

A. Milieu group
B. Psychoeducational recovery group
C. Coping skills group
D. Counseling group
E. Specialized group

Correct Answer: C.

Explanation: Skill groups are aimed at helping people develop or improve their intrapersonal and interpersonal skills. For example, these groups teach problem-solving methods and stress management, cognitive, and relapse prevention strategies. Relapse prevention strategies help people identify and manage early signs of relapse (the relapse "process"), identify and manage high-risk factors, or learn steps to take to intervene in a lapse or relapse.

A. Milieu groups are offered in residential and hospital programs and usually involve a group meeting to start and/or end the day. A morning group may review the upcoming day's schedule, whereas an evening group may review the day's treatment and recovery activities and allow participants to reflect on their experiences that day.
B. Psychoeducational recovery groups provide information about specific topics related to addiction and recovery and help people begin to learn how to cope with the challenges of recovery. These groups use a combination of lectures, discussions, educational videos, behavioral rehearsals, and completion of written assignments such as a recovery workbook or personal journal.
C. Counseling groups (also called therapy groups, problem-solving groups, or process groups) are less structured and give the participants an opportunity to create their own agenda in terms of problems, conflicts, or struggles to

work on during group sessions. These groups focus more on gaining insight and raising self-awareness than on education or skill development.

D. Specialized groups may be based on developmental stage (adolescents, young adults, adults, older adults), gender, different clinical populations (pregnant women or women with small children addicted to opioids, or anyone involved in the criminal justice system), or groups addressing specific issues or populations (parenting issues, anger or mood management, or trauma).

Reference: Group therapies. In: Ries RK, editor. The ASAM principles of addiction medicine. 5th ed. Philadelphia: Wolters Kluwer Health; 2014. p. 847–8.

4. A primary care clinician referred her 31-year-old patient to you for addiction consultation. When you call the patient, she is already attending AA meetings and SUD/Relapse Prevention Group once a week and has found them useful. She is willing to stay sober. You start by identifying the stages of change. Which stage is this patient most likely in?

   A. Relapse
   B. Precontemplation
   C. Contemplation
   D. Preparation
   E. Action

   Correct Answer: E.

   Explanation: The action stage is the phase in the change process where an individual has made the decision to change their behavior and is actively taking steps toward achieving that change. This stage is marked by a commitment to action and the implementation of specific strategies to make and sustain the desired behavior change.

   A. Relapse is not the patient's stage of change. It is only after several relapses that the person discovers what recovery from an addiction means.
   B. Precontemplation is the stage where the person does not see their SUD as significant as compared to the benefits. Characteristics of this stage are a lack of interest in change and having no plan or intention to change. We might describe this person as unaware.
   C. Contemplation stage refers to a phase in the change process where an individual is aware of a problem and is considering the possibility of making a change but has not yet committed to acting. This stage is characterized by ambivalence—meaning the person feels conflicted or uncertain about whether to change. They may see both the benefits and the drawbacks of changing and may struggle with the decision.
   D. Preparation is a stage where the person accepts responsibility for changing her or his behavior. She evaluates and selects techniques for behavioral change. Characteristics of this stage include developing a plan to make the needed changes, building confidence and commitment to change, and having the intention to change within a period. We might describe this person as willing to change and anticipating the benefits of change.

Reference: Miller WR, Rollnick S. Motivational interviewing: helping people change. 3rd ed. New York: Guilford Press; 2013.

5. A 47-year-old man decided to taper off his buprenorphine treatment a year ago after 13 years of full abstinence. The patient was actively involved in your clinic where he was attending CBT/SUD groups weekly in addition to following up monthly with you. After 12 months, the patient came back to you describing an intense desire to use opioids after he started working in a bar and ran into a "source" he knew from the past. The patient then noticed along with his intense desire to use opioids, a more subtle desire to run into the person again so that he could ask him where he could get a "hit of fentanyl." How do you define what this person is experiencing?

   A. Withdrawal
   B. Urge
   C. Triggers
   D. Drug craving
   E. Conditioned positive reinforcement

   Correct Answer: D.

   Explanation: Drug cravings are a longing for or desire to use a substance, varying in intensity from mild to very strong. Cravings can be a desire for the euphoric effects of the substance, or a means to avoid or escape unpleasant emotions or physical symptoms such as those associated with withdrawal.

   A. Withdrawal: A group of symptoms of variable clustering and degree of severity that occur on cessation or reduction of use of a psychoactive substance that has been taken repeatedly, usually for a prolonged period and/or in high doses. The syndrome may be accompanied by signs of physiological disturbance. A withdrawal syndrome is one of the indicators of a dependence syndrome. It is also the defining characteristic of the narrower psycho-pharmacological meaning of dependence.
   B. Urge: An urge is an intention to use a substance once the individual is experiencing cravings. There can be a strong craving with very little intention to use, or the intention to use can be quite high, making the individual more vulnerable to relapse unless the person then utilizes active coping strategies to manage these cravings and urges.
   C. Triggers: Triggers are external or internal events that instigate thoughts or emotions related to the substance use process. Triggers often induce cravings. The goal of identifying the trigger is to learn management of external factors (people, places, events, experiences, or objects) or internal (feelings or thoughts).
   D. Conditioned positive reinforcement: This involves the addition of a reinforcing stimulus following a behavior that makes it more likely that the behavior will occur again in the future. When a favorable outcome, event, or reward occurs after an action, that particular response or behavior will be strengthened.

Reference: Koob GF, Moal ML. Neurobiology of addiction. London: Elsevier AP; 2011.

6. A 33-year-old woman in recovery attended a party for the first time after completing 8 months of sobriety. She had struggled with alcohol use for several years and, prior to beginning Cognitive Behavioral Therapy (CBT), had attempted to quit drinking multiple times but relapsed each time. In the past, she reported in these situations feeling overwhelmed by cravings and doubted her ability to stay sober, often thinking, *"I can't handle this without drinking. I'll never be able to quit for good."* Through CBT, she learned to recognize this type of thinking, known as self-doubt. When a person at the party offered her an alcoholic beverage, she reframed her thoughts, replacing the negative self-talk with: *"I've handled stress before without drinking. I have the skills to cope, even if it feels tough right now."* She then politely responded to the person, saying, "I have a medical condition, and I cannot drink. Could you please offer me a non-alcoholic beverage instead?" Afterward, she chose a soda for herself and joined her supportive friends. According to the original Cognitive-Behavioral Model of Relapse, which of the following factors helped her decrease the chance of relapse?

   A. Ineffective coping response and positive outcome expectancy
   B. Abstinence violation effect and high-risk situation
   C. Cognitive restructuring, application of coping skills, assertive communication, seeking support from sober friends, avoiding triggers and high-risk situations
   D. Lack of motivation and poor emotional regulation
   E. Peer pressure and self-doubt

   Correct Answer: C.

   Explanation: The original CBT model of relapse begins with the individual presented with a high-risk situation (B), defined as a situation in which the individual's attempt to refrain from substance use is challenged. The individual may then respond with either an ineffective coping response (A) or an effective coping response. An individual who utilizes an ineffective coping response will tend to cave to temptation or pressure, possibly carried along by their positive outcome expectancies (A) of the initial effects of using the substance. This leads to the initial use, or lapse. The lapse can be followed by the abstinence violation effect (B), in which the individual experiences guilt and demotivation, focusing excessively on blaming themselves for their failure, to the detriment of their previous commitment to sobriety ("why even bother anymore, when I've already messed up"). She used to have poor coping skills to manage peer pressure and self-doubt. (E) The end result of all these steps is an overall increased likelihood of relapse. The only response that does not follow this is (C) Cognitive restructuring (reframing negative self-talk to a more positive and empowering thought); Application of coping skills (using new skills to manage stress and cravings); Assertive communication (setting boundaries and requesting non-alcoholic beverages); Seeking support from sober friends (engaging with supportive people in her network) and Avoiding triggers and high-risk situations (actively choosing non-alcoholic options and distancing herself from temptation). The successful maintenance of abstinence reinforces the individual's confidence that they will succeed again in similar situations, and their risk of relapse is lowered. In turn they increase their ability to remain sober.

Reference: Witkiewitz K, Marlatt GA. Relapse prevention for alcohol and drug problems: that was Zen, this is Tao. Am Psychol. 2004;59(4):224–35.

7. Karol is a 29-year-old woman who has been sober for two months after a long struggle with alcohol use. Throughout her recovery, she has attended therapy and group support meetings. While she is proud of her sobriety, Karol reports experiencing occasional urges to drink, especially when she feels stressed or anxious. She describes these moments: "I felt tightness in my chest, and my heart was racing. I felt overwhelmed and unsure of how to calm down." These urges typically arise in high-pressure situations, such as work deadlines or family gatherings, and are accompanied by thoughts like, "I can't handle this stress without drinking," or "I'll never be able to enjoy social events without alcohol." Karol also struggles with staying present in the moment, often getting caught up in past regrets or future worries, which only increases her anxiety. In therapy, Karol and her counselor have been working on understanding and integrating her thoughts, emotions, and bodily sensations in the present moment. What are the main components of this therapeutic approach, and what is it called?

   A. Affirmation/Core Beliefs: Motivational Interviewing
   B. Problem Solving/CBT
   C. Mindfulness Meditation, Cognitive restructuring, Awareness of Thought Patterns and Relapse Prevention/ MBCT
   D. Safety/Seeking Safety
   E. Cognitive restructuring/CPT

   Correct Answer: C.

   Explanation: Mindfulness-Based Cognitive Therapy (MBCT) is an integrative therapeutic approach that combines elements of Cognitive Behavioral Therapy (CBT) and Mindfulness Meditation. Originally developed to prevent relapse in depression, MBCT has since been adapted to address SUDs. The therapy emphasizes focusing attention on the present moment—whether that be on the breath, physical sensations, or emotions—without judgment. This practice helps individuals become more aware of their thoughts, feelings, and physical reactions, enabling them to respond thoughtfully rather than react impulsively. MBCT includes several key components: Cognitive Restructuring: This involves identifying automatic negative thoughts (ANTs) and cognitive distortions that contribute to emotional distress or maladaptive behavior. Awareness of Thought Patterns: Individuals become more aware of ruminative thought patterns, such as self-criticism, catastrophizing, or all-or-nothing thinking, which can trigger distress, cravings, and relapse and Relapse Prevention: MBCT teaches individuals how to respond to cravings, negative emotions, or stress in mindful, nonjudgmental ways to prevent relapse.

Other therapeutic approaches that complement or are used alongside MBCT in treating SUDs include the other ones mentioned: Motivational Interviewing (MI) (A); Cognitive Behavioral Therapy (CBT) (B); Seeking Safety (D): A trauma-informed therapy that integrates treatment for co-occurring disorders, particularly trauma and substance use and Cognitive Processing Therapy (CPT) (E): A trauma-focused therapy designed to help individuals process and cope with traumatic experiences.

Reference: Kabat-Zinn, J., & Hanh, T. N. (2009). Mindfulness-Based Cognitive Therapy: A New Approach to Relapse Prevention. Guilford Press.

References

1. Center for Substance Abuse Treatment. Chapter 2: How stimulants affect. In: Treatment for stimulant use disorder. Treatment improvement protocols (TIP) series no. 33. Rockville: Substance Abuse and Mental Health Services Administration; 2001. p. 13–33.
2. Daley DC, Marlatt GA. Overcoming your alcohol or drug problem: effective recovery strategies: Therapist guide. 2nd ed. Oxford: Oxford University Press; 2006. p. 181–93.
3. Dutra L, Stathopoulou G, Basden SL, Leyro TM, Powers MB, Otto MW. A meta-analytic review of psychosocial interventions for substance use disorders. Am J Psychiatry. 2008;165(2):179–87.
4. Deak JD, Johnson EC. Genetics of substance use disorders: a review. Psychol Med. 2021;51(13):2189–2200. https://doi.org/10.1017/S0033291721000969. Epub 2021 Apr 21. Erratum in: Psychol Med. 2022 Mar;52(4):800. doi:10.1017/S0033291722000629. PMID: 33879270; PMCID: PMC8477224.
5. Stone AL, Becker LG, Huber AM, Catalano RF. Review of risk and protective factors of substance use and problem use in emerging adulthood. Addict Behav. 2012;37(7):747–75.
6. Drake RE, O'Neal EL, Wallach MA. A systematic review of psychosocial research on psychosocial interventions for people with co-occurring severe mental and substance use disorders. J Subst Abus Treat. 2008;34(1):123–38.
7. Prochaska JO, Velicer WF. The transtheoretical model of health behavior change. Am J Health Promot. 1997;12(1):38–48. https://doi.org/10.4278/0890-1171-12.1.38. PMID: 10170434
8. Betty Ford Institute Consensus Panel. What is recovery? A working definition from the Betty Ford Institute. J Subst Abus Treat. 2007;33(3):221–8.
9. Substance Abuse and Mental Health Services Administration: Recovery from Substance Use and Mental Health Problems Among Adults in the United States. Publication No. PEP23-10-00-001. Rockville: Office of Recovery, Substance Abuse and Mental Health Services Administration, 2023.
10. White WL. Addiction recovery: Its definition and conceptual boundaries. J Subst Abus Treat. 2007;33(3):229–41.
11. Substance Abuse and Mental Health Services Administration. 2023 National Survey on Drug Use and Health (NSDUH). 2023. U.S. Department of Health and Human Services. https://www.samhsa.gov/data/
12. SAMHSA. Key substance use and mental health indicators in the United States: Results from the 2017 National Survey on Drug Use and Health (NSDUH Series H-53, HHS Publication No. SMA, Issue 18–5068) Center for Behavioral Health Statistics and Quality – Substance Abuse and Mental Health Services Administration. 2018. https://www.samhsa.gov/data/
13. SAMHSA. Key substance use and mental health indicators in the United States: Results from the 2018 National Survey on Drug Use and Health (NSDUH Series H-54, HHS Publication

No., Issue PEP19–5068) Center for Behavioral Health Statistics and Quality – Substance Abuse and Mental Health Services Administration. 2019. https://www.samhsa.gov/data/

14. Paquette CE, Daughters SB, Witkiewitz K. Expanding the continuum of substance use disorder treatment: Nonabstinence approaches. Clin Psychol Rev. 2022;91:102110. https://doi.org/10.1016/j.cpr.2021.102110. Epub 2021 Nov 26. PMID: 34864497; PMCID: PMC8815796.
15. Miller WR. Motivational factors in addictive behaviors. In Rethinking substance abuse: What the science shows, and what we should do about it. The Guilford Press; 2006. p. 134–50.
16. Gumbley SJ. Recovery in the 21st century: from shame to strength. J Addict Nurs. 2016;27:143–7. https://doi.org/10.1097/JAN.0000000000000125.
17. White W, Cloud W. Recovery capital: a primer for addictions professionals. Counselor. 2008;9(5):22–7.
18. Best D, Hennessy EA. The science of recovery capital: Where do we go from here? Addiction. 2022;117(4):1139-1145. https://doi.org/10.1111/add.15732. Epub 2021 Dec 1. PMID: 34729852; PMCID: PMC9209877.
19. Hennessy EA. Recovery capital: a systematic review of the literature. Addict Res Theory. 2017;25(5):349–60.
20. Gudin JA, Mogali S, Jones JD, Comer SD. Risks, management, and monitoring of combination opioid, benzodiazepines, and/or alcohol use. Postgrad Med. 2013;125(4):115–30. [PMC free article] [PubMed]
21. Melemis SM. Relapse prevent and the five rules of recovery. Yale J Biol Med. 2015;88(3):325–32.
22. Witkiewitz K, Marlatt GA. Relapse prevention for alcohol and drug problems: That was Zen, this is Tao. Am Psychol. 2004;59(4):224–35.
23. Cummings C, Gordon JR, Marlatt GA. The addictive behaviors: Treatment of alcoholism, drug abuse, smoking, and obesity. Oxford: Pergamon; 1980. Relapse: Strategies of prevention and prediction; pp. 291–321
24. Grant S, Colaiaco B, Motala A, Shanman R, Booth M, Sorbero M, et al. Mindfulness-based relapse prevention for substance use disorders: a systematic review and meta-analysis. J Addict Med. 2017;11(5):386–96.

Part II

Addictions and Their Treatments

Nicotine

7

Stephanie L. Hsia and Javad J. Fatollahi

High-Yield Review Points

- Tobacco use continues to be the leading preventable cause of morbidity and mortality in the United States.
- Nicotine is a nicotinic receptor agonist that produces stimulant effects, reduces anxiety, and stimulates the dopamine reward pathway through the release of several neurotransmitters.
- The combination of behavioral and pharmacological treatment for tobacco use disorder is more effective than either intervention alone.
- Cognitive behavioral therapy in individual and group settings is a first-line behavioral treatment for tobacco use disorder.
- Combination nicotine replacement therapy, bupropion SR, and varenicline are first-line pharmacotherapies for tobacco use disorder.
- Electronic Nicotine Delivery Systems (ENDS) deliver nicotine in concentrations comparable to conventional cigarettes, making them a potential tool for smoking cessation, but they also pose significant risks due to increased nicotine dependence and dual use with traditional cigarettes.

S. L. Hsia (✉)
Department of Clinical Pharmacy, University of Southern California Alfred E. Mann School of Pharmacy and Pharmaceutical Sciences, Los Angeles, CA, USA
e-mail: shsia@usc.edu

J. J. Fatollahi
Department of Psychiatry, University of California San Diego, La Jolla, CA, USA
e-mail: jfatollahi@ucsd.edu

C. Marienfeld, M. Soltani (eds.), *AAAP Review of Addiction Psychiatry*,
https://doi.org/10.1007/978-3-032-24174-0_7

Introduction

Epidemiology

The prevalence of tobacco dependence has been steadily declining since the Surgeon General's report in 1964 that linked smoking with lung cancer. The rate of smoking in the United States has dropped from 42% in 1964 to 14% in 2017 and 11.5% in 2021. Certain subpopulations are at a higher risk of smoking than others. In 2021, the prevalence of cigarette smoking was greater in individuals who were male, aged 5–64, non-Hispanic White, non-Hispanic Black, or other non-Hispanic, uninsured or insured by Medicaid, had no diploma or a General Education Development (GED) Certificate, identified as lesbian, gay, or bisexual, low income, lived in the Midwest or South, or had a disability [1]. Additionally, individuals who reported regularly having feelings of severe psychological distress, were ever told by a healthcare provider that they had depression, and those with other mental illnesses (e.g., schizophrenia, mood and anxiety disorders, and substance use disorders) have elevated rates of smoking compared to the general population. In fact, people with mental illness and/or substance use disorder consume 40% of cigarettes sold in the United States [2].

While the prevalence of tobacco use has declined, the prevalence of nicotine vaping has been increasing. The rate of past-month nicotine vaping in the United States in people aged 12 or older increased from 8.3% in 2022 to 9.4% in 2023. In 2023, the percentage of people who vaped was greater in individuals who were aged 18 to 25, American Indian or Alaska Native, Multiracial, or White. [46, 47] The use of ENDS among youth in the United States has also been an area of concern. From 2011 to 2018, the past 30-day use of ENDS by high school students exponentially increased from 1.5% in 2011 to 20.8% in 2018.[48] This has since decreased to 7.8% in 2024. [49]

Consequences of Use

According to the Surgeon General Report, smoking is the leading preventable cause of morbidity and mortality in the United States, resulting in 490,000 deaths annually [3]. Smoking damages nearly every organ in the body, with the most common severe medical complications being cancer, respiratory diseases, cardiovascular disease, diabetes, immune and autoimmune disorders, eye disease, and reproductive and developmental effects [3]. On average, cigarette smokers die 10 years earlier than people who have never smoked [4]. In addition, primary and second-hand smoke expose people to more than 7000 chemicals, some of which are carcinogenic. Smoking costs the United States more than $600 billion per year, with more than $240 billion for medical care and another $180 billion lost in productivity due to premature death [5]. The long-term health effects of the use of ENDS are not yet known, given that they have only been widely used in the past decade. Based on physiological mechanisms that are understood about ENDS components (such as nicotine and solvents such as propylene glycol) and limited studies, there may potentially be increased cardiovascular and pulmonary risk with chronic ENDS use; however, more research and long-term data is needed to better understand these potential risks [48]. Studies have demonstrated that the decrease in smoking prevalence over the past 50 years has led to the avoidance of almost 4 million deaths from lung cancer [53]. Given the detrimental effects of cigarettes on both individual health and society, the increasing use of ENDS, and the population health benefits of reducing smoking, it is vital to better understand tobacco, tobacco-related products, and tobacco use disorder, nicotine-containing products, and nicotine use disorder in greater detail.

Pharmacology

Pharmacokinetics

Nicotine is a weak base ($pK_a = 8.0$), which requires a slightly alkaline pH to absorb across physiological membranes and into circulation. The two primary routes of delivery of nicotine are inhalation and buccal. In cigarettes, pipes, and cigars, tar droplets produced from the burning of tobacco deliver nicotine directly to the lungs. In ENDS, a liquid solution containing nicotine is heated or atomized to generate a nicotine aerosol for inhalation. Since inhalation bypasses first-pass metabolism, smoked or inhaled nicotine is rapidly absorbed into the circulation and reaches high concentrations in the brain within 10–20 seconds. On average, smoking 1 cigarette delivers approximately 1 mg of nicotine. In chewing tobacco, snuff, and nicotine gum/lozenges, nicotine is buffered in a slightly alkaline pH, which facilitates absorption through buccal membranes. Compared to inhalation, buccal absorption is slower, and nicotine concentrations in the brain increase more gradually, reaching peak concentrations in 30 min. This slower absorption is less reinforcing for the dopamine reward pathways. Nicotine is also readily absorbed through the skin, though at a slower rate than buccal and inhaled administration. After absorption, nicotine readily distributes through bodily tissues and is metabolized by CYP2A6 in the liver to its primary metabolite, cotinine. Cotinine is partially excreted unchanged by the kidney and metabolized to further metabolites, which are then eliminated.

The polycyclic aromatic hydrocarbons present in cigarette *smoke* are strong inducers of CYP1A2 and, therefore, may increase metabolism and lead to *lower* plasma levels of drugs that are metabolized through this enzyme [6, 50]. Two examples of medications that are metabolized by CYP1A2 are the atypical antipsychotics of clozapine and olanzapine. Especially since tobacco use is a prevalent comorbidity in individuals with mental illness, this can be a clinically significant interaction. Studies have suggested that clozapine plasma levels could decrease by up to 30% in a patient who begins to smoke [51]. Conversely, when a patient stops smoking, their drug plasma levels can increase, and the dose may need to be decreased. Other medications that may be affected by smoking are caffeine, fluvoxamine, tacrine, and theophylline [50]. Healthcare professionals should consider smoking status when prescribing these medications, being sure to monitor for changes in efficacy or side effects and potentially empirically adjusting the dose when patients report changes in smoking.

Pharmacodynamics

Nicotine is a nicotinic acetylcholinergic receptor (nAChR) agonist. When nicotine activates the nAChR, it facilitates the release of several neurotransmitters, including dopamine, norepinephrine, acetylcholine, serotonin, glutamate, γ-aminobutyric acid (GABA), and endorphins. These neurotransmitters are responsible for the physiological and addictive effects of nicotine. The release of norepinephrine and acetylcholine leads to its stimulant effects, namely, increases in heart rate and blood pressure and appetite suppression. The release of GABA and endorphins leads to reduction of anxiety and tension. Chronic administration of nicotine causes the release of dopamine in the mesolimbic area, corpus striatum, and prefrontal cortex, and neuroadaptive changes occur, which form the pharmacological basis of nicotine addiction. With chronic administration, the number of nACHRs in the brain increases and nACHRs are desensitized, leading to tolerance and withdrawal symptoms [7].

Pathogenesis

Intoxication

As the doses of nicotine found in most commercially available products are quite low, nicotine intoxication is rarely seen. However, nicotine toxicity has been reported with oral ingestion of liquid nicotine that is used for electronic cigarettes as these liquids can contain lethal doses of nicotine if ingested inappropriately [8, 9]. At commercially available doses, nicotine administration produces stimulant effects, such as increased heart rate and blood pressure, arousal, and reduction of anxiety. At high doses, nicotine can produce bradycardia, hypotension, and depressed mental status due to ganglionic blockade [7]. Symptoms of nicotine overdose can develop within 15–90 min of exposure and include gastrointestinal upset, nausea, vomiting, respiratory depression, and seizures. Treatment of nicotine intoxication occurs primarily in cases of poisoning or overdose. Primary treatment consists of activated charcoal to remove nicotine from the gastrointestinal tract and supportive treatments and care (e.g., benzodiazepines for seizures, fluids/vasopressors for hypotension) [10].

Withdrawal

Nicotine withdrawal symptoms can occur as early as 30–40 min after smoking a cigarette. The rapid onset of withdrawal symptoms and desire to alleviate them is one of the primary reasons people use tobacco and why nicotine has such addictive potential [7]. Common symptoms of nicotine withdrawal are irritability, restlessness, anxiety, difficulty concentrating, increased appetite, insomnia, and depressed mood [11]. Withdrawal symptoms typically peak within 2–3 days after quitting, and last 2–4 weeks, but may persist for months in some individuals. Effective treatments for nicotine withdrawal include first-line therapies for tobacco use disorder: nicotine replacement therapy, bupropion, and varenicline [12]. These pharmacological options are discussed further below.

Tobacco Use Disorder

For the purposes of this chapter, we will focus on the treatment of Tobacco Use Disorder (TUD) since most studies are addressing this, though we will provide some information on treatment for Nicotine Use Disorder (NUD) as available.

Diagnosis

Diagnostic criteria for Tobacco Use Disorder (TUD), as defined in the *Diagnostic and Statistical Manual for Mental Disorders, fifth edition* (DSM-5), are similar to those of other substance use disorders (i.e., tolerance, withdrawal, and criteria about problems resulting from use) [11]. A diagnosis of TUD is common among individuals who use tobacco daily, but uncommon among those who do not use tobacco daily or who solely use nicotine-containing products. Tolerance to tobacco is often indicated by the absence of dizziness and/or nausea after tobacco intake. Substance use diagnostic criteria that are uncommon in TUD include spending excessive time obtaining tobacco (as it is readily and legally available), spending time recovering from tobacco (since intoxication is rare), and recurrent tobacco use resulting in failure to fulfill major role obligations. The presence of these criteria may indicate more severe TUD [11].

Assessment

The first step in treating TUD is to screen for and assess an individual's tobacco use. The 5 As, Ask, Advise, Refer (AAR), and Ask-Advise-Connect (AAC) are three useful frameworks for brief smoking cessation interventions. The 5As is the gold standard method for brief intervention and consists of five steps: (1) Ask every patient about their smoking status; (2) Advise the patient to quit; (3) Assess the patient's readiness to quit; (4) Assist the patient with their quit attempt if they are ready; and (5) Arrange for follow-up. "Ask, Advise, Refer" is a briefer intervention and consists of three steps: (1) Ask the patient about their smoking status; (2) Advise the patient to quit; and (3) Refer the patient to evidence-based smoking cessation strategies. AAC is like AAR, but instead of referring the patient, the provider directly connects the individual to a resource such as a tobacco cessation program or quit line. Some students have suggested that AAC may be more effective than AAR in reaching and engaging people who smoke [3, 12, 13].

Table 7.1 Heaviness of smoking index for nicotine dependence [14]

	Response	Point value
Items		
How soon after waking do you smoke your first cigarette?	<5 min	3 points
	5–30 min	2 points
	31–60 min	1 point
	>60 min	0 points
How many cigarettes do you smoke each day?	>30 cigarettes	3 points
	21–30 cigarettes	2 points
	11–20 cigarettes	1 point
	≤10 cigarettes	0 points
Scoring		
Nicotine dependence score	0 points	No dependence
	1–2 points	Low dependence
	3–4 points	Moderate dependence
	5–6 points	High dependence

Appropriate assessment of a patient's nicotine and tobacco use is an integral component of treating TUD. To help guide treatment, the patient's level of nicotine dependence should be determined. One brief and validated scale which may be used to assess a patient's nicotine dependence is the Heaviness of Smoking Index (HSI), an abbreviated version of the Fagerström Test for Nicotine Dependence [14]. The HSI (Table 7.1) assesses a patient's dependence based on their time to first cigarette and total daily cigarette intake. Of note, one pack contains 20 cigarettes.

Treatment of Tobacco Use Disorder

Overview of Treatment

Once an individual's level of nicotine dependence has been assessed, treatment should be initiated based on the person's level of motivation. If the individual is ready and willing to attempt to quit, the provider should work with him/her to plan for and set a quit date—the day the individual stops all tobacco. Since nicotine addiction includes behavioral and physiological dependence, treatment of TUD should involve behavioral as well as pharmacological interventions. The combination of medication and counseling has been shown to be more effective in helping patients remain tobacco-free compared to either intervention alone [12]. Though cigarette smoking is the most common form of tobacco use, it is also important to ask and assist individuals who use non-cigarette tobacco products [15]. Electronic cigarettes have become more frequently used and are discussed in more detail below. Behavioral interventions should be recommended for all tobacco users; however, evidence-based recommendations for pharmacological treatment of non-cigarette tobacco users are limited [16].

Nonpharmacological Treatment

Psychotherapy is a commonly used first-line treatment for TUD. Both individual and group therapy are effective for treating TUD and are associated with abstinence rates of about 20–25% [12, 17, 18]. Among the many psychotherapies that are used to treat TUD, cognitive-behavioral therapy (CBT) adapted for smoking cessation is the most widely studied and used modality [12]. CBT typically includes (1) education about nicotine dependence, withdrawal, and relapse; (2) recognizing danger situations (triggers) that could lead to relapse; (3) developing coping skills, such as avoiding temptation, coping with negative affective states, reducing overall stress, and distracting attention from smoking urges with other activities (i.e., relapse prevention techniques); (4) social support (both within and outside of treatment); and (5) encouragement to taper off all tobacco products. At each session, CBT and other psychotherapies usually include questioning about recent cigarette usage and monitoring of exhaled carbon monoxide (CO) levels, with levels of ≤4 parts per million (ppm) being consistent with no cigarette usage within the past 24 h [19]. CBT (and other psychotherapies) can be done in a group or individual format.

During psychotherapy for smoking cessation, and in other settings with tobacco users who are not yet ready to quit, motivational interviewing (MI) techniques are often used. These techniques are designed to encourage patient engagement in active behavior change and include exploring self-ratings of the importance of quitting and confidence in quitting using open-ended questions and reflection. MI can include the "5 R's," which consist of determining the "Relevance" of quitting to the tobacco user, discussing "Risks" of continued tobacco use, exploring "Rewards" of quitting, examining "Roadblocks" to quitting, and "Repetition" of the tobacco cessation discussion [20]. MI has consistently been found to increase the number of quit attempts and to be effective for engaging smokers with mental illness.

In addition to in-person therapies, Internet-based, mobile phone text message-based, printed self-help, and telephone-based interventions have been shown to be more effective than non-active control conditions in helping smokers achieve abstinence. Ongoing research is focused on improving the delivery of these treatments and tailoring treatments to specific subgroups of smokers (e.g., smokers with mental illness) [21].

Pharmacological Treatment

FDA-approved treatments for TUD are nicotine replacement therapy (NRT), bupropion, and varenicline. All three treatments are recommended by the guidelines as first-line pharmacological options for TUD. Meta-analysis has suggested that both combination NRT and varenicline may be more effective than bupropion or NRT monotherapy [22]. Selection of an agent should be based on patient-specific characteristics [12, 13].

Nicotine Replacement Therapy

Nicotine replacement therapy (NRT) is a first-line recommended treatment for TUD. NRT's primary mechanism of action is as a nicotinic agonist at nAChR [7]. Since the absorption of nicotine from NRTs is much slower than that of cigarettes, NRTs carry a minimal risk of dependence/addiction while still achieving sufficient concentrations to relieve withdrawal symptoms. NRTs do not produce the peak in concentration and subsequent "rush" that smokers get from rapid absorption of nicotine through cigarettes, thereby reducing positive reinforcement from nicotine [7]. NRT can be categorized into two groups: long-acting and short-acting. The only currently FDA-approved long-acting form of NRT is the transdermal nicotine patch. The nicotine patch provides a steady amount of nicotine throughout the day and reduces nicotine dependence by relieving background cravings and reducing withdrawal [23]. The nicotine patch is typically administered once daily (approximately every 24 h), though some remove the patch at bedtime to prevent side effects such as intense dreams. There are several forms of short-acting NRT: nicotine gum, lozenge, nasal spray, and oral inhaler. While the nicotine patch relieves background cravings, short-acting NRT relieves breakthrough cravings and provides sensory stimulation (e.g., hand-to-mouth motion) [23]. The different formulations of short-acting NRT primarily differ in their method of use and pharmacokinetics. Of the four forms, the nicotine nasal spray has the fastest absorption and, therefore, has the highest risk of perpetuating physiological dependence. Similarly, the nicotine inhaler most closely resembles a cigarette in terms of appearance and use and may perpetuate behavioral smoking habits. Therefore, the nasal spray and inhaler are not typically used as first-line options but may be preferred in certain patients who are unable to use oral NRT [23].

Combination NRT

Studies have shown that combination NRT (use of a long-acting with a short-acting formulation) is more effective than monotherapy NRT. The use of long- and short-acting formulations together provides relief of both background and breakthrough cravings without increasing incidence of adverse effects [12, 20]. Though combination NRT is recommended as first-line therapy, there is no official dosing recommendation, and the dosing used in studies has varied [23]. The initial nicotine patch dose should be based on the patient's nicotine dependence (Table 7.2). Most patients can initially start on the 2 mg dose of short-acting NRT (e.g., gum or lozenge), though patients who are highly dependent or who smoke less than 30 min after waking may start on the 4 mg dose (Table 7.2). As general guidance for tapering, patients may remain on their initial dose of the nicotine patch for 6 weeks and then step down to the next patch for 2 weeks [24]. It is important to realize that package insert tapering recommendations should only serve as general guidance and that tapering of NRT should be individualized and based on the patient's progress (e.g., a patient should not step down to the next patch strength if s/he is still experiencing significant cravings or has had a recent slip). NRT has been studied in extended treatment

Table 7.2 Package insert and guideline dosing recommendations for combination NRT[a]

	Nicotine patch strength	Nicotine gum/lozenge strength
High dependence	21 mg/day × 6 weeks 14 mg/day × 2 weeks 7 mg/day × 2 weeks	Smokes < 30 min after waking: 4 mg Smokes ≥ 30 min after waking: 2 mg 1 piece q1–2 h prn cravings × 6 weeks 1 piece q2–4 h prn cravings × 2 weeks 1 piece q4–8 h prn cravings × 2 weeks
Moderate dependence	21 mg/day × 6 weeks 14 mg/day × 2 weeks 7 mg/day × 2 weeks	2 mg strength 1 piece q1–2 h prn cravings × 6 weeks 1 piece q2–4 h prn cravings × 2 weeks 1 piece q4–8 h prn cravings × 2 weeks
Low dependence	14 mg/day × 6 weeks 7 mg/day × 2 weeks	2 mg strength 1 piece q1–2 h prn cravings × 6 weeks 1 piece q2–4 h prn cravings × 2 weeks 1 piece q4–8 h prn cravings × 2 weeks

[a]Dosing from package insert recommendations, tapering schedule should still be individualized to each patient and extended if clinically indicated

for up to 6 months; therefore, extending NRT treatment past the recommended 10 weeks is safe [12]. The recommended maximum daily dosages of the gum and lozenge are 24 pieces and 20 pieces, respectively [25]. Initially, it may be beneficial for patients to use at least 6 pieces of short-acting NRT daily as cravings are typically strongest within the first few weeks after quitting [23].

Common adverse effects with NRT are similar to those of nicotine and include increased heart rate, blood pressure, headache, stomach upset (if incorrectly swallowed), insomnia, and nervousness. For the nicotine patch, patients may experience irritation or redness at the application site, or, uncommonly, allergic reactions. If a patient has any signs of an allergic reaction (edema, hives, shortness of breath), s/he should discontinue use immediately [24, 25]. NRT has been shown to be safe to use in patients with cardiovascular disease. Caution should be exercised when using NRT in patients with a recent (<2 weeks) myocardial infarction, serious arrhythmias, or serious angina. However, it is also important to note that NRT is, in general, still safer than cigarette smoking in these at-risk patients [12].

Counseling on how to properly use NRT is crucial to its efficacy. For the nicotine patch, patients should be instructed to apply the patch to a clean, dry patch of skin on the chest, back, stomach, or upper arm. They should wash their hands after application and rotate application sites daily to minimize skin irritation. Patches should only be worn for a maximum of 24 h, though if the patient experiences abnormal dreams or has difficulty sleeping, s/he may remove the patch before bedtime. Patches should be properly disposed of out of reach of children or animals [24].

For the nicotine gum, patients should be instructed on the "chew and park" method. Patients should be instructed to chew the gum until they experience a tingling sensation or peppery taste in their mouth. Once they do, they should "park" the piece of gum between their gum and cheek (as this is where the nicotine absorbs). After the tingling/taste stops, they should repeat, but "park" the piece in a different area between their gum and cheek. They should repeat this process until the tingle/taste no longer occurs (approximately 30 min per piece of gum) [25].

For the nicotine lozenge, patients should be instructed to suck on the lozenge and let it dissolve in their mouth gradually over 30 min. They should move the lozenge to different sides and areas of their mouth to minimize skin irritation. They should not chew the lozenge as this may affect nicotine release and cause irritation. For both the gum and lozenge, patients should also be instructed to avoid swallowing the nicotine and eating, or drinking at least 15 min before or after or during use of the gum since it requires physiological pH to absorb. Patients should also be instructed not to swallow the nicotine gum or lozenge as doing so may cause significant stomach upset.

Bupropion (Zyban®)

Bupropion SR (Zyban®) is an antidepressant that is FDA-approved for the treatment of TUD. Its proposed mechanisms of action are the inhibition of dopamine and norepinephrine reuptake and antagonism of nAChR [12]. Bupropion should be initiated 1–2 weeks before the target quit date. The dosing for TUD is 150 mg daily for 3 days and then increase to 150 mg twice daily for 7–12 weeks [12]. Bupropion is contraindicated in patients at risk for seizure (i.e., with a history of seizure or eating disorders) and in patients who have taken a monoamine oxidase inhibitor (MAOI) in the past 14 days. Since bupropion is an antidepressant and can have effects on mood, its psychiatric effects should be considered when used in the psychiatric population. Common adverse effects of bupropion include insomnia, dry mouth, increased blood pressure, and weight loss. Bupropion is a strong CYP2D6 inhibitor and is extensively metabolized in the liver. Therefore, drug–drug interactions should be considered, and dose reduction may be required in patients with hepatic dysfunction [26].

Varenicline (Chantix®)

Varenicline (Chantix®) is a partial α_4 β_2 nicotinic acetylcholine receptor agonist. It prevents nicotine withdrawal and cravings by partially stimulating the nicotine receptor to a degree lower than that of cigarettes and below the threshold for the dopamine reward pathway responsible for addiction. Varenicline should be initiated 1 week before the target quit date. The dosing for varenicline is 0.5 mg once daily for 3 days, then 0.5 mg twice daily for 4 days, then 1 mg twice daily for 3 months. Serious neuropsychiatric adverse effects (suicidal ideation, depression, aggression, changes in behavior) have been reported with the use of varenicline. Therefore, patients should be monitored for changes in mood/behavior, and caution should be exercised in psychiatric patients. The FDA removed the black box warning regarding neuropsychiatric events after a study demonstrated that use of varenicline in stable psychiatric patients (defined as clinically stable and receiving treatment for 6 months) was not associated with an increased incidence of neuropsychiatric events [27]. Other significant warnings include an increased risk of seizure and an increased effect of alcohol. Patients should be educated to reduce the amount of alcohol they consume until they know how varenicline affects them. The most common adverse effect of varenicline is nausea, which can be minimized if the medication is taken after meals on a full stomach. Other common side effects include insomnia and abnormal dreams. Varenicline is primarily eliminated by the kidneys and, therefore, requires dose adjustment in patients with renal dysfunction [28].

Off-Label Treatments

Clonidine and nortriptyline have also been studied and shown some effectiveness for TUD. However, there are significant adverse effects associated with the use of these medications and variable dosing in studies for TUD. Therefore, clonidine and nortriptyline are only recommended as second-line treatment options for patients who have failed or are not candidates for first-line pharmacotherapy options [12].

Electronic Nicotine Delivery Systems (ENDS)

Background and Formulations

ENDS, often called "e-cigs," "e-hookahs," "mods," "vape pens," "vapes," "tank systems," or "electronic cigarettes" are often small inhalers that simulate cigarette smoking by producing an aerosol that is inhaled [29]. Typical ENDS use a battery-powered heating coil to aerosolize a liquid solution known as e-liquid or "eJuice." These e-liquids usually contain a mixture of nicotine, flavoring agents, and a diluent (typically propylene glycol and/or vegetable glycerin) [30]. E-liquids can be offered in several different strengths of nicotine. For example, one ENDS brand offers pods that contain either 3% (23 mg) or 5% (40 mg) nicotine by weight. Electromechanically, current e-cigarette technology employs a coil of resistive wire around a wick material positioned across the axis of a narrow flow tube through which the user draws in a mouthful of aerosol. ENDS usage leads to peak plasma nicotine concentrations similar to conventional cigarette usage, making it a possible alternative [31].

The use of ENDS has rapidly proliferated, with a rise in adjusted national sales from $11.6 million in 2010 to $2.763 billion in 2021 [32, 33]. While smoking cessation and harm reduction are the primary reasons people report using ENDS, almost 1/3 of users are nonsmokers who initiate nicotine usage with ENDS [34, 35]. Because ENDS do not contain tobacco, they appear to be less harmful than conventional cigarettes, which deliver thousands of chemicals. Harmful chemicals and particulate matter in e-cigarettes are ~9–450 times lower than those found in conventional cigarettes, and similar to levels found in the FDA-approved nicotine inhaler [36, 37]. Currently, ENDS are not approved by the US Food and Drug Administration for the treatment of tobacco use disorder.

Current Evidence

Despite the growing popularity of ENDS, research on their efficacy as an aid for smoking cessation is not unanimous. One review of relevant studies found evidence that people are more likely to stop smoking for at least 6 months using ENDS than using nicotine replacement therapy or e-cigarettes without nicotine [38]. Included in this review was the finding that ENDS may also help more people to stop smoking than no support or behavioral support only. Another review analyzed relevant studies published between 2003 and 2017 and found that ENDS were moderately effective with regard to smoking reduction (48–59%) and cessation (13–23%), with frequent reports of non-severe adverse events that diminished with time (i.e., throat irritation, anxiety, and insomnia) [39]. A recent randomized trial looked at the effectiveness of ENDS compared to nicotine replacement therapy for smoking cessation. What this study found was that ENDS were more effective for smoking cessation than nicotine replacement therapy when both products were accompanied by behavioral support [52]. Overall, the literature points toward cautious optimism for smoking reduction; however, more evidence is needed to fully understand how ENDS facilitate smoking cessation.

Risks/Disadvantages

Significant concerns have been raised about dependence on nicotine delivered by the introduction of ENDS into the marketplace. Usage by young adults and adolescents is on the rise, which raises concern that ENDS function as a gateway to nicotine and/or tobacco dependence. In a study of US high school juniors and seniors, students who used ENDS were 6 times more likely to initiate conventional cigarette use during a 16-month follow-up period, and 40% of them did so, indicating that ENDS usage may lead to nicotine dependence [34, 40, 41].

In addition, many ENDS users have trouble weaning themselves off nicotine delivered via the devices, and a large online survey of ENDS users demonstrated that these devices ended up being used for longer durations than typical nicotine replacement therapies [42–44]. Not surprisingly, this combination of factors has led to the most common pattern of usage being dual use of ENDS and conventional cigarettes [45]. Given the growing and widespread use of ENDS as both a treatment for TUD and for recreational use, further studies are needed for an improved understanding of the impact of these devices on health and smoking behavior.

Treatment for individuals with nicotine use disorder who use ENDS is an emerging area of research. While traditional cessation therapies—like nicotine replacement therapy, bupropion, and varenicline—are well-established for tobacco use disorder, there is limited but growing evidence to guide their use in ENDS users. First-line pharmacotherapies like combination nicotine replacement therapy (e.g., patch plus gum or lozenge), bupropion, and varenicline remain standard clinical options and are sometimes adapted for ENDS users based on individual dependence and history. Clinical judgment is essential, especially since some users may struggle with dual use of cigarettes and ENDS or find it difficult to stop using ENDS due to persistent nicotine cravings. While no formal guidelines exist specifically for treating nicotine use disorder from ENDS, applying evidence-based treatments used for tobacco cessation, along with behavioral interventions such as cognitive-behavioral therapy or motivational interviewing, is considered the best practice until more targeted data are available.

Chapter Review Questions

1. CK is a 46-year-old Chinese American female with a history of hyperlipidemia and hypertension who presents to your primary care clinic for her yearly check-up. Which of CK's demographic characteristics has been associated with a higher prevalence of smoking?

   A. Gender
   B. Age
   C. History of hyperlipidemia
   D. History of hypertension
   E. Ethnicity

   Correct Answer: B

   Explanation: Males, aged 45–64, non-Hispanic White, non-Hispanic Black, or other non-Hispanic, uninsured or insured by Medicaid, had no diploma or a General Education Development (GED) Certificate, identified as lesbian, gay, or bisexual, low income, lived in the Midwest or South, or had a disability, have a higher prevalence of smoking. The category CK falls into is age (45–64).

2. AH is a 52-year-old male with no prior medical history who is ambivalent regarding treatment for his tobacco use disorder. Which of the following non-pharmacological therapies would be most appropriate for the treatment of AH's tobacco use disorder?

   A. Acceptance and commitment therapy (ACT)
   B. Motivational Interviewing (MI)
   C. Dialectical behavioral therapy (DBT)
   D. Exposure therapy
   E. Mindfulness-based therapy

   Correct Answer: B

   Explanation: Motivational Interviewing (MI) is a nonpharmacological therapy that can be used when working with tobacco users who are not yet ready to quit smoking. These techniques are designed to encourage patient engagement in active behavior change and include exploring self-ratings of the importance of quitting and confidence in quitting using open-ended questions and reflection. Since AH is ambivalent regarding his tobacco use, MI would be the most appropriate as a first-line therapy.

3. LK is a 37-year-old male with a history of major depressive disorder and tobacco use disorder who was discharged 1 week ago after being hospitalized for suicidal ideation. He smokes 1 pack of cigarettes per day and smokes his first cigarette within 5 min after waking up. He has tried combination nicotine replacement therapy (nicotine patch + nicotine gum) in the past for smoking cessation, but it was ineffective. Which would be the most appropriate pharmacological treatment option for LK?

   A. Nicotine patch monotherapy
   B. Nicotine gum monotherapy
   C. Bupropion
   D. Varenicline
   E. Clonidine

   Correct Answer: C

   Explanation: Bupropion is the most appropriate choice since it is a first-line pharmacological therapy and the safest option for this patient. Since this patient has already failed treatment with combination nicotine replacement (nicotine patch + nicotine gum), a monotherapy trial would not be indicated as combination therapy is superior. Since this patient was recently hospitalized for suicidal ideation, varenicline would not be appropriate either since it has only been shown to be safe in patients who have had stable psychiatric symptoms for 6 months. Clonidine is not considered a first-line treatment for TUD due to its risk of significant adverse effects and variable dosing in past studies.

4. TL is a 28-year-old female with tobacco use disorder. She smokes 2 packs of cigarettes per day and smokes her first cigarette 30 min after waking up. Which strength of nicotine patch and nicotine lozenge would be most appropriate to initiate in TL based on her level of tobacco dependence?

   A. 21 mg nicotine patch with 4 mg nicotine lozenge
   B. 21 mg nicotine patch with 2 mg nicotine lozenge
   C. 14 mg nicotine patch with 4 mg nicotine lozenge
   D. 14 mg nicotine patch with 2 mg nicotine lozenge
   E. 7 mg nicotine patch with 2 mg nicotine lozenge

   Correct Answer: A

   Explanation: Using the HIS, TL has 5 points (2 points for smoking 5–30 min after waking and 3 points for smoking 40 cigarettes/day) and high tobacco dependence. Therefore, she should be initiated on the 21 mg nicotine patch with the 4 mg nicotine lozenge.

5. SH is a 30-year-old female who is interested in using nicotine electronic cigarettes (e-cigarettes) to quit smoking and presents to your clinic to learn more about them. Which of the following statements would be the most accurate for you to tell SH regarding nicotine e-cigarettes?

   A. Studies show that you are more likely to quit smoking cigarettes for at least 6 months using nicotine e-cigarettes over nicotine replacement therapy.
   B. Electronic cigarettes are regulated by the FDA.

C. Electronic cigarettes are FDA-approved for the treatment of tobacco use disorder.
D. Electronic cigarette use does not carry a risk for nicotine dependence.
E. Only previous/current smokers use electronic cigarettes.

Correct Answer: A

Explanation: Nicotine e-cigarettes appear to be more effective in helping people quit smoking for at least 6 months when compared to nicotine replacement therapy. Nicotine e-cigarettes are not regulated by the FDA, are not FDA-approved for treatment of tobacco use disorder and carry a risk for nicotine dependence. Nicotine e-cigarettes are increasingly used among youth/adolescents and may serve as a gateway to conventional cigarettes.

References

1. Cornelius ME, Loretan CG, Jamal A, et al. Tobacco product use among adults—United States, 2021. MMWR Morb Mortal Wkly Rep. 2023;72:475–83.
2. Lasser K, Boyd JW, Woolhandler S, Himmelstein DU, McCormick D, Bor DH. Smoking and mental illness: a population-based prevalence study. JAMA. 2000;284:2606–10.
3. U.S. Department of Health and Human Services. Eliminating tobacco-related disease and death: addressing disparities—a report of the surgeon general. Atlanta: U.S. Department of Health and Human Services, Centers for Disease Control and Prevention, National Center for Chronic Disease Prevention and Health Promotion, Office on Smoking and Health; 2024.
4. Jha P, Ramasundarahettige C, Landsman V, Rostron B, Thun M, Anderson RN, et al. 21st-century hazards of smoking and benefits of cessation in the United States. N Engl J Med. 2013;368:341–50.
5. CDC. Economic trends in tobacco. Smoking and tobacco use. 2024. https://www.cdc.gov/tobacco/php/data-statistics/economic-trends/index.html. Accessed 17 Apr 2025.
6. Benowitz NL, Hukkanen J, Jacob P. Nicotine chemistry, metabolism, kinetics and biomarkers. Handb Exp Pharmacol. 2009;192:29–60.
7. Benowitz NL. Clinical pharmacology of nicotine: implications for understanding, preventing, and treating tobacco addiction. Clin Pharmacol Ther. 2008;83:531–41.
8. Cameron JM, Howell DN, White JR, Andrenyak DM, Layton ME, Roll JM. Variable and potentially fatal amounts of nicotine in e-cigarette nicotine solutions. Tob Control. 2014;23:77–8.
9. Solarino B, Rosenbaum F, Rießelmann B, Buschmann CT, Tsokos M. Death due to ingestion of nicotine-containing solution: case report and review of the literature. Forensic Sci Int. 2010;195:e19–22.
10. Nicotine Poisoning | California Poison Control System | UCSF [Internet]. [cited 2019 Jan 4]. Available from: https://calpoison.org/news/nicotine-poisoning.
11. Substance-Related and Addictive Disorders. Diagnostic and statistical manual of mental disorders [Internet]. Arlington: American Psychiatric Association; 2013. [cited 2019 Jan 4]. Available from. https://doi.org/10.1176/appi.books.9780890425596.dsm16.
12. Panel TU and DG. Treating tobacco use and dependence: 2008 update. Rockville: US Department of Health and Human Services; 2008.
13. Siu AL. Preventive Services Task Force US. Behavioral and pharmacotherapy interventions for tobacco smoking cessation in adults, including pregnant women: U.S. Preventive Services Task Force recommendation statement. Ann Intern Med. 2015;163:622–34.
14. John U, Meyer C, Schumann A, Hapke U, Rumpf H-J, Adam C, et al. A short form of the Fagerström Test for Nicotine Dependence and the Heaviness of Smoking Index in two adult population samples. Addict Behav. 2004;29:1207–12.
15. O'Connor RJ. Non-cigarette tobacco products: what have we learned and where are we headed? Tob Control. 2012;21:181–90.

16. Ebbert JO, Elrashidi MY, Stead LF. Interventions for smokeless tobacco use cessation. Cochrane Database Syst Rev. 2015:CD004306.
17. Lancaster T, Stead LF. Individual behavioural counselling for smoking cessation. Cochrane Database Syst Rev. 2017;3:CD001292.
18. Stead LF, Carroll AJ, Lancaster T. Group behaviour therapy programmes for smoking cessation. Cochrane Database Syst Rev. 2017;3:CD001007.
19. Perkins KA, Karelitz JL, Jao NC. Optimal carbon monoxide criteria to confirm 24-hr smoking abstinence. Nicotine Tob Res. 2013;15:978–82.
20. Clinical Practice A. Guideline for treating tobacco use and dependence: 2008 update. Am J Prev Med. 2008;35:158–76.
21. Kerr S, Woods C, Knussen C, Watson H, Hunter R. Breaking the habit: a qualitative exploration of barriers and facilitators to smoking cessation in people with enduring mental health problems. BMC Public Health. 2013;13:221.
22. Cahill K, Stevens S, Perera R, Lancaster T. Pharmacological interventions for smoking cessation: an overview and network meta-analysis. Cochrane Database Syst Rev [Internet]. 2013; [cited 2019 Mar 1]; Available from: https://www.cochranelibrary.com/cdsr/doi/10.1002/14651858.CD009329.pub2/abstract
23. Hsia SL, Myers MG, Chen TC. Combination nicotine replacement therapy: strategies for initiation and tapering. Prev Med. 2017;97:45–9.
24. DailyMed – NICODERM CQ- nicotine patch, extended release [Internet]. [cited 2019 Jan 6]. Available from: https://dailymed.nlm.nih.gov/dailymed/drugInfo.cfm?setid=93b2d1b9-83c1-40b5-b6af-90c38c8d6cef.
25. DailyMed – NICOTINE GUM- nicotine polacrilex gum, chewing [Internet]. [cited 2019 Jan 6]. Available from: https://dailymed.nlm.nih.gov/dailymed/drugInfo.cfm?setid=3872c622-1a30-459c-b878-61648bb30627.
26. GlaxoSmithKline. ZYBAN (bupropion hydrochloride) sustained-release tablets [package insert]. Research Triangle Park: GlaxoSmithKline; 2017.
27. Anthenelli RM, Benowitz NL, West R, St Aubin L, McRae T, Lawrence D, et al. Neuropsychiatric safety and efficacy of varenicline, bupropion, and nicotine patch in smokers with and without psychiatric disorders (EAGLES): a double-blind, randomised, placebo-controlled clinical trial. Lancet. 2016;387:2507–20.
28. Pfizer Labs. CHANTIX (varenicline tartrate) [package insert]. New York, NY: Pfizer Labs; 2019. Available from: http://labeling.pfizer.com/showlabeling.aspx?id=557
29. Health CO on S and. Smoking and tobacco use; electronic cigarettes [Internet]. Atlanta: Centers for Disease Control and Prevention; 2018. [cited 2019 Jan 17]. Available from: https://www.cdc.gov/tobacco/basic_information/e-cigarettes/index.htm
30. Hutzler C, Paschke M, Kruschinski S, Henkler F, Hahn J, Luch A. Chemical hazards present in liquids and vapors of electronic cigarettes. Arch Toxicol. 2014;88:1295–308.
31. Marsot A, Simon N. Nicotine and cotinine levels with electronic cigarette: a review. Int J Toxicol. 2016;35:179–85.
32. Cantrell J, Huang J, Greenberg M, Willett J, Hair E, Vallone D. History and current trends in the electronic nicotine delivery systems retail marketplace in the United States: 2010–2016. Nicotine Tob Res. 2018;20(7):845–54. https://doi.org/10.1093/ntr/nty214.
33. E-Cigarette Report for 2021 [Internet]. Federal Trade Commision. 2024 [cited 2024 Oct 1]. Available from: https://www.ftc.gov/system/files/ftc_gov/pdf/E-CigaretteReportfor2021.pdf. Accessed 02 Oct 2024.
34. Grana RA, Ling PM, Benowitz N, Glantz S. Electronic cigarettes. Cardiology patient page. Circulation. 2014;129:e490–2.
35. McMillen RC, Gottlieb MA, Shaefer RMW, Winickoff JP, Klein JD. Trends in electronic cigarette use among U.S. adults: use is increasing in both smokers and nonsmokers. Nicotine Tob Res. 2015;17:1195–202.
36. Goniewicz ML, Knysak J, Gawron M, Kosmider L, Sobczak A, Kurek J, et al. Levels of selected carcinogens and toxicants in vapour from electronic cigarettes. Tob Control. 2014;23:133–9.

37. Ruprecht AA, De Marco C, Pozzi P, Munarini E, Mazza R, Angellotti G, et al. Comparison between particulate matter and ultrafine particle emission by electronic and normal cigarettes in real-life conditions. Tumori. 2014;100:e24–7.
38. Hartmann-Boyce J, Lindson N, Butler AR, et al. Electronic cigarettes for smoking cessation. Cochrane Database Syst Rev. 2022;11(11):CD010216. Published 2022 Nov 17. https://doi.org/10.1002/14651858.CD010216.pub7.
39. Liu X, Lu W, Liao S, Deng Z, Zhang Z, Liu Y, et al. Efficiency and adverse events of electronic cigarettes: a systematic review and meta-analysis (PRISMA-compliant article). Medicine (Baltimore). 2018;97:e0324.
40. Barrington-Trimis JL, Urman R, Berhane K, Unger JB, Cruz TB, Pentz MA, et al. E-cigarettes and future cigarette use. Pediatrics. 2016;138:e20160379.
41. Dutra LM, Glantz SA. Electronic cigarettes and conventional cigarette use among U.S. adolescents: a cross-sectional study. JAMA Pediatr. 2014;168:610–7.
42. Farsalinos KE, Romagna G, Tsiapras D, Kyrzopoulos S, Voudris V. Evaluating nicotine levels selection and patterns of electronic cigarette use in a group of "vapers" who had achieved complete substitution of smoking. Subst Abuse. 2013;7:139–46.
43. Dawkins L, Turner J, Roberts A, Soar K. "Vaping" profiles and preferences: an online survey of electronic cigarette users. Addiction. 2013;108:1115–25.
44. Etter J-F, Bullen C. A longitudinal study of electronic cigarette users. Addict Behav. 2014;39:491–4.
45. QuickStats: Cigarette smoking status among current adult E-cigarette users, by age group — National Health Interview Survey, United States, 2015. MMWR Morbidity Mortality Weekly Report [Internet]. 2016 [cited 2019 Jan 17];65. Available from: https://www.cdc.gov/mmwr/volumes/65/wr/mm6542a7.htm.
46. Substance Abuse and Mental Health Services Administration. Key substance use and mental health indicators in the United States: results from the 2023 National Survey on Drug Use and Health, HHS Publication No. PEP24-07-021, NSDUH Series H-59. Rockville: Center for Behavioral Health Statistics and Quality, Substance Abuse and Mental Health Services Administration; 2024. https://www.samhsa.gov/data/report/2023-nsduh-annual-national-report
47. Substance Abuse and Mental Health Services Administration. Key substance use and mental health indicators in the United States: results from the 2022 National Survey on Drug Use and Health, HHS Publication No. PEP23-07-01-006, NSDUH Series H-58. Center for Behavioral Health Statistics and Quality, Substance Abuse and Mental Health Services Administration; 2023. https://www.samhsa.gov/data/report/2022-nsduh-annual-national-report
48. Rose JJ, Krishnan-Sarin S, Exil VJ, et al. Cardiopulmonary impact of electronic cigarettes and vaping products: a scientific statement from the American Heart Association. Circulation. 2023;148(8):703–28. https://doi.org/10.1161/CIR.0000000000001160.
49. Products C for T. Results from the Annual National Youth Tobacco Survey. FDA. Published online March 14, 2025. https://www.fda.gov/tobacco-products/youth-and-tobacco/results-annual-national-youth-tobacco-survey. Accessed 17 Apr 2025.
50. Kroon LA. Drug interactions with smoking. Am J Health Syst Pharm. 2007;64(18):1917–21. https://doi.org/10.2146/ajhp060414.
51. Wagner E, McMahon L, Falkai P, Hasan A, Siskind D. Impact of smoking behavior on clozapine blood levels – a systematic review and meta-analysis. Acta Psychiatr Scand. 2020;142(6):456–66. https://doi.org/10.1111/acps.13228. Epub 2020 Sep 27
52. Berry KM, Fetterman JL, Benjamin EJ, et al. Association of electronic cigarette use with subsequent initiation of tobacco cigarettes in US youths. JAMA Netw Open. 2019;2(2):e187794. https://doi.org/10.1001/jamanetworkopen.2018.7794.
53. Islami F, Nargis N, Liu Q, et al. Averted lung cancer deaths due to reductions in cigarette smoking in the United States, 1970–2022. CA Cancer J Clin. 2025;75(3):216–25. https://doi.org/10.3322/caac.70005.

Alcohol

8

Matthew E. Sloan, Angela Praecht, Robert B. Werner, Stephanie Yarnell-MacGrory, and Ismene Petrakis

High-Yield Review Points

- Risk factors for alcohol use disorder include family history of alcoholism, male sex, and early onset of alcohol use.
- Individuals with specific polymorphisms in the genes coding for alcohol dehydrogenase and aldehyde dehydrogenase, the two main enzymes involved in alcohol metabolism, are at decreased risk of alcohol use disorder.
- Alcohol withdrawal can lead to a range of symptoms including seizures and delirium. The most commonly used instrument to assess withdrawal symptoms is the Clinical Institute Withdrawal Assessment for Alcohol, Revised (CIWA-Ar).

M. E. Sloan (✉)
Addictions Division, Centre for Addiction and Mental Health, Toronto, ON, Canada

Department of Psychiatry, Temerty Faculty of Medicine, University of Toronto, Toronto, ON, Canada
e-mail: matthew.sloan@camh.ca

A. Praecht
Addictions Division, Centre for Addiction and Mental Health, Toronto, ON, Canada
e-mail: a.praecht@mail.utoronto.ca

R. B. Werner · S. Yarnell-MacGrory
Department of Psychiatry, Yale University School of Medicine, New Haven, CT, USA
e-mail: dr.werner@blakewernermd.com; stephanie.yarnell@yale.edu

I. Petrakis
Department of Psychiatry, Yale University School of Medicine, New Haven, CT, USA

VA Connecticut Healthcare System, West Haven, CT, USA
e-mail: ismene.petrakis@yale.edu

C. Marienfeld, M. Soltani (eds.), *AAAP Review of Addiction Psychiatry*, https://doi.org/10.1007/978-3-032-24174-0_8

- Benzodiazepines are the most commonly used pharmacotherapy for alcohol withdrawal, though phenobarbital and certain anticonvulsants may be used depending on withdrawal severity, the treatment setting, and response to benzodiazepines.
- There are three FDA-approved pharmacotherapies for alcohol use disorder: naltrexone, a mu-opioid receptor antagonist; acamprosate, a modulator of glutamatergic neurotransmission; and disulfiram, a medication that causes adverse reactions to alcohol by inhibiting aldehyde dehydrogenase, an enzyme involved in alcohol metabolism.
- Topiramate and gabapentin are commonly used off-label for alcohol use disorder. Topiramate reduces excitatory neurotransmission by acting on AMPA and kainate receptors and increases inhibitory neurotransmission through activating $GABA_A$ receptors; gabapentin targets voltage-gated calcium channels.
- Laboratory markers are used to monitor alcohol consumption. Direct markers are products of alcohol metabolism and include ethyl glucuronide, ethyl sulfate, and phosphatidylethanol. Indirect markers reflect alcohol's effects on organ systems and cellular function and include GGT, AST, ALT, CDT, and MCV.

Epidemiology

Alcohol use remains one of the most important risk factors for death and disability worldwide [1] and was directly responsible for 49,061 deaths in the United States in 2020 [2]. Alcohol-related mortality has been gradually increasing over the past decade [3]. Findings from the National Epidemiologic Survey on Alcohol and Related Conditions (NESARC) indicate that the 12-month prevalence of alcohol use disorder (AUD) is 13.9%, with higher rates in males than females (17.6% vs. 10.4%) [4]. This survey also found that the prevalence of alcohol use, risky drinking, and alcohol use disorders is increasing [5]. In 2023, the National Survey on Drug Use and Health (NSDUH) found that approximately 135 million individuals aged 12 and older were current alcohol users. Among them, 28.9 million were diagnosed with AUD, yet only 4.5 million received treatment [6]. The COVID-19 pandemic appears to have been an additional risk factor for alcohol misuse, contributing to an observed increase in alcohol sales and mortality. For example, alcohol-related deaths increased by approximately 25% between 2019 and 2020 [7, 8].

There are important sex differences in both the prevalence and progression of alcohol use disorder. An earlier iteration of NESARC found that alcohol use disorder was 2.5 times more prevalent in men compared to women [9]. These sex differences appear to be diminishing over time as the most recent NESARC findings indicate that the male-to-female ratio for alcohol use disorder is 1.7:1 [4]. Research suggests that alcohol use is rising in women but not in men. For example, a meta-analysis of six different U.S. surveys found that between 2002 and 2016, alcohol consumption and binge drinking increased in women by 6% and 14%, respectively, whereas consumption decreased by 0.2% in men and binge drinking only increased by 0.5% over the same period [9–11]. Additional findings from the 2015-2017 Behavioral Risk Factor Surveillance System indicate that 11.5% of pregnant women consumed alcohol and 3.9% engaged in binge drinking in the past 30 days (with an average of 4.5 episodes of binge drinking) [12]. Women also tend to experience a more rapid progression from first alcohol exposure to development of an alcohol use disorder when compared to men, a somewhat controversial phenomenon known as telescoping [13] and are at higher risk of experiencing certain alcohol-related sequelae than men including alcohol-induced cardiovascular disease and certain cancers [9]. Women who develop problematic alcohol-related behaviors should therefore be closely monitored for progression and offered appropriate counseling.

Binge drinking, defined by the National Institute on Alcohol Abuse and Alcoholism (NIAAA) as consuming five or more drinks for men or four or more drinks for women in a single occasion, peaks in young adulthood and then gradually declines with age [14]. This aligns with the 12-month prevalence of AUD, which also peaks during young adulthood and declines with age [4]. Age of onset of alcohol use is thought to be an important risk factor for AUD; individuals who start drinking at a younger age are at greater risk [15]. Therefore, it is concerning that according to school surveys, alcohol use is starting at an alarmingly early age regardless of gender, often beginning before the age of 15, with a prevalence rate of 50-70% in this age group [16].

The Genetics of Alcohol Use Disorder

Family history of alcoholism is an established risk factor for alcohol use disorder and is listed under the genetic and physiological risk factors in the Diagnostic and Statistical Manual of Mental Disorders, Fifth Edition (DSM-5-TR) [17]. Individuals with a family history of alcoholism may have an inherent preference for ethanol. For example, there is evidence that healthy social drinkers with a family history of alcoholism consume substantially more alcohol in laboratory settings [18]. Aggregated data from twin studies suggest that alcoholism is approximately 50% heritable [19]. The largest multi-ancestry Genome-wide Association Study (GWAS) for alcohol misuse confirms the polygenic nature of AUD. This study had over 1 million individuals, including 165,952 AUD cases and found 85 independent risk variants in participants with European ancestry and 110 variants that were associated with problematic alcohol use in either within-ancestry or cross-ancestry meta-analyses [20].

Polymorphisms in genes involved in alcohol metabolism have been most consistently linked with alcohol use disorder. Ethanol is metabolized in a two-step process: alcohol dehydrogenase converts ethanol to acetaldehyde and then aldehyde dehydrogenase metabolizes acetaldehyde to acetate. A variant of the alcohol dehydrogenase 1B gene leads to rapid alcohol metabolism and decreases the risk of alcohol use disorder in individuals of European and Asian ancestry [21–23], whereas a different polymorphism in the same gene has a similar effect in individuals of African ancestry [22]. Alterations in the second step of alcohol metabolism can also affect AUD risk. In individuals of Asian ancestry, a less functional variant of aldehyde dehydrogenase 2 protects against alcoholism by causing a buildup of acetaldehyde during drinking, which may induce flushing, nausea, and tachycardia [21, 24]. Individuals who are heterozygous for this allele but continue to consume alcohol are at increased risk of esophageal cancer, as acetaldehyde is also a known carcinogen [25]. Patients with a history of alcohol-induced flushing should therefore be counseled to limit their alcohol intake.

Pharmacokinetics

Alcohol is absorbed primarily by passive diffusion in the duodenum and the jejunum and to a lesser degree in the stomach [26]. As a result, the rate of gastric emptying plays an important role in the rate of absorption. The presence of food in the stomach slows down the rate of gastric emptying, which greatly reduces absorption [27]. When advising patients about alcohol use, it is always helpful to caution against drinking on an empty stomach.

Alcohol is primarily eliminated in the liver and to a lesser degree in the gastrointestinal (GI) tract. In the first step of metabolism, alcohol is metabolized to acetaldehyde by alcohol dehydrogenase, and then, in the second step, acetaldehyde is oxidized to acetate by the enzyme aldehyde dehydrogenase. Alcohol is also metabolized to a lesser extent by a cytochrome P450-dependent ethanol-oxidizing system.

In general, after consuming a single standard drink, the amount of alcohol in a drinker's blood peaks within 30–45 min (a "standard drink" is defined by NIAAA as containing 14 grams of pure ethanol, typically about 1.5 ounces of distilled spirits, 5 ounces of wine, or 12 ounces of beer) [28]. However, absorption and metabolism vary according to a person's age, height, sex, weight, liver function, and recent food consumption. In addition to metabolism in the liver, alcohol is oxidized by certain isoforms of alcohol dehydrogenase in the stomach. Certain medications inhibit gastric alcohol dehydrogenase activity, such as the H2 blockers cimetidine and ranitidine [28]. The activity of gastric alcohol dehydrogenase is also reported to be lower in women [27], which may explain in part why women have greater blood alcohol levels compared to men following a fixed dose of alcohol. Females also tend to have a greater percentage of body fat and less total body water than males, which is another important reason for this phenomenon [27].

Pharmacodynamics

Alcohol has pharmacodynamic effects on a wide range of neurotransmitter systems. For the sake of simplicity, this chapter will focus on two systems: the GABAergic system and the glutamatergic system.

Gamma-aminobutyric acid (GABA) is the major inhibitory neurotransmitter in the brain and consists of two main receptor subtypes: $GABA_A$ and $GABA_B$. $GABA_A$ receptors are ligand-gated ion channels that, when activated, allow the inflow of negative chloride ions (Cl−), which hyperpolarize the neuron, whereas $GABA_B$ is a metabotropic G-coupled receptor. Acute alcohol intake increases $GABA_A$ activity through direct effects on the receptor and indirect effects such as increased presynaptic GABA release [29]. Chronic alcohol intake leads to several neuroadaptations within the GABAergic system that are thought to play a role in the development of physiologic dependence.

Glutamate is the most abundant excitatory neurotransmitter in the human brain. Glutamate receptors include three major classes of ionotropic receptors: α-amino-3-hydroxy-5-methylisoxazole-4-propionic acid (AMPA) receptors, *N*-methyl-D-aspartate (NMDA) receptors, and kainate receptors. NMDA receptors are typically inhibited by acute ingestion of ethanol [30]. Conversely, chronic ethanol exposure upregulates NMDA receptors, enhances their functionality, and increases NMDA receptor-mediated glutamatergic synaptic transmission [31]. It is thought that alcohol withdrawal-related hyperexcitability is due to increases in NMDA receptor transmission; this may also explain the enhanced susceptibility to seizures during withdrawal [31]. The mechanisms by which chronic ethanol consumption enhances NMDA receptor function are still not fully understood.

Alcohol Intoxication

Alcohol intoxication occurs when alcohol accumulates in the bloodstream, with signs and symptoms varying depending upon the type and amount of alcohol consumed, rate of intake, and the frequency and pattern of use. In individuals who do not drink heavily or frequently, the clinical effects of alcohol intoxication are relatively predictable, with neurologic, gastrointestinal, and cardiovascular effects that are usually related to blood alcohol concentration (BAC). Conversely, after chronic alcohol use, individuals can develop tolerance. When tolerance develops, the effects of alcohol can become unpredictable, with some showing little or no signs of intoxication even with high BACs.

Among individuals who do not consume alcohol heavily and chronically, associated symptoms with each BAC range are as follows [32, 33]:

- BAC between 10 mg/dl and 100 mg/dl: relaxation, mild impairment of attention or memory, increased talkativeness, mild deficits in coordination.
- BAC between 100 mg/dl and 200 mg/dl: ataxia, greater deficits in attention, slurred speech, prolonged reaction time, nystagmus, impaired judgment, behavioral changes.
- BAC between 200 mg/dl and 300 mg/dl: lack of coordination, severely impaired attention, amnesia, dysarthria, hypothermia, nausea, vomiting.
- BAC exceeding 300 mg/dl: stupor, loss of consciousness, coma, respiratory depression, death.

Management of Alcohol Intoxication

The treatment for isolated, acute alcohol intoxication is primarily supportive. Management for clinically significant intoxication typically occurs in the emergency department. Initial evaluation should include an airway assessment, observation of respiratory function, and measurement of vital signs. The patient should be placed in a lateral position to prevent aspiration [34]. Individuals should also be carefully assessed for traumatic injuries and should be asked whether they have ingested or otherwise taken other drugs or potentially harmful substances. Obtaining history from the patient can be difficult, so additional information may need to be collected from paramedics, witnesses at the scene, friends, and family members, and by objective means [35]. A toxicology screen can be helpful to determine whether other substances were co-ingested [36]. If co-ingestion of methanol, ethylene glycol, or other substances is suspected, treatment should be modified to address these substances.

Patients with moderate to severe ethanol intoxication may present with volume depletion, malnutrition, and electrolyte abnormalities. Since an altered mental status can be caused by hypoglycemia, a finger-stick glucose test should be performed [35]. Intravenous fluids should be administered to correct fluid and electrolyte abnormalities, but in those with suspected or potential thiamine deficiency, intravenous thiamine should be given prior to glucose administration to prevent the precipitation of Wernicke's encephalopathy [34]. If the patient is experiencing nausea or vomiting, the use of antiemetic drugs may be indicated [34]. Individuals should be closely monitored with serial examinations until clinical sobriety has been achieved. Any acute changes in clinical status or alteration in the level of consciousness should be immediately investigated.

Alcohol Withdrawal

Alcohol withdrawal is a potentially life-threatening condition. Symptoms of alcohol withdrawal usually begin 6 to 24 h after the cessation of drinking and may develop while patients still have an elevated blood alcohol concentration [37]. Withdrawal symptoms are thought to be due to central nervous system hyperactivity and may include anxiety, irritability, agitation, tremor, headache, diaphoresis, insomnia, nausea, and vomiting [37, 38]. Elevated blood pressure and tachycardia can occur. Severe alcohol withdrawal syndromes (AWS) include alcohol withdrawal seizures, alcoholic hallucinosis, and delirium tremens (DTs), which are discussed individually below.

Withdrawal seizures are typically generalized tonic-clonic seizures that occur within 6–48 h after the last alcoholic drink [38]. While status epilepticus is rare, multiple seizures can occur [39]. Untreated withdrawal seizures may progress to delirium tremens in nearly one-third of patients [40]. Therefore, irrespective of the measured withdrawal severity scores, the occurrence of seizures during the alcohol withdrawal period is indicative of severe alcohol withdrawal and merits aggressive treatment.

Alcoholic hallucinosis refers to hallucinations that typically develop within 12–24 h of abstinence [38]. Hallucinations can be visual, auditory, or tactile in nature. The presence of hallucinations with normal vital signs and a clear sensorium is a hallmark of this disorder [40]. Because individuals know they are hallucinating, this condition can be quite distressing. Most cases typically resolve within 48 h [38]. Alcoholic hallucinosis is not synonymous with delirium tremens. Though hallucinations may be present in both, alcoholic hallucinosis presents with a clear sensorium and normal vital signs.

The most severe form of alcohol withdrawal is delirium tremens (DTs), in which persons who have recently abstained from alcohol or reduced their alcohol intake develop symptoms of withdrawal and delirium (an acute-onset disturbance in attention, awareness, and cognition that fluctuates in intensity during the day) [41]. Delirium tremens may present with tachycardia, hypertension, hyperthermia, and diaphoresis [42]. This syndrome typically begins 48–96 h after the last drink but may appear over a week later. DTs may last 7–10 days, although most cases resolve within 2–3 days [42–44]. There are several risk factors for developing delirium tremens, including a previous history of delirium tremens, a history of withdrawal seizures, older age, comorbid medical illnesses, and Clinical Institute Withdrawal Assessment for Alcohol, revised (CIWA-Ar) scores greater than 15 [41]. Delirium tremens is a life-threatening condition; the present-day mortality ranges between 1 and 4% in hospitalized patients [41]. Death most commonly occurs due to arrhythmias, hyperthermia, or complications due to comorbid conditions [41].

Management of Alcohol Withdrawal

Early identification of withdrawal symptoms is critical. For patients who are using alcohol regularly and heavily, their risk for developing AWS should be assessed even in the absence of signs or symptoms [44]. The Prediction of Alcohol Withdrawal Severity Scale (PAWSS) can be utilized to predict withdrawal severity before symptoms begin. The PAWSS score ranges from 0 to 10. A score of 4 or higher indicates a high risk for moderate to severe alcohol withdrawal [45]. The PAWSS had a 93.1% sensitivity for prospectively identifying inpatients admitted to general medicine or surgery units who would experience severe alcohol withdrawal [45].

The primary goals of managing alcohol withdrawal are alleviation of symptoms, prevention of progression, and identification and correction of metabolic derangements. Correction of fluid and electrolyte abnormalities should be performed using intravenous fluids and nutritional supplementation. In those with an extensive drinking history, thiamine should be administered prior to glucose to prevent precipitation of Wernicke's encephalopathy. Vital signs should be closely monitored.

Medication management is needed in individuals with a history of severe withdrawal (e.g., seizures or delirium tremens) and those who demonstrate moderate to severe symptoms of withdrawal at presentation or are at risk of developing such symptoms [37]. Benzodiazepines are the first-line treatment of alcohol withdrawal because of their well-documented effectiveness in reducing the signs and symptoms of withdrawal, including seizures and delirium. Benzodiazepines can be given using a fixed-schedule or symptom-triggered approach [38]. In the symptom-triggered approach, the Clinical Institute Withdrawal Assessment for Alcohol, Revised (CIWA-Ar), a 10-item scale with scores ranging from 0 to 67, is typically utilized to assess the severity of alcohol withdrawal symptoms [38]. Benzodiazepines are then given to the patient when severity scores exceed a certain threshold. As an example of a symptom-triggered treatment regimen, the CIWA-Ar could be administered every hour and then 2–4 mg of lorazepam could be given when the CIWA-Ar score is greater than or equal to 10 [38]. Although symptom-triggered regimens lead to the administration of less medication and shorten the duration of treatment [38], they require monitoring by a healthcare professional and are not recommended for outpatient detoxification [37]. In a fixed-schedule dosing regimen, benzodiazepines are given at fixed intervals even in the absence of active symptoms of withdrawal. Fixed-schedule dosing should be used in individuals with a history of withdrawal seizures regardless of CIWA-Ar score [37]. Long-acting benzodiazepines such as diazepam and chlordiazepoxide are commonly used with both approaches, particularly in outpatient settings. Treatment with lorazepam and oxazepam is more common in inpatient settings and is preferable in the elderly and patients with liver disease [38].

For patients experiencing moderate to severe withdrawal symptoms, benzodiazepines are the first-line treatment. Gabapentin or carbamazepine can be used as an alternative for mild to moderate withdrawal. Phenobarbital can be used as an alternative for severe withdrawal in inpatient settings but should only be used with extensive monitoring and by clinicians experienced with its use, given its narrow therapeutic window and risk for respiratory depression [44].

While treating alcohol withdrawal is crucial, it is important to underscore that withdrawal management should not be the sole treatment goal. Instead, it should be a component of the broader process of initiating and engaging patients in treatment for AUD [44].

Management of Withdrawal Seizures

Alcohol withdrawal seizures are a medical emergency. A thorough evaluation is necessary to rule out other causes of seizures, including electrolyte disturbances and traumatic brain injury. Individuals with withdrawal seizures should be treated with an intravenous benzodiazepine [37]. The patient should then be monitored and appropriately treated for other symptoms of withdrawal [37]. Most withdrawal seizures do not require treatment with non-benzodiazepine anticonvulsant medications long-term.

Management of Delirium Tremens

Individuals with delirium tremens should be closely observed and their vital signs should be frequently monitored. This should ideally be done in a quiet room with good lighting and environmental cues such as a calendar and clock. Those with severe delirium tremens may need to be placed in an intensive care unit for continuous monitoring [36]. Physical restraints may be temporarily required in cases of severe agitation for the protection of both the patient and staff [42]. A thorough evaluation should be performed to rule out concurrent medical conditions and other causes of delirium. Fluid and electrolyte abnormalities, hyperthermia, and high blood pressure should be appropriately managed [37] and intravenous thiamine should be administered [41]. Sedative-hypnotic medications are recommended as the mainstay treatment; intravenous benzodiazepines are most commonly used [42]. The goal of treatment is to give sufficient medication to achieve and maintain light somnolence, a state in which the patient falls asleep unless stimulated but is easily aroused [42].

Laboratory Screening for Alcohol Use

Direct biomarkers are products of ethanol metabolism and include ethyl glucuronide (EtG), ethyl sulfate (EtS), and phosphatidylethanol (PEth).

- *Ethyl glucuronide (EtG)* is a metabolite of alcohol that is formed by enzymatic conjugation of ethanol with glucuronic acid. It can be collected from a variety of bodily fluids and tissues but is most commonly and easily measured in the urine. Although urine EtG can remain positive for up to 5 days following heavy alcohol consumption [46], its sensitivity is highest within the first 24 h after drinking [47, 48].
- *Ethyl sulfate (EtS)* is an alcohol metabolite formed by the enzymatic conjugation of activated sulfate and ethanol. The time course for its detection in the urine following ethanol consumption is similar to EtG [46].
- *Phosphatidylethanol (PEth)* refers to a group of ethanol metabolites formed through a phospholipase D-mediated reaction of ethanol with phosphatidylcholine [49]. PEth is measured in whole blood and is used to detect heavy alcohol consumption, approximately 50 g of alcohol per day, for up to 3 weeks after abstinence [50].

Indirect biomarkers reflect the toxic effects of ethanol on organs, tissues, or body biochemistry. These include gamma-glutamyltransferase (GGT), aspartate aminotransferase (AST) and alanine aminotransferase (ALT), carbohydrate-deficient transferrin (CDT), and mean corpuscular volume (MCV).

- *Gamma-glutamyltransferase (GGT)* is an enzyme in liver cells released into the blood with cell inflammation and death, which can be elevated after several weeks of heavy drinking [51]. GGT levels may increase significantly in response to alcohol use, though GGT is not specific for alcohol use, as levels can be elevated in other conditions such as viral hepatitis and liver injury due to hepatotoxins [37, 52]. Levels typically return to normal after 2–6 weeks of abstinence [51].
- *Aspartate aminotransferase (AST) and alanine aminotransferase (ALT)* are enzymes that are elevated secondary to hepatic injury. An AST/ALT ratio of greater than 2 may be indicative of alcohol-related liver disease [51].

- *Carbohydrate-deficient transferrin (CDT)* refers to isoforms of transferrin that are deficient in sialic acid due to alcohol use. CDT levels are elevated following consumption of 60–80 grams of alcohol per day for 2–3 weeks and return to normal after 2–4 weeks of abstinence [51]. Although false positives can occur, CDT is far more specific than GGT for detecting alcohol use [51].
- *Mean corpuscular volume (MCV)* is a measure of red blood cell size and can be altered due to the direct effect of alcohol on erythroblast development [51]. It has low sensitivity and can take several months to return to normal following abstinence [51], so it has limited utility as an indicator of relapse.

Diagnosing Alcohol Use Disorder

Screening

There are a range of screening tools for alcohol use disorder. Some commonly used instruments include: The Alcohol Use Disorders Identification Test (AUDIT), the AUDIT Consumption (AUDIT-C), and the CAGE questionnaire. The AUDIT is a 10-item screening tool developed by the World Health Organization. It has three domains which assess consumption ("hazardous alcohol use"), dependence symptoms, and consequences of drinking ("harmful alcohol use") [53]. Responses to each of the ten items are scored from 0–4, with total scores ranging from 0–40; scores of 8 points or more are usually used as an indicator of problematic drinking [53]. The AUDIT-C is a brief alcohol screening instrument and consists of the first 3 questions of the full 10-item AUDIT. It is scored on a scale from 0 to 12, with higher scores indicating excessive alcohol use. A score of 3 or higher for women and 4 or higher for men is considered positive [54, 55]. The CAGE questionnaire is a four-item acronym questionnaire evaluating a person's history of cutting down on drinking, annoyance at others` concern about their drinking, guilt related to drinking and using alcohol first thing in the morning to cope with withdrawal symptoms or a hangover (an "eye-opener"). Scores of 2 or more are considered a positive screening [56] and indicate that the patient warrants further assessment for alcohol use disorder.

Diagnosis

The DSM-5 defines alcohol use disorder as "a problematic pattern of alcohol use leading to clinically significant impairment or distress" [17]. The manual requires that individuals meet at least 2 of 11 diagnostic criteria within the same 12-month period to be diagnosed with the disorder. The severity of the diagnosis is based on symptom counts. Individuals with 2–3 symptoms have mild AUD, those with 4–5 symptoms have moderate AUD, and individuals with 6 or more symptoms have severe AUD [17]. Alcohol use disorder is defined as being in early remission if no criteria (except craving) have been met for at least 3 months but less than 12 months and in sustained remission if no criteria have been met (except craving) for 12 months or longer [17].

Psychotherapy for Alcohol Use Disorder

Both psychotherapy and pharmacotherapy are effective treatments for alcohol use disorder [57]. In clinical practice, these two modalities are often used in tandem. Evidence-based psychotherapy options for AUD include cognitive behavioral therapy (CBT), motivational enhancement therapy, and 12-step facilitation [58]. The Project MATCH study, the largest psychotherapy trial for AUD, found no superiority among these interventions [59]. Furthermore, the COMBINE study, another large treatment trial, found no differences between CBT and naltrexone, nor any benefit of adding naltrexone to CBT alone [60]. Psychotherapies for substance use disorders are described elsewhere in this volume; the remainder of this chapter will focus on pharmacotherapy.

Pharmacotherapy for Alcohol Use Disorder

FDA-Approved Pharmacotherapies

There are currently three pharmacotherapies approved by the Food and Drug Administration (FDA) for alcohol use disorder: disulfiram, naltrexone, and acamprosate (for dosages and common side effects, see Table 8.1).

- *Naltrexone* is a nonselective opioid receptor antagonist that has been shown to reduce relapse to drinking including heavy drinking, percentage of drinking days, and return to binge drinking at the 50 mg/d oral dose compared to placebo [61]. It is available in both oral and long-acting injectable formulations, but fewer data are available for the injectable formulation. A recent meta-analysis found that oral naltrexone treatment led to significant improvements in alcohol consumption outcomes (e.g., reduced percentage of drinking days). The number needed to treat (NNT) to prevent return to any drinking was 18 and to prevent return to heavy drinking was 11 [62]. Given that naltrexone blocks mu-opioid receptors, individuals who are prescribed naltrexone should be screened for recent opioid use and naltrexone should not be administered if opioids have been used within the past 7–10 days due to the risk of precipitated withdrawal. Naltrexone should also be avoided if opioid administration is anticipated in the near future (e.g., an upcoming surgery requires opioid analgesia). Dizziness, nausea, and vomiting are common side effects [62]. The FDA has issued a black box warning for hepatotoxicity, although this tends to be associated with higher doses of naltrexone than the typical dose used clinically [63] and some risk has been attributed to comorbid conditions [64]. Nonetheless, liver function tests should be measured at baseline and monitored periodically [63].

Table 8.1 FDA-approved pharmacotherapies for alcohol use disorder [51, 52, 54]

	Disulfiram	Naltrexone	Acamprosate
Dose	250–500 mg PO daily	50 mg PO daily (oral) 380 mg IM q28 days (IM)	666 mg PO TID
Absolute contraindications	Use of metronidazole, paraldehyde, or alcohol-containing products Hypersensitivity to disulfiram Severe cardiac disease Psychosis	Acute hepatitis/liver failure Active opioid use, failed naloxone challenge, positive urine drug screen for opioids, or acute opioid withdrawal Hypersensitivity to naltrexone	Severe renal impairment (CrCl <30 ml/min) Hypersensitivity to acamprosate
Relative contraindications	Hepatic disease Diabetes Seizures Pregnancy	Active liver disease Serum aminotransferases 5 times upper levels Pregnancy Bleeding or coagulation disorder (IM formulation)	Pregnancy
Common side effects	Drowsiness Fatigue Acne Allergic dermatitis Headache Impotence Metallic or garlic aftertaste	Nausea Vomiting Dizziness Headache Somnolence Fatigue Injection site reactions (IM formulation)	Diarrhea Flatulence Nausea Vomiting Anxiety Pruritis Somnolence
Serious side effects	Hepatotoxicity Optic neuritis Peripheral neuropathy Psychosis Seizures	Precipitated withdrawal Hepatotoxicity Depression and suicidality	Suicidality
Baseline laboratory tests	Liver function tests Pregnancy test Breathalyzer (if clinically indicated)	Urine toxicology screen Liver function tests Pregnancy test	Renal function tests Pregnancy test
Clinical notes	Patients must abstain from alcohol for >12 h prior to initiation. Avoid products containing alcohol, reactions can occur up to 14 days after the last use of disulfiram. Monitor liver function tests	Blocks effects of opioid analgesics. Patients should be opioid free for a minimum of 7–10 days. Provide patients with documentation stating that they are taking naltrexone. Monitor liver function tests	Can be used in patients with hepatic impairment. Modify dose in patients with moderate renal impairment (CrCl 30–50 ml/min)

- *Acamprosate* is a medication that is thought to modulate glutamatergic neurotransmission [65]. A meta-analysis found that acamprosate reduces alcohol consumption compared to placebo. Acamprosate was also effective at preventing the return to any drinking with an NNT of 11 but, unlike naltrexone, was not effective at preventing return to heavy drinking [62]. Most clinical trials suggest that acamprosate may be more efficacious in patients who have attained abstinence from alcohol prior to initiating treatment. Thus, acamprosate is typically initiated after at least 3–5 days of abstinence but can be used safely in patients actively consuming alcohol [63, 66]. This medication is typically well tolerated; diarrhea is the most common side effect. Prior to initiation of acamprosate, it is important to obtain baseline renal function tests as it is excreted exclusively by the kidneys. Due to the lack of hepatic metabolism, it can be used safely in individuals with hepatic impairment or severe liver disease [63]. A meta-analysis of 4 randomized clinical trials comparing acamprosate and naltrexone did not find statistically significant differences in alcohol outcomes between the two medications [62].

- *Disulfiram* was the first available FDA-approved pharmacotherapy for the treatment of alcohol use disorder [67]. It inhibits the enzyme aldehyde dehydrogenase, leading to a buildup of acetaldehyde that can cause nausea, vomiting, flushing, sweating, tachycardia, palpitations, hypotension, hyperventilation, and rarely serious cardiovascular issues [63, 68]. Disulfiram functions as a form of aversion therapy; patients avoid drinking due to fear of a disulfiram-ethanol reaction. Findings related to the effectiveness of disulfiram are mixed. Findings from a recent meta-analysis including three randomized controlled trials (RCTs) revealed no significant differences between disulfiram and placebo in preventing relapse to drinking [67]. Another meta-analysis reported that disulfiram significantly reduced alcohol use in open-label studies but not in blinded trials, suggesting that its efficacy may be influenced by placebo effects [69]. There is a substantial amount of evidence indicating that disulfiram is most effective when medication adherence is closely supervised, highlighting the importance of monitoring in its clinical use [69–71]. Its efficacy largely relies on the patient consistently taking the medication and being aware of the consequences of drinking alcohol while taking disulfiram. Due to the potential for adverse effects, disulfiram is not a first-line treatment and should only be used in patients that are currently abstinent and wish to remain abstinent from alcohol. Patients should wait at least 12 h since their last drink before starting disulfiram (but may need to wait longer than this depending on their level of consumption) [63]. As disulfiram binds irreversibly to aldehyde dehydrogenase, it can take up to 2 weeks after discontinuation before the patient can drink without inducing a disulfiram-ethanol reaction [63]. Due to the potential for hepatotoxicity, it is recommended to obtain baseline liver function tests prior to initiating treatment and repeat testing 2 weeks after starting the medication [63]. Liver function tests should then be monitored monthly for the first 6 months of treatment and every 3 months thereafter [63].

Non-FDA-Approved Pharmacotherapies

There are multiple medications that are used as off-label treatments for alcohol use disorder. We will discuss three of the most commonly used medications: topiramate, gabapentin, and baclofen (for dosages and common side effects, see Table 8.2). Additionally, the opioid antagonist nalmefene is approved for the treatment of

Table 8.2 Off-label medications for alcohol use disorder [62, 63]

	Topiramate	Gabapentin	Baclofen
Dose	25 mg PO daily—150 mg PO BID	300 mg PO TID—600 mg PO TID	5–20 mg PO TID Maximum: 20 mg PO QID
Absolute contraindications	None	Hypersensitivity to gabapentin	Hypersensitivity to baclofen
Relative contraindications	Pregnancy (increased risk of cleft lip and/or palate)	Severe renal impairment (CrCl <30 ml/min) Pregnancy	Severe renal impairment Pregnancy
Common side effects	Cognitive dysfunction Paresthesias Taste abnormalities Anorexia Weight loss Nervousness Fatigue Somnolence Dizziness	Dizziness Somnolence Fatigue Ataxia Nystagmus Peripheral edema	Drowsiness Dizziness Weakness Confusion Headache Nausea Insomnia/Sleepiness Numbness
Serious side effects	Nephrolithiasis Hyperammonemia Suicidality Metabolic acidosis Hyperthermia Acute myopia/glaucoma	Anaphylaxis and angioedema Suicidality Drug reaction with eosinophilia and systemic symptoms (DRESS)	Severe withdrawal (symptoms can include seizures, hallucinations, hyperpyrexia and death)
Baseline laboratory tests	Renal function tests Serum bicarbonate Pregnancy test	Renal function tests Pregnancy test	Renal function tests Pregnancy test
Clinical notes	Primarily excreted unchanged in the urine. Dose should be modified in patients with renal impairment (CrCl <70 ml/min). Slowly taper to discontinuation to prevent withdrawal seizures	Almost exclusively eliminated renally. Dose should be modified in patients with renal impairment	Excreted primarily through the kidneys. Dose modifications may be necessary in individuals with renal impairment. Slowly taper to discontinuation to prevent withdrawal

alcohol use disorder in Europe, but it is not approved for use in the U.S. and is not discussed here.

- Topiramate is an FDA-approved treatment for epilepsy and migraine. There is meta-analytic evidence from randomized controlled trials that treatment with topiramate is associated with decreased drinking days, drinks per drinking day, and heavy drinking days when compared with placebo [61]. Topiramate decreases excitatory neurotransmission by acting on AMPA and kainate receptors and increases inhibitory neurotransmission by enhancing GABA-A conduction [72]. Topiramate also inhibits carbonic anhydrase and acts on several other types of receptors, including L-type calcium channels and voltage-dependent sodium channels [72].

- Gabapentin targets voltage-gated calcium channels and is FDA-approved as a treatment for postherpetic neuralgia and as an adjunctive therapy for epilepsy. The evidence for its effectiveness is promising, but mixed. Research indicates that gabapentin is particularly effective in reducing the frequency of heavy drinking days [73], decreasing the number of drinks consumed per drinking day [74], and alleviating cravings [75–77]. Additionally, it has been shown to prolong the time to relapse, with notably greater success observed among individuals experiencing more severe withdrawal symptoms prior to treatment [78, 79]. Overall, gabapentin may be most effective for treating heavy drinking days and treating AUD in individuals with a history of more severe withdrawal [77, 81]. There is also evidence from one trial that a combination of gabapentin and naltrexone in the first 6 weeks after drinking cessation performed better than naltrexone alone at preventing relapse to heavy drinking [82]. However, a large multicenter alcohol use disorder trial investigating gabapentin enacarbil extended-release, a longer-acting prodrug formulation of gabapentin, showed no effect on any drinking outcome measure [80]. Gabapentin has been demonstrated to have some potential for misuse [83], so adherence with the prescribed dosage should be closely monitored.
- Baclofen is a selective $GABA_B$ receptor agonist that is FDA-approved for the treatment of spasticity associated with multiple sclerosis and spinal cord diseases. Baclofen is more frequently used in some European countries as an off-label medication for alcohol use disorder. However, the evidence for baclofen's efficacy is mixed [84]. Although three meta-analyses reported increased abstinence days after treatment with baclofen [62, 85, 86], the strength of evidence was low given substantial heterogeneity in effect sizes [62, 86]. A meta-analysis by Bschor and colleagues [87] reported no significant superiority of baclofen over placebo. While some physicians prescribe baclofen to patients who are actively drinking, there is an increased risk of side effects in individuals who consume alcohol while taking baclofen and most trials have tested baclofen in abstinent patients [88]. One RCT found that patients with AUD and liver cirrhosis randomized to baclofen had higher rates of abstinence than patients assigned to placebo, suggesting that baclofen could be useful in patients with both conditions [89], although additional studies are needed.

Chapter Review Questions

1. A 67-year-old man with a long history of alcohol use disorder presents to the emergency room with moderate symptoms of alcohol withdrawal and a CIWA-Ar score of 15. His medical history is significant for cirrhosis. Which of the following is the most appropriate management strategy for this patient?

   A. Initiate symptom-triggered withdrawal management with diazepam until symptoms abate and the CIWA-Ar score is less than 10.

B. Start fixed-schedule dosing with diazepam to prevent withdrawal seizures, irrespective of the CIWA-Ar score.
C. Start symptom-triggered withdrawal management with lorazepam using the CIWA-Ar.
D. Begin fixed-schedule dosing with lorazepam.
E. Begin fixed-schedule dosing with diazepam.

Correct Answer: C.

Explanation: In patients with liver cirrhosis and the elderly, benzodiazepines such as lorazepam and oxazepam do not undergo extensive hepatic metabolism and are therefore preferred due to their safer pharmacokinetic profile. Chlordiazepoxide and diazepam are long-acting benzodiazepines that are extensively metabolized by the liver, making them less appropriate in an elderly patient with cirrhosis. A symptom-triggered regimen is appropriate in the emergency room where monitoring is available. Symptom-triggered approaches have been found to shorten the duration of treatment and reduce the overall dose of benzodiazepines required. Since there is no mention of a history of withdrawal seizures, there is no need to initiate a seizure-prevention protocol.

2. Alcohol use is a significant public health concern. Which of the following statements reflects current trends and risk factors associated with alcohol use in the United States?

A. The prevalence of alcohol use among pregnant women has steadily declined over the past decade, with less than 5% reporting alcohol use.
B. While alcohol use in men has always been higher than in women, recent data suggests that binge drinking in men significantly decreased over the past 10 years while it increased in women.
C. Binge drinking, defined by the NIAAA as five or more drinks in a single occasion for men and four drinks or more for women, has remained largely stable across all age groups, with no significant variation by sex or age.
D. Although alcohol use disorder remains more prevalent in men, recent data suggest a narrowing of the gender gap, with women showing an increase in both alcohol consumption and binge drinking over the past decade.
E. As a result of alcohol screening programs, the majority of individuals with alcohol use disorder receive pharmacological or psychotherapeutic treatment.

Correct Answer: D.

Explanation: Alcohol use during pregnancy is associated with an increased risk of fetal alcohol spectrum disorders (FASDs) and other developmental abnormalities. While 3.9% of pregnant women report binge drinking, the overall prevalence of alcohol use among pregnant women remains concerning, with more than 10% of pregnant women reporting alcohol use. Recent data indicate that while AUD is still more prevalent in men, the gap is narrowing as alcohol use and binge drinking have increased in women but stayed relatively stable in men. The current male-to-female ratio for AUD is 1.7:1. Despite alcohol screening programs, only a small percentage of those diagnosed are receiving pharmacological or psychotherapeutic interventions. Many barriers, including stigma, lack of awareness, or limited access to care, prevent individuals from seeking treatment.

3. A 49-year-old patient who has a long history of alcohol use is on a stable dose of naltrexone for 7 weeks. He mentions that he tolerates the medication well and reports less desire for alcohol. However, he has not been drinking for the past two days and complains about tremors and agitation. Which of the following best explains the neurobiological mechanism underlying alcohol withdrawal-related hyperexcitability?

   A. Acute alcohol intake enhances GABAergic transmission by increasing $GABA_A$ receptor activity, contributing to sedation and leading to enhanced inhibitory neurotransmission.
   B. Chronic alcohol exposure upregulates NMDA receptors. During alcohol withdrawal, GABA activity is decreased and there is increased glutamatergic transmission, contributing to hyperexcitability during withdrawal.
   C. Acute alcohol intake increases activity at both NMDA and $GABA_B$ receptors. Alcohol withdrawal leads to a downregulation of GABA receptors, increasing the risk for seizures.
   D. Chronic alcohol use increases activity at $GABA_A$ receptors and decreases kainate receptor function, enhancing inhibitory neurotransmission and reducing seizure risk during withdrawal.
   E. Chronic alcohol use decreases $GABA_A$ and NMDA receptor function, leading to seizures.

   Correct Answer: B.

   Explanation: Chronic alcohol exposure leads to an upregulation of NMDA receptors. This upregulation causes increased excitatory neurotransmission during alcohol withdrawal, resulting in hyperexcitability and an elevated risk of seizures. While acute alcohol intake inhibits NMDA receptors and enhances $GABA_A$ receptor function, chronic exposure produces the neuroadaptations that contribute to withdrawal symptoms.

4. A 52-year-old male with a 20-year history of AUD has been abstinent for 3 months. He is currently taking naltrexone to help reduce alcohol cravings but expresses concerns about potential relapse due to stress at work. He reports that his cravings have decreased but not completely disappeared.

   Which of the following statements describes the mechanisms of action and clinical use of medications in the treatment of AUD?

   A. Naltrexone is an opioid receptor agonist that reduces alcohol cravings by enhancing dopamine release in the nucleus accumbens, thereby reducing the reward response to alcohol.
   B. Acamprosate is thought to reduce alcohol cravings by modulating glutamatergic neurotransmission and restoring the balance between excitatory and inhibitory pathways disrupted by chronic alcohol use.
   C. Disulfiram acts primarily as an alcohol dehydrogenase inhibitor, leading to a buildup of acetaldehyde and functions as a form of aversion therapy.

D. Naltrexone and acamprosate are equally effective in preventing relapse, with both medications enhancing GABAergic neurotransmission to reduce cravings and decrease withdrawal symptoms.
E. Topiramate, an off-label anti-craving medication, exerts its effects by acting as a $GABA_A$ receptor agonist, reducing alcohol cravings by decreasing inhibitory neurotransmission.

Correct Answer: B.

Explanation: Naltrexone is a nonselective opioid receptor antagonist and acts by reducing the rewarding effects of alcohol. While the specific mechanisms through which acamprosate works to treat AUD remain under investigation, it is thought to reduce alcohol cravings by modulating glutamatergic neurotransmission. Disulfiram is an aldehyde (not alcohol) dehydrogenase inhibitor, leading to a buildup of acetaldehyde and functions as a form of aversion therapy, as patients avoid drinking due to the fear of disulfiram-ethanol reaction. Topiramate is an FDA-approved treatment for epilepsy and migraine. Topiramate decreases excitatory neurotransmission by acting on AMPA and kainate receptors and increases inhibitory neurotransmission by enhancing GABA-A conduction.

5. A 55-year-old man has been an inpatient at a residential treatment center for the past 6 days. He was intoxicated upon admission and has a long history of daily heavy alcohol use. He has no other health conditions. Which of the following biomarker profiles is most likely for this patient at this point in recovery?

	Ethyl glucuronide (EtG)	Gamma-glutamyl tranferase (GGT)	Mean corpuscular volume (MCV)	Phophatidylethanol (PEth)
A.	Negative	Elevated	Elevated	Positive
B.	Positive	Elevated	Elevated	Positive
C.	Negative	Normal	Normal	Positive
D.	Positive	Normal	Elevated	Positive
E.	Negative	Elevated	Elevated	Negative

Correct Answer: A.

Explanation: Ethyl glucuronide (EtG) is a direct biomarker that is most likely to test positive 24 h after alcohol consumption but can remain positive for up to 5 days following heavy consumption. Since this patient has not consumed alcohol for 6 days, his urine EtG will likely be negative. Phosphatidylethanol (PEth) may still test positive after 6 days and can remain detectable in whole blood for up to 2 weeks following heavy consumption. Gamma-glutamyltransferase (GGT) may be elevated after several weeks of heavy drinking and typically returns to normal after 2–6 weeks of abstinence. Mean corpuscular volume (MCV) is a measure of red blood cell size and can take several months to return to normal following alcohol use cessation.

References

1. Stanaway JD, Afshin A, Gakidou E, Lim SS, Abate D, Abate KH, et al. Global, regional, and national comparative risk assessment of 84 behavioural, environmental and occupational, and metabolic risks or clusters of risks for 195 countries and territories, 1990–2017: a systematic analysis for the Global Burden of Disease Study 2017. Lancet (London, England). 2018;392(10159):1923–94.
2. Kochanek KD, Murphy SL, Xu JQ, Arias E. Deaths: final data for 2020. Natl Vital Stat Rep. 2023;72(10):1–92. https://stacks.cdc.gov/view/cdc/131355
3. QuickStats: age-adjusted death rates* attributable to alcohol-induced causes, (dagger) by race/ethnicity – United States, 1999–2015. MMWR Morb Mortal Wkly Rep. 2017;66(18):491.
4. Grant BF, Goldstein RB, Saha TD, Chou SP, Jung J, Zhang H, et al. Epidemiology of DSM-5 alcohol use disorder: results from the National Epidemiologic Survey on Alcohol and Related Conditions III. JAMA Psychiat. 2015;72(8):757–66.
5. Grant BF, Chou SP, Saha TD, Pickering RP, Kerridge BT, Ruan WJ, et al. Prevalence of 12-month alcohol use, high-risk drinking, and DSM-IV alcohol use disorder in the United States, 2001–2002 to 2012–2013: results from the National Epidemiologic Survey on Alcohol and Related Conditions. JAMA Psychiat. 2017;74(9):911–23.
6. Substance Abuse and Mental Health Services Administration. Key substance use and mental health indicators in the United States: results from the 2023 National Survey on Drug Use and Health, HHS Publication No. PEP24-07-021, NSDUH Series H-59. Center for Behavioral Health Statistics and Quality, Substance Abuse and Mental Health Services Administration; 2024. https://www.samhsa.gov/data/report/2023-nsduh-annual-national-report
7. White AM, Castle IP, Powell PA, Hingson RW, Koob GF. Alcohol-related deaths during the COVID-19 pandemic. JAMA. 2022;327(17):1704–6. https://doi.org/10.1001/jama.2022.4308. PMID: 35302593; PMCID: PMC8933830
8. MacKillop J, Cooper A, Costello J. National retail sales of alcohol and cannabis during the COVID-19 pandemic in Canada. JAMA Netw Open. 2021;4(11):e2133076. https://doi.org/10.1001/jamanetworkopen.2021.33076.
9. White AM. Gender differences in the epidemiology of alcohol use and related harms in the United States. Alcohol Res. 2020;40(2):01. https://doi.org/10.35946/arcr.v40.2.01. PMID: 33133878; PMCID: PMC7590834
10. Hasin DS, Stinson FS, Ogburn E, Grant BF. Prevalence, correlates, disability, and comorbidity of DSM-IV alcohol abuse and dependence in the United States: results from the National Epidemiologic Survey on Alcohol and Related Conditions. Arch Gen Psychiatry. 2007;64(7):830–42.
11. Grucza RA, Sher KJ, Kerr WC, Krauss MJ, Lui CK, McDowell YE, Hartz S, Virdi G, Bierut LJ. Trends in adult alcohol use and binge drinking in the early 21st-century United States: a meta-analysis of 6 National Survey Series. Alcohol Clin Exp Re. 2018;42:1939–50. https://doi.org/10.1111/acer.13859.
12. Denny CH, Acero CS, Naimi TS, Kim SY. Consumption of alcohol beverages and binge drinking among pregnant women aged 18–44 years – United States, 2015–2017. MMWR Morb Mortal Wkly Rep. 2019;68(16):365–8. https://doi.org/10.15585/mmwr.mm6816a1. PMID: 31022164; PMCID: PMC6483284
13. Brady KT, Randall CL. Gender differences in substance use disorders. Psychiatr Clin North Am. 1999;22(2):241–52.
14. Kanny D, Naimi TS, Liu Y, Lu H, Brewer RD. Annual total binge drinks consumed by U.S. adults, 2015. Am J Prev Med. 2018;54(4):486–96.
15. Grant BF, Dawson DA. Age at onset of alcohol use and its association with DSM-IV alcohol abuse and dependence: results from the National Longitudinal Alcohol Epidemiologic Survey. J Subst Abus. 1997;9:103–10.
16. Substance Abuse and Mental Health Services Administration. Key substance use and mental health indicators in the United States: results from the 2020 National Survey on Drug Use and Health, HHS Publication No. PEP21-07-01-003, NSDUH Series H-56. Rockville: Center

for Behavioral Health Statistics and Quality, Substance Abuse and Mental Health Services Administration; 2021. Retrieved from https://www.samhsa.gov/data/
17. American Psychiatric Association. Diagnostic and statistical manual of mental disorders. 5th ed., text rev. https://doi.org/10.1176/appi.books.9780890425787
18. Gowin JL, Sloan ME, Stangl BL, Vatsalya V, Ramchandani VA. Vulnerability for alcohol use disorder and rate of alcohol consumption. Am J Psychiatry. 2017;174(11):1094–101.
19. Verhulst B, Neale MC, Kendler KS. The heritability of alcohol use disorders: a meta-analysis of twin and adoption studies. Psychol Med. 2015;45(5):1061–72.
20. Zhou H, Kember RL, Deak JD, Xu H, Toikumo S, Yuan K, Lind PA, Farajzadeh L, Wang L, Hatoum AS, Johnson J, Lee H, Mallard TT, Xu J, Johnston KJA, Johnson EC, Nielsen TT, Galimberti M, Dao C, Levey DF, Overstreet C, Byrne EM, Gillespie NA, Gordon S, Hickie IB, Whitfield JB, Xu K, Zhao H, Huckins LM, Davis LK, Sanchez-Roige S, Madden PAF, Heath AC, Medland SE, Martin NG, Ge T, Smoller JW, Hougaard DM, Børglum AD, Demontis D, Krystal JH, Gaziano JM, Edenberg HJ, Agrawal A, Million Veteran Program, Justice AC, Stein MB, Kranzler HR, Gelernter J. Multi-ancestry study of the genetics of problematic alcohol use in over 1 million individuals. Nat Med. 2023;29(12):3184–92. https://doi.org/10.1038/s41591-023-02653-5. Epub 2023 Dec 7. PMID: 38062264; PMCID: PMC10719093
21. Edenberg HJ, McClintick JN. Alcohol dehydrogenases, aldehyde dehydrogenases, and alcohol use disorders: a critical review. Alcohol Clin Exp Res. 2018;42(12):2281–97.
22. Walters RK, Polimanti R, Johnson EC, McClintick JN, Adams MJ, Adkins AE, et al. Transancestral GWAS of alcohol dependence reveals common genetic underpinnings with psychiatric disorders. Nat Neurosci. 2018;21(12):1656–69.
23. Li D, Zhao H, Gelernter J. Strong association of the alcohol dehydrogenase 1B gene (ADH1B) with alcohol dependence and alcohol-induced medical diseases. Biol Psychiatry. 2011;70(6):504–12.
24. Tawa EA, Hall SD, Lohoff FW. Overview of the genetics of alcohol use disorder. Alcohol Alcohol (Oxford, Oxfordshire). 2016;51(5):507–14.
25. Brooks PJ, Enoch MA, Goldman D, Li TK, Yokoyama A. The alcohol flushing response: an unrecognized risk factor for esophageal cancer from alcohol consumption. PLoS Med. 2009;6(3):e50.
26. Cederbaum AI. Alcohol metabolism. Clin Liver Dis. 2012;16(4):667–85.
27. National Institute on Alcohol Abuse and Alcoholism. Alcohol alert: alcohol metabolism. No. 35, PH 371. Bethesda: The Institute; 1997.
28. Hernandez-Munoz R, Caballeria J, Baraona E, Uppal R, Greenstein R, Lieber CS. Human gastric alcohol dehydrogenase: its inhibition by H2-receptor antagonists, and its effect on the bioavailability of ethanol. Alcohol Clin Exp Res. 1990;14(6):946–50.
29. Kumar S, Porcu P, Werner DF, Matthews DB, Diaz-Granados JL, Helfand RS, et al. The role of GABA(A) receptors in the acute and chronic effects of ethanol: a decade of progress. Psychopharmacology. 2009;205(4):529–64.
30. Lovinger DM, White G, Weight FF. Ethanol inhibits NMDA-activated ion current in hippocampal neurons. Science. 1989;243(4899):1721–4.
31. Gass JT, Olive MF. Glutamatergic substrates of drug addiction and alcoholism. Biochem Pharmacol. 2008;75(1):218–65.
32. Vonghia L, Leggio L, Ferrulli A, Bertini M, Gasbarrini G, Addolorato G. Acute alcohol intoxication. Eur J Intern Med. 2008;19(8):561–7.
33. National Institute on Alcohol Abuse and Alcoholism. Understanding the dangers of alcohol overdose; 2018. Available from: https://www.niaaa.nih.gov/publications/brochures-and-fact-sheets/understanding-dangers-of-alcohol-overdose.
34. Jung YC, Namkoong K. Alcohol: intoxication and poisoning – diagnosis and treatment. Handb Clin Neurol. 2014;125:115–21.
35. Marco CA, Kelen GD. Acute intoxication. Emerg Med Clin North Am. 1990;8(4):731–48.
36. Allison MG, McCurdy MT. Alcoholic metabolic emergencies. Emerg Med Clin North Am. 2014;32(2):293–301.

37. Center for Substance Abuse Treatment. Detoxification and substance abuse treatment, Treatment Improvement Protocol (TIP) Series, No. 45. HHS publication no. (SMA) 15-4131. Rockville: Center for Substance Abuse Treatment; 2006.
38. Bayard M, McIntyre J, Hill KR, Woodside J Jr. Alcohol withdrawal syndrome. Am Fam Physician. 2004;69(6):1443–50.
39. Rathlev NK, Ulrich AS, Delanty N, D'Onofrio G. Alcohol-related seizures. J Emerg Med. 2006;31(2):157–63.
40. Tovar R. Diagnosis and treatment of alcohol withdrawal. JCOM. 2011;18(8):361–70.
41. Schuckit MA. Recognition and management of withdrawal delirium (delirium tremens). N Engl J Med. 2014;371(22):2109–13.
42. Mayo-Smith MF, Beecher LH, Fischer TL, Gorelick DA, Guillaume JL, Hill A, et al. Management of alcohol withdrawal delirium. An evidence-based practice guideline. Arch Intern Med. 2004;164(13):1405–12.
43. Saddichha S, Manjunatha N, Prasad Sinha BN, Khess CRJ. Delayed-onset delirium tremens – a diagnostic and management challenge. Acta Neuropsychiatrica. 2008;20(3):152–6. https://doi.org/10.1111/j.1601-5215.2008.00285.x.
44. The ASAM Clinical Practice Guideline on Alcohol Withdrawal Management. J Addict Med. 2020;14(3S Suppl 1):1–72. https://doi.org/10.1097/ADM.0000000000000668. Erratum in: J Addict Med. 2020 Sep/Oct;14(5):e280. doi:10.1097/ADM.0000000000000731
45. Maldonado JR, Sher Y, Das S, Hills-Evans K, Frenklach A, Lolak S, Talley R, Neri E. Prospective validation study of the Prediction of Alcohol Withdrawal Severity Scale (PAWSS) in medically ill inpatients: a new scale for the prediction of complicated alcohol withdrawal syndrome. Alcohol Alcohol. 2015;50(5):509–18. https://doi.org/10.1093/alcalc/agv043. Epub 2015 May 21
46. Helander A, Bottcher M, Fehr C, Dahmen N, Beck O. Detection times for urinary ethyl glucuronide and ethyl sulfate in heavy drinkers during alcohol detoxification. Alcohol Alcohol. 2009;44(1):55–61.
47. Jatlow PI, Agro A, Wu R, Nadim H, Toll BA, Ralevski E, et al. Ethyl glucuronide and ethyl sulfate assays in clinical trials, interpretation, and limitations: results of a dose ranging alcohol challenge study and 2 clinical trials. Alcohol Clin Exp Res. 2014;38(7):2056–65.
48. Wojcik MH, Hawthorne JS. Sensitivity of commercial ethyl glucuronide (ETG) testing in screening for alcohol abstinence. Alcohol Alcohol (Oxford, Oxfordshire). 2007;42(4):317–20.
49. Hansson P, Caron M, Johnson G, Gustavsson L, Alling C. Blood phosphatidylethanol as a marker of alcohol abuse: levels in alcoholic males during withdrawal. Alcohol Clin Exp Res. 1997;21(1):108–10.
50. Harris JC, Leggio L, Farokhnia M. Blood biomarkers of alcohol use: a scoping review. Curr Addict Rep. 2021;8(4):500–8. https://doi.org/10.1007/s40429-021-00402-7. Epub 2021 Oct 15. PMID: 37274945; PMCID: PMC10237590
51. Allen JP, Sillanaukee P, Strid N, Litten RZ. In: Allen JP, Wilson VB, editors. Biomarkers of heavy drinking. Bethesda: U.S. Department of Health and Human Services; 2003. p. 37–53.
52. Rafaqat S, Sattar A, Khalid A, Rafaqat S. Role of liver parameters in diabetes mellitus – a narrative review. Endocr Regul. 2023;57(1):200–20. https://doi.org/10.2478/enr-2023-0024.
53. Babor TF, Higgins-Biddle JC, Saunders JB, Monteiro MG. The alcohol use disorders identification test. Guidelines for use in primary health care. Geneva: World Health Organization; 1992.
54. Bush K, Kivlahan DR, McDonell MB, Fihn SD, Bradley KA, for the Ambulatory Care Quality Improvement Project (ACQUIP). The AUDIT alcohol consumption questions (AUDIT-C): an effective brief screening test for problem drinking. Arch Intern Med. 1998;158(16):1789–95. https://doi.org/10.1001/archinte.158.16.1789.
55. Bradley KA, Bush KR, Epler AJ, et al. Two brief alcohol-screening tests from the Alcohol Use Disorders Identification Test (AUDIT): validation in a female veterans affairs patient population. Arch Intern Med. 2003;163(7):821–9. https://doi.org/10.1001/archinte.163.7.821.
56. Mayfield D, McLeod G, Hall P. The CAGE questionnaire: validation of a new alcoholism screening instrument. Am J Psychiatry. 1974;131(10):1121–3.

57. Anton RF, O'Malley SS, Ciraulo DA, Cisler RA, Couper D, Donovan DM, et al. Combined pharmacotherapies and behavioral interventions for alcohol dependence: the COMBINE study: a randomized controlled trial. JAMA. 2006;295(17):2003–17.
58. Kranzler HR. Overview of alcohol use disorder. Am J Psychiatry. 2023;180(8):565–72. https://doi.org/10.1176/appi.ajp.20230488.
59. Matching Alcoholism Treatments to Client Heterogeneity. Project MATCH posttreatment drinking outcomes. J Stud Alcohol. 1997;58(1):7–29. https://doi.org/10.15288/jsa.1997.58.7.
60. Anton RF, O'Malley SS, Ciraulo DA, Cisler RA, Couper D, Donovan DM, Gastfriend DR, Hosking JD, Johnson BA, JS LC, Longabaugh R, Mason BJ, Mattson ME, Miller WR, Pettinati HM, Randall CL, Swift R, Weiss RD, Williams LD, Zweben A, COMBINE Study Research Group. Combined pharmacotherapies and behavioral interventions for alcohol dependence: the COMBINE study: a randomized controlled trial. JAMA. 2006;295(17):2003–17. https://doi.org/10.1001/jama.295.17.2003.
61. Jonas DE, Amick HR, Feltner C, Bobashev G, Thomas K, Wines R, et al. Pharmacotherapy for adults with alcohol use disorders in outpatient settings: a systematic review and meta-analysis. JAMA. 2014;311(18):1889–900.
62. McPheeters M, O'Connor EA, Riley S, Kennedy SM, Voisin C, Kuznacic K, Coffey CP, Edlund MD, Bobashev G, Jonas DE. Pharmacotherapy for alcohol use disorder: a systematic review and meta-analysis. JAMA. 2023;330(17):1653–65. https://doi.org/10.1001/jama.2023.19761. PMID: 37934220; PMCID: PMC10630900
63. Center for Substance Abuse Treatment. Incorporating alcohol pharmacotherapies into medical practice, Treatment Improvement Protocol (TIP) series 49. HHS publication no. (SMA) 09-4380. Rockville: Substance Abuse and Mental Health Services Administration; 2009.
64. Singh D, Saadabadi A. Naltrexone. In: StatPearls [Internet]. Treasure Island: StatPearls Publishing; 2025. [Updated 2023 May 30]. Available from: https://www.ncbi.nlm.nih.gov/books/NBK534811/.
65. Kalk NJ, Lingford-Hughes AR. The clinical pharmacology of acamprosate. Br J Clin Pharmacol. 2014;77(2):315–23.
66. Kampman KM, Pettinati HM, Lynch KG, Xie H, Dackis C, Oslin DW, Sparkman T, Sharkoski T, O'Brien CP. Initiating acamprosate within-detoxification versus post-detoxification in the treatment of alcohol dependence. Addict Behav. 2009;34(6-7):581–6. https://doi.org/10.1016/j.addbeh.2009.03.014. Epub 2009 Mar 24. PMID: 19345510; PMCID: PMC2729436
67. Stokes M, Patel P, Abdijadid S. Disulfiram. In: StatPearls [Internet]. Treasure Island: StatPearls Publishing; 2024. [Updated 2024 Mar 21]. Available from: https://www.ncbi.nlm.nih.gov/books/NBK459340/.
68. Kranzler HR, Soyka M. Diagnosis and pharmacotherapy of alcohol use disorder: a review. JAMA. 2018;320(8):815–24.
69. Skinner MD, Lahmek P, Pham H, Aubin HJ. Disulfiram efficacy in the treatment of alcohol dependence: a meta-analysis. PLoS One. 2014;9(2):e87366.
70. Fuller RK, Branchey L, Brightwell DR, Derman RM, Emrick CD, Iber FL, James KE, Lacoursiere RB, Lee KK, Lowenstam I, et al. Disulfiram treatment of alcoholism. A Veterans Administration cooperative study. JAMA. 1986;256(11):1449–55.
71. Jonas DE, Amick HR, Feltner C, Bobashev G, Thomas K, Wines R, Kim MM, Shanahan E, Gass CE, Rowe CJ, Garbutt JC. Pharmacotherapy for adults with alcohol-use disorders in outpatient settings [Internet]. Rockville: Agency for Healthcare Research and Quality (US); 2014. Report No.: 14-EHC029-EF
72. Kenna GA, Lomastro TL, Schiesl A, Leggio L, Swift RM. Review of topiramate: an antiepileptic for the treatment of alcohol dependence. Curr Drug Abuse Rev. 2009;2(2):135–42.
73. Mason BJ, Quello S, Goodell V, Shadan F, Kyle M, Begovic A. Gabapentin treatment for alcohol dependence: a randomized clinical trial. JAMA Intern Med. 2014;174(1):70–7. https://doi.org/10.1001/jamainternmed.2013.11950. PMID: 24190578; PMCID: PMC3920987
74. Furieri FA, Nakamura-Palacios EM. Gabapentin reduces alcohol consumption and craving: a randomized, double-blind, placebo-controlled trial. J Clin Psychiatry. 2007;68(11):1691–700. https://doi.org/10.4088/jcp.v68n1108.

75. Mason BJ, Light JM, Williams LD, Drobes DJ. Proof-of-concept human laboratory study for protracted abstinence in alcohol dependence: effects of gabapentin. Addict Biol. 2009;14(1):73–83. https://doi.org/10.1111/j.1369-1600.2008.00133.x. Epub 2008 Oct 9. PMID: 18855801; PMCID: PMC2758315
76. Pani PP, Trogu E, Pacini M, Maremmani I. Anticonvulsants for alcohol dependence. Cochrane Database Syst Rev. 2014;2014(2):CD008544. https://doi.org/10.1002/14651858.CD008544.pub2. PMID: 24523233; PMCID: PMC10585425
77. Mason BJ, Quello S, Shadan F. Gabapentin for the treatment of alcohol use disorder. Expert Opin Investig Drugs. 2018;27(1):113–24.
78. Burnette EM, Nieto SJ, Grodin EN, Meredith LR, Hurley B, Miotto K, Gillis AJ, Ray LA. Novel agents for the pharmacological treatment of alcohol use disorder. Drugs. 2022;82(3):251–74. https://doi.org/10.1007/s40265-021-01670-3. Epub 2022 Feb 8. PMID: 35133639; PMCID: PMC8888464
79. Anton RF, Latham P, Voronin K, Book S, Hoffman M, Prisciandaro J, Bristol E. Efficacy of gabapentin for the treatment of alcohol use disorder in patients with alcohol withdrawal symptoms: a randomized clinical trial. JAMA Intern Med. 2020;180(5):728–36. https://doi.org/10.1001/jamainternmed.2020.0249. PMID: 32150232; PMCID: PMC7063541
80. Falk DE, Ryan ML, Fertig JB, Devine EG, Cruz R, Brown ES, et al. Gabapentin Enacarbil extended-release for alcohol use disorder: a randomized, double-blind, placebo-controlled, multisite trial assessing efficacy and safety. Alcohol Clin Exp Res. 2019;43(1):158–69.
81. Andrade C. Gabapentin for alcohol-related disorders: critical appraisal of the symptom-driven approach. J Clin Psychiatry. 2020;81(6):20f13775. https://doi.org/10.4088/JCP.20f13775.
82. Anton RF, Myrick H, Wright TM, Latham PK, Baros AM, Waid LR, et al. Gabapentin combined with naltrexone for the treatment of alcohol dependence. Am J Psychiatry. 2011;168(7):709–17.
83. Evoy KE, Morrison MD, Saklad SR. Abuse and misuse of pregabalin and gabapentin. Drugs. 2017;77(4):403–26.
84. de Beaurepaire R, Sinclair JMA, Heydtmann M, Addolorato G, Aubin HJ, Beraha EM, et al. The use of baclofen as a treatment for alcohol use disorder: a clinical practice perspective. Front Psych. 2018;9:708.
85. Pierce M, Sutterland A, Beraha EM, Morley K, van den Brink W. Efficacy, tolerability, and safety of low-dose and high-dose baclofen in the treatment of alcohol dependence: a systematic review and meta-analysis. Eur Neuropsychopharmacol. 2018;28(7):795–806. https://doi.org/10.1016/j.euroneuro.2018.03.017. Epub 2018 Jun 20
86. Rose AK, Jones A. Baclofen: its effectiveness in reducing harmful drinking, craving, and negative mood. A meta-analysis. Addiction. 2018;113(8):1396–406. https://doi.org/10.1111/add.14191. Epub 2018 Mar 24
87. Bschor T, Henssler J, Müller M, Baethge C. Baclofen for alcohol use disorder-a systematic meta-analysis. Acta Psychiatr Scand. 2018;138(3):232–42. https://doi.org/10.1111/acps.12905. Epub 2018 Jun 10
88. Agabio R, Sinclair JM, Addolorato G, Aubin HJ, Beraha EM, Caputo F, et al. Baclofen for the treatment of alcohol use disorder: the Cagliari statement. Lancet Psychiatry. 2018;5(12):957–60.
89. Addolorato G, Leggio L, Ferrulli A, Cardone S, Vonghia L, Mirijello A, Abenavoli L, D'Angelo C, Caputo F, Zambon A, Haber PS, Gasbarrini G. Effectiveness and safety of baclofen for maintenance of alcohol abstinence in alcohol-dependent patients with liver cirrhosis: randomised, double-blind controlled study. Lancet. 2007;370(9603):1915–22. https://doi.org/10.1016/S0140-6736(07)61814-5.

9 Benzodiazepines and Other Sedatives, Hypnotics, and Anxiolytics

Christine LaGrotta and Anil Thomas

High-Yield Review Points

- The incidence of benzodiazepine use, both prescribed and non-prescribed, has been increasing in the past two decades, and the risk of interaction between opioids and benzodiazepines is becoming more important because of concerns about high rates of concurrent use, synergistic effects with concurrent use, and high rates of concurrent use in fatal opioid overdoses.
- Sedative, hypnotic, and anxiolytic intoxication must be evaluated to determine risk for toxicity, overdose, and withdrawal complications, as well as assessing for other causes of altered mental status such as co-ingestion with additional CNS depressants.
- Withdrawal from sedatives, hypnotics, and anxiolytics can be a medical emergency that can lead to seizures and death.
- Barbiturates, though less commonly prescribed than benzodiazepines, have a narrower therapeutic index and are more lethal in overdose than other sedative-hypnotics.
- Selective benzodiazepine receptor medications, also known as nonbenzodiazepine "Z"-drugs, are prescribed for insomnia, but can have adverse effects that need to be recognized by clinicians, such as withdrawal, hallucinations, amnesia, parasomnias, coma, and death.

C. LaGrotta (✉)
Department of Psychiatry, James J. Peters Bronx VA Hospital, Bronx, NY, USA

A. Thomas
Department of Psychiatry, NYU Grossman School of Medicine, New York, NY, USA
e-mail: Anil.Thomas@nyulangone.org

C. Marienfeld, M. Soltani (eds.), *AAAP Review of Addiction Psychiatry*,
https://doi.org/10.1007/978-3-032-24174-0_9

Epidemiology

The 2023 National Survey on Drug Use and Health (NSDUH) showed the incidence of prescription tranquilizer or sedative misuse in the United States was 1.7% of people aged 12 and older, representing about 4.7 million people. The NSDUH included benzodiazepines, muscle relaxants, barbiturates and Z-drugs in these statistics. In 2023, the percentage of people aged 12 and older who misused prescription tranquilizers or sedatives was highest among Multiracial and White people (2.2% and 1.9%, respectively) [1]. Between 1996 and 2013, the percentage of adults filling a benzodiazepine prescription increased from 4.1% to 5.6% with an annual percentage change of 2.5%. During that time period (1996–2013), the overdose rate increased from 0.58 to 3.07 per 100,000 adults (with a plateau from 2010 onward) [2]. Between 2000 and 2019, there was a total of 118,208 benzodiazepine involved overdose deaths in the United States. In 83.5% of these deaths, opioids were co-involved. During this same time period, benzodiazepine involved overdose deaths increased among all racial groups and both sexes [3]. Another study showed that among US adults, between 2015 and 2016, 12.5% of the population used benzodiazepines, 2.1% misused benzodiazepines at least once, and 0.2% had a benzodiazepine use disorder [4]. Rates of use worldwide appear to be similar to those reported in the United States [5].

In the past few years, especially with the current increased problems with opioids, even more attention is being given to benzodiazepines because of concerns about high rates of concurrent use, synergistic effects with concurrent use, and high rates of concurrent use in fatal opioid overdoses. Nonmedical benzodiazepine use is common in those with opioid use disorder, which is concerning because of the synergistic risk for overdose when opioids and benzodiazepines are combined. The number of deaths involving benzodiazepines, in combination with other synthetic narcotics, has been steadily increasing since 2014, while the number of deaths involving benzodiazepines without any opioids has remained steady. Between 2007 and 2017 there was a 1.7-fold increase in deaths involving benzodiazepines only, while there was a 2.8-fold increase in deaths involving benzodiazepine and any opioids and an 11.2-fold increase in death involving benzodiazepines and other synthetic narcotics [6]. A potential explanation for the co-occurring nonmedical use of benzodiazepines and opioids is that nonmedical use of these medications might help reduce anxiety, sleep disruption, or an acute protracted withdrawal associated with opioid use [7].

Benzodiazepines

Risk Factors

The main risk factors for diagnosis of a benzodiazepine use disorder include participation in a self-help group for medication dependence, younger age, longer duration of benzodiazepine use, higher dose of benzodiazepine, the interaction of higher benzodiazepine dose with longer duration of benzodiazepine use, lower level of education, non-native cultural origin and outpatient treatment for alcohol and/or drug dependence. Less predictive risk factors are a short benzodiazepine half-life and higher levels of depression and anxiety [8].

Mechanism of Action

Benzodiazepines, as well as barbiturates and "Z-drugs," work on the gamma-aminobutyric acid (GABA) system in the body. GABA is synthesized by the neurotransmitter glutamate and is the primary inhibitory neurotransmitter in both the brain and spinal cord. There are three different types of GABA receptors: two ionotropic (GABA-A and GABA-C) and one metabotropic, G-protein-coupled receptor (GABA-B). When GABA binds the ionotropic receptor, ion channels open and an influx of negative chloride (Cl-) ions results in inhibition of the neuron. Benzodiazepines, barbiturates, and alcohol all bind GABA-A receptors. Benzodiazepines act as positive allosteric modulators at the GABA-A receptor, specifically binding in a pocket created by the alpha and gamma subunits, thus causing a conformational change that allows GABA to bind. There are two benzodiazepine receptor subunits: benzodiazepine subunit 1 (BZD1) and benzodiazepine subunit 2 (BZD2). BZD1 receptors are highly concentrated in the cortex, thalamus, and cerebellum and are responsible for the sedative effects and anterograde amnesia caused by benzodiazepines. BZD2 receptors are highly concentrated in the limbic system, motor neurons and dorsal horn of the spinal cord and are responsible for the anxiolytic effects of benzodiazepines [9].

Benzodiazepines increase the *frequency* of GABA-A receptor openings, while barbiturates increase the *duration* of opening, both resulting in an increase in Cl- ions into the neuron, causing further inhibition. GABA-B receptors are thought to be important in pain, mood, and memory, while the function of GABA-C receptors is not known. With chronic exposure to benzodiazepines, there is both a decreased GABA-A receptor response as well as a change in the expression of this receptor subtype. Because of this, there is less of an inhibitory response and physical dependence emerges. With chronic exposure there is an increased expression of excitatory glutamatergic neurons and, upon withdrawal, this increase in unopposed excess glutamatergic activity leads to some of the clinical symptoms of benzodiazepine withdrawal (see below).

Similar to other substances that are misused, benzodiazepines increase dopamine (DA) in the mesolimbic dopaminergic reward system. The ventral tegmental area (VTA) contains GABA interneurons (as well as glutamate and dopamine neurons). When benzodiazepines bind to the GABA interneurons, the neurons are hyperpolarized, and then no longer inhibit DA neurons, thus removing a control on their activity. Since GABA is inhibitory, there is subsequently more dopamine released (less inhibition).

Pharmacokinetics

The onset and duration of action of benzodiazepines is largely determined by three factors: half-life, rate of absorption, and lipophilicity. Half-life is determined by how quickly the drug is metabolized and the presence of active metabolites. The greater the lipophilicity of a drug, the quicker it crosses the blood–brain barrier, causing a more rapid effect. This rapid effect leads to a DA spike in the DA reward pathways that is more reinforcing or rewarding than a slower onset. Benzodiazepines can be divided into three categories based on onset of action: short acting (15–30 min; with rapid acting being within 15 min), intermediate acting (30–60 min), and long acting (1+ h). See Table 9.1 for the characteristics of common benzodiazepines. All benzodiazepines are metabolized by the liver, though certain ones (oxazepam, temazepam and lorazepam) only undergo hepatic conjugation and then do not have any active metabolites. The rest of the benzodiazepines also undergo CYP-mediated oxidation, and many have active metabolites and thus longer duration of action [12].

Diagnosis

Diagnosis of a use disorder is made using DSM-5-TR criteria under the heading of Sedative, Hypnotic, or Anxiolytic Use Disorder. As with other substances, the severity of the use disorder is classified based on the number of criteria met. The criteria are the same as other substance use disorders and as reported elsewhere in this book. The diagnosis for intoxication and withdrawal is discussed below.

Tapering Benzodiazepines

Discontinuing benzodiazepines can be challenging, especially because physical dependence is expected with long term use. Care must be taken in the benzodiazepine tapering process because abrupt discontinuation can lead to dangerous withdrawal symptoms, including death. Discontinuation or a short taper can be considered when

Table 9.1 Pharmacology of commonly used benzodiazepines [10, 11]

Drug	Relative potency (mg)	Onset of action[a]	Peak onset (h)	Elimination half-life[b] (h)
Alprazolam	0.5	Intermediate	0.5–1.5	6–20[c]
Chlordiazepoxide	10	Intermediate	2-4	3–100
Clonazepam	0.25–0.5	Intermediate	1–4	18–40
Diazepam	5	Rapid	0.5–1	40–120[d]
Lorazepam	1	Intermediate	2–4	10–20
Oxazepam	15	Slow	2–3	5–20

[a]Rapid = 15 min, Intermediate = 15–30 min, Slow = 30–60 min
[b]Includes metabolites
[c]Varies with age, hepatic functioning, and weight
[d]Increased in older age, renal, or hepatic impairment

the risk of physical dependence is thought to be low or not existent, but if it is thought that the patient is physically dependent, a taper should occur. When deciding if a patient who is on chronic benzodiazepines should be tapered, a risk/benefit analysis should be done every 3 months (which should include but not be limited to the state's PDMP). This should be done in conjunction with the patient whenever possible [13].

If possible, if there are no contraindications, it should be considered to switch to a long-acting benzodiazepine. Initially, a taper of about 5%–10% should be considered, with no more than 25% reduction every 2 weeks [13].

Intoxication

Clinical Syndrome

According to the DSM-5-TR signs of benzodiazepine intoxication include one or more of the following (developing during or shortly after use): slurred speech, incoordination, unsteady gait, nystagmus, impairment in cognition (attention or memory), and stupor or coma. The impairment in memory that occurs during intoxication is most often characterized by anterograde amnesia [14].

Overdose

Benzodiazepine overdose most commonly presents as central nervous system (CNS) depression with normal vital signs, and the patient is often able to provide a history. Benzodiazepines have a relatively large therapeutic index, and thus, on their own, overdoses will usually exhibit relatively mild CNS symptoms [15]. There is concern with co-ingestion with other substances, most often alcohol, and now opioids. Respiratory compromise is unlikely, unless co-ingestion with another CNS depressant has occurred (alcohol or opioids commonly). Respiratory compromise also depends on other factors, such as tolerance, weight, age, and genetics. The clinical presentation is similar to other depressants including ethanol, barbiturates, gamma hydroxybutyrate (GHB), and chloral hydrate. A differential diagnosis of benzodiazepine overdose can include other substances, hypoglycemia, carbon monoxide poisoning, stroke, meningitis, and encephalitis. The workup should include glucose levels, acetaminophen and salicylate levels, a pregnancy test, an EKG, and ethanol levels. Head CT and cerebrospinal analysis should be considered if clinically indicated.

Laboratory/Diagnostic Evaluation

Urine immunoassay drug screens typically do not detect for the parent compound; rather they test for metabolites like nordiazepam and oxazepam. Oxazepam is a metabolite of diazepam, temazepam, and chlordiazepoxide. Other benzodiazepines have a low cross-reactivity in the immunoassay, so that several routinely ingested benzodiazepines are often missed if taken in low doses, including clonazepam, lorazepam, alprazolam, or midazolam. Immunoassays used can vary across labs and may have different cross-reactants. False negatives can occur due to limited cross-reactivity, but false positives can occur with medications like sertraline [16]. Confirmatory testing, using gas or liquid chromatography and mass spectrometry, can be helpful to differentiate benzodiazepine drugs, as well as identify those less reactive to the typical immunoassays.

Treatment

Treatment of intoxication starts with stabilization of the airway, breathing, and circulation. Once the diagnosis of benzodiazepine overdose or intoxication is established, targeted treatment can occur. Using activated charcoal as a gastrointestinal decontaminant is not recommended due to increased risk of aspiration. Flumazenil is a specific and competitive antagonist at the benzodiazepine receptor that reverses the effects of agonists. It is given as 0.1–0.3 mg IV over 30 s. This dose can be repeated if necessary. Usually, response will occur with doses <1.0 mg in pure benzodiazepine overdose and <2.0 mg in a mixed overdose. Due to the short half-life of flumazenil, re-sedation may occur after administration, requiring re-administration. Controversy exists over the use of flumazenil in clinical situations, particularly in those with a history of seizures (especially withdrawal seizures) or who were given benzodiazepines for seizure control, as it can precipitate seizures in those with benzodiazepine tolerance. Caution should be used if a patient's EKG is indicative of tricyclic antidepressant overdose, in patients taking drugs that could cause seizures in overdose, and in patients taking MAOIs, lithium, and arrhythmogenic drugs [17].

Withdrawal

Clinical Syndrome

Individuals can become tolerant to benzodiazepines in a few weeks, and physical dependence can occur quickly, putting the person at risk for withdrawal. Benzodiazepine withdrawal is named in the DSM-5-TR as Sedative, Hypnotic, or Anxiolytic Withdrawal and is defined as cessation in (or reduction in) sedative, hypnotic, or anxiolytic use that has been prolonged. Two or more of the following must be present: (1) autonomic hyperactivity (e.g., sweating or pulse rate > 100 bpm), (2) hand tremor, (3) insomnia, (4) nausea or vomiting, (5) transient visual, tactile, or auditory hallucinations or illusions, (6) psychomotor agitation, (7) anxiety, and (8) grand mal seizures [14].

Though the DSM-5-TR lists the eight symptoms above, this is not an exhaustive list. Withdrawal symptoms can be divided into psychological and physical. Psychological symptoms can include increased anxiety, excitability, insomnia and nightmares, panic attacks and agoraphobia, social phobia, perceptual distortions, depersonalization, derealization, hallucinations, misperceptions, depression, obsessions, paranoid thoughts, irritability, and poor memory and concentration. Physical symptoms can include headache, body pain/stiffness, seizure, tingling, numbness, altered sensation, weakness, fatigue, influenza-like symptoms, muscle twitches, jerks, tics, electric shock-like sensations, tremor, dizziness, light-headedness, tinnitus, hypersensitivity (to light, sounds, tough, taste and smell), gastrointestinal symptoms (nausea, vomiting, diarrhea, constipation, pain, distension, difficulty swallowing), appetite or weight change, dry mouth, and metallic taste or an unusual smell [18].

Treatment

The mainstay for treatment of benzodiazepine withdrawal and benzodiazepine use disorder is to use benzodiazepines themselves to help control withdrawal symptoms. The goal is to eliminate withdrawal symptoms without causing excessive sedation or respiratory depression. A Cochrane systematic review noted that when withdrawing or tapering a person from benzodiazepines, a longer withdrawal (10 weeks) was preferred to a shorter time period because of a higher dropout rate in those being tapered too quickly. This specific review did not find much benefit in switching from a short-acting to a long-acting benzodiazepine. There was no evidence to support the use of propranolol, buspirone, progesterone, or hydroxyzine in terms of managing benzodiazepine withdrawal or improving abstinence. There was some evidence that carbamazepine might have been used as an adjunctive medication for benzodiazepine withdrawal, especially in individuals receiving the equivalent of 20 mg/day or more of diazepam [19].

Barbiturates

Mechanism of Action

Barbiturates, like benzodiazepines, have action at the GABA-A receptor. However, barbiturates increase the *duration* of opening of the GABA receptors while benzodiazepines increase the *frequency* of opening of the GABA receptors. In general, the barbiturates are well absorbed after oral administration. They are metabolized by the liver and excreted by the kidneys. The half-lives range from 1 to 120 h, depending on the substance.

Clinical Uses

Barbiturates are used less in the clinical setting since the development and increased popularity of benzodiazepines and other hypnotics. However, they still have some use in clinical practice. The barbiturate methohexital is used as an anesthetic agent for ECT as well as to abort prolonged seizures in ECT or to limit postictal agitation.

Phenobarbital is the most commonly used barbiturate for the treatment of seizures (including status epilepticus, generalized tonic-clonic, and simple partial seizures), and it is used for alcohol withdrawal, most commonly in emergency room settings or for persons refractory to benzodiazepine treatment for alcohol withdrawal. Butalbital is one ingredient in the pain medication Fioricet. The barbiturate amobarbital has historically been used to help in the diagnosis of different psychiatric conditions such as conversion disorder, catatonia, and unexplained muteness. On occasion, barbiturates can also be used for sleep as they reduce sleep latency and the number of awakenings per night. They are rarely used, however, as tolerance to these effects usually develops in about 2 weeks and discontinuation of the barbiturates can lead to rebound worsening of insomnia and serious withdrawal symptoms [20].

Adverse Effects

Barbiturates and benzodiazepines have many overlapping adverse effects. However, there are some that are more specific to barbiturates. These can include the development of Stevens-Johnson syndrome, megaloblastic anemia, and neutropenia. Barbiturates can also precipitate acute porphyria reactions. One of the biggest differences between benzodiazepines and barbiturates is the low therapeutic index of barbiturates, making fatal overdose more likely [20].

Intoxication with barbiturates is like that of benzodiazepines and includes delirium, confusion, and CNS and respiratory depression. Respiratory depression is more likely when there is co-ingestion of another CNS depressant.

Treatment

The treatment of barbiturate intoxication, withdrawal, and barbiturate use disorders are similar to that of benzodiazepines. There are also instances in which the treatment of the two differs.

Intoxication: As stated above, barbiturates have a narrower therapeutic index than benzodiazepines and so in the treatment of acute intoxication, one must be even more vigilant to assess airway, breathing, and circulation. In addition, since flumazenil binds to the benzodiazepine receptor, it will not reverse the effects of a barbiturate overdose [21].

Withdrawal: Treatment of withdrawal from barbiturates is like that of benzodiazepines. Though barbiturates can be used to treat withdrawal, because of the narrow therapeutic index, benzodiazepines are often used in a similar fashion to treat benzodiazepine withdrawal for barbiturate withdrawal.

Barbiturate Use Disorder: Falling also under the DSM-5-TR classification of Sedative, Hypnotic, or Anxiolytic Use Disorders, treatment is both pharmacologically and psychosocially similar to that of benzodiazepine use disorder.

Benzodiazepine Derivatives/"Z"-Drugs

Other sedative-hypnotics include the nonbenzodiazepine sleeping agents, more commonly referred to as "Z-drugs." The most common of these drugs in the US are zolpidem (Ambien), eszopiclone (Lunesta), and zaleplon (Sonata). These drugs also work at the GABA-A receptor, though they selectively have a high affinity for the alpha-1 subunit associated with the hypnotic-inducing effects of the benzodiazepine GABA-A receptor, with less affinity for the benzodiazepine 2 receptor, which is associated with ataxia and coordination impacts, as well as anxiolysis. They were introduced into the market in the 1990s and have only been FDA-approved for insomnia.

Pharmacology

Zolpidem is an imidazopyridine agent that acts mainly on the alpha-1 GABA-A receptor, with minimal effect on the alpha 2, 3, and 5 subunits. It is considered a potent sedative-hypnotic with little anxiolytic efficacy. The standard dose of the immediate release form (most commonly prescribed) is 10 mg in men and 5 mg in women (due to a recommendation from the FDA in 2013 stemming from increased duration of action in women), and a lower dose should be considered in the elderly. It is available in both an immediate-release and an extended-release preparation. It is metabolized by the CYP450 system (predominantly CYP3A4), thus requiring a lower dose in those with hepatic impairment [22].

Eszopiclone is a cyclopyrrolone drug that is the s-enantiomer of the racemic mixture zopiclone (only eszopiclone is available in the United States). Eszopiclone has affinity for the alpha 2 and 3 subunits at the GABA-A receptor. Note that zopiclone requires dose reduction in those with renal impairment, though there is no such recommendation for eszopiclone [22].

Zaleplon is a pyrazolopyrimidine drug that exerts its effects by selectively binding to the alpha-1 subunit of the benzodiazepine receptor with low affinity at the alpha 2 and 3 subunits. It is short-acting, which gives it the benefit of being able to be taken after trying to fall asleep or for a middle-of-the-night awakening. It is not useful in sleep maintenance. It has low bioavailability due to extensive first-pass hepatic metabolism and thus dosage decrease is recommended in patients with hepatic impairment [22]. See Table 9.2 for the pharmacology of commonly used "Z-drugs."

Adverse Effects

The most common adverse effects of the "Z-drugs" are headache, GI distress, and dizziness, though they are generally well tolerated. Ten to thirty-five percent of people taking zopiclone/eszopiclone noted a bitter or unpleasant taste that was bad enough to lead to cessation of the drug. All three drugs are on a list that was released

Table 9.2 Pharmacology of commonly used "Z-drugs" [22–25]

Generic name	Main clinical effect	Time to onset of effects (h)	Half-life (h)	Maximum daily dose
Zolpidem IR	Sleep initiation	1.6	1.4–4.5	5 mg for females 10 mg for males
Zolpidem ER	Sleep initiation and sleep maintenance	1.5	1.4–4.5	6.25 mg for females 12.5 mg for males
Eszopiclone	Sleep initiation and sleep maintenance	~1	~6	3 mg
Zaleplon	Sleep initiation	~1	~1	20 mg

by the FDA in 2007 as having a potential risk of increased sleep-related behaviors such as eating or driving while sleeping (this is especially concerning with the more commonly prescribed zolpidem). Daytime residual effects on cognition and psychomotor performance are a concern. They influence the next day's performance of body balance, reaction times, and ability to multitask [22]. In addition, among patients receiving prescription opioids, concomitant treatment with "Z-drugs" was associated with an increased risk of overdose [26].

There is also a concern for tolerance, dependence, and withdrawal from all the "Z-drugs"; however, this appears to be less common and less severe than with benzodiazepines. After cessation of the drug, especially higher doses of zolpidem, rebound insomnia can occur. The withdrawal from the drugs is similar to the withdrawal from other benzodiazepines and includes insomnia, delirium, craving, anxiety, tremor, palpitations, and rarely, seizures and psychosis [22].

Chapter Review Questions

1. A 26-year-old medical student would like to take a medication at night to help with anxiety and sleep but is worried that they will be groggy the next morning if the medication lasts too long in their system. The duration of action of a benzodiazepine is based on which of the following:

   A. The drug itself.
   B. The drug itself and all metabolites, both active and inactive.
   C. The drug itself and inactive metabolites.
   D. The drug itself and its active metabolites.
   E. Only the drug's active metabolites.

   Correct Answer: D.

   Explanation: The duration of action of a benzodiazepine is based on the drug itself and its active metabolites. Inactive metabolites do not have clinical effects and thus do not contribute to the duration of action of the benzodiazepine.

   Reference: Sankar [27].

2. A 35-year-old woman is found unconscious on the street when EMS is called. EMS arrives with both naloxone and flumazenil. Which of the following is true of flumazenil?

   A. If there is a suspected co-ingestion with opioids, naloxone should be given prior to flumazenil.
   B. There are no scales that can be used to monitor the effect of flumazenil.
   C. Once awoken with flumazenil, there is no need for readministration.
   D. It is metabolized by the kidney.
   E. Flumazenil can be given without consideration for a history of seizures.

   Correct Answer: A.

   Explanation: If there is a suspected co-ingestion with opioids, naloxone should be given prior to flumazenil as it is better tolerated and has a better safety profile. Flumazenil is metabolized by the liver. The Glasgow coma scale can be used to monitor the effects of flumazenil. Flumazenil has a short duration of action and may need to be readministered. The history of seizures should be considered before giving flumazenil in patients, particularly those with benzodiazepine dependence who are at risk for withdrawal seizures.

   Reference: Weinbroum et al. [17].

3. A 38-year-old male with a sedative hypnotic use disorder runs out of alprazolam and asks a friend for some of his. His friend says that he has a medication that is similar to alprazolam, but he heard that it may have some different side effects. Which of the following is a possible adverse effect of barbiturate use?

   A. Cough suppression
   B. Increased immune response
   C. Loss of appetite
   D. Constipation
   E. Stevens-Johnson syndrome

   Correct Answer: E.

   Explanation: Stevens-Johnson syndrome is an adverse effect of barbiturate use; others include the development of acute intermittent porphyria attacks, neutropenia, and megaloblastic anemia. The other answers are not adverse effects of barbiturate use.

   Reference: Sadock and Sadock [20].

4. A 36-year-old female is requesting a medication for anxiety in preparation for an upcoming overseas flight and is curious about the mechanism of action of the different medications. The binding of benzodiazepines and barbiturates to the GABA-A receptor allows for the influx of which of the following:

   A. Sodium
   B. Bicarbonate
   C. Chloride

D. Potassium
E. Glutamate

Correct Answer: C.

Explanation: The binding of benzodiazepines and barbiturates to the GABA-A receptor allows for the influx of negatively charged chloride ions. The other answers are simply distractors.

Reference: Twyman et al. [28].

5. A psychiatry resident is studying for his upcoming board examination and is curious about the difference in the mechanism of action of the different medications that he has been studying. Which of the following is a correct statement regarding benzodiazepines and barbiturates and the receptors they act upon?

   A. Barbiturates have a more dangerous withdrawal syndrome because of their binding to the GABA-C receptor.
   B. The alpha-1 subunit of the GABA-A receptor mediates sleep.
   C. Barbiturates bind to the GABA-B receptor.
   D. Benzodiazepines are less safe in overdose compared to barbiturates.
   E. There is no cross-tolerance between barbiturates and benzodiazepines.

   Correct Answer: B.

   Explanation: It is the alpha-1 subunit of the GABA-A receptor that is involved in mediating sleep (which is why the nonbenzodiazepine "Z-drugs" that act on the alpha-1 subunit are involved in promoting sleep). Barbiturates do have a dangerous withdrawal syndrome, but they act on the GABA-A receptor, making answer choices a and b incorrect. Barbiturates are more dangerous in overdose compared to benzodiazepines and there is cross-tolerance between barbiturates and benzodiazepines.

   Reference: Sadock and Sadock [20].

6. A 30-year-old male was recently admitted to an inpatient rehabilitation center for a sedative hypnotic use disorder and wonders about when he can consider himself in remission. According to the DSM-V-TR, for how long should a person *not* meet any criteria for sedative, hypnotic, or anxiolytic use disorder (except for craving) in order to be considered in early remission?

   A. As soon as they stop using the substance
   B. 3 months
   C. 1 month
   D. 2 weeks
   E. 12 months.

   Correct Answer: B.

   Explanation: This is a definition question from the DSM. Early remission is defined as at least 3 months while sustained remission is 12 months.

   Reference: American Psychiatric Association [14].

References

1. SAMHSA. The national survey on drug use and health. Substance Abuse and Mental Health Services Administration; 2023. https://www.samhsa.gov/data/sites/default/files/reports/rpt47095/National%20Report/National%20Report/2023-nsduh-annual-national.pdf.
2. Bachhuber MA, Hennessy S, Cunningham CO, Starrels JL. Increasing benzodiazepine prescriptions and overdose mortality in the United States, 1996–2013. Am J Public Health. 2016;106(4):686–8.
3. Kleinman RA, Weiss RD. Benzodiazepine-involved overdose deaths in the USA: 2000–2019. J Gen Intern Med. 2022;37(8):2103–9.
4. Blanco C, Han B, Jones CM, Johnson K, Compton WM. Prevalence and correlates of benzodiazepine use, misuse, and use disorders among adults in the United States. J Clin Psychiatry. 2018;79, 18m12174(6)
5. Votaw VR, Geyer R, Rieselbach MM, McHugh RK. The epidemiology of benzodiazepine misuse: a systematic review. Drug Alcohol Depend. 2019;200:95–114.
6. Drugabuse.gov. Overdose Death Rates. [online]. 2019. Available at: https://www.drugabuse.gov/related-topics/trends-statistics/overdose-death-rates. Accessed 9 May 2019.
7. McHugh RK, Votaw VR, Bogunovic O, Karakula SL, Griffin ML, Weiss RD. Anxiety sensitivity and nonmedical benzodiazepine use among adults with opioid use disorder. Addict Behav. 2017;65:283–8.
8. Kan CC, Hilberink SR, Breteler MH. Determination of the main risk factors for benzodiazepine dependence using a multivariate and multidimensional approach. Compr Psychiatry. 2004;45(2):88–94.
9. Griffin CE, Kaye AM, Bueno FR, Kaye AD. Benzodiazepine pharmacology and central nervous system–mediated effects. Ochsner J. 2013;13(2):214–23.
10. Msp.scdhhs.gov. [online]. 2019. Available at: https://msp.scdhhs.gov/tipsc/sites/default/files/tipSC%20Mar%202018%20benzoequivtable%2042018.pdf. Accessed 10 May 2019.
11. Vhpharmsci.com. Comparison of Benzodiazepines. [online]. 2019. Available at: http://www.vhpharmsci.com/vhformulary/tools/benzodiazepines-comparison.htm. Accessed 10 May 2019.
12. Mihic SJ, Harris RA. Chapter 17. Hypnotics and sedatives. In: Chabner BA, Knollmann BC, editors. Goodman & Gilman's the pharmacological basis of therapeutics. 12nd ed. New York: McGraw-Hill; 2011.
13. Team ASAM. Joint clinical practice guideline on benzodiazepine tapering, considerations when benzodiazepine risks outweigh benefits. J Gen Intern Med. 2025;40:2814–59.
14. American Psychiatric Association. Diagnostic and statistical manual of mental disorders, fifth edition, text revision. Arlington: American Psychiatric Association; 2022.
15. Gaudreault P, Guay J, Thivierge RL, Verdy I. Benzodiazepine poisoning. Drug Saf. 1991;6(4):247–65.
16. Nasky KM, Cowan GL, Knittel DR. False-positive urine screening for benzodiazepines: an association with sertraline?: a two-year retrospective chart analysis. Psychiatry (Edgmont). 2009;6(7):36.
17. Weinbroum AA, Flaishon R, Sorkine P, Szold O, Rudick V. A risk-benefit assessment of flumazenil in the management of benzodiazepine overdose. Drug Saf. 1997;17(3):181–96.
18. Schöpf J. Withdrawal phenomena after long-term administration of benzodiazepines a review of recent investigations. Pharmacopsychiatry. 1983;16(01):1–8.
19. Denis C, Fatseas M, Lavie E, Auriacombe M. Pharmacological interventions for benzodiazepine mono-dependence management in outpatient settings. Cochrane Database Syst Rev. 2006;3:CD005194.
20. Sadock BJ, Sadock VA. Kaplan and Sadock's synopsis of psychiatry: behavioral sciences/clinical psychiatry. Philadelphia: Lippincott Williams & Wilkins; 2015.
21. Sivilotti ML. Flumazenil, naloxone and the 'coma cocktail'. Br J Clin Pharmacol. 2016;81(3):428–36.

22. Gunja N. The clinical and forensic toxicology of Z-drugs. J Med Toxicol. 2013;9(2):155–62.
23. Salvà P, Costa J. Clinical pharmacokinetics and pharmacodynamics of zolpidem. Clin Pharmacokinet. 1995;29(3):142–53.
24. Brielmaier BD. Eszopiclone (Lunesta): a new nonbenzodiazepine hypnotic agent. In: Baylor University Medical Center proceedings, vol. 19 (no. 1). Taylor & Francis; 2006. p. 54–9.
25. Dooley M, Plosker GL. Zaleplon Drugs. 2000;60(2):413–45.
26. Szmulewicz A, Bateman BT, Levin R, Huybrechts KF. The risk of overdose with concomitant use of Z-drugs and prescription opioids: a population-based cohort study. Am J Psychiatry. 2021;178(7):643–50.
27. Sankar R. GABA(A) receptor physiology and its relationship to the mechanism of action of the 1,5-benzodiazepine clobazam. CNS Drugs. 2012;26(3):229–44. https://doi.org/10.2165/11599020.
28. Twyman RE, Rogers CJ, Macdonald RL. Differential regulation of γ-aminobutyric acid receptor channels by diazepam and phenobarbital. Ann Neurol. 1989;25(3):213–20.

Cannabinoids

10

Joao P. De Aquino, Julio C. Nunes, and Bachaar Arnaout

High-Yield Summary Points

- The psychoactive components and activity of cannabis and cannabinoid products vary widely, and most safety data come from studies involving products less potent than those currently available for public consumption.
- Cannabinoids have dose-dependent, often biphasic (i.e., low and high doses can have very different effects on symptoms such as anxiety, concentration, and analgesia), and time-dependent effects.
- While the medical use of cannabinoids may benefit a select group of patients, systematic scientific evidence supporting most claims remains limited.
- With increased accessibility and changes in cannabis laws, a growing number of patients are using cannabinoid products for medical purposes. Chronic pain is the most common indication, but currently, there is no high-quality evidence to routinely support this use.

Disclosures: Dr. De Aquino is supported by the grants K23DA052682, R21DA057240, and R01DA600066 from the National Institute on Drug Abuse (NIDA). Dr. De Aquino has been supported in clinical trials by Jazz Pharmaceuticals, specifically through medication provisions. Additionally, he has been a compensated consultant for Boehringer Ingelheim. Dr. Nunes is supported by a National Institute of Health (NIH) Research Training grant R25MH071584.

J. P. De Aquino (✉) · J. C. Nunes
Department of Psychiatry, Yale School of Medicine, New Haven, CT, USA

Department of Psychiatry, West Haven Veteran Affairs, West Haven, CT, USA
e-mail: joao.deaquino@yale.edu

B. Arnaout
Department of Psychiatry, Yale School of Medicine, New Haven, CT, USA

C. Marienfeld, M. Soltani (eds.), *AAAP Review of Addiction Psychiatry*,
https://doi.org/10.1007/978-3-032-24174-0_10

- Due to tolerance, patients may gradually require higher doses of cannabinoids to achieve the desired effect, and abrupt discontinuation may precipitate withdrawal.
- Cannabinoids may impair cognition, with effects potentially exacerbated when combined with other psychoactive substances, including opioids, benzodiazepines, and alcohol, or when used by those with neurocognitive disorders.
- Individuals with major psychiatric disorders and adolescents may be more prone to developing adverse effects from cannabinoids.
- New onset or worsening of anxiety, mood disturbance, cognitive impairment, or psychosis should prompt clinical evaluation to determine whether cannabinoids are a contributing factor.

Introduction

Epidemiology and Recent Trends in Cannabinoid Use

Cannabis is one of the most widely used substances in the United States. According to the 2023 National Survey on Drug Use and Health (NSDUH), about 145 million individuals—approximately 51% of Americans aged 12 years or older—used cannabis in their lifetime [1]. In 2021 alone, 62 million individuals reported using cannabis [1]. From 1992 until 2012, the proportion of Americans regularly using cannabis increased by roughly 60%. Several factors may account for this, such as the increased perception of cannabis as "benign" and higher social acceptability, especially among adolescents, as well as flexibilization of cannabis-related legislation across the country [2]. Of the 3 million individuals using cannabis for the first time in 2016, most were under the age of 18. Consistent with this, since the Monitoring the Future (MTF) survey of 12th graders began in 1975, the perceived risk of cannabis use has declined, and use prevalence has increased, with 31% of 12th graders reporting any cannabis use in the past 12 months in 2021 and 2022 [3].

Medical and Recreational Cannabinoid Use Policy

In recent years, there have been several changes to legislation surrounding the use of cannabinoids, with several U.S. states and other jurisdictions in Europe and South and Central America moving toward legalization.

In the U.S., medical cannabis programs began as compassionate care initiatives for terminally ill patients, ensuring their right to use cannabis for conditions such as nausea, cachexia, or spasticity. Initially adopted by a few states between 1979 and 1991, these programs have since expanded significantly. By early 2024, 37 states and the District of Columbia had authorized medical cannabis use or established agencies to regulate its production and distribution. Physicians in over 33 U.S. states and Washington D.C. can now recommend and authorize cannabis for medical purposes to patients with qualifying conditions, especially since it has been rescheduled as a Schedule III substance under federal law on May 21, 2024. However, there is significant inconsistency between states regarding qualifying conditions and a considerable discrepancy between what is allowed under state law and the scientific evidence base. In many states, individuals receive cannabis recommendations from physicians they see for a single visit, with no regular follow-up.

Despite the discrepancies in medical cannabis programs, physicians had been enlisted as gatekeepers to legal access—potentially paving the way for broader legalization. At the time of writing, Canada, 25 U.S. states, and the District of Columbia have fully legalized cannabis for recreational use by adults over 21. With these rapid societal changes, understanding the impact of cannabinoid use on mental health has become an urgent public health priority.

Pharmacology

Overview of the Endocannabinoid System

The endocannabinoid (eCB) system is one of the most widespread in the central nervous system (Fig. 10.1). It consists of receptors, endogenous transmitters (eCBs), and enzymes that synthesize and degrade eCBs, including fatty acid amide hydrolase (FAAH) and monoacylgycerol lipase (MAGL). The two main receptors are the G-protein–coupled receptors cannabinoid-1 receptor (CB1R) and cannabinoid-2 receptor (CB2R). Additionally, some cannabinoids engage transient receptor potential (TRP) channels and peroxisome proliferator-activated receptors (PPARs). The two most well-studied eCBs are the lipid ligands anandamide (AEA) and 2-arachidonoylglycerol (2-AG). CB1Rs are densely expressed in the brain and are critical in mediating the psychoactive effects of cannabis, as they are the targets of tetrahydrocannabinol (THC), a partial agonist at these receptors. CB2Rs, in contrast, are mostly expressed peripherally (in the immune, gastrointestinal, and peripheral nervous systems) [4].

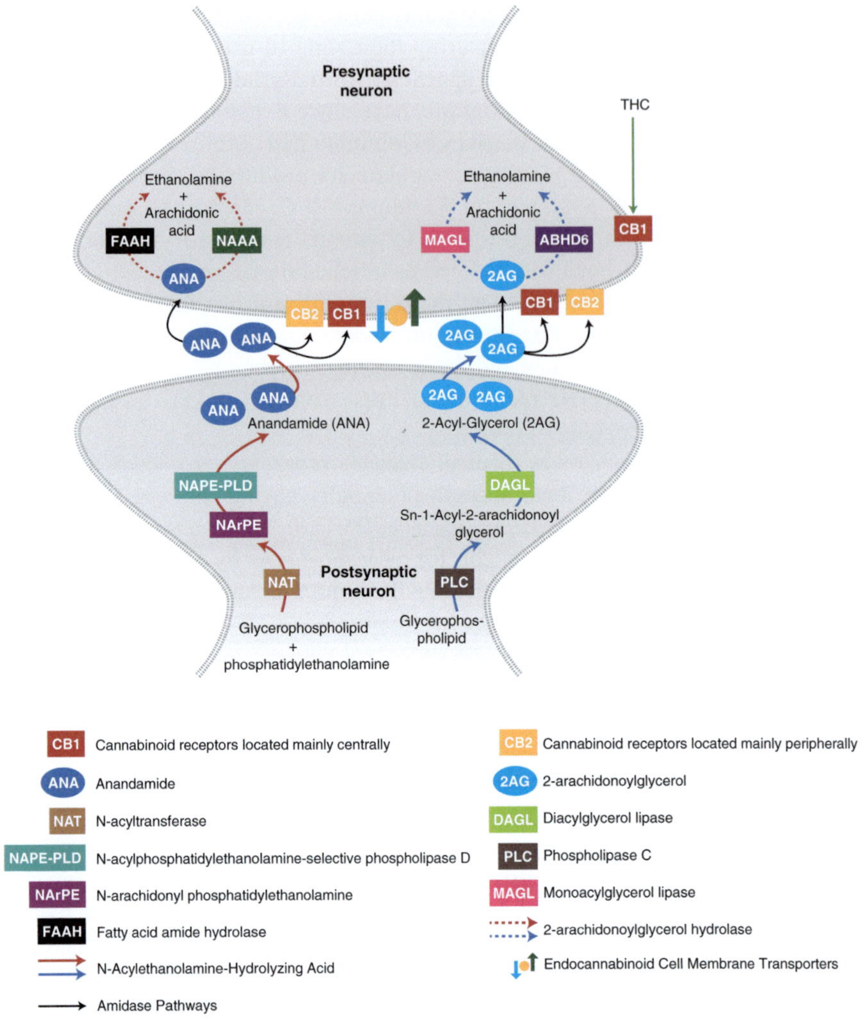

Fig. 10.1 The endocannabinoid system

Plant-Based Cannabinoids

Cannabis is a complex and highly variable mixture containing approximately 400 or more chemical compounds, including plant-based cannabinoids (or phytocannabinoids), terpenoids, and flavonoids, which produce individual and interactive effects. Delta-9-tetrahydrocannabinol (THC) is the principal psychoactive constituent, but there are around 70 other known phytocannabinoids with their own effects. For example, cannabidiol (CBD) may exhibit anxiolytic and antipsychotic-like effects that counterbalance the anxiety and psychotomimetic effects induced by THC. Preclinical studies suggest that the individual effects of phytocannabinoids are multi-phasic and dose-dependent, as illustrated by the anxiolytic effects of THC at lower doses and anxiogenic effects at higher doses. [5].

Beyond THC and CBD, there are also "minor cannabinoids," such as cannabinol (CBN), cannabichromene (CBC), cannabigerol (CBG), cannabidioloic acid (CBDA), cannabigerolic acid (CBGA), cannabinolic acid (CBNA), cannabidivarin (CBDV), cannabigerovarin (CBGV), and cannabichromevarin (CBCV), tetrahydrocannabinolic acid (THCA), and tetrahydrocannabivarin (THCV), among others [6, 7]. Some of these compounds, such as CBDV and THCV have unique pharmacological properties, binding at both cannabinoid and non-cannabinoid receptors [8]. Notably, none of these compounds have been demonstrated to have psychoactive properties [8]. Although understudied, they are receiving growing attention as potential pharmacotherapies. For example, CBN isolates have shown potential in reducing myofascial pain in preclinical models and may have anti-inflammatory and analgesic properties [9]. CBN may also function as an appetite stimulant [10] and sleep-inducing substance [11]. However, as of 2024, no clinical trials have investigated these uses. Nonetheless, these compounds present as promising targets for new pharmacotherapeutics given their action on cannabinoid receptors without psychoactive side effects.

Synthetic Cannabinoids

Synthetic cannabinoids (SC) originated from basic research on cannabinoid agonists. They are full CB1R receptor agonists and can be up to 800 times more potent than plant-based cannabinoids [12]. Products sold as "spice" or "K2" often contain a diverse array of compounds, resulting in effects that are generally more pronounced than those of cannabis. Users may experience heightened anxiety, psychotomimetic effects, hypertension, and tachycardia. Some products also contain stimulant cathinones (commonly known as "bath salts") combined with SCs, leading to life-threatening or fatal effects, such as seizures, toxic hepatitis, cardiac ischemia, and stroke. Acute intoxications and deaths related to synthetic cannabinoid use have increased in the United States and Europe, representing a public health concern [13, 14]. Withdrawal symptoms are similar to those of cannabis but tend to be more pronounced, often involving somatic symptoms such as nausea and vomiting.

SC use is more prevalent among individuals who use cannabis, users of other synthetic drugs, and those seeking to avoid detection by standard drug urine screens that typically only test for THC (e.g., individuals on probation, in the military, or in workplaces that utilize drug testing).

Clinical Significance (What Psychiatrists Should Know About) of Cannabinoids

Cannabis, cannabis-derived products, and synthetic cannabinoids (SCs) vary widely in cannabinoid content and composition (Table 10.1). In the U.S., the average concentration of delta-9-tetrahydrocannabinol (THC)—the primary psychoactive component of cannabis—has increased substantially over the past few decades, rising from approximately 4% in 1995 to 12% in 2014, with some contemporary products exceeding 50% THC by weight [4]. The THC-to-CBD ratio has also shifted markedly, with many commonly used forms now characterized by high THC and minimal cannabidiol (CBD) content [4]. To better reflect these trends, the National Institute on Drug Abuse (NIDA) Drug Supply Program has expanded its offerings to include cannabis flower with potencies up to 20% THC [15]. Nonetheless, most federally funded research over the past decade has used cannabis with THC concentrations ranging from 5% to 10%, which may not accurately represent the potency or diversity of products available in the community.

Table 10.1 Currently available cannabinoid products

Cannabinoid product	Description	Method of use
Smoked products	Dried cannabis leaves and flowers	Smoked in hand-rolled cigarettes ("joints," "blunts"), pipes with filtration systems ("bong," "hookah"), or vaporizers
Hashish	Concentrated trichomes with higher THC concentration than other parts of the plant	Smoked or mixed with food.
Kief	Powder extracted from THC-rich trichomes (resin glands)	Smoked or compressed into hashish "cakes"
Hash oil	A mixture of essential oils and resins extracted from the cannabis plants using solvents, such as ethanol or butane	The solvent is evaporated, leaving a THC-rich oil that can be smoked, vaporized, or mixed with food
Edibles	Food products infused with cannabis	Directly added cannabis, or cannabis butter or oil. Can be alcoholic beverages
Tincture	Cannabinoids extracted using alcohol	Liquid form, absorbed through the mucous membranes (oral mucosa or sublingually)
Topicals	Oils infused with cannabis	Applied topically as salve or cream
Skunk	*Cannabis* strains that are strong-smelling and THC-rich	Smoked
Shatter	A cannabis concentrate with a transparent, amber appearance that looks glassy when cold, and like thick honey when warm	"Dabbing" (special pipe) or vaporizing
Wax	Opaque cannabis concentrate with a buttery appearance. Different wax consistencies are created using varying oil textures and different moisture and heat levels.	"Dabbing" (special pipe) or vaporizing

THC:Delta-9-tetrahydrocannabinol

In community settings, cannabis products encompass a broad spectrum of formulations beyond dried flower, including high-potency concentrates such as wax, shatter, and oils (often exceeding 70–90% THC), as well as edibles like gummies and baked goods, tinctures, vapes, and topicals. These products differ not only in potency but also in route of administration, onset, and duration of effect—factors that may influence patterns of use, dependence potential, and associated health risks. As such, the growing disconnect between research-grade cannabis and commercially available products presents challenges for translating findings to real-world use.

Vaping cannabis products has gained substantial popularity, particularly among adolescents and young adults, contributing to a nationwide outbreak of vaping-associated pulmonary injury (VAPI), also referred to as EVALI (e-cigarette or vaping product use-associated lung injury). This condition has been linked to inhalation of vitamin E acetate, a diluent commonly found in low-cost cannabis-derived cartridges. However, emerging evidence suggests additional contributors to pulmonary toxicity, including the type of metal used in heating coils and the power levels at which vaping devices are operated, both of which may influence the production of toxic aerosols. Between 2019 and 2020, over 3,000 individuals in the United States were hospitalized due to VAPI, with approximately 70 confirmed deaths.

Acute Intoxication

The onset of cannabinoid effects depends on the route of administration, with effects emerging within minutes after inhalation but taking 60–90 min following oral consumption [16]. The duration of effects is highly variable but usually lasts from 2 (for inhaled cannabis) to 4 h (for oral consumption). The acute effects of cannabinoids are likely to be more pronounced with higher doses, a higher THC/CBD ratio, and with full agonists such as SCs. It is not fully understood why some healthy individuals are more vulnerable to the acute effects of cannabinoids. Individuals who use cannabinoids regularly may show blunted responses due to tolerance.

Mood/Anxiety Cannabis has acute, transient effects on mood. The "high" produced by cannabis includes a combination of effects such as relaxation, euphoria, relaxed inhibitions, and an overall sense of well-being. While cannabis is generally anxiolytic, especially at lower doses, the higher concentration of THC found in recent years has probably led to an increase in reports of panic-like effects. THC has been reported to increase anxiety when administered alone, especially at high doses and under stressful conditions, while co-administration with CBD can counter THC-induced anxiety [17].

There are observational reports of elevated mood and reduced depressive symptoms following short-term consumption of cannabis, and these effects are blocked by CB1R antagonists. However, it is challenging to differentiate this from the euphoria induced by cannabis intoxication. Additionally, the administration of a

CB1R inverse agonist (rimonabant) to healthy individuals has been shown to increase anxiety, depression, and suicidal ideation. The evidence for the antidepressant effects of herbal cannabis remains contradictory, as brief dysphoric reactions are also well-recognized consequences of acute cannabis use, especially to those who are cannabis naïve [18].

Psychosis Cannabis intoxication is associated with transient psychosis-like effects, including depersonalization, derealization, ideas of reference, grandiose and paranoid delusions, flight of ideas, disorganized thinking, and auditory and visual hallucinations. These effects have been increasingly reported with high-THC strains of cannabis and SCs. Individuals with a predisposition to psychotic disorders or a family history of psychosis are more prone to experiencing psychotomimetic effects [18].

Cognitive Effects Cannabis can acutely impair various cognitive domains. The acute effects of cannabis on cognition may depend on the THC/CBD ratio, with higher concentrations of CBD reducing cognitive deficits [19].

Attention Cannabis can induce deficits in selective, focused, and divided attention tasks. Additionally, acute administration of both cannabis and THC has been shown to impair attention allocation in healthy individuals. Impaired performance on a divided attention task was observed in occasional, but not heavy, users, indicating tolerance [19].

Memory Cannabis may impact spatial working memory, procedural memory, verbal learning and recall, and associative learning. Deficits in verbal learning and memory are recognized as the most robust impairments associated with acute cannabis use. THC has been shown to interfere with the encoding, but not retrieval, of verbal memory, suggesting that learning information prior to cannabis use is not likely to disrupt its recall. Whether THC impairs encoding of non-verbal information and memory consolidation remains to be elucidated [20]. The activation of CB1Rs, especially in the hippocampus, which contains a high density of these receptors, may interfere with short-term memory and impair memory consolidation [21].

Inhibitory Control Impairment of inhibitory control has been observed following acute cannabis intoxication, with THC and CBD potentially exerting opposite effects on response inhibition in "Go/NoGo" tasks. It has been proposed that the eCB system may modulate dopaminergic tone in the prefrontal cortex and nucleus accumbens, which contributes to incentive salience and impulsivity. THC is thought to disrupt these physiological mechanisms, affecting inhibitory and decision-making processes [22].

Analgesia Cannabinoids are commonly believed to have analgesic properties by both prescribers and patients, leading to frequent use in pain management, either self-prescribed or recommended by a healthcare professional. However, human laboratory studies on the analgesic effects of cannabis and cannabinoid agonists (e.g., THC, dronabinol, nabilone) have produced mixed results among healthy populations [23]. Recent reviews have concluded that there is insufficient evidence to confidently support the use of cannabinoids for treating acute or chronic pain conditions [24]. Despite this, chronic pain is a qualifying condition for medical cannabis use in most U.S. states and is the most common diagnosis used to justify a medical indication for cannabis. Some suggest that cannabis may reduce the affective quality of chronic pain (i.e., the negative emotional response to pain) without significantly altering the intensity of the pain itself [23]. Although current evidence does not justify the routine recommendation of cannabinoids for pain management, further research into the complex nature of pain and multimodal treatment approaches may reveal if these substances are valuable adjuvant options.

Motoric Effects and Relevance for Driving Ability Consistent with the known distribution of CB1Rs in areas involved in cognitive and motor processes (e.g., brain cortex, basal ganglia, cerebellum), driving simulation studies collectively suggest that cannabinoids produce acute impairments in driving ability. These impairments are exemplified by an increase in lateral position errors, lane deviation, steering instability, braking distance, and collisions [25].

Effects of Chronic Use: Cognitive Effects

The chronic cognitive effects of cannabinoids are more complex and controversial than their acute effects, appearing to be related to the level of use and the age at which use began [20]. The evidence is stronger for impairments in verbal learning and memory, as well as working memory and attention, with mixed evidence for effects on decision-making. Whether these impairments are permanent is not fully understood.

In one of the largest and longest prospective studies controlling for premorbid function, Meier *et al.* reported that cannabis use before the age of 18 resulted in greater decline in intelligence by age 38, persisting even after cessation or reduction of use in the past year. A recent meta-analysis, conversely, found that only small magnitude effects are apparent in the first few weeks of abstinence (of the order of $d = 0.25$ to 0.35), and these become non-significant with extended abstinence (to around $d = 0.15$) [26]

Cannabis Use Disorder

Cannabis use disorder (CUD) is the most prevalent substance use disorder (SUD) in the U.S. population after alcohol and tobacco use disorders. Approximately 1 in 10 individuals who use cannabis progress to compulsive use at the CUD level. According to the National Epidemiologic Survey on Alcohol and Related Conditions-III (NESARC-III), the lifetime prevalence of CUD is 6.3% [27]. The lifetime rates of CUD in those who begin use in adolescence have been reported to be close to 17% [27].

Importantly, participants in the NESARC-III with CUD experienced significant disability in various domains. Their level of disability correlated with the frequency of cannabis use and was higher than the corresponding levels associated with alcohol use disorder [27]. Notably, chronic pain is a risk factor for developing CUD [28]. It remains unclear whether medical cannabis use is associated with lower or higher levels of CUD. Some evidence suggests the latter, as states where medical cannabis is legal had higher rates of CUD diagnoses among veterans in 2002, 2008, and 2009 [29].

Some evidence suggests that regular cannabinoid use may be implicated in the development of SUDs other than CUD (i.e., the "gateway hypothesis" of cannabis). Approximately 1 in 10 cannabis users develop an SUD other than CUD, with higher rates among adolescents [30]. In a large nationally representative sample, cannabis use was prospectively associated with increased prevalence and incidence of alcohol and other SUDs, even after adjusting for several covariates that predicted cannabis use. It has also been proposed that the neurocircuitry involved in mediating the effects of cannabis overlaps with that involved in other substances. However, it remains unclear whether this overlap leads to cross-sensitization to other substances or reflects a common underlying vulnerability across distinct substances [30]. Conflicting data exist regarding the transition from cannabis use to other SUDs. For instance, a meta-analysis found no statistical association between cannabis use and risk of nonmedical opioid use among patients receiving treatment for opioid use disorder [31]. As with many other clinical considerations regarding cannabis use, the evidence remains limited.

Cannabis Withdrawal

Recognized in DSM-5 as a distinct entity, cannabis withdrawal is characterized by anger, aggression, appetite changes, weight loss, irritability, anxiety, restlessness, sleep disturbances, cannabis cravings, and physical discomfort [32]. Less common symptoms include chills, depressed mood, stomach pain, and diaphoresis. Most symptoms appear within 1 day of abstinence, peak within 2–3 days, and resolve within 1–3 weeks. However, some studies suggest that withdrawal symptoms, particularly sleep disturbances, may persist for longer than 4 weeks [33].

Associations with Other Psychiatric Disorders

Adolescent Psychiatric Disorders In general, the adolescent brain differs from the adult brain in that it is more susceptible to external influences. As a result, adolescents are more likely to develop psychiatric consequences from prolonged cannabis use. The mesolimbic dopaminergic system and the hypothalamic pituitary-adrenal axis (HPA) develop earlier than the prefrontal cortex (PFC), which remains less mature during adolescence. The eCB system regulates developmental processes throughout the brain, including pyramidal cell specification, interneuron migration and morphogenesis, neuronal connectivity, and synaptic plasticity, all of which contribute to the PFC's maturation. The influence of exogenous cannabinoids may interfere with these processes, increasing the risk of psychiatric disorders [34].

Psychotic Disorders Transient, cannabis-induced psychosis is often clinically indistinguishable from a primary psychotic disorder and can outlast the period of acute intoxication, sometimes persisting for up to 30 days. Although most people who use cannabis do not experience psychosis, the link between cannabis and psychosis may be stronger in those with predisposing genetic and environmental factors. As with other negative effects of cannabis, the risk of psychosis appears to be heightened by heavy and early use. Cannabis use has also been shown to exacerbate the course of illness in individuals with established psychotic disorders [19]. With the rising potency of cannabis strains and more frequent use, there is some evidence that the age of onset of first-episode psychosis is decreasing. Among substance-induced psychotic disorders, cannabis-induced psychosis is the most likely to persist as a chronic, primary psychotic disorder after cessation of use (about 1 in 3 people) [35].

Anxiety Disorders Long-term cannabis use can exacerbate anxiety, trigger panic attacks, and worsen the neuroendocrine response to stress. While individuals with anxiety disorders often use cannabis with the aim of alleviating their symptoms, it is unclear whether cannabis use provides relief or contributes to worsening anxiety symptoms. Chronic cannabis use has also been associated as a risk factor for social anxiety disorder [36].

Mood Disorders Cannabis use is associated with a worse clinical course of mood disorders, including more frequent hospitalizations, longer and more frequent manic episodes, and a higher prevalence of psychotic symptoms in individuals with bipolar disorder [36]. There is also preliminary evidence that cannabis use may increase the risk of developing bipolar and depressive disorders. Conversely, both unipolar and bipolar mood disorders appear to increase rates of cannabis use and CUD in prospective studies.

Attention-Deficit/Hyperactivity Disorder (ADHD) Preliminary data indicate that ADHD is a risk factor for developing cannabis misuse in adulthood. However, the impact of cannabis use on the course of ADHD is not fully understood. Though data are sparse, chronic and particularly early cannabis use appears to be associated with negative outcomes in ADHD, including further attention deficits and reduced responsiveness to pharmacological treatment [37, 38].

Sleep Disorders The relationship between cannabis use and sleep is complex, influenced by time-dependent effects, as well as intoxication and withdrawal.

Overall, cannabis use is associated with reduced rapid eye movement (REM) sleep, shortened sleep-onset latency, and increased stage 4 sleep. Sedation following cannabis exposure may persist into the following day. Additionally, insomnia and vivid dreams are common during cannabis withdrawal, particularly among heavy users. Preliminary evidence also suggests that childhood-onset sleep disorders may predict cannabis and alcohol use in adolescence and early adulthood [39].

Posttraumatic Stress Disorder (PTSD) Individuals with PTSD have higher rates of cannabis use, as well as SUDs in general, compared to the general population. However, there is no evidence thus far that cannabis use is a risk factor for developing PTSD. Although cannabis is increasingly being offered as a treatment for PTSD, systematic reviews indicate that the evidence regarding its benefits and individuals with this disorder remains conflicting and incomplete [40].

Treatment of Cannabis Use Disorder

Assessment of Cannabis Use

Individuals seeking treatment for cannabis use typically report nearly daily use for over a decade and multiple attempts (around 7) to quit [18]. A small minority specifically seeks addiction treatment for cannabis misuse. More commonly, individuals present to general psychiatric or primary care settings with symptoms such as depression, anxiety, fatigue, impaired concentration, irritability, or relationship stress. Those with high-intensity use may present to emergency departments with acute anxiety, psychotomimetic effects, psychosis, or altered mental status. Adolescents may exhibit declining school performance, while adults may experience impaired job performance [18].

Several screening tools are available to assist clinicians in assessing cannabis use, including the Cannabis Use Disorder Identification Test-Revised (CUDIT-R) [41], the Severity of Dependence Scale (SDS) [42], and the Cannabis Problems Questionnaire [43]. It is important for clinicians to have a broad understanding of cannabis consumption methods and the variety of products available, as terminology and strain names can vary regionally (Table 10.1).

Pharmacological Interventions

Currently, no FDA-approved medications exist for the treatment of CUD. However, there is growing interest in developing pharmaceutical treatments, spurred by the recognition of cannabis withdrawal and a better understanding of the physical and societal impacts of cannabis misuse.

A large 12-week randomized controlled trial (RCT) found that dronabinol (20 mg twice daily) did not significantly improve abstinence during a 2-week maintenance phase (17.7% abstinence in the dronabinol group vs. 15.6% in the placebo group, though the dronabinol group had better treatment retention and relief of withdrawal symptoms. Similarly, a two-site RCT investigating nabiximols—a spray formulation with a 1:1 ratio of THC and CBD—found no significant difference in self-reported cannabis us after 28 days between the treatment and placebo groups [44].

Preliminary data suggest potential for gabapentin [45], cannabinoid degradative enzyme inhibitors such as fatty acid amide hydrolase (FAAH) inhibitors [46], and glutamate modulators like N-acetylcysteine [47] in reducing cannabis use. Notably, N-acetylcysteine has been shown to reduce cannabis use in non-treatment-seeking adolescents but not in adults [47]. Lofexidine, an FDA-approved medication for opioid withdrawal, has also shown promise in reducing symptoms of cannabis withdrawal [48]. An ongoing multi-site RCT with 230 participants is currently exploring the efficacy of FAAH (ClinicalTrials.gov ID: NCT03386487). Antidepressants, buspirone, divalproex sodium, and lithium do not appear to be particularly effective for treating CUD, and there is little research to guide a rational pharmacological approach to co-occurring psychiatric disorders.

Despite the current limitations in the literature, findings from basic science and human laboratory studies offer optimism that further clinical trials will yield meaningful pharmacotherapeutic interventions for CUD and cannabis withdrawal.

Psychosocial Interventions

Research on psychosocial treatments for CUD shows some evidence of efficacy. These interventions aim to help individuals reduce or stop cannabis use, with cognitive behavioral therapy (CBT) focusing on skills development and motivational enhancement therapy (MET) designed to strengthen motivation to change. Evidence suggests that individuals receiving CBT or MET tend to have improved outcomes, including reduced frequency of use and better psychosocial functioning [49]. However, various methodological limitations highlight the need for further research on the efficacy of these interventions.

Recently, there has been growing interest in software-based interventions, which aim to increase access to evidence-based treatments and reduce costs by offering them outside traditional clinical settings. Various placebo-controlled studies suggest that web-based interventions show promise in treating CUD [49].

Medical Use of Cannabinoids: Indications, Formulations, and Adverse Effects

The U.S. Food and Drug Administration (FDA) has approved 1 cannabis-derived drug: Epidiolex (cannabidiol), and 3 synthetic cannabis-related products: Marinol (dronabinol), Syndros (dronabinol), and Cesamet (nabilone). Dronabinol and nabilone are FDA-approved for the treatment of chemotherapy-induced nausea and vomiting; dronabinol is also approved for AIDS-associated anorexia. The FDA approved CBD, in a formulation called Epidiolex, for treating seizures associated with 2 rare pediatric epileptogenic syndromes, Lennox-Gastaut syndrome and Dravet syndrome [50]. Nabiximols, a THC/CBD formulation administered as a spray containing THC and CBD in a 1:1 ratio, has been approved in Canada for treating cancer-related pain and multiple sclerosis-related spasticity, and a U.S. phase 3 trial is planned to test this drug for the latter indication.

Regarding adverse effects, the FDA cautions that "Information from adverse event reports regarding cannabis use is extremely limited; the FDA primarily receives adverse event reports for approved products" [50]. Given the rarity and limited approved indications of these formulations, real-world data is scarce. Available studies indicate that the most common side effects (occurring in more than 3% of patients) include dizziness, fatigue, dry mouth, light-headedness, abdominal pain, nausea, and euphoria. More severe but rarer adverse effects (occurring in less than 1% of patients) include physical dependence, cognitive impairment, psychosis, anxiety, hypertension, syncope, tachycardia, seizures, and cannabinoid hyperemesis syndrome. The latter is defined as a paradoxical syndrome characterized by cyclic nausea, severe vomiting, and abdominal pain that can last for days and recur periodically; it may persist even after discontinuation of cannabis and can result in hospitalization due to dehydration and hypernatremia [50].

Interactions of Cannabinoids with Other Drugs

Cannabis may interact in clinically significant ways with certain pharmaceuticals, including antiplatelet and anticoagulant agents, chemotherapy agents, antivirals, barbiturates, and some antibiotics. When combined with antidepressants, cannabis can induce mood changes, and it may have synergistic effects with alcohol and other central nervous system depressants (Table 10.2) [51].

Genetic Factors

Genetic variation partially contributes to the risk of initiating and maintaining cannabis use. A meta-analysis of twin studies estimated heritability at approximately 40%, with a range of 12–70% for lifetime use and 33–76% for CUD [52]. However, another meta-analysis of genome-wide association studies found that no genetic variant reached genome-wide significance, and that only about 6% of cannabis use initiation could be attributed to common genetic variants [53]. While it is plausible that CUS carries some degree of genetic variability, genetic factors alone do not fully explain the risk.

Table 10.2 Cannabis-pharmaceutical interactions

Mechanism	Drugs
Antiestrogenic effect	Contraceptive medications Hormone replacement therapy
Competition with metabolism, leading to increased drug levels	Barbiturates (phenobarbital, pentobarbital, secobarbital)
Inhibition of platelet aggregation	Nonsteroidal anti-inflammatory drugs Anticoagulants (warfarin) Antiplatelet agents (clopidogrel)
Induction of cytochrome P450 2E1, leading to decreased levels of substrate drugs	Acetaminophen, ethanol, theophylline, anesthetics (enflurane, halothane, isoflurane)
Inhibition of cytochrome P450 3A4, leading to increased levels of substrate drugs	Lovastatin, cyclosporine, diltiazem, indinavir, triazolam, clarithromycin
Inhibition of P-glycoproteins, leading to increased levels of substrate drugs	Chemotherapy agents (etoposide, paclitaxel, vinblastine, vincristine, vindesine) Antifungals (ketoconazole, itraconazole) Protease inhibitors (amprenavir, nelfinavir, saquinavir, indinavir) Histamine H2 antagonists (cimetidine, ranitidine) Calcium channel blockers (diltiazem, verapamil) Corticosteroids Others (quinidine, cyclosporine, loperamide, quinidine, erythromycin, fexofenadine)
Additive/synergistic effects	Ethanol Other central nervous system depressants

Adapted from: Compton, M. T. (Ed.). (2016). *Marijuana and mental health*. American Psychiatric Pub.

Influence of Biological Sex

Although limited, some clinical and preclinical studies have explored sex-based differences in the acute and chronic effects of cannabis. Most of these studies are observational or retrospective and vary in methodologies (e.g., smoked, vaporized, or oral routes of administration) or lack appropriate demographic matching between male and female participants. However, preliminary data suggest clinically relevant sex differences in areas such as age of first exposure, time to development of CUD, the influence of hormonal status on cannabis effects, and the degree and type of exposure (dose, frequency, and duration).

For example, a clinical-laboratory investigation of healthy, chronic cannabis users found that men were more sensitive to its analgesic effects [54], a finding aligned with preclinical evidence [55]. Regarding withdrawal symptoms, several studies suggest that these are more severe in women than in men, also consistent with preclinical data [56]. Another clinical-laboratory study indicated that women rated their experience of acute psychotomimetic effects (i.e., feeling "high") as more intense than men, even when demographically matched and given the same THC dose [57]. In summary, while cannabis and its derivatives may affect people differently based on their sex, with women potentially more vulnerable to these effects, further research is needed to better understand these differences.

Chapter Review Questions

1. A 21-year-old woman started using cannabis at age 15 and escalated to daily use by age 17 to achieve the same desired effect. When she stops using cannabis, she feels "jittery and depressed" and struggles to fall asleep, so she continues to use it to prevent these symptoms. She was an above-average student in junior high school, but her performance and grades subsequently declined, and she often felt unmotivated to do homework. Despite wanting to pursue a college education, she missed several application deadlines. She took a job at a local coffee shop because the short work shifts allowed more time to use cannabis alone at home. Which of the following diagnoses best describes this presentation?

   A. Cannabis hyperemesis syndrome
   B. Cannabis withdrawal
   C. Chronic cannabis syndrome
   D. Cannabis use disorder
   E. Non-disordered cannabis use

   Correct Answer: D.

   Explanation: This individual has symptoms consistent with cannabis use disorder, including tolerance, withdrawal, and significant impairment in major role obligations. Cannabis hyperemesis syndrome is characterized by cyclical nausea and vomiting, which is not described here. Cannabis withdrawal involves symptoms after cessation but does not fully account for the broader pattern of problematic use and impairment seen in this case, which are also not compatible with non-disordered cannabis use. Chronic cannabis syndrome is not a recognized DSM-5 diagnostic entity.
2. A 34-year-old man has been smoking hashish daily for the past 12 months. He was stopped by the police for driving while intoxicated and held in custody over the weekend until a court hearing on Monday. While unable to use hashish, which of the following sets of symptoms is he most likely to experience?

   A. Muscle twitches, lacrimation, rhinorrhea, and diarrhea
   B. Hallucinations, tachycardia, and hypertension
   C. Slurred speech, vomiting, ataxia, and hypotension
   D. Nausea, headache, irritability, vomiting, and insomnia
   E. He is unlikely to develop any symptoms, as cannabis withdrawal is uncommon

   Correct Answer: D.

   Explanation: This person is likely to experience symptoms consistent with cannabis withdrawal, likely to occur after abrupt discontinuation of cannabis after prolonged daily use. Symptoms may include nausea, headache, irritability, vomiting, and insomnia. Muscle twitches, lacrimation, rhinorrhea, and diarrhea are more typical of opioid withdrawal. Hallucinations, tachycardia, and hypertension are common in severe alcohol withdrawal. Slurred speech, ataxia, vomiting, and hypotension are associated with opioid intoxication.

3. A 20-year-old man develops paranoid delusions and dissociative symptoms over 7 months, culminating in hospitalization for behavioral dysregulation. He reports smoking several joints of cannabis daily since the age of 13. He is diagnosed with an unspecified psychotic disorder and started on antipsychotic medication. Which of the following best describes the current scientific consensus regarding the relationship between cannabis use and psychotic disorders?

   A. Though the relationship between psychosis and cannabis use is complex, cannabis does appear to be a risk factor for the development of psychosis
   B. Schizophrenia is caused by early cannabis use
   C. Prodromal psychotic symptoms are temporarily relieved by cannabis
   D. The development of a psychotic disorder is independent of cannabis use
   E. Cannabis has not been indicated as a potential risk factor for the development of psychosis

   Correct Answer: A.

   Explanation: Cannabis use is recognized as a risk factor for psychosis, though it is neither necessary nor sufficient to cause it. In this scenario, prolonged and heavy cannabis use may have contributed to the onset of the psychotic disorder. Among substance-induced psychotic disorders, cannabis-induced psychosis has a higher likelihood (about 1 in 3) of persisting as a chronic, primary psychotic disorder even after cessation of use. There is no evidence to support the idea that prodromal symptoms of psychosis are relieved by cannabis use.

4. A 22-year-old man presents to the emergency department with complaints of shortness of breath, cough, and chest pain that have been worsening over the past 3 weeks. He also reports low-grade fever, nausea, and fatigue. His symptoms began gradually and progressively worsened. He denies any recent travel, sick contacts, or history of asthma or other chronic respiratory conditions. The patient reports vaping THC cartridges daily for the past 2 years, with increased use over the past few months. He does not smoke cigarettes or use any other substances. On physical examination, the patient appears moderately distressed with a respiratory rate of 24 breaths per minute, oxygen saturation of 88% on room air, and bilateral inspiratory crackles on lung auscultation. His heart rate is 110 beats per minute, and his temperature is 37.8°C (100°F). A chest X-ray reveals bilateral patchy infiltrates. Laboratory results show the following: white blood cell count of 12,500/mm^3, C-reactive protein of 60 mg/L, arterial blood gas (ABG) with pH 7.45, PaO2 of 58 mmHg, PaCO2 of 35 mmHg, HCO3- of 22 mEq/L. What is the most likely diagnosis in this patient?

   A. Bacterial pneumonia
   B. Viral pneumonia

C. Pulmonary embolism
D. Vaping-associated pulmonary injury (VAPI)
E. Congestive heart failure

Correct Answer: D.

Explanation: This patient's history of daily vaping, combined with his respiratory symptoms (shortness of breath, cough, and chest pain), physical findings (bilateral inspiratory crackles), and radiologic findings (bilateral rather than unilateral or consolidated patchy infiltrates), strongly suggests VAPI. The elevated white blood cell count, and C-reactive protein indicate inflammation. The gradual onset and lack of recent travel or sick contacts make bacterial or viral pneumonia less likely. There are no signs of congestive heart failure or risk factors for pulmonary embolism noted in the history.

References

1. Substance Abuse and Mental Health Services Administration. Results from the 2023 National Survey on Drug Use and Health. 2023. Available at: https://www.samhsa.gov/data/data-we-collect/nsduh-national-survey-drug-use-and-health/datafiles. Accessed on 14 Apr 2025.
2. Azofeifa A. National estimates of marijuana use and related indicators—National Survey on Drug Use and Health, United States, 2002–2014. MMWR Surveillance Summaries. 2016;65:1–28.
3. Johnston LD, O'Malley PM, Miech RA, et al. Monitoring the future national survey results on drug use, 1975–2022: secondary school students. Ann Arbor: Institute for Social Research; 2023.
4. ElSohly MA, Mehmedic Z, Foster S, et al. Changes in cannabis potency over the last 2 decades (1995–2014): analysis of current data in the United States. Biol Psychiatry. 2016;79(7):613–9.
5. Rey AA, Purrio M, Viveros MP, et al. Biphasic effects of cannabinoids in anxiety responses: CB1 and GABA(B) receptors in the balance of GABAergic and glutamatergic neurotransmission. Neuropsychopharmacology. 2012;37(12):2624–34.
6. Hanuš LO, Meyer SM, Muñoz E, et al. Phytocannabinoids: a unified critical inventory. Nat Prod Rep. 2016;33(12):1357–92.
7. Gülck T, Møller BL. Phytocannabinoids: origins and biosynthesis. Trends Plant Sci. 2020;25(10):985–1004.
8. Walsh KB, McKinney AE, Holmes AE. Minor cannabinoids: biosynthesis, molecular pharmacology and potential therapeutic uses. Front Pharmacol. 2021;12:777804.
9. Wong H, Cairns BE. Cannabidiol, cannabinol and their combinations act as peripheral analgesics in a rat model of myofascial pain. Arch. Oral Biol. 2019;104:33–9.
10. Farrimond JA, Whalley BJ, Williams CM. Non-Δ^9tetrahydrocannabinol phytocannabinoids stimulate feeding in rats. Behav. Pharmacol. 2012b;23:113–7.
11. Yoshida H, Usami N, Ohishi Y, et al. Synthesis and pharmacological effects in mice of halogenated cannabinol derivatives. Chem. Pharm. Bull. (Tokyo). 1995;43:335–7.
12. Roque-Bravo R, Silva RS, Malheiro RF, et al. Synthetic cannabinoids: a pharmacological and toxicological overview. Annu Rev Pharmacol Toxicol. 2023;63:187–209.
13. European Monitoring Center for Drugs and Drug Addiction. (EMCDDA). European drug report 2021: trends and developments. Luxembourg: Publications Office of the European Union; 2021.
14. Riederer AM, Campleman SL, Carlson RG, et al. Acute poisonings from synthetic cannabinoids — 50 U.S. Toxicology Investigators Consortium Registry Sites, 2010–2015. MMWR Morb Mortal Wkly Rep. 2016;65:692–5.

15. National Institute on Drug and Alcohol Abuse. Drug supply program ordering guidelines. 2016. Available at: https://nida.nih.gov/research/research-data-measures-resources/nida-drug-supply-program-dsp/nida-drug-supply-program-dsp-ordering-guidelines/marijuana-plant-material-available. Accessed on July 18 2024
16. ElSohly M, Gul W. Constituents of *Cannabis sativa*. In: Pertwee RG, editor. Handbook of cannabis. Oxford: Oxford University Press; 2014. p. 3–22.
17. Karila L, Roux P, Rolland B, et al. Acute and long-term effects of cannabis use: a review. Curr Pharm Des. 2014;20(25):4112–8.
18. Jefsen OH, Erlangsen A, Nordentoft M, et al. Cannabis use disorder and subsequent risk of psychotic and nonpsychotic unipolar depression and bipolar disorder. JAMA Psychiatry. 2023;80(8):803–10.
19. Volkow ND, Swanson JM, Evins AE, et al. Effects of cannabis use on human behavior, including cognition, motivation, and psychosis: a review. JAMA Psychiatry. 2016;73(3):292–7.
20. Ranganathan M, D'souza DC. The acute effects of cannabinoids on memory in humans: a review. Psychopharmacology. 2006;188(4):425–44.
21. Meier MH, Caspi A, Knodt AR, et al. Long-term cannabis use and cognitive reserves and hippocampal volume in midlife. Am J Psychiatry. 2022;179(5):362–74.
22. Borgwardt SJ, Allen P, Bhattacharyya S, et al. Neural basis of Δ-9-tetrahydrocannabinol and cannabidiol: effects during response inhibition. Biol Psychiatry. 2008;64(11):966–73.
23. De Vita MJ, Moskal D, Maisto SA, et al. Association of cannabinoid administration with experimental pain in healthy adults: a systematic review and meta-analysis. JAMA Psychiatry. 2018;75(11):1118–27.
24. Häuser W, Petzke F, Fitzcharles MA. Efficacy, tolerability and safety of cannabis-based medicines for chronic pain management—an overview of systematic reviews. Eur J Pain. 2018;22(3):455–70.
25. Simmons SM, Caird JK, Sterzer F, et al. The effects of cannabis and alcohol on driving performance and driver behaviour: a systematic review and meta-analysis. Addiction. 2022;117(7):1843–56.
26. Meier MH, Caspi A, Ambler A, et al. Persistent cannabis users show neuropsychological decline from childhood to midlife. Proc Natl Acad Sci U S A. 2012;109(40):E2657–64.
27. National Institute on Alcohol Abuse and Alcoholism. National Epidemiologic Survey on Alcohol and Related Conditions-III (NESARC-III). 2021. Available on https://www.niaaa.nih.gov/research/nesarc-iii. Accessed on 18 July 2024.
28. Hasin DS, Shmulewitz D, Cerdá M. U.S. adults with pain, a group increasingly vulnerable to nonmedical cannabis use and cannabis use disorder: 2001–2002 and 2012–2013. Am J Psychiatry. 2020;177(7):611–8.
29. Bonn-Miller MO, Harris AH, Trafton JA. Prevalence of cannabis use disorder diagnoses among veterans in 2002, 2008, and 2009. Psychol Serv. 2012;9(4):404–16.
30. Blanco C, Hasin DS, Wall MM, et al. Cannabis use and risk of psychiatric disorders: prospective evidence from a US national longitudinal study. JAMA psychiatry. 2016;73(4):388–95.
31. Costa GPA, Nunes JC, Heringer DL, et al. The impact of cannabis on non-medical opioid use among individuals receiving pharmacotherapies for opioid use disorder: a systematic review and meta-analysis of longitudinal studies. Am J Drug Alcohol Abuse. 2024;50(1):12–26.
32. Hasin DS, O'Brien CP, Auriacombe M, et al. DSM-5 criteria for substance use disorders: recommendations and rationale. Am J Psychiatry. 2013;170(8):834–51.
33. Gates P, Albertella L, Copeland J. Cannabis withdrawal and sleep: a systematic review of human studies. Subst Abus. 2016;37(1):255–69.
34. Scheyer AF, Laviolette SR, Pelissier AL, et al. Cannabis in adolescence: lasting cognitive alterations and underlying mechanisms. Cannabis Cannabinoid Res. 2023;8(1):12–23.
35. Ganesh S, Cortes-Briones J, Ranganathan M, et al. Psychosis-relevant effects of intravenous delta-9-tetrahydrocannabinol: a mega analysis of individual participant-data from human laboratory studies. Int J Neuropsychopharmacol. 2020;23:559–70.

36. Gobbi G, Atkin T, Zytynski T, et al. Association of cannabis use in adolescence and risk of depression, anxiety, and suicidality in young adulthood: a systematic review and meta-analysis. JAMA Psychiatry. 2019;76(4):426–34.
37. Sibley MH, Pelham WE Jr, Molina BS, et al. The role of early childhood ADHD and subsequent CD in the initiation and escalation of adolescent cigarette, alcohol, and marijuana use. J Abnorm Psychol. 2014;123(2):362.
38. Bidwell L, Henry E, Willcutt E, et al. Childhood and current ADHD symptom dimensions are associated with more severe cannabis outcomes in college students. Drug Alcohol Depend. 2014;135:88–94.
39. Schierenbeck T, Riemann D, Berger M, et al. Effect of illicit recreational drugs upon sleep: cocaine, ecstasy and marijuana. Sleep Med Rev. 2008;12(5):381–9.
40. Bedard-Gilligan M, Lehinger E, Cornell-Maier S, et al. Effects of cannabis on PTSD recovery: review of the literature and clinical insights. Curr Addict Rep. 2022;9(3):203–16.
41. Adamson SJ, Kay-Lambkin FJ, Baker AL, et al. An improved brief measure of cannabis misuse: the Cannabis Use Disorders Identification Test-Revised (CUDIT-R). Drug Alcohol Depend. 2010;110(1-2):137–43.
42. Rotermann M. Using the severity of dependence scale to examine cannabis consumers with impaired control in Canada. Health Rep. 2023;34(6):3–16.
43. Copeland J, Gilmour S, Gates P, et al. The Cannabis Problems Questionnaire: factor structure, reliability, and validity. Drug Alcohol Depend. 2005;80(3):313–9.
44. Levin FR, Mariani JJ, Brooks DJ, et al. Dronabinol for the treatment of cannabis dependence: a randomized, double-blind, placebo-controlled trial. Drug Alcohol Depend. 2011;116(1–3):142–50.
45. Mason BJ, Crean R, Goodell V, et al. A proof-of-concept randomized controlled study of gabapentin: effects on cannabis use, withdrawal and executive function deficits in cannabis-dependent adults. Neuropsychopharmacology. 2012;37(7):1689–98.
46. D'Souza DC, Cortes-Briones J, Creatura G, et al. Efficacy and safety of a fatty acid amide hydrolase inhibitor (PF-04457845) in the treatment of cannabis withdrawal and dependence in men: a double-blind, placebo-controlled, parallel group, phase 2a single-site randomised controlled trial. Lancet Psychiatry. 2019;6(1):35–45.
47. Tomko RL, Jones JL, Gilmore AK, et al. *N*-acetylcysteine: a potential treatment for substance use disorders. Curr Psychiatr. 2018;17(6):30–6. 41–42, 55
48. Haney M, Hart CL, Vosburg SK, et al. Effects of THC and lofexidine in a human laboratory model of marijuana withdrawal and relapse. Psychopharmacology. 2008;197(1):157–68.
49. Gates PJ, Sabioni P, Copeland J, et al. Psychosocial interventions for cannabis use disorder. Cochrane Database Syst Rev. 2016;2016(5):CD005336.
50. Food and Drug Administration. FDA regulation of cannabis and cannabis-derived products, including cannabidiol (CBD). 2024. Available at: https://www.fda.gov/news-events/public-health-focus/fda-regulation-cannabis-and-cannabis-derived-products-including-cannabidiol-cbd#:~:text=22.,years%20of%20age%20and%20older. Accessed on 19 July 2024.
51. Antoniou T, Bodkin J, Ho JM. Drug interactions with cannabinoids. CMAJ. 2020;192(9):E206.
52. Verweij KJH, Vink JM, Abdellaoui A, et al. The genetic aetiology of cannabis use: from twin models to genome-wide association studies and beyond. Transl Psychiatry. 2022;12:489.
53. Johnson EC, Demontis D, Thorgeirsson TE, et al. A large-scale genome-wide association study meta-analysis of cannabis use disorder. Lancet Psychiatry. 2020;7(12):1032–45.
54. Cooper ZD, Haney M. Investigation of sex-dependent effects of marijuana in daily marijuana smokers. Drug Alcohol Depend. 2014;136:85–91.
55. Wakley AA, Wiley JL, Craft RM. Sex differences in antinociceptive tolerance to THC. Drug Alcohol Depend. 2014;143:22–8.
56. Cooper ZD, Craft RM. Sex-dependent effects of cannabis and cannabinoids: a translational perspective. Neuropsychopharmacology. 2018;43(1):34–51.
57. Aghaei AM, Spillane LU, Pittman B, et al. Sex differences in the acute effects of oral THC: a randomized, placebo-controlled, crossover human laboratory study. Psychopharmacology. 2024;241(10):2149–60.

Opioids

11

Marina Tsoy-Podosenin and Anil Thomas

High-Yield Review Points

- The diagnosis of OUD is based on the presence of two or more (three or more in the setting of prescribed opioids) criteria related to loss of control, risky use, social problems, and physical dependence within the same 12-month period. Detailed drug and medical history and presence of characteristic signs of drug use on medical evaluation play an important role in the diagnosis of OUD.
- Opioid intoxication may result in overdose and death. The risk of overdose increases if opioid use is combined with other sedatives, e.g., alcohol, benzodiazepines, and barbiturates, as well as in persons who recently completed detoxification or after a period of prolonged abstinence (e.g., former inmates) due to reduced tolerance. Naloxone hydrochloride for intranasal, intravenous, intramuscular, and subcutaneous use effectively reverses opioid overdose.
- Opioid withdrawal, although generally not life-threatening, and opioid craving are often the main drivers in the continuation of opioid use. Medical management of opioid withdrawal involves the use of full (methadone) or partial opioid agonists (buprenorphine), alpha-2 adrenergic agonists, and medications providing symptomatic relief.

M. Tsoy-Podosenin (✉)
Catholic Health Services of Long Island, Long Island, NY, USA
e-mail: marina.tsoy-podosenin@chsli.org

A. Thomas
Department of Psychiatry, NYU Grossman School of Medicine, New York, NY, USA
e-mail: anil.thomas@nyulangone.org

C. Marienfeld, M. Soltani (eds.), *AAAP Review of Addiction Psychiatry*,
https://doi.org/10.1007/978-3-032-24174-0_11

- Maintenance treatment for OUD includes a combination of pharmacological agents (opioid agonists or antagonists) with counseling and psychosocial support. All medications approved for OUD decrease illicit or problematic opioid use and improve function. Specific indications, availability of pharmacological agents, and a person's motivation and health condition should be taken into consideration.

Introduction

Epidemiology of Opioid Use

More than half a million people in the United States have died from an overdose involving opioids since 1999, including prescription and illicit opioids. Increased prescription of opioid medications in the 1990s contributed to widespread misuse of both prescription and non-prescription opioids. The total estimated number of U.S. opioid-related overdose deaths in 2024 was 54,743. This is a notable decrease from the estimated 83,140 opioid-involved deaths in 2023 [1]. Synthetic opioids (primarily illegally manufactured fentanyl (IMF)) were involved in 48,422 estimated deaths. Introduction of IMFs as adulterants of or replacements for heroin led to a sharp rise in overdose deaths due to their high potency and rapid onset of their effects. Carfentanil, a fentanyl analog 100 times more potent than fentanyl, was detected in 513 overdose deaths during January 2021–June 2024 [2]. Among people aged 12 and older in 2023, 2.0% (or 5.7 million people) had opioid use disorder in the past year [3]. Among them, only 18.0% (or 1.0 million people) received medication for OUD in the past year. Most adults who needed OUD treatment either did not perceive that they needed it (42.7%) or received treatment without medications (30%) [4]. OUD is often associated with other substance use disorders, particularly those involving tobacco, alcohol, cannabis, stimulants, and benzodiazepines, which are frequently taken to reduce the symptoms of opioid withdrawal or the craving for opioids, or to enhance the effects of administered opioids. Additional consequences of high rates of OUD include a rising incidence of infants born with neonatal opioid withdrawal syndrome (NOWS) because their mothers used these substances during pregnancy and increased spread of infectious diseases, such as HIV and hepatitis C.

Definition of Opiate Versus Opioid

Opiates are alkaloids derived from the poppy plant *Papaver Somniferum*. Morphine, codeine, and thebaine are examples of natural opiates. The term *opioid* refers to the entire class of compounds that bind to one or more types of opioid receptors, including endogenous peptides (β-endorphin, enkephalins, and dynorphins), natural

Table 11.1 Generic name, trade name, and street name of commonly abused opioids

Generic name	Trade name	Street name
Codeine	Tylenol #3	Cody, Captain, Schoolboy, Syrup
Morphine	MS-Contin, Avinza, Depodur, Duramorph, Infumorph, Astramorph, Kadian, Roxanol, Oramorph	M, Monkey, Good Fella, Miss Emma, Morph
Heroin (illicit drug)	N/A	H, White Horse, Junk, Dope, Black, Brown Sugar, Skunk, Tar, Black Tar
Oxycodone	Percocet, Percodan, Oxycontin, Roxicodone	Oxys, Percs, Cotton, Orange County, Killers, OC
Hydrocodone	Vicodin, Lorcet, Lortab, Norco, Hycodan, Co-Gesic	Vics, Hydros, Lorris, Watsons
Hydromorphone	Dilaudid, Exalgo	Hospital Heroin, Dust, Juice, Dillies, M2s
Oxymorphone	Opana	Blue Haven, Octagons, Biscuits, Pink Lady, Stop Signs
Meperidine	Demerol	Dust, Juice, Demmies
Tramadol	Ultram, Ultracet	Trammies, Chill Pills, Ultras
Fentanyl	Abstral, Fentora, Subsys, Onsolis, Sublimaze, Duragesic (transdermal)	Apache, TNT, China Girl, China White, Goodfella, Jackpot, Tango and Cash
Methadone	Methadose, Dolophine	Chocolate Chip Cookies, Fizzies, Saliva, Wafers
Buprenorphine	Buprenex, in combination with naloxone—Suboxone, Zubsolv, Bunavail, Cassipa	Box, Stops, Subs

alkaloids (opiates), and all semisynthetic and synthetic drugs that mimic the actions of opiates [5]. Examples of semisynthetic opioids include oxycodone, buprenorphine, and heroin (diacetylmorphine). Methadone, fentanyl, tramadol, and meperidine are synthetic opioids. Most opioids are categorized under Schedule II of the United States Controlled Substances Act, which indicates that these drugs have a high potential for abuse, with use potentially leading to severe psychological or physical dependence. Buprenorphine is categorized as a Schedule III drug, which means it has moderate-to-low potential for physical dependence or high potential for psychological dependence. Commonly misused prescribed and illicit opioids are listed in Table 11.1.

Pharmacology of Opioids

The endogenous opioid system consists of opioid receptors and endogenous opioid peptide ligands. The endogenous opioid system plays an important role in response to pain, stress regulation involving the hypothalamic-pituitary-adrenal axis, regulation of reward, mood, learning, and memory, as well as reproductive, gastrointestinal, cardiovascular, and pulmonary function [5, 6]. Opioid receptors belong to a family of 7-transmembrane G-protein-coupled receptors. To date, five types of opioid receptors have been identified and cloned—mu (MOR), kappa (KOR), delta (DOR), zeta (ZOR), and nociception or opioid receptor-like-1 (OPRL-1) receptor [7, 8]. Three types of endogenous opioids—beta-endorphins, enkephalins, and dynorphins—have a degree of selectivity for mu, delta, and kappa receptors, respectively. Exogenous opioids act primarily as agonists or partial agonists at mu receptors.

Heroin is a potent agonist of mu-opioid receptors; it has a half-life of 30 minutes but a duration of action of 4–5 hours due to active metabolites, including morphine. Heroin is more lipid-soluble than morphine, allowing it to rapidly cross the blood-brain barrier for rapid onset (resulting in a dopamine surge in the reward pathways) and to reach high levels in the brain. Fentanyl is another potent synthetic opioid, approximately 100 times more potent than morphine. Fentanyl is hepatically metabolized via the CYP3A4 enzyme primarily into norfentanyl and other metabolites. Fentanyl is highly lipophilic, which explains its rapid onset and short duration of action. Illegally manufactured fentanyl (IMF) initially was being used as an adulterant or additive to heroin and cocaine and sold as counterfeit Xanax pills. Because users of these substances were often opioid-naïve, the risk of overdose and death may be higher [9]. IMF is commonly the most widely available and preferred illicit opioid [2].

Illicit Opioid Contaminants, Adulterants, and Additives

When discussing illicit drugs, the terms "contaminants," "additives," and "adulterants" refer to substances found within the drug product that are not the primary psychoactive substance themselves. While sometimes used interchangeably, these terms have nuanced distinctions, often related to the intent (or lack thereof) behind their presence and their potential effects. Contaminants are substances present in an illicit drug unintentionally. They are typically introduced accidentally during the manufacturing, processing, storage, or transportation of the drug. Examples include environmental contamination, pesticides, heavy metals, and cross-contamination with other drugs. Additives ("cutting or bulking agents") are substances intentionally mixed with an illicit drug to increase its volume (sugar, talc, starch, etc.) or to make the drug easier to use (e.g., caffeine might be added to heroin to help it vaporize when smoked). Adulterants are substances intentionally added to an illicit drug to alter effects (mimic, enhance) or mask quality. Adulterants may include drugs with similar effects (e.g., local anesthetics might be added to cocaine to mimic its numbing effect), more potent drugs (IMF, veterinary tranquilizer Xylazine, potent veterinary sedative medetomidine), and drugs with different psychoactive effects (examples include benzodiazepines added to illicit opioids, PCP or synthetic cannabinoids added to cannabis). IMF supply is increasingly being found adulterated with a range of other dangerous substances. Veterinary tranquilizers Xylazine and medetomidine are potent synthetic alpha-2 adrenergic agonists. They can cause profound sedation, hypotension, bradycardia, and necrotic skin wounds. Naloxone does not reverse the effects of Xylazine or medetomidine. Other synthetic opioids, e.g., carfentanil, nitazenes, dipyanone, are significantly more potent than fentanyl and dramatically increase the risk of overdose [2].

Laboratory Diagnosis

A standard opiate immunoassay test detects the use of opiates such as morphine, codeine, and heroin. It has variable sensitivity for semisynthetic opioids oxycodone, hydrocodone, and hydromorphone. Synthetic opioids, such as meperidine, fentanyl, and methadone, and the semisynthetic buprenorphine, will not be detected and require confirmatory testing using gas or liquid chromatography and mass spectrometry [10]. Fentanyl and its primary metabolite, norfentanyl, can be detected in urine up to 72 hours. With heavy chronic use, the detection window may extend up to 5–7 days due to accumulation of metabolites. Ingestion of poppy seeds can result in positive urine opiate screens for codeine and morphine for 48 hours at the common cutoff of 300 mg/ml [11]. Heroin is metabolized to 6-monoacetylmorphine (6-MAM), which then is hydrolyzed to morphine. Detection of 6-MAM in urine unequivocally proves heroin use.

Diagnosis and Management of Opioid Use Disorder

OUD is defined by the DSM-5-TR as two or more (three or more in the setting of prescription opioid use) of the following within the same 12-month period [12]:

- Using larger amounts of opioids or over a longer period than was intended
- Persistent desire to cut down or unsuccessful efforts to control use
- A great deal of time spent obtaining, using, or recovering from use
- Craving, or a strong desire or urge to use substance
- Failure to fulfill major role obligations at work, school, or home due to recurrent opioid use
- Continued use despite recurrent or persistent social or interpersonal problems caused or exacerbated by opioid use
- Giving up or reducing social, occupational, or recreational activities due to opioid use
- Recurrent opioid use in physically hazardous situations
- Continued opioid use despite physical or psychological problems caused or exacerbated by its use
- Tolerance (marked increase in amount; marked decrease in effect)
- Withdrawal syndrome as manifested by cessation of opioids or use of opioids (or a closely related substance) to relieve or avoid withdrawal symptoms.

Tolerance and withdrawal criteria are not considered to be met for those taking opioids solely under appropriate medical supervision.

The severity of OUD is categorized as mild (presence of 2–3 symptoms), moderate (4–5 symptoms), or severe (6 or more symptoms).

Remission of OUD is categorized as follows:

- In early remission: none of the criteria for OUD have been met for at least 3 months but for less than 12 months (except for craving, or a strong desire or urge to use opioids), but full criteria for opioid use disorder were previously met.
- In sustained remission: none of the criteria for OUD have been met at any time during a period of 12 months or longer (except for craving, or a strong desire or urge to use opioids), but full criteria for opioid use disorder were previously met.

Opioid Intoxication and Overdose

Diagnostic criteria for opioid intoxication [12]:

A. Recent use of an opioid.
B. Clinically significant problematic behavioral or psychological changes (e.g., initial euphoria followed by apathy, dysphoria, psychomotor agitation or retardation, impaired judgment) that developed during or shortly after opioid use.
C. Pupillary constriction (or pupillary dilation due to anoxia from severe overdose) and one (or more) of the following signs or symptoms developing during or shortly after opioid use:
   (a) Drowsiness or coma.
   (b) Slurred speech.
   (c) Impairment in attention or memory.
D. The signs or symptoms are not attributable to another medical condition and are not better explained by another mental disorder, including intoxication with another substance.

The level of tolerance to opioids can have a significant effect on an individual's risk of opioid overdose. Tolerance to respiratory depression is lower than tolerance to euphoric effects, which explains why overdose often occurs even among "experienced" opioid users [13]. Recently detoxified persons or people with long periods of abstinence (such as those recently released or received treatment with opioid antagonists) are at higher risk for overdose.

Acute opioid use significantly reduces the responsiveness of the brainstem respiratory centers to carbon dioxide and reduces peripheral chemoreceptor response to hypoxia, thought primarily to be mediated by mu-opiate receptors.

Diagnosis of opioid overdose [14, 15]:

A. Classic "triad": coma, pinpoint pupils, respiratory depression (respiratory rate <12/min).
B. History of opioid use (ask about drug, amount, and time of last use). Polydrug use (high mortality if combined with opioids and benzodiazepines, alcohol, or cocaine) may indicate the need for additional therapy (e.g., flumazenil to reverse benzodiazepine effect).
C. Use of collateral information.

D. Circumstantial evidence of opioid use (i.e., needle marks or cellulitis).
E. Laboratory tests: toxicology screens for opioids and other drugs, rule out hypoglycemia, acidosis, and electrolyte abnormalities.

The risk of opioid overdose is increased with concurrent use of alcohol, benzodiazepines, barbiturates, other sedatives, and amphetamines. Atypical presentation and unusual complications may be the result of contamination of drugs with additives or adulterants—substances used to "cut" street drugs, including dextromethorphan, lidocaine, scopolamine, and levamisole.

Management of opioid overdose involves the administration of an opioid antagonist naloxone (prepacked nasal spray Narcan or injectable naloxone for intravenous, intramuscular, or subcutaneous administration), to reverse the effects of opioids. The initial dose of 0.4–0.8 mg may be repeated at 2–3-minute intervals. Overdose with opioids that are more potent and have high receptor binding affinity (e.g., fentanyl) or longer acting (e.g., methadone) may require higher doses of naloxone given over longer periods. If a person does not respond to multiple doses of naloxone, consider alternative causes—intoxication with non-opioid drugs (e.g., benzodiazepines or barbiturates) or medical causes (hypoglycemia, acidosis, electrolyte abnormalities, head trauma, or subarachnoid hemorrhage) [15].

Opioid Withdrawal

Opioid withdrawal is a combination of self-reported and observed symptoms when an individual who developed physical dependence as a result of chronic exposure to opioids discontinues or reduces opioid use. Opioid withdrawal is a direct result of neuroadaptations that occur in response to chronic opioid exposure, regardless of the purpose of use. The severity of opioid withdrawal varies with the specific opioid used, route of administration, dose, and duration of drug use. The half-life of the drug determines the onset and duration of acute withdrawal. Thus, withdrawal may begin 4–6 hours after the use of heroin and subside substantially within 5–7 days. Fentanyl is a potent, short-acting opioid. Withdrawal symptoms can begin very quickly after the last dose, within 6–12 hours after the last use. Initial withdrawal signs might appear as early as 2–4 hours for some individuals, especially with frequent, high-dose use. Symptoms typically peak within 1–3 days, and last for about 5–7 days. With methadone withdrawal, in contrast, the onset of withdrawal may be delayed up to 36 hours after the last use of methadone, but the symptoms may not subside for 14–21 days. Intermittent drug use usually does not cause severe withdrawal. Although opioid withdrawal generally includes no life-threatening complications in adults, it causes marked discomfort, prevents many persons from entering treatment, and often is a factor in the continuation of opioid use to relieve suffering. A protracted abstinence syndrome that can last months has been described, which may include continuous craving, insomnia, fatigue, dysphoria, and irritability, all of which increase the likelihood of relapse [14].

Diagnostic criteria for opioid withdrawal [12]:

A. Presence of either of the following:
   (a) Cessation of (or reduction in) opioid use that has been heavy and prolonged (i.e., several weeks or longer).
   (b) Administration of an opioid antagonist after a period of opioid use.
B. Three (or more) of the following, developing within minutes to several days after Criterion A:
   (a) Dysphoric mood, nausea or vomiting, muscle aches, lacrimation or rhinorrhea, pupillary dilation, piloerection, or sweating, diarrhea, yawning, fever, and insomnia.
C. The signs or symptoms in Criterion B cause clinically significant distress or impairment in social, occupational, or other important areas of functioning.
D. The signs and symptoms are not attributable to another medical condition and are not better explained by another mental disorder, including intoxication or withdrawal from another substance.

Several clinical tools are available to assess the severity of opioid withdrawal. The most widely used are the Clinical Opioid Withdrawal Scale (COWS), designed to be administered by clinicians, and the Subjective Opiate Withdrawal Scale (SOWS), designed to be completed by patients. Both scales quantify the severity of opioid withdrawal and monitor these symptoms over time. Opioid withdrawal can be managed in inpatient or outpatient settings. Several factors, including severity of withdrawal, presence and severity of underlying medical and psychiatric comorbidities, failure to complete outpatient detoxification in the past, availability of social supports, and access to methods of detoxification may determine the treatment approach (slow vs. rapid detoxification) and a choice of the treatment setting [16].

Management of opioid withdrawal involves a combination of general supportive measures (safe environment and adequate nutrition) and specific pharmacologic therapies such as the use of full (methadone) or partial opioid agonists (buprenorphine), alpha-2 adrenergic agonists (clonidine, guanfacine, and lofexidine (Lucemyra)), and medications providing symptomatic relief (nonsteroidal anti-inflammatory agents, ondansetron, dicyclomine, loperamide, benzodiazepines, trazodone, etc.). Existing guidelines on the treatment of OUD do not recommend short-term medically supervised withdrawal alone due to a high risk of relapse [17]. Opioid maintenance treatment with medications for OUD should always be recommended.

Methadone, a long-acting full mu-opioid agonist, effectively controls opioid withdrawal and reduces craving for opioids. The use of methadone has been restricted to inpatient settings or specialized licensed Opioid Treatment Programs (OTPs). In pre-fentanyl era, the initial methadone dose was limited to 30 mg over the first 24 hours, in 5- to 10-mg increments [16, 18]. For persons with higher opioid tolerance presenting in moderate-to-severe withdrawal, the initial methadone dose of up to 50 mg on the first day may be reasonable [24–26]. Dose adjustment can then be made based on objective signs of opioid withdrawal rather than on subjective complaints alone. Methadone tapering can be accomplished in 5–7 days in an inpatient setting, whereas outpatient detoxification is often extended to minimize withdrawal symptoms and to decrease the likelihood of relapse [16].

Buprenorphine is a high-affinity, long-acting partial mu-opioid agonist with a lower risk of respiratory depression and sedation compared to methadone, which is effective for the treatment of opioid withdrawal and maintenance treatment of OUD [19]. Buprenorphine may displace opioid agonists with similar or lower binding affinity (i.e., heroin, oxycodone, and fentanyl) from mu-opioid receptors and precipitate opioid withdrawal in persons with recent opioid usage. It has been suggested that inducting persons dependent on short-acting opioids (i.e., heroin, oxycodone) should occur after an emergence of mild to moderate withdrawal symptoms (6–12 hours after the last heroin use). Various strategies for buprenorphine induction are discussed in the opioid maintenance treatment section.

Buprenorphine taper may be completed in 5–7 days in an inpatient setting, whereas outpatient detoxification is often gradual and may take 2–8 weeks.

Both opioids and alpha-2 adrenergic agonists can suppress the activity of the locus coeruleus, a major noradrenergic center in the brain that is hyperactive during opioid withdrawal. Clonidine, the alpha-2 adrenergic agonist, has been used off-label to facilitate opioid withdrawal in both inpatient and outpatient settings. Clonidine has mild analgesic properties, and at dosages of 0.6–1.2 mg/day, it reduces many of the autonomic components of the opioid withdrawal syndrome, although craving, muscle aches, insomnia, and irritability are not well suppressed but can be ameliorated by other adjunct treatments. Benzodiazepines can be used short-term to treat insomnia and muscle aches but should be given with caution due to their misuse potential and interaction with opioids, especially in the outpatient setting.

Clonidine has some advantages over the use of opioid agonists: it has no addictive properties, is available to general physicians, and facilitates the transition to maintenance treatment with opioid antagonists. Sedation and dizziness from orthostatic hypotension have been reported as the most common side effects of clonidine. Persons should be cautioned about driving, and operating equipment during the first few days. A history of psychosis, cardiac arrhythmias, pregnancy, and use of tricyclic antidepressants within 3 weeks precludes the use of clonidine [15]. In 2018, the US Food and Drug Administration (FDA) approved a non-opioid agent, lofexidine hydrochloride (Lucemyra) for the mitigation of withdrawal symptoms. Lofexidine is a selective alpha-2 adrenergic agonist associated with a lower risk of hypotension and sedation compared to clonidine.

Agents other than opioid agonists and alpha-2 adrenergic agonists have been investigated for the treatment of opioid withdrawal. Various alternatives to current detoxification strategies, including the use of N-methyl-D-aspartate (NMDA) receptor antagonist memantine, 5HT-1A partial agonist buspirone, gabapentin, tramadol, ibogaine, acupuncture, and others, require further study. Anesthesia-Assisted Ultra Rapid Opioid Detoxification has revealed little benefit while leading to significant adverse events [15].

Opioid Maintenance Treatment

The current mainstay of treatment for OUD is the use of medications for opioid use disorder (MOUD) in combination with counseling and psychosocial support. The FDA approved three pharmacological agents for the treatment of OUD: full mu-opioid agonist methadone, partial mu-opioid agonist buprenorphine, and opioid antagonist naltrexone (Vivitrol) [15, 16, 18]. All three of these treatments have been demonstrated to be safe and effective in reducing opioid use, the transmission of infectious disease, and crime [17, 18, 20]. There is no maximum recommended duration of maintenance treatment, and, for some persons, treatment may continue indefinitely. The treatment goals include prevention or reduction of medical, psychiatric, and other consequences of OUD, and improvement of functioning, quality of life, and overall well-being of persons [16].

Opioid Agonists

Treatment with an opioid agonist—methadone or buprenorphine—at an adequate dose suppresses craving and withdrawal symptoms, attenuates the euphoric effects of illicit opioids due to cross-tolerance, allows persons to improve psychosocial functioning, and reduces criminal activity and transmission of infectious diseases. Oral or sublingual route of administration leads to a relatively slow rate of increase in plasma level and thus is less euphorigenic and reinforcing. A longer half-life allows for the prevention of withdrawal and stabilizes fluctuations in mood and level of consciousness found with the use of short-acting opioids [15].

Methadone

Methadone has proven efficacy in reducing illicit opioid use and reducing the mortality and morbidity associated with OUD in numerous studies since methadone was approved for use in the United States in 1947. Both methadone and buprenorphine are included in the World Health Organization List of Essential Medicines, the most effective and safe medicines needed in a health system [21]. Methadone for maintenance treatment of OUD is only available in specialized and licensed OTP programs. Methadone as a full mu-opioid receptor agonist carries a higher risk of misuse, and can cause potentially fatal respiratory depression or lethal overdose in accidental ingestion. Methadone use is also associated with QT-interval prolongation and serious arrhythmia (torsades de pointes), particularly at higher doses. Providers should be aware of substantial inter-individual pharmacokinetic variability and numerous drug interactions. Most significant medication interactions with methadone are presented in Table 11.2.

Table 11.2 Medication interactions with methadone [22, 23]

Medications that may reduce methadone clearance and increase risk of potential toxicity and cardiac arrhythmia (torsades de pointes)	Antiarrhythmics: amiodarone, diltiazem, verapamil, quinidine Macrolide antibiotics: clarithromycin, erythromycin, ciprofloxacin Antifungals: fluconazole, ketoconazole, voriconazole, terbinafine SSRI: sertraline, paroxetine, fluvoxamine Urinary alkalinizers (sodium bicarbonate decreases methadone excretion by kidneys) Other: Disulfiram, Dihydroergotamine, Ethanol, Moclobemide, Metronidazole, grapefruit juice
Medications that may accelerate metabolism of methadone and increase risk of opioid withdrawal	Antiepileptics: carbamazepine, phenobarbital, phenytoin Antiretrovirals: efavirenz, nevirapine, darunavir/ritonavir, lopinavir/ritonavir, nelfinavir, tipranavir/ritonavir Other: rifampin, St. John's wort
Medications associated with QT-interval prolongation	Anesthetics, muscle relaxants, antiemetics (ondansetron, granisetron), antipsychotics (chlorpromazine, ziprasidone, aripiprazole, quetiapine), SSRI (citalopram, fluoxetine, paroxetine, sertraline), tricyclic antidepressants, some anticholinesterase inhibitors
Pharmacodynamic synergistic interaction resulting in increased sedation and potentially lethal respiratory depression	Alcohol, benzodiazepines, barbiturates, opioids, and other CNS depressants

Methadone Induction

Original guidelines recommended "starting low and going slow." Methadone has a relatively long half-life (24–36 hours or longer) and significant genetic variability in metabolism; therefore, a person will not feel the full effect of the initial dose for 4 or more days. The risk of overdose is highest in the first 2–4 weeks of methadone treatment. The initial suggested dose was limited to 30 mg [18]. In Feb 2024, SAMHSA updated regulations to allow a day 1 dosage of methadone up to 50 mg [24]. The rapid initiation algorithm allows titration of methadone to 80 mg on day 3 and increase the dose to 100 mg on day 6 [24, 25]. The potential benefits include alleviation of withdrawal symptoms, decreased illicit opioid use, faster time to a "blocking dose," and improved retention in treatment [26]. The potential risks of a rapid induction include the risk of sedation and overdose, particularly if methadone is combined with illicit opioids or other sedatives. Dosing must be individualized based on patient response.

Slow methadone detoxification is used for termination of methadone maintenance treatment to avoid long residual withdrawal symptoms from methadone withdrawal. Persons who choose not to continue MOUD should be tapered off methadone slowly over a 3- to 6-month period or longer.

Buprenorphine

Buprenorphine has a unique pharmacological and safety profile, which makes it an attractive treatment for persons with OUD and a popular option for office-based treatment. The Consolidated Appropriations Act of 2023 (CAA 2023) has amended the Controlled Substances Act and eliminated the Drug Addiction Treatment Act of 2000 (DATA 2000). As of June 2023, providers are no longer required to obtain DATA 2000 Waiver to prescribe buprenorphine for OUD. However, when applying for registration, providers are required to complete a one-time attestation confirming that they have fulfilled the CAA 2023 training requirements, which include 8 hours of training on identifying and treating addiction, or belong to a group of exempt professionals, such as those with board certification in addiction psychiatry or addiction medicine [24].

As a partial agonist at the mu-opioid receptor, buprenorphine has a very high affinity and low intrinsic activity. Therefore, it displaces full opioid agonists without stimulating the receptor at full opioid activity. It has lower misuse potential compared to methadone, lower level of physical dependence, less withdrawal discomfort, and a ceiling effect at higher doses (flattening of the dose-effect curve for respiratory depression and sedation) [27]. Buprenorphine is less likely to cause fatal respiratory depression in comparison with a full opioid agonist, and is therefore much less likely to result in opioid overdose unless combined with other central nervous system (CNS) depressants.

Buprenorphine Induction Strategies

The standard conventional approach is to administer buprenorphine 2–4 mg sublingually and another 2–4 mg dose of buprenorphine approximately 60–90 minutes later, depending on the person's comfort level, with a total of 8–12 mg of buprenorphine on day 1 to sufficiently relieve withdrawal symptoms [18].

In emergency or inpatient settings, high-dose and low-dose approaches have been tested to accommodate a person's needs and substance use patterns, including use of high-potency synthetic opioids like fentanyl. Persons with high tolerance to opioids, persons with moderate-severe withdrawal, including those who have recently been administered naloxone for overdose, may benefit from a high-dose ("Quick Start") protocol. After the initial administered buprenorphine dose of 8–16 mg (for persons with very high tolerance to opioids, some protocols suggest starting with up to 32 mg), the person is observed for 30–60 minutes. If withdrawal symptoms persist, an additional dose of 8–16 mg of buprenorphine is administered. The total dose on the first day can be up to 32 mg, and, in some cases higher, to control symptoms. The typical maintenance daily dose is between 16 and 24 mg [28].

Buprenorphine low-dose induction, first described in 2010, is being used in both inpatient and outpatient settings. For persons on high doses of opioids, persons with chronic pain, or those who are unable to tolerate withdrawal required for traditional buprenorphine induction, a low-dose cross-tapering strategy has been shown as a safe and effective way to avoid withdrawal and uncontrolled pain [29, 30]. Buprenorphine low-dose cross-tapers are conducted with sublingual, buccal, and transdermal formulations. Intravenous buprenorphine has been used as well. Repetitive administration of small doses of buprenorphine, typically 0.5 mg or less every 12 hours, does not precipitate withdrawal. Over time, buprenorphine accumulates and replaces full opioid agonist without causing unpleasant symptoms of withdrawal [43].

As with any drug stimulating mu-opioid receptor, buprenorphine has the potential for misuse and diversion. To decrease the potential for misuse, the buprenorphine/naloxone combination in a 4:1 ratio (Suboxone) has been developed. Sublingual naloxone has relatively low oral and sublingual bioavailability; however, in case of injection or intranasal use of the combination product, the mu-opioid receptor antagonist naloxone has greater availability and can precipitate withdrawal syndrome [19]. Buprenorphine is metabolized by CYP 450 3A4; therefore, agents that inhibit or induce CYP 3A4 enzyme can increase or reduce the plasma concentration of buprenorphine. In therapeutic doses, buprenorphine does not cause clinically significant QT-interval prolongation. Buprenorphine can cause respiratory depression if co-administered with other CNS depressants, i.e., alcohol, benzodiazepines [22].

To improve retention in treatment and minimize the risk of diversion, extended-release injectable formulations of buprenorphine for treatment of moderate and severe OUD have been developed. Sublocade is a monthly extended-release buprenorphine injection administered subcutaneously in the abdominal region by a healthcare provider. It is available in 100 and 300 mg dosage forms. The recommended starting dose is 300 mg monthly for 2 months, followed by a maintenance dose of 100 mg monthly. The maintenance dose can be increased to 300 mg monthly in case of unsatisfactory clinical response [31]. Brixadi is another extended-release buprenorphine injection, available for monthly and weekly subcutaneous administration. Brixadi has a more flexible dosing range equal to SL buprenorphine 6–24 mg; therefore, it may be a better choice for persons who require higher doses [32].

Opioid Antagonists

Naltrexone, a long-acting mu-opioid antagonist, provides blockade of mu-opioid receptors, thus blocking the reinforcing properties of opioids, which theoretically makes it an ideal maintenance agent for persons with OUD. Poor adherence and increased risk of overdose after discontinuation of treatment significantly limited the use of *oral* naltrexone for OUD [33]. Nevertheless, in the situation when medication use can be supervised, and for certain highly motivated persons with OUD, such as healthcare professionals, business executives, pilots, commercial drivers, and probation referrals, for whom there is an external incentive to comply with naltrexone therapy and to remain opioid abstinent, naltrexone has been very effective [34]. As an example, naltrexone has been a routine adjunct for the treatment of anesthesiologists who are addicted to opioids [14]. In 2010, an extended-release injectable naltrexone (XR-NTX) Vivitrol was FDA-approved for prevention of relapse to opioid dependence following opioid detoxification as part of an individualized comprehensive management program that includes psychosocial support [35].

XR-NTX can be given in various clinical settings, including primary care and criminal justice systems. Persons treated with XR-NTX have better treatment adherence, lower rates of opioid use, and reduced craving as compared with persons treated with placebo [36]. Persons on probation or parole who were randomly assigned to open-label treatment with XR-NTX compared with treatment as usual had significantly lower rates of relapse, longer relapse-free survival, lower rates of heroin use, and fewer overdoses over a 24-week treatment period, with a loss of effect seen at 28 and 54 weeks after the end of treatment [34]. Recent studies directly comparing the efficacy of XR-NTX and buprenorphine/naloxone show that among persons who successfully initiated treatment with medications, treatment outcomes were comparable [37, 38].

All persons who discontinue agonist or antagonist therapy and resume opioid use should be made aware of the increased risks associated with an opioid overdose, especially the increased risk of death. A comparison of commonly used opioid agonist and antagonist therapies is presented in Table 11.3.

Table 11.3 Comparison of opioid agonists and antagonists used for maintenance treatment of OUD [5, 16, 18]

	Full opioid agonist	Partial opioid agonist/antagonist	Opioid antagonist
Generic (trade) name	Methadone (Dolophine)	Buprenorphine (Subutex) Buprenorphine/ naloxone (Suboxone, Zubsolv), Extended-release subcutaneous buprenorphine (Sublocade, Brixadi)	Extended-release injectable naltrexone (Vivitrol)
Mechanism of action	Mu-opioid receptor agonist, weak N-methyl-D-aspartate (NMDA) receptor antagonist	Mu-opioid receptor partial agonist, kappa-opioid receptor antagonist, delta-opioid receptor antagonist	Mu-opioid receptor antagonist, partial kappa-opioid receptor agonist
Pharmacokinetics	Extensively metabolized by CYP 3A4, 2B6, 2D6, and 2C19. Autoinduction of metabolism. Elimination half-life is highly variable, for 12–150 hours	Metabolized by CYP 3A4 and 2C8. Elimination half-life of sublingual buprenorphine is 24–42 hours	Metabolized by dihydrodiol dehydrogenase and not by the CYP450 system. Elimination half-life of injectable naltrexone is 5–10 days

(continued)

Table 11.3 (continued)

	Full opioid agonist	Partial opioid agonist/antagonist	Opioid antagonist
Adverse effects	Sedation, dizziness, orthostatic hypotension, headache, constipation, sweating, nausea, vomiting, reduced libido, erectile dysfunction, urinary retention, dry mouth, peripheral edema, respiratory depression, QT-interval prolongation, cardiac arrhythmias, coma	Headache, drowsiness, constipation, nausea, vomiting, sweating, orthostatic hypotension, oral hypoesthesia, peripheral edema, blurred vision, reduced libido, injection site reactions (pruritus)	Nausea, headache, decreased appetite, pharyngitis, anxiety, insomnia, diarrhea, liver function abnormalities (<1%), injection site reactions (pain, tenderness, induration, swelling, erythema, or bruising)
Initial dose	10–30 mg (up to 50 mg in rapid induction)	Conventional protocol: 2–4 mg, may be increased in increments of 2–4 mg for a total dose up to 12 mg on day 1 Quick Start protocol: initial dose 8–16 mg, may be increased up to 32 mg on day 1 Low Dose protocol: Day 1: 0.5 mg SL qday Day 2: 0.5 mg BID Day 3: 1 mg SL BID Day 4: 2 mg SL BID Day 5: 3 mg SL BID Day 6: 4 mg SL BID Day 7: 6 mg SL BID Day 8: 8 mg SL BID (Stop opioid agonist)	380 mg deep intramuscular injection in the gluteal muscle
Average effective dose	60–120 mg daily Persons using fentanyl may need a dose >100 mg	16–24 mg daily	380 mg every 4 weeks
Risk of overdose	Increased risk of overdose and death during the initial 2 weeks of methadone induction. High genetic variability in metabolism rate. Concomitant use of medications interfering with methadone metabolism or sedatives (alcohol, benzodiazepines) increases the risk of overdose	Partial agonist properties produce a ceiling effect and reduce the risk of overdose. Low risk of QT-interval prolongation	Increased risk of overdose on illicit opioids if treatment was interrupted and there was use of high potency opioids in the setting of low tolerance

(continued)

Table 11.3 (continued)

	Full opioid agonist	Partial opioid agonist/antagonist	Opioid antagonist
Special considerations to start medication	Use caution in persons with co-use of other CNS depressants	Persons should experience mild to moderate opioid withdrawal before taking the first dose to reduce the risk of precipitated withdrawal	Absence of physical dependence from opioid agonists: at least 7 days between the last dose of heroin and the first dose of naltrexone, or 10–14 days between the last dose of methadone or buprenorphine/naloxone and the first dose of naltrexone; naloxone challenge may be useful
Psychosocial treatment	Required	Recommended	Recommended
Habit forming/ Risk of diversion	Yes	Yes	No
Frequency of visits	Determined by federal guidelines; daily visits during stabilization	Weekly during stabilization, then advance commensurate with stability	No specific requirements; injections are given monthly
Barriers for treatment	Stigma Requires specialized Opioid Treatment Program Adverse effects and interaction with other agents Fear of physical withdrawal upon treatment cessation	Persons unable to tolerate withdrawal symptoms prior to or during start may benefit from low-dose induction Fear of physical withdrawal upon treatment cessation	Difficulty initiating treatment Low penetration into formularies Limited knowledge among professionals
Transition to other medication	To buprenorphine: persons on low dose of methadone (30–40 mg or less), wait until developing mild to moderate withdrawal To naltrexone: stop methadone for up to 14 days to avoid withdrawal; naloxone challenge may be useful	To methadone: no required time delay To naltrexone: 7–14 days between the last dose of buprenorphine and the first dose of naltrexone to avoid precipitated withdrawal; naloxone challenge may be useful	Switching from naltrexone to a full agonist or partial agonist is less complicated, with no risk of precipitated withdrawal. Consider lower initial dose of full agonist or partial agonist
Discontinuation of treatment	Slow taper over several months; abrupt discontinuation causes prolonged opioid withdrawal	Slow taper over several weeks to months; abrupt discontinuation causes opioid withdrawal	Taper not necessary

Treatment of OUD in Pregnant Women

Pregnant women with untreated OUD are more likely to seek prenatal care late in pregnancy, miss appointments, experience poor weight gain, or exhibit signs of withdrawal or intoxication. The fluctuating levels of opioids in the blood of mothers misusing opioids expose the fetus to repeated periods of withdrawal, which can also harm the function of the placenta and increase the risk of intrauterine complications, preterm labor, and fetal death [39, 43]. Pregnant women are also at risk of untreated maternal infections such as HIV, malnutrition, and poor prenatal care, and dangers conferred by engaging in drug use, including violence and incarceration. Although there are no medications approved by the FDA for the treatment of OUD in pregnant women, methadone remains the standard of care for pregnant women with OUD. Methadone enhances the likelihood of the woman participating in prenatal care and addiction treatment. A stable methadone dose reduces the fluctuations in maternal opioid levels that can occur with illicit opioid use, and this stabilization is hypothesized to reduce stress on the fetus. Treatment with methadone should be initiated as early as possible. Providers should be aware that with advancing gestational age, plasma levels of methadone progressively decrease, and clearance increases. Therefore, increased or divided doses are often needed during pregnancy, and the needs may change as the pregnancy advances. After childbirth, doses may need to be adjusted. During pregnancy, the use of buprenorphine monoproduct (Subutex) has been historically preferred to prevent prenatal naloxone exposure, which is hypothesized to precipitate withdrawal and potentially cause maternal and fetal hormonal changes. However, switching medications for someone stable on buprenorphine-naloxone combination is not necessary. A recently published observational study demonstrated similar maternal and neonatal outcomes for pregnancies exposed to buprenorphine combined with naloxone compared with buprenorphine alone [40]. The pharmacokinetics of buprenorphine does not change significantly during pregnancy, and the need to adjust the dosing of buprenorphine during pregnancy is less than that of methadone. Flexible twice-a-day dosing may reduce withdrawal symptoms and craving to use illicit drugs. Several studies demonstrated strong evidence for improved neonatal outcomes with buprenorphine compared with methadone, including lower risk of preterm birth, greater birth weight, and less severe neonatal abstinence syndrome (NAS) [41, 42]. Mothers receiving methadone and buprenorphine monoproduct for the treatment of opioid use disorders should be encouraged to breastfeed if the mother is not using other drugs. Data on the use of long-acting injectable naltrexone for OUD during pregnancy is limited, but emerging evidence from small studies suggests it is a viable option for select patients, particularly those already stable on the medication prior to pregnancy. While associated with a significantly lower risk of neonatal opioid withdrawal syndrome compared to opioid agonists, its initiation during pregnancy is challenging due to the required detoxification period and risk of relapse [43]. Due to the lack of robust safety data, opioid agonists like methadone and buprenorphine remain the recommended standard of care for pregnant individuals with opioid use disorder [44].

Chapter Review Questions

1. A 38-year-old woman with a history of schizophrenia and OUD, treated with buprenorphine/naloxone 8 mg/2 mg, inquired about starting a new medication for treatment of schizophrenia, which contains olanzapine and samidorphan. What would you recommend?

   A. Start olanzapine 5 mg/samidorphan 10 mg per patient request
   B. Suggest an alternative antipsychotic without samidorphan
   C. Suggest switching to methadone
   D. Switch to Sublocade and start olanzapine 5 mg/samidorphan 10 mg
   E. Discontinue buprenorphine/naloxone 8 mg/2 mg, immediately initiate Vivitrol, and start olanzapine 5 mg/samidorphan 10 mg

   Correct Answer: B. Suggest an alternative antipsychotic

   Explanation: Samidorphan is a mu-opioid antagonist that may cause precipitated withdrawal if used concomitantly with partial mu-opioid agonist buprenorphine or full mu-opioid agonist methadone [44].

2. A 28-year-old male treated with buprenorphine/naloxone 24 mg/6 mg continues to report withdrawal and drug-related urges. He inquires about increasing the dose. When you review the results of his urine toxicology, you notice that the levels of buprenorphine and norbuprenorphine significantly fluctuate. Please select the best next step:

   A. Increase buprenorphine/naloxone to 32 mg/8 mg to alleviate the craving.
   B. Switch to injectable extended-release buprenorphine to minimize the risk of diversion and interdose withdrawal.
   C. Confront the patient and discharge from the program.
   D. Educate the patient about the risk of withdrawal if he misses the dose. Discuss alternative options to improve adherence to recommended treatment.
   E. Discontinue the buprenorphine/naloxone 24 mg/6 mg and inform the patient that moving forward, he will only receive Vivitrol.

   Correct Answer: D

   Explanation: Although switching to injectable extended-release buprenorphine is a viable option, the first step is to educate the patient and discuss existing options.

3. A 27-year-old, 24-week pregnant person presents to the methadone clinic complaining of nausea, diarrhea, runny nose, and muscle aches that peak in the morning before she comes to the clinic. For pregnant women with OUD taking methadone during the second trimester, the dose of methadone most likely will need to be

   A. Reduced to prevent NOWS.
   B. Increased to control opioid withdrawal and prevent relapse.
   C. Unchanged to prevent the fetus from developing withdrawal syndrome.
   D. Reduced to avoid cardiovascular complications.
   E. Unchanged to minimize the risk of QTC prolongation.

Correct Answer: B

Explanation: Increased fluid volume and metabolism rate during pregnancy will affect distribution and accelerate metabolism of methadone, which may lead to precipitated opioid withdrawal and require dose adjustment by increasing the dose or dividing the dose.

4. An anesthesiologist with OUD wants to discuss non-opioid options for maintenance treatment. Which statement regarding the extended-release injectable naltrexone (XR-NTX) is correct?

   A. In 1990, XR-NTX was FDA-approved for the maintenance treatment of opioid use disorder.
   B. XR-NTX demonstrated worse adherence to treatment compared to oral naltrexone.
   C. CYP 450 enzymes do not primarily metabolize XR-NTX.
   D. XR-NTX requires a special license to be prescribed.
   E. XR-NTX is the most effective treatment for opioid use disorder.

   Correct Answer: C

   Explanation: Naltrexone is extensively metabolized in humans. Production of the primary metabolite, 6 β-naltrexol, is mediated by dihydrodiol dehydrogenase, a cytosolic family of enzymes in the liver. The cytochrome P450 system is not involved in naltrexone metabolism. Naltrexone and its metabolites are also conjugated to form glucuronide products. XR-NTX was FDA-approved for treatment of OUD in 2010. XR-NTX demonstrated better adherence to treatment compared to oral naltrexone. XR-NTX does not require a special license to be prescribed. Methadone and buprenorphine are more effective in reducing opioid-related deaths and retaining people in treatment.

5. A 65-year-old man taking a high dose of benzodiazepine for anxiety developed OUD due to long-standing treatment with oxycodone for chronic pain. He wants to discuss treatment options for OUD. His psychiatrist suggests a partial mu-opioid receptor antagonist buprenorphine. A "ceiling effect" of buprenorphine means that

   A. At low doses, buprenorphine acts as an opioid antagonist and does not cause euphoria.
   B. Buprenorphine at higher doses is less likely to cause fatal respiratory depression in comparison with a full opioid agonist.
   C. When abruptly stopped, buprenorphine does not cause opioid withdrawal.
   D. Buprenorphine, as a mixed agonist/antagonist, has no misuse potential, and when injected, buprenorphine precipitates opioid withdrawal.
   E. Injecting buprenorphine will not result in intoxication.

   Correct Answer: B

   Explanation: Buprenorphine as a partial mu-opioid receptor agonist has very high affinity and low intrinsic activity. The flattening of the dose-effect curve indicates that buprenorphine has a lower risk of producing respiratory depression and sedation. If injected, buprenorphine may cause euphoria; therefore, it has a misuse potential. Abrupt discontinuation of buprenorphine will result in opioid withdrawal.

References

1. Centers for Disease Control and Prevention. National Vital Statistics System Provisional counts of drug overdose deaths. National Center for Health Statistics, Centers for Disease Control and Prevention; 2025.
2. Tanz LJ, Stewart A, Gladden RM, Ko JY, Owens L, O'Donnell J. Detection of illegally manufactured fentanyl and carfentanil in drug overdose deaths — United States, 2021–2024. MMWR Morb Mortal Wkly Rep. 2024;73:1099–105.
3. Substance Abuse and Mental Health Services Administration. Key substance use and mental health indicators in the United States: Results from the 2023 National Survey on Drug Use and Health (HHS Publication No. PEP24-07-021, NSDUH Series H-59). Center for Behavioral Health Statistics and Quality, Substance Abuse and Mental Health Services Administration; 2024. https://www.samhsa.gov/data/report/2023-nsduh-annual-national-report.
4. Centers for Disease Control and Prevention (CDC). Treatment for opioid use disorder: population estimates — United States, 2022. MMWR Morb Mortal Wkly Rep. 2024;73(25):591–8. Published June 27, 2024.
5. Pathan H, Williams J. Basic opioid pharmacology: an update. Br J Pain. 2012;6(1):11–6.
6. Drolet G, Dumont E, Gosselin I, Kinkead R, Laforest S, Trottier J. Role of endogenous opioid system in the regulation of the stress response. Prog Neuro-Psychopharmacol Biol Psychiatry. 2001;25(4):729–41.
7. Valentino R, Volkow N. Untangling the complexity of opioid receptor function. Neuropsychopharmacology. 2018;43:2514–20.
8. Rosenbaum D, Rasmussen S, Kobilka B. The structure and function of G-protein-coupled receptors. Nature. 2009;459(7245):356–63.
9. Comer S, Cahill C. Fentanyl: receptor pharmacology, abuse potential, and implications for treatment. Neurosci Biobehav Rev. 2019;106:49–57.
10. Stolbach A, Connors N, Nelson L, Kulig K. ACMT position statement: interpretation of urine opiate and opioid tests. J Med Toxicol. 2022;18(2):176–9.
11. Hayes L, Krasselt W, Mueggler P. Concentrations of morphine and codeine in serum and urine after ingestion of poppy seeds. Clin Chem. 1987;33(6):806–8.
12. American Psychiatric Association. Diagnostic and statistical manual of mental disorders. 5th ed., text rev. American Psychiatric Association Publishing; 2022.
13. Pattinson K. Opioids and the control of respiration. Br J Anaesth. 2008;100(6):747–58.
14. Fiellin D, Miller S, Saitz R. The ASAM principles of addiction medicine. 5th ed. Lippincott Williams & Wilkins; 2014.
15. Galanter M, Kleber H, Brady K. The American Psychiatric Publishing textbook of substance abuse treatment. 5th ed. American Psychiatric Publishing; 2014.
16. Kampman K, Jarvis M. American Society of Addiction Medicine (ASAM) national practice guideline for the use of medications in the treatment of addiction involving opioid use. J Addict Med. 2015;9:358–67.
17. Nunes E, Gordon M, Friedmann P, Fishman M, Lee J, Chen D, Hu M, Boney T, Wilson D, O'Brien C. Relapse to opioid use disorder after inpatient treatment: protective effect of injection naltrexone. J Subst Abus Treat. 2018;85:49–55.
18. Substance Abuse and Mental Health Services Administration. Treatment improvement protocol (TIP) series, No. 63. Medications for opioid use disorder. HHS Publication No. PEP21-02-01-002. Rockville: Substance Abuse and Mental Health Services Administration (SAMHSA); 2021.
19. Center for Substance Abuse Treatment. Clinical guidelines for the use of buprenorphine in the treatment of opioid addiction. In: Treatment improvement protocol (TIP) series 40. DHHS Publication No. (SMA) 07-3939. Rockville: Substance Abuse and Mental Health Services Administration; 2004.
20. Hser Y, Evans E, Huang D, Weiss R, Saxon A, Carroll K, Woody G, Liu D, Wakim P, Matthews A, Hatch-Maillette M, Jelstrom E, Wiest K, McLaughlin P, Ling W. Long-term outcomes after

randomization to buprenorphine/naloxone versus methadone in a multi-site trial. Addiction. 2016;111(4):695–705.
21. World Health Organization. WHO model list of essential medicines (19th List) (PDF). 2015. http://www.who.int/medicines/publications/essentialmedicines/EML_2015_FINAL_amended_NOV2015.pdf?ua=1.
22. McCance-Katz E, Sullivan L, Nallani S. Drug interactions of clinical importance among the opioids, methadone and buprenorphine, and other frequently prescribed dedications: a review. Am J Addict. 2010;19(1):4–16.
23. Saber-Tehrani A, Bruce R, Altice F. Pharmacokinetic drug interactions and adverse consequences between psychotropic medications and pharmacotherapy for the treatment of opioid dependence. Am J Drug Alcohol Abuse. 2011;37:1–11.
24. Substance Abuse and Mental Health Services Administration. Federal guidelines for opioid Treatment programs. Rockville: Substance Abuse and Mental Health Services Administration; 2024.
25. Bromley L, Kahan M, Regenstreif L, Srivastava A, Wyman J. Methadone treatment for people who use fentanyl: recommendations. Toronto: META:PHI; 2021. www.metaphi.ca.
26. Casey S, Regan S, Gale E, Adams ZM, Lambert E, Omede FO, Wakeman SE. Rapid methadone induction in a general hospital setting: a retrospective, observational analysis. Subst Abus. 2023;44(3):177–83. https://doi.org/10.1177/08897077231185655.
27. Walsh S, Eissenberg T. The clinical pharmacology of buprenorphine: extrapolating from the laboratory to the clinic. Drug Alcohol Depend. 2003;70:S13–27.
28. Snyder H, Chau B, Kalmin MM, et al. High-dose buprenorphine initiation in the emergency department among patients using fentanyl and other opioids. JAMA Netw Open. 2023;6(3):e231572. https://doi.org/10.1001/jamanetworkopen.2023.1572.
29. Raheemullah A, Benhamou O, Kuo J, Lembke A. Buprenorphine microdosing cross tapers: a time for change. Int J Environ Res Public Health. 2022;19(24):16436.
30. Quirk K, Stevenson M. Buprenorphine microdosing for the pain and palliative care clinician. J Palliat Med. 2022;25(1):145–54.
31. Clinical Review Report: buprenorphine extended-release injection (Sublocade): (Indivior Canada, Ltd.): Indication: for the management of moderate-to-severe opioid use disorder in adult patients who have been inducted and clinically stabilized on a transmucosal buprenorphine-containing product [Internet]. Ottawa: Canadian Agency for Drugs and Technologies in Health; 2019. Executive Summary.
32. Lofwall M, Walsh S, Nunes E, et al. Weekly and monthly subcutaneous buprenorphine depot formulations vs daily sublingual buprenorphine with naloxone for treatment of opioid use disorder: a randomized clinical trial. JAMA Intern Med. 2018;178(6):764–73.
33. Minozzi S, Amato L, Vecchi S, Davoli M, Kirchmayer U, Verster A. Oral naltrexone maintenance treatment for opioid dependence. Cochrane Database Syst Rev. 2011;2011(4):CD001333.
34. Bisaga A, Mannelli P, Sullivan M, Vosburg S, Compton P, Woody G, Kosten T. Antagonists in the medical management of opioid use disorders: historical and existing treatment strategies. Am J Addict. 2018;27:177–87.
35. Krupitsky E, Nunes E, Ling W, Illeperuma A, Gastfriend D, Silverman B. Injectable extended-release naltrexone for opioid dependence: a double-blind, placebo-controlled, multicenter randomized trial. Lancet. 2011;377(9776):1506–13.
36. Nunes E, Krupitsky E, Ling W, Zummo J, Memisoglu A, Silverman B, Gastfriend D. Treating opioid dependence with injectable extended-release naltrexone (XR-NTX): who will respond? J Addict Med. 2015;9:238–43.
37. Lee J, Nunes E, Novo P, Bachrach K, Bailey G, Bhatt S, Farkas S, Fishman M, Gauthier P, Hodgkins C, King J, Lindblad R, Liu D, Matthews A, May J, Peavy K, Ross S, Salazar D, Schkolnik P, Shmueli-Blumberg D, Stablein D, Subramaniam G, Rotrosen J. Comparative effectiveness of extended-release naltrexone versus buprenorphine-naloxone for opioid relapse prevention (X:BOT): a multicenter, open-label, randomized controlled trial. Lancet. 2018;91(10118):309–18.

38. Tanum L, Solli KK, Latif ZE, Benth JŠ, Opheim A, Sharma-Haase K, Krajci P, Kunøe N. Effectiveness of injectable extended-release naltrexone vs daily buprenorphine-naloxone for opioid dependence: a randomized clinical noninferiority trial. JAMA Psychiatry. 2017;74(12):1197–205.
39. Kaltenbach K, Berghella V, Finnegan L. Opioid dependence during pregnancy: effects and management. Obstet Gynecol Clin N Am. 1998;25(1):139–51.
40. Straub L, Bateman BT, Hernández-Díaz S, Zhu Y, Suarez EA, Vine SM, Jones HE, Connery HS, Davis JM, Gray KJ, Lester B, Terplan M, Zakoul H, Mogun H, Huybrechts KF. Comparative safety of in utero exposure to buprenorphine combined with naloxone vs buprenorphine alone. JAMA. 2024;332(10):805–16.
41. Tran T, Griffin B, Stone R, Vest K, Todd T. Methadone, buprenorphine and naltrexone for the treatment of opioid use disorder in pregnant women. Pharmacotherapy. 2017;37(7):824–39.
42. Zedler B, Mann A, Kim M, Amick H, Joyce A, Murrelle E, Jones H. Buprenorphine compared with methadone to treat pregnant women with opioid use disorder: a systematic review and meta-analysis of safety in the mother, fetus and child. Addiction. 2016;111:2115–28.
43. Hulse G, O'Neill G. A case series of continuing injectable extended-release naltrexone during pregnancy. J Clin Psychopharmacol. 2017;37(6):720–2.
44. CA Bridge Treatment Protocols. Buprenorphine hospital start: low-dose bup initiation with opioid continuation. 2024. https://bridgetotreatment.org/resource/low-dose-buprenorphine-initiation-with-opioid-continuation/.

Stimulants: Cocaine, Amphetamines, and Other Stimulants

12

Jeffrey J. DeVido

High-Yield Review Points

- The DSM-5 allows for formal diagnoses of Stimulant Intoxication, Stimulant Withdrawal, Other Stimulant-Induced Disorder, Unspecified Stimulant-Related Disorder, and Stimulant Use Disorder (addiction) with the categories of stimulants being amphetamine-type substances, cocaine, and other or unspecified stimulants (e.g., *khât*, cathinone derivatives). The DSM-5 also allows for Caffeine-Induced Disorders (e.g., anxiety and panic) as well as a characteristic Caffeine Withdrawal Syndrome.
- Cocaine is a potent reuptake blocker of catecholamines, while amphetamine and most amphetamine-type stimulants both block reuptake *and* function as transporter substrates that cause a greater release of intracellular catecholamines.
- There are no FDA-approved pharmacotherapies for cocaine use disorder and for amphetamine and amphetamine-type stimulant use disorders.
- There is limited evidence for the possible effectiveness of some off-label pharmacotherapies for the treatment of cocaine or amphetamine and amphetamine-type stimulant use disorders in certain populations of individuals. Bupropion (with or without combination with naltrexone),

J. J. DeVido (✉)
Addiction Services, Behavioral Health and Recovery Services, Marin County California, Department of Health and Human Services, San Rafael, CA, USA

Partnership HealthPlan of California, Fairfield, CA, USA

Department of Psychiatry and Behavioral Sciences, Weill Institute for Neurosciences, University of California San Francisco, San Francisco, CA, USA

C. Marienfeld, M. Soltani (eds.), *AAAP Review of Addiction Psychiatry*,
https://doi.org/10.1007/978-3-032-24174-0_12

topiramate, mirtazapine, modafinil, and even prescription psychostimulants all have limited evidence showing some potential effectiveness.

- Psychosocial and behavioral therapies remain the mainstay of treatment for cocaine use disorder and for amphetamine and amphetamine-type stimulant use disorders, with cognitive behavioral therapies and contingency management (voucher-based reinforcement therapy) approaches having demonstrated efficacy.
- Caffeine's psychostimulatory effects are generally less than that of classical psychostimulants, and its effects are the result of A_1 and A_{2A} adenosine receptor antagonism.

Introduction

Stimulants is a term that describes a diverse range of naturally occurring and synthetic substances that are used for medical and non-medical purposes. Naturally occurring stimulants have been consumed for millennia and are found in various species of plants grown naturally and cultivated throughout the world including coca (cocaine), *khât* (cathinone), ephedra (ephedrine and pseudoephedrine), tea and coffee (caffeine), and tobacco (nicotine). Synthetic stimulants are myriad, and include amphetamine, methylphenidate, methamphetamine, methylenedioxymethamphetamine (MDMA), modafinil and r-modafinil, benzphetamine, diethylpropion, mazindol, phendimetrazine, phenmetrazine, phentermine, and the cathinone derivatives ephedrone and mephedrone. While many stimulants are ingested orally, they are also widely ingested via inhalation, injection, and intranasal, topical, and transrectal routes of administration. In the US, some stimulants are legally available over the counter (i.e., caffeine), while others are available via prescription for medical purposes (i.e., methylphenidate), and still others are found in the illicit drug market (i.e., cathinones, MDMA), or some combination thereof.

There are many medical uses of stimulants including the treatment of attention-deficit hyperactivity disorder (ADHD), nasal sinus congestion, migraine headaches, sleep disorders, obesity, and altitude sickness, as well as a topical/oral anesthetic. Stimulants are also used to improve cognitive performance and enhance wakefulness, and sometimes as a depressive disorder augmenting pharmacotherapy.

As a class, stimulants act pharmacologically in both the central and peripheral nervous systems where they primarily enhance the transmission of the catecholamine neurotransmitters norepinephrine and dopamine, creating the characteristic hedonic, reinforcing and sympathomimetic effects attributed to stimulants: for example, euphoria, increased libido, decreased appetite, increased attention and wakefulness, tachycardia and hypertension, and hyperthermia. Stimulants can also secondarily affect additional neurotransmitter systems (adenosine, serotonergic, and alpha- and beta-adrenergic systems, and neuronal sodium channel systems; they also inhibit monoamine oxidase function), which contributes to the variety of physiological and psychiatric effects attributed to stimulants.

The Diagnostic and Statistical Manual, fifth Edition (DSM-5), describes several disorders related to stimulants, which are divided into the following rubrics: intoxication, withdrawal, use disorder (addiction), other induced disorders, and unspecified stimulant-related disorders [1]. In this chapter, the main focus will be on intoxication, withdrawal, and use disorders related to stimulants. When relevant, other induced disorders and unspecified stimulant-related disorders will be highlighted, but it is sufficient to understand more broadly that other induced disorders and unspecified stimulant-related disorders represent the following: (1) other induced disorders are syndromes that resemble primary psychiatric disorders; however, the cause is stimulant-related (e.g., caffeine-induced anxiety disorder, methamphetamine-induced psychotic disorder) and (2) unspecified stimulant-related disorders are syndromes wherein stimulant use results in clinically significant distress and/or impairment without meeting full diagnostic criteria for intoxication, withdrawal, or use disorder (e.g., unspecified caffeine-related disorder) [1].

Significantly, some stimulants have a high potential for non-medical use as well as use disorder (addiction) and are widely misused for their hedonic and reinforcing effects, temporary cognitive and sexual enhancement, and/or augmentation of alertness and energy. It is difficult to definitively pinpoint the proportion of those who use stimulants who will go on to develop a stimulant use disorder (addiction). Previous national surveys of individuals not in treatment and those seeking treatment estimate that 15–50%, respectively, of those misusing stimulants will develop characteristics of a use disorder [2, 3]. Factors that increase the likelihood of developing a stimulant use disorder include using via routes of administration that favor more rapid delivery to the brain (e.g., inhalation, injection), and greater amounts used [3]. More generally, genetic and environmental factors (and their interactions) can increase the likelihood of developing a use disorder. For example, early life stress (such as neglect or trauma) can result in epigenetic changes that favor development of substance use disorders, and exposure to substance use prior to full maturation of prefrontal cortical circuitry (mid 20 s) has also been tied to increased risk [4].

The prevalence of non-medical stimulant use has been increasing over the past decade, with US surveys revealing that in 2022 10.2 million people 12 and older reported misuse of cocaine, amphetamines, and/or prescription stimulants (an increase from 9.4 million in 2021) [5]. This increase in prevalence has also corresponded with an increase in overdose/poisoning deaths in which stimulants have been involved: from less than 1% in 2010 to 32% in 2021 [6]. The rates of stimulant-related deaths are increasing among all racial and ethnic groups but are particularly pronounced among certain demographic groups. For instance, cocaine-related deaths were highest among black populations, and methamphetamine-related deaths were highest among American Indian/Alaska Native populations [7]. Lesbian/gay/bisexual/transgender individuals, people experiencing homelessness, and people with mental illnesses also report particularly elevated rates of stimulant use and stimulant use disorder [6, 8]. Data suggest that even among pregnant individuals stimulant use is increasing, with California alone noting an increase in stimulant use diagnoses in pregnancy increasing from 554 to 747 diagnoses per 100,000 deliveries during 2012–2020 [9].

Stimulants are also associated with various deleterious psychiatric consequences such as mood disorders, psychosis, aggression, impulse control disorders, and panic attacks. The negative physiologic effects of stimulant misuse are numerous, and every organ system can be impacted. Negative psychiatric and physiological consequences result from either direct effect of the stimulant (e.g., the excessive dopamine release and consequent psychosis and movement disorders seen in methamphetamine use), or indirect stimulant effects (e.g., organ ischemia due to vasoconstriction). Additional negative consequences of stimulant misuse include trauma sustained while intoxicated, as well as the full range of social/economic/relational/legal consequences typical of all addictive disorders. While adulteration of illicit stimulant supplies with potentially toxic "fillers" and additives is not new, recent experience supports the increasingly widespread presence of highly potent synthetic opioids, such as fentanyl, in illicit stimulant supplies, resulting in an explosion of opioid overdose/poisoning deaths in those individuals using stimulants (whether knowingly or not). Often called the "fourth wave" of the US opioid epidemic/overdose crisis, deaths involving *both* highly potent synthetic opioids and stimulants have skyrocketed from 0.6% of the total number of overdose deaths in 2010 to 32.3% in 2021 ($N = 34{,}429$) [5, 10].

In this chapter, particular focus will be on cocaine, amphetamines, and caffeine. Nicotine and MDMA will be considered in separate chapters. Over-the-counter stimulants and the wakefulness enhancers modafinil and r-modafinil will not be considered further in this chapter.

Diagnostic Considerations for Cocaine and Other Stimulants

The DSM-5-TR consolidates the diagnostic criteria for all non-caffeine/tobacco stimulants around 3 categories of substances: (1) amphetamine-type substances, (2) cocaine, and (3) other or unspecified stimulants (e.g., *khât*, cathinone derivatives). DSM-5-TR diagnoses in relation to stimulants parallel those of caffeine described above: Stimulant Intoxication, Stimulant Withdrawal, Other Stimulant-Induced Disorder, Unspecified Stimulant-Related Disorder, and Stimulant Use Disorder (addiction). For each diagnostic entity, the diagnostic criteria are shared, but the specific stimulant is specified (e.g., Cocaine Use Disorder, Methamphetamine Intoxication, and *khât* withdrawal) [1]. While there are substance-specific considerations, it is efficient and clinically useful to consolidate (as the DSM-5 does) all non-caffeine/tobacco stimulant-related disorders. Therefore, in this section, the broad category of stimulant-related disorders will be outlined, followed by sections specifically highlighting unique considerations for cocaine, amphetamine, and amphetamine-type stimulants, in turn.

The DSM-5-TR diagnosis of Stimulant Intoxication is marked by clinically significant problematic behavioral or psychological changes such as hallucinations, agitation, euphoria, delusions (e.g., paranoia), and two or more of the following: tachycardia or bradycardia; pupillary dilation; elevated or lowered blood pressure; perspiration or chills; nausea or vomiting; evidence of weight loss; psychomotor agitation or retardation; muscle weakness, respiratory depression, chest pain, or cardiac arrhythmias; confusion, seizures, hyperpyrexia, dyskinesias, dystonias, or coma [1]. Psychomotoric activation and vital sign elevation typically predominate, with psychomotoric retardation and bradycardia/hypotension seen less frequently and if seen are more likely witnessed in chronic heavy stimulant users.

There are several acute medical complications of stimulant intoxication that are worth specifically highlighting. Stimulants are known to decrease seizure threshold, with case series describing generalized tonic-clonic seizures in individuals with no previously evident seizure disorder, and neurocognitive impairments resulting from chronic use are also documented [11, 12]. Hyperthermia and trauma resulting from the combination of psychomotoric activation and altered mentation (psychosis and/or delirium) resulting from acute stimulant ingestion can also be life-threatening. Cerebral and cardiac vasoconstriction can be marked with stimulant intoxication and ongoing use and can lead to hypertensive crises, atherosclerotic disease, cardiac arrhythmias, heart failure, stroke, and myocardial infarction [13, 14]. Pulmonary edema, hemorrhage, pneumothorax, pulmonary arterial hypertension (especially with methamphetamine use), and pneumomediastinum have all been documented with stimulant inhalation and ongoing use (especially intravenous use). A combination of intramuscular artery vasoconstriction, direct toxic effects of stimulants, and/or muscle damage secondary to seizures or hyperthermia can result in renal damage through ischemia and/or rhabdomyolysis [14, 15]. Gastrointestinal and other organ ischemia are also possible through the potent vasoconstrictive effects of stimulants [15]. Therefore, appropriate medical work-up of the stimulant-intoxicated individual is essential to diagnosing acute, life-threatening, complications and making sure that they are appropriately managed in a timely fashion.

Psychiatrically, psychosis is common among stimulant-intoxicated individuals and can be profound. Hallucinations may be auditory, visual, or somatosensory (especially tactile hallucinations of bugs crawling under the skin known as formication). The presence of visual or somatosensory hallucinations is less common in schizophrenia, which is marked by predominance of auditory hallucinations and negative affective and cognitive symptoms, making this a potentially useful way of attempting to distinguish between these two oft-conflated disease entities. Paranoid delusions are also common in stimulant intoxication and may contribute to aggressive or violent behavior [16–19]. Unfortunately, psychotic symptoms may persist long after stimulant intoxication, especially in the use of methamphetamine, in which the psychosis may last for a year or longer after discontinuation [20, 21]. In part related to psychosis generated by stimulant use, an increased risk of violence has been associated with cocaine and amphetamine and amphetamine-type (AAT) stimulant intoxication (even between episodes of intoxication [22]), but the association with methamphetamine use is well documented [17, 23].

Treatment of stimulant intoxication involves a combination of environmental modifications to ensure safety as well as pharmacologic interventions to treat symptoms. Behavioral interventions are centered on decreasing environmental stimuli and providing calm reassurance and support. Physical restraints are a measure of last resort, since these may contribute to hyperthermia and rhabdomyolysis. Pharmacologically, sedative-hypnotics such as benzodiazepines are preferred, particularly those that are available through oral, intravenous, and intramuscular routes of administration. Diazepam [10–30 mg PO or 2–10 mg IM or IV] or lorazepam [2–4 mg PO or 1–2 mg IM or IV] are commonly used [24]. In the very agitated or psychotic stimulant-intoxicated individual, antipsychotic medications are used. Much has been written about the potential compounding risks of antipsychotic medications alongside stimulant intoxication, given that these medications may lower the seizure threshold, as well as exacerbate hyperthermia. However, studies have also demonstrated that use of antipsychotics (either alone or in combination with benzodiazepines) can be safe and effective, and that the concerns related to seizure threshold lowering and hyperthermia may be exaggerated [25–27]. Therefore, high-potency antipsychotics are preferred, such as haloperidol, since these high-potency neuroleptics are less likely to have anticholinergic side effects that are particularly implicated in the development of the risks highlighted above. Common antipsychotic regimens include haloperidol 5 mg IM or 0.2–0.67 mg/kg, olanzapine 2.5–10 mg every 2 hours, ziprasidone 20 mg, and quetiapine 50–100 mg as needed to achieve behavioral control. Monitoring of QTc (via EKG) regularly when providing antipsychotics is prudent. In addition, for hyperadrenergic states, clonidine 0.1–0.2 mg every 4 hours as needed, or intravenous dexmedetomidate (0.2–0.4 mg/kg/h titrated up to maximum of 1.5 mg/kg/h) or nitroprusside (0.5–4 mg/kg/minute) can be considered in an appropriately monitored acute setting (i.e., intensive care unit or equivalent). Finally, the NMDA-receptor antagonist ketamine (1–5 mg/kg IM) can be considered in the setting of severe agitation in an appropriate acute setting (i.e., emergency department) [28].

The use of beta-blocker medications in the setting of stimulant intoxication (especially in those presenting concurrently with stimulant intoxication and evidence of myocardial infarction) is controversial and therefore worth mentioning here. Beta-blockers are potentially attractive pharmacotherapeutics for managing the adrenergic hyperactivity often seen in individuals intoxicated on stimulants. Use of beta-blockers in this context has been largely shunned, though, based on both the theoretical risk of harmful vasoconstriction resulting from "unopposed alpha-receptor stimulation," and early studies that supported this theoretical risk and consequently shaped future guidance. Beta-1 receptor stimulation results in increased heart rate and cardiac contractility, whereas beta-2 receptor stimulation results in smooth muscle relaxation. Alpha-1 receptor stimulation causes vasoconstriction. Therefore, theoretically, selective blockage of beta-1 and 2 receptors could result in alpha-1 receptor-induced vasoconstriction in the absence of beta-2 receptor corresponding vasodilation. On account of these concerns, the American Heart Association's 2014 guidelines on the management of non-ST elevation myocardial infarction (NSTEMI) advises against using beta-blockers in individuals with evidence of stimulant intoxication, as there is potentially a risk of harmful vasoconstriction. On the other hand, subsequent studies and systematic reviews have not universally supported the risks of vasoconstriction posited by the early research. Furthermore, a 2020 systematic review found no evidence of harm from maintenance treatment of cardiac conditions with beta-blocker medications in those who use stimulants. If beta-blocking medications are to be considered in these individuals, preference should perhaps be given to those beta-blocking medications that also have some alpha-1 receptor antagonism activity as well (i.e., labetalol, carvedilol) [29–31].

Prolonged use of stimulants can lead to the development of physiological tolerance, and upon abrupt discontinuation or dose reduction a clinically significant stimulant withdrawal syndrome can develop. Stimulant withdrawal is not typically life-threatening, and manifests characteristically as the opposite of intoxication, namely a clinically distressing or impairing dysphoric mood and 2+ of the following: fatigue, vivid unpleasant dreams, insomnia or hypersomnia, increased appetite, psychomotor retardation, or agitation [1]. Individual variability is significant, but onset of stimulant withdrawal is typically between several hours to days after last use and can last for several days, with some symptoms such as psychosis (see above) persisting even longer.

There are no specific FDA-approved pharmacologic treatments for stimulant withdrawal. Generally, stimulant withdrawal is marked by minimal physiological distress, and targeted symptomatic treatment of non-specific musculoskeletal pain, tremors, chills, and other symptoms can be helpful. Psychiatric sequalae of stimulant withdrawal such as disproportionate dysphoria or low-level psychosis can be treated with antidepressants or antipsychotic medications, respectively, in line with usual dosing approaches for these pharmacotherapies. Continuing to monitor for emergence of suicidality, especially in the context of withdrawal-related dysphoria, is prudent. In addition, small studies of the mood stabilizer/antiepileptic topiramate (up to 300 mg per day) have shown some potential benefit (i.e., fewer cocaine-positive urine screens) in those cocaine-using individuals who experience severe withdrawal symptoms (as measured by the Cocaine Selective Severity Assessment (CSSA)), especially in those with co-occurring alcohol use disorder [32–35]. However, topiramate does have significant potential side effect burden (i.e., Steven Johnson Syndrome, kidney stones, word finding difficulty, peripheral neuropathies, drowsiness), which should be monitored as per routine.

Other Stimulant-Induced Disorders include those disorders that mimic other primary psychiatric disorders but are precipitated by the use of particular substances. In particular, in methamphetamine-induced psychotic disorder significantly distressing or impairing delusions or hallucinations predominate the clinical presentation, and by history, physical exam, or laboratory findings, these symptoms are temporally related to intoxication or withdrawal from methamphetamine use.

There are several approaches to screening for stimulant use and stimulant use disorders. Patient self-report has been demonstrated to be reasonably accurate, so long as there are not competing motivations for misrepresentation of use (e.g., legal ramifications) [36]. Other validated easy-to-use screening tools for stimulant use include the 3-question Tobacco, Alcohol, Prescription Medication, and Other Substance Use screening instrument [37], the single question screening test [38], and the 10-item Drug Abuse Screening Test [39], while the Screen of Drug Use can be effective in detecting stimulant use disorder [40]. For detection of stimulant use during pregnancy (in addition to other substances and alcohol), the 4Ps Plus is a 5-item, validated screen that is easy to use [41].

The 2024 ASAM/AAAP Clinical Practice Guideline on the Management of Stimulant Disorder provides additional consensus recommendations/considerations for the assessment of individuals with stimulant use disorders. In short, the guidelines recommend obtaining comprehensive clinical biopsychosocial history, including the use of collateral information when available, as well as physical exam, laboratory studies based on clinical judgment (considering, at a minimum, pregnancy screen, toxicology screen, CBC with Differential, CMP, HIV and hepatitis testing), and the offering of vaccines for hepatitis B and other infectious diseases [28].

Cocaine

Cocaine is a classical stimulant and analgesic alkaloid chemical that is present in the leaves of the *Erythroxylum* (coca) bush endemic to the higher altitude (1500–6000 feet) regions of the Andes Mountains in South America. For thousands of years, preparations using the coca plant have been used by local populations to stave off altitude sickness and enhance energy and performance in addition to the treatment of a wide range of physical disorders. Since then, cocaine has developed both medical and non-medical uses. Medically, in the United States, cocaine is a schedule II substance with FDA indication for local and topical analgesia. Historically, cocaine has found particular medical usage as anesthesia for dental, ophthalmologic, and nasal surgical procedures. However, due to the development of other synthetic local anesthetics with more favorable side effect profiles, cocaine is rarely used in modern medical practice. In the latter part of the nineteenth century, cocaine was also added to various consumer products such as alcoholic beverages and soft drinks (e.g., Coca-Cola), a practice which ended in the early 1900s.

Cocaine exerts its psychomotor and reinforcing effects primarily through augmentation of transmission of the catecholamines dopamine and norepinephrine. This is achieved through the blockade of transporters that would otherwise clear previously released catecholamines from the extracellular space. In other words, cocaine acts as a *reuptake* blocker that enables dopamine and norepinephrine to spend greater time in the extracellular space, where they can continue to activate psychostimulatory pathways to a greater extent than would be otherwise naturally possible. In particular, cocaine potently augments dopamine neurotransmission in the mesocorticolimbic pathway involved in reward processing which accounts for its extraordinarily rewarding and reinforcing effect. Secondarily, cocaine also blocks neuronal sodium channels, which accounts for its anesthetic properties [42].

Cocaine exists in two chemical forms, salt and base, each of which has unique characteristics that drive use patterns. Illicit cocaine is extracted in bulk from the coca leaf, and concentrated, purified, and converted chemically into its salt form through acidification. As a salt, cocaine is readily absorbable through mucous membranes making it ideal for intranasal use (insufflation). The salt is also readily dissolvable in water making it thereby available for injection. However, cocaine salt has a high melting point which provides little margin between the vaporization point and "burning" point of the chemical. Since burning cocaine renders it pharmacologically useless, cocaine salt is therefore not ideal for vaporized inhalation. However, converting the cocaine salt into its base form through alkalization drops the melting point significantly and allows for vaporization that facilitates easy ingestion through inhalation. The base form, conversely, is poorly dissolvable making it less ideal for injection and insufflated administration. The so-called "freebase" cocaine results in what has been commonly known as "crack," the use of which reached epidemic proportions in the 1980s. While it is often referred to as being "smoked," technically freebase cocaine is vaporized, not burned, unlike other smoked substances such as tobacco.

Ingested orally the onset of effect is relatively slower (30–45 minutes) than via insufflation (1–5 minutes), intravenous (4–7 minutes), or vaporized inhalation (6–8 seconds) routes of administration, with times to peak effect being 60–90 minutes, 20–30 minutes, 3–5 minutes, and 3–5 minutes, respectively. Correspondingly, the duration of action is longer for cocaine ingested orally (3 hours), via insufflation (1 hour), than via intravenous or inhalation (15–30 minutes) routes of administration [43]. When consumed with alcohol a new compound, cocaethylene, is formed with less potency than cocaine but with a longer half-life, as well as the potential to cause cardiac arrhythmias [44, 45].

Cocaine is primarily metabolized via ester bond hydrolysis in the liver to benzoylecgonine which is readily detectable via routine immunoassay in urine for 2–3 days in non-daily users, but upwards of 2 weeks in those who use cocaine heavily.[1] Cocaine may also be detected through hair, blood, sweat (via patches), and oral fluid samples, with varying times of positivity (up to 12 hours in blood and oral fluids, weeks for sweat, to months-years in hair, although hair testing results may vary significantly based on race/ethnicity, location of hair sample, and the presence of hair treatments) [46].

While a urine assay positive for benzoylecgonine is reliably indicative of cocaine use, test positivity does not, in-and-of itself, indicate the presence of a cocaine use disorder (addiction). Rather, cocaine use disorder is diagnosed through screening for the range of behavioral and physical criteria described in the DSM-5-TR for all other substance use disorders (described elsewhere in this text).

In 2023, 16.4%, 1.9%, and 0.7% of US residents 18 years and older reported use of cocaine in their lifetime, in the past year, and in the past month, respectively. The predominance of 18+ year-old past year users are male (2.5% vs. 1.3% female),

[1] Windows of detection are dependent on a number of factors, including the relative cut-off levels of the individual tests. For example, a test with a lower cut-off level could potentially detect both a smaller amount of substance used as well as detect the presence of a substance for a longer period of time following exposure.

white (1.9%), or American Indian or Alaska Native (AIAN) (2.1%) unemployed men with some college education (2.2%) [6]. Past-year crack "freebase" cocaine use remains more common, however, among black and AIAN populations (0.8% and 0.9%, respectively, relative to 0.4% in non-Hispanic white populations) [6]. Historically, most cocaine users use relatively infrequently (58% report using only 12 times a year), in what is typically described as a "binge" involving long periods of little or no use punctuated by short periods of heavy use. Cocaine users frequently describe symptoms of depression and anxiety and are likely to use other substances (in particular tobacco and alcohol) to mediate or enhance the effects of intoxication or withdrawal [47].

In addition to the medical and psychiatric sequelae discussed above for stimulants in general, cocaine use is associated with several specific consequences, acute and chronic: cognitive impairment [48], suicidality and suicide attempts [49–51], and increased risk of infections such as hepatitis and HIV (by any route of administration) [52]. Insufflated cocaine can cause perforation of the nasal septum, while cocaine use via any route of administration can cause acute and chronic movement disorders such as choreoathetosis, dystonia (especially in conjunction with neuroleptic medications), and akathisia [53]. Vaporized cocaine is also associated with a severe pulmonary syndrome characterized by fever, hypoxemia, hemoptysis, respiratory failure, and eosinophilic alveolar infiltrates—the so-called "crack lung" [54].

Cocaine ingestion in pregnancy has been associated with several deleterious consequences (either as a direct result of cocaine use, or due to other environmental factors associated with its use), including vaginal bleeding, abruptio placenta, placenta previa, premature rupture of membranes, premature birth, decreased head circumference, low birth weight, and autonomic instability [55]. In addition, cocaine is found in breastmilk and infants breastfed from mothers using cocaine may demonstrate irritability, sleep difficulty, and tremors, which is exacerbated by newborn infants lacking enzymes necessary for metabolism of cocaine [56].

For the treatment of cocaine use disorder, randomized trials have examined the roles of novel cocaine vaccines, as well as stimulant replacement medication strategies, dopamine agonists, various antidepressants (e.g., fluoxetine, desipramine, bupropion), GABAergic medications (e.g., topiramate, vigabatrin), cholinergic medications (e.g., galantamine), ondansetron, and disulfiram. None of these pharmacotherapies have demonstrated consistent efficacy in treating cocaine use disorder. However, of out of these trials, the most promising results have been with dopamine agonist agents (i.e., long-acting mixed amphetamine salts) and modafinil (200–400 mg/day), as well as with GABA agonists/glutamate antagonists, such as topiramate (100–150 mg twice daily) [57, 58]. Moreover, the 2024 ASAM/AAAP Clinical Practice Guideline on the Management of Stimulant Disorder further provides conditional recommendation of consideration of either bupropion (typically 150–300 mg/day of XL formulation) or topiramate (200–300 mg/day), especially if patients present with co-occurring tobacco use disorder or alcohol use disorder, respectively. The Practice Guideline also provides additional conditional considerations when considering dopamine agonist treatment: limiting prescribing of Schedule II prescription stimulants (not modafinil) to physician specialists who are board-certified in addiction medicine or addiction psychiatry; and physicians with commensurate training, competencies, and capacity for close patient monitoring (i.e., pill counts, drug testing, more frequent clinical contact, more frequent Prescription Drug Monitoring Program (PDMP) checking). Typical dopamine agonist dosing in representative studies for cocaine use disorder has been extended-release mixed amphetamine salts 60–80 mg/day, sustained release dextroamphetamine 60 mg/day, or, less so, methylphenidate extended-release 18–180 mg/day [28].

Relative to pharmacotherapeutic interventions, behavioral treatment strategies have met with greater success in the treatment of cocaine use disorder [58, 59]. Behavioral therapies represent a wide array of interventions that target various aspects of the challenges inherent in addictive disorders, from helping to explore and resolve ambivalence around usage (motivational interviewing (MI), motivational enhancement therapy (MET)), enhancing coping strategies (cognitive behavioral therapy (CBT)), altering thought processes around use (cognitive therapy (CT), CBT), learning how to utilize techniques to avoid/prevent triggers (CBT), changing the environmental reinforcing contingencies (contingency management (CM) often referred alternatively as voucher-based reinforcement therapy (VBRT)), community reinforcement approach (CRA), to promoting a sense of detachment from cravings, thoughts, and emotions that contribute to relapse (mindfulness/meditation therapies). A 2008 meta-analysis of psychosocial/behavioral treatments for multiple substance use disorders showed medium to large effect sizes in impacting cocaine use ($d = 0.62$) [60]. More recently, a 2024 Cochrane Review demonstrated that behavioral treatments (CBT, VBRT, motivational interviewing (MI), psychodynamic psychotherapy, and twelve step facilitation (TSF)) for stimulant use disorders showed superiority over treatment as usual (TAU) in one particular outcome measure: treatment retention [61]. Additionally, a 2024 systematic review examining predictors of cocaine use disorder treatment outcomes concluded that "Younger age, more years of cocaine use, and higher craving levels were significant predictors of relapse and treatment dropout. By contrast, fewer withdrawal symptoms, greater baseline abstinence, and more self-efficacy were all predictive of longer duration of abstinence" [62]. In addition, additional studies have demonstrated the effectiveness of MI/MET [63], especially when coupled with CBT treatment [64]. Mindfulness-based treatments such as Acceptance and Commitment Therapy (ACT), Dialectical Behavioral Therapy (DBT), Mindfulness-Based Stress Reduction (MBSR), and Transcendental Meditation (TM) are used widely in substance use treatment, but the data evaluating these in individuals using cocaine are comparatively limited [65].

Behavioral treatments are delivered in an array of different formats of varying intensity. While most cocaine use disorder treatment is delivered in a "standard" outpatient drug treatment format (i.e., once or twice per week), higher intensity treatment formats such as intensive outpatient treatment (i.e., up to 9 hours of outpatient treatment per week) are perhaps more effective [66, 67]. Nonetheless, whatever the intensity of behavioral treatment delivered, individuals with cocaine use disorder have high treatment dropout rates, with one notable exception mentioned above: VBRT, in which participants receive gift cards or other monetary incentives for providing urine toxicology screens negative for stimulants [68]. Despite its demonstrated effectiveness, widespread adoption of VBRT in general clinical settings is limited, due to a combination of federal limitations on annual amounts of money ($75) as well as logistic challenges related to needing to have often multiple encounters with patients each week. In 2024, California received a federal 1115 waiver to pilot widespread rollout of VBRT throughout the state's Medicaid system in which participants are eligible to receive monetary vouchers up to $599/year through the first-of-its-kind 24-week VBRT "Recovery Incentives Program" [69]. Data from this pilot program is forthcoming but may set the blueprint for national policy changes if the program proves effective.

Twelve-step fellowships (e.g., alcoholics anonymous, narcotics anonymous, cocaine anonymous) are ubiquitously available abstinence-based substance use treatment programming, often employed alone or in tandem with other treatment approaches, and have been shown to be helpful for some with cocaine use, especially those who actively participate in the fellowship programming and when twelve-step participation is formally reinforced in treatment settings (i.e., TSF) [61, 70].

Amphetamine and Amphetamine-Type Stimulants

Amphetamine and amphetamine-type (AAT) stimulants are a diverse array of compounds (amphetamine, methamphetamine, dextroamphetamine) that are either structurally related to a parent phenethylamine chemical compound or have similar effects but are structurally unrelated (methylphenidate, *Ephedra*, *cathinone*). Unlike cocaine, AAT stimulants continue to be widely used in medical practice for the treatment of a wide array of FDA-approved indications, making them readily available through licit supply chains. Diversion of AAT stimulants from these licit sources, in combination with a robust illicit manufacture and supply chain, contributes to their widespread availability. National surveys indicate that non-medical use (NMU) of stimulants has been increasing, with emergency department visits relating to NMU of stimulants increasing 200% from 2005 to 2010 [71], and secondary school data suggesting rates of NMU of stimulants ranging from 0% to 75% with schools in which a larger proportion of students are being prescribed stimulants having higher rates of NMU as well [72]. 2014 surveys highlight that 0.6% of the population ages 12 or older reports current NMU of stimulants (0.2% methamphetamine, specifically), which represents an increase over most years between 2005 and 2013 [65]. In 2023, of the 9.7 million people in the US who reported using stimulants, 2.8 million reported NMU of prescription stimulants exclusively [6].

Ephedrine-containing *Ephedra* plants have been used in Chinese medicine for thousands of years and continued to be used widely in weight loss products until being banned from the US market in 2006 due to ephedrine's association with serious cardiac side effects. α-methylphenethylamine (amphetamine) was first synthesized in 1887 but lay fallow until 1927 when G.A. Alles brought the chemical to mainstream medicine while he was seeking a synthetic substitute for ephedrine [73]. Methamphetamine was first synthesized from ephedrine in Japan in 1897 but found significant widespread use during World War II where it was broadly distributed by German military leadership to enhance wakefulness and combat performance. More recently, illicit amphetamine use has been tied to a significant increase in overdose deaths, in part related to the adulteration of illicit methamphetamine (in particular) with high potency synthetic opioids such as fentanyl. This is often described as the "fourth wave" of the opioid epidemic, and unlike the typical natural history of illicit drug manufacturing and distribution, illicit methamphetamine drug supplies are demonstrating *increasing* purity [74].

Amphetamine exists in two optically active isomers, dextro (or *d*-) and levo- (or *l*-), with the d-isomer (trade name, Dexedrine) being significantly more potent. Like amphetamine, methamphetamine exists in two isomers (*l*- and *d*-) with *d*-methamphetamine being a highly potent stimulant, while *l*-methamphetamine has virtually no intrinsic psychoactivity. Both *l*- and *d*-amphetamine and *d*-methamphetamine are Schedule II medications in the United States (indicative of their high abuse potential), while *l*-methamphetamine is available over the counter as a decongestant nasal spray.

Methamphetamine exists in both base and salt forms, with the former being liquid at room temperature and the latter being a clear crystal at room temperature (e.g., "crystal methamphetamine"). The crystalline form of methamphetamine is readily dissolved in water and injected or vaporized and inhaled in a manner similar to crack cocaine. Anecdotally, methamphetamine is felt to be a more potent and dangerous psychostimulant than amphetamine; however, rat and human studies have not consistently supported this assertion [75]. However, it is conceivable that these anecdotal differences are based on actual chemical differences. For example, methamphetamine is more lipophilic than amphetamine and therefore more readily crosses the blood–brain barrier leading to more rapid onset of action which can have potent reinforcing effects. Additionally, methamphetamine may be more resistant to enzymatic degradation, thereby enhancing its effect through prolongation of action ($t_{1/2}$ upwards of 30 hours) [76].

Like cocaine, AAT are ingested through several routes of administration, and the clinical presentations of use disorder, intoxication, and withdrawal are all similar to those of cocaine. Some significant differences are worth noting. Some AAT, such as methamphetamine, have a significantly longer duration of action (as above, $t_{1/2}$ upwards of 30 hours) relative to cocaine's relatively short duration of action ($t_{1/2}$ around 1.5 hours) [77]. In addition, chronic use of methamphetamine is particularly correlated with significant xerostomia which can lead to noteworthy dental pathology (e.g., "meth mouth"). Chronic AAT use is also tied to increased risk of stroke even in younger individuals [78], significant cognitive deficits and long-lasting psychotic symptoms, both of which are attributable to amphetamine's different mechanism of action (see below) relative to cocaine [11, 19, 21, 79].

Methamphetamine is metabolized into amphetamine which is then further metabolized via three different metabolic pathways in the liver, unlike cocaine's primary hepatic hydrolytic metabolic pathway. Amphetamine is readily detectable in urine, hair, sweat, blood, and oral fluids. As above, detection windows are dependent on several factors, but generally amphetamines are detectable in urine and oral fluids for 2–4 days post exposure, and up to 90 days in hair. The detection window for amphetamines in blood may be only several hours, depending on the amount taken. False-positive test results have been documented on amphetamine immunoassays, especially in individuals also taking bupropion, certain tricyclic antidepressant medications, quetiapine, *l*-methamphetamine nasal inhalers, or ephedrine/pseudoephedrine-containing cold medications. Confirmatory testing via gas or liquid chromatography can provide definitive results when false positives may be suspected [46].

While cocaine exerts its pharmacological effect by blocking reuptake of catecholamines, AATs (particularly *d*-amphetamine and *d*-methamphetamine both) block reuptake *and* stimulate direct release of catecholamines. Both amphetamine and *d*-methamphetamine achieve this added pharmacologic effect on catecholaminergic neurons by a complex pathway that involves (1) co-transportation alongside sodium ions into the neuronal cytoplasm, (2) disruption of monoamine vesicular storage causing an intracellular release of catecholamine stores, and (3) increased release of synaptic catecholamines resulting from the increased intracellular availability of these chemicals. Therefore, amphetamine and *d*-methamphetamine are referred to as "transporter substrates" [80], that, in sum, result in relatively higher synaptic release of catecholamines than cocaine. This substantial synaptic and intracellular catecholamine release may have neuronal toxic effects, which has been tied to the prolonged psychosis and significant cognitive impairments that are associated with chronic amphetamine and *d*-methamphetamine use [11, 48, 79]. In addition, chronic use of amphetamine and *d*-methamphetamine has been tied to decreased brain serotonin receptor density, which, in animal models, has been associated with increased aggression or violence [81]. Other AATs, however, such as methylphenidate, function pharmacologically more similarly to cocaine (reuptake blockade), whereas *khât* (cathinone) and its synthetic derivatives (e.g., mephedrone) possess catecholamine transporter substrate and reuptake blockade activity (particularly dopamine) and also enhance synaptic serotonin release [82, 83]. Together, these findings highlight the vast diversity of compounds and their respective mechanisms of action that make up this class of drugs.

Stimulants are the second most misused illicit substance during pregnancy, and data suggest that their use is increasing in the US: methamphetamine use during pregnancy, for example, hospitalization for methamphetamine use during pregnancy doubled between 1988 and 2004 [84, 85]. AAT use during pregnancy can present a complex set of considerations. For example, prescription psychostimulants (amphetamine, methylphenidate) can cross the placental barrier, but those used *as directed* have not been shown to have clinically significant associations with preeclampsia, placental abruption, small-for-gestational-age neonates, and preterm delivery, despite concerns about vasoconstrictive effects of these medications on placental circulation [86]. On the other hand, pregnant users of illicit methamphetamine have been shown to have greater risks of preeclampsia and gestational hypertension, fetal demise, abortion, and preterm labor [87–89]. When taken as prescribed, methylphenidate and amphetamine levels in breastmilk are very low and risk-benefit of continued use should be discussed carefully with nursing individuals. However, amphetamine use may inhibit prolactin release which could decrease milk production, and while overall levels of amphetamine in breastmilk are low, amphetamine levels in breastmilk can be 2.8–7.5 times higher than in maternal serum [89]. While some studies indicate that use of prescribed psychostimulants during breastfeeding is potentially safe [87], other guidelines suggest more caution (and also recommend against breastfeeding in those individuals actively using illicit methamphetamine) [89].

Like the situation with cocaine use disorder, studies of various pharmacotherapies for the treatment of amphetamine and methamphetamine use disorders have not shown significant universal efficacy. Prescription psychostimulants, tricyclic antidepressants, SSRIs, ondansetron, topiramate, naltrexone, mirtazapine, bupropion, antipsychotics, and amlodipine (among others) have all been trialed in the treatment of stimulant use disorders [90]. Of these pharmacotherapies, some have demonstrated better potential efficacy than others, especially among certain subpopulations. In reviewing the extant literature, the clinical consensus committee that developed the ASAM/AAAP Clinical Practice Guideline on the Management of Stimulant Use Disorder provided conditional recommendations to consider the following pharmacotherapeutic approaches for methamphetamine use disorder: bupropion (sustained release 150 mg twice daily or XL 300 mg once daily) for individuals with low-moderate frequency of use (i.e., less than 18 days/month) and those with co-occurring depressive disorder and/or tobacco use disorder; bupropion and ER injectable naltrexone combination (450 mg daily, 380 mg monthly or every 3 weeks, respectively), and those with co-occurring depressive disorder, and/or tobacco use disorder, and/or alcohol use disorder; topiramate (200 mg/day) especially in those with co-occurring alcohol use disorder and those who perhaps are able to achieve abstinence prior to initiation of medication; mirtazapine (30 mg/day) and those with co-occurring depressive disorders (the two studies investigating this pharmacotherapy focused on individuals who had relatively severe methamphetamine use disorder and were also men who have sex with men (MSM)) [28]. Regarding the use of psychostimulants for the treatment of AAT, the ASAM/AAAP Guideline recommendations are consistent with those described above for cocaine use disorder; namely, that in appropriately monitored contexts, under the supervision of appropriately trained/boarded physicians, this treatment pathway can be considered. Specifically for AAT, the consensus guideline committee advised considering the preferential use of long-acting methylphenidate preparations (i.e., methylphenidate ER 54 mg/day), and in individuals with moderate to higher frequency amphetamine use (i.e., >10 days/month) [28].

Behavioral/psychosocial therapies for the treatment of AAT stimulant use disorders span the same gamut as those described above for cocaine. Of those outlined above for cocaine use disorder, however, those with supportive evidence specifically in the treatment of AAT include CBT and VBRT (as described above for cocaine use disorder), with the latter considered first line behavioral therapy for AAT use disorders [91]. For some patients, the structure and programmatic organization of an intensive outpatient therapy program for stimulant use disorder may be beneficial. Systematically operationalizing these varied treatment approaches has been studied through use of the manualized Matrix Model, which incorporates educational materials on the effects of stimulant use, family education, 12-Step program participation, and positive reinforcement for behavior change and treatment compliance [92]. In addition, the community reinforcement approach (CRA) model in which clinicians work with patients to adjust aspects of their lives that interfere with a healthy lifestyle has been shown to be modestly effective, with slight improvements noted when combined with VBRT. However, CRA can be resource-intensive and as such lacks widespread adoption [28].

Caffeine

Caffeine is an alkaloid chemical that is consumed orally through food, drink, and dietary supplements and is present in over 60 distinct species of plants, such as tea, guarana, cacao, and yerba maté. Orally, caffeine is 100% bioavailable, and effects are experienced between 45 minutes and 2 hours after ingestion. In addition to adenosine receptor antagonism that promotes wakefulness, caffeine ingestion can also result in vascular smooth muscle relaxation and vasodilation (which may account for its effectiveness in relieving migraine headache) [93, 94]. Caffeine has also become incorporated into cosmetic products under the auspices of facilitating hair growth (with limited preclinical evidence) [95, 96]. Caffeine is the most widely used psychoactive substance in the world, with an estimated 69% of the US population 2 years old and older consuming one or more caffeinated beverage a day. Individuals aged 50–64 years old consume the greatest amount of daily caffeine, and coffee (70%) is the most common source of consumed caffeine, with carbonated soft drinks, tea, and energy drinks following behind (14.9%, 8.7%, 6%, respectively) [97, 98]. Caffeine use is generally not associated with significant deleterious health consequences when used in moderation, and caffeine ingestion has been proposed to potentially provide some health benefits by enhancing athletic performance, decreasing inflammation, preventing Parkinson's disease, liver cirrhosis, some cancers, and certain forms of dementia and depression, although the data on these effects are currently inconclusive [99–102].

Caffeine is used medically in conjunction with various analgesics such as acetaminophen and ibuprofen to enhance the pain-mitigating effects of these analgesics, to treat caffeine withdrawal, and to treat apnea in neonates and infants [103–105]. Outside of medical indications, caffeine is widely consumed to improve alertness and enhance wakefulness and is commonly added in varying amounts to weight loss and energy products, sometimes in conjunction with alcohol.

Endogenous adenosine activity is responsible for escalating sleepiness following periods of prolonged wakefulness and also is implicated in several other aspects of sleep homeostasis. Caffeine's psychomotor-reinforcing effects and hyperarousal are the result of the antagonism of central A_1 and A_{2A} adenosine receptors. Compared to classical psychostimulants such as cocaine and amphetamine, caffeine has comparatively less augmentation effect on dopaminergic and catecholaminergic neurotransmission. Nonetheless, caffeine ingestion increases both systolic and diastolic blood pressures, causes head and neck vasoconstriction as well as bronchodilation, and has diuretic and colonic stimulatory effects [106].

The ubiquity and relative minor health or psychological impact of caffeine makes it difficult to pinpoint specific caffeine-related disorders and problems. The DSM-5-TR describes Caffeine-Related Disorders as Caffeine Intoxication, Caffeine Withdrawal, Other Caffeine-Induced Disorders, and Unspecified Caffeine-Related Disorders [1]. Caffeine Use Disorder (addiction) is listed as a condition for further study in DSM-5-TR.

Affecting an estimated 7% of the US population, caffeine intoxication is marked by recent use of caffeine, typically in doses in excess of 250 mg, and 5 or more of the following factors, causing significant distress or impairments in social, occupational, or other important areas of functioning: restlessness, nervousness, excitement, insomnia, flushed face, diuresis, gastrointestinal disturbance, muscle twitching, rambling flow of thought and speech, tachycardia or cardiac arrhythmia, periods of inexhaustibility, and/or psychomotor agitation. Symptoms usually resolve without lasting consequence within 24 hours of onset, consistent with caffeine's 4–6-hour half-life. However, deaths have been reported following extremely high-dose ingestions, as well as the potential need for hemodialysis (5–25 g) [1, 93]. The U.S. Poison Control Center reports that calls related to caffeine ingestion in youth (under age 20) increased 24.2% from 2022 to 2023, which is especially tied to the increased availability of high-caffeine energy drinks [107].

Frequent ingestion of caffeine can reliably result in the development of physiological tolerance. Development of tolerance is, in part, the result of adenosine A_1 receptor upregulation in chronic caffeine exposure. Abrupt discontinuation or marked reduction in amount of consumed caffeine in a tolerant individual can result in a clinically significant withdrawal syndrome characterized by 24 hours of 3 or more of the following symptoms causing significant distress and impairments in social, occupational, or other important areas of functioning: headache; marked fatigue or drowsiness; dysphoric mood, depressed mood, or irritability; difficulty concentrating; flu-like symptoms such as nausea, vomiting, or muscle pain/stiffness. Headache is a particularly common symptom, affecting upwards of 50% of those with caffeine withdrawal. Most symptoms resolve within 2–9 days [1].

In part due to the difficulty in defining a caffeine use disorder (addiction), treatment of problematic caffeine use is poorly studied. One study utilized a combination of manualized cognitive behavioral therapy (CBT) in conjunction with caffeine down taper over 5 weeks and showed significant caffeine intake reduction that was successfully maintained at the 1-year follow-up timepoint [108]. A similar study also showed positive effects through a combination of 6 week down taper informed by manualized instructions for this down taper [109].

Tobacco cigarette smokers and alcohol-dependent individuals have been shown to consume significantly higher amounts of caffeine than individuals without these disorders [110]. Caffeine has also been shown to have a potentiating effect on other classical psychostimulants [111]. Furthermore, caffeine has been shown to decrease the metabolism of the atypical antipsychotic clozapine and lithium toxicity has been documented during withdrawal from caffeine related to changes in renal clearance of lithium following discontinuation of caffeine [112, 113].

Caffeine readily crosses the placenta, and meta-analytic data suggest that maternal caffeine consumption during pregnancy has a small but significant association with adverse pregnancy outcomes such as increased rates of spontaneous abortion, stillbirth, low birth weight, and small for gestational age (SGA) in a dose-response pattern [114]. However, the thresholds for risk increase are uncertain and several studies have presented conflicting conclusions about this association [115, 116]. As a result, the American College of Obstetrics and Gynecology, the American Pregnancy Association, and the March of Dimes recommend that pregnant individuals limit their caffeine intake, to 200 mg or less daily [117–119]. The half-life of caffeine may increase significantly late in pregnancy [120], increasing the risk of toxicity. A small amount of caffeine is found in breastmilk of nursing individuals. The Centers for Disease Control and Prevention indicates that low-to-moderate caffeine consumption is safe during breastfeeding (<300 mg/day, or 2–3 cups of coffee), and other studies have also demonstrated that consumption in excess of 2–3 cups of coffee per day (300 mg) has been associated with irritability and poor sleeping patterns in nursing infants [121–123].

Chapter Review Questions

1. A 27-year-old female doctoral student has been regularly consuming caffeine-containing energy drinks as she rushes to complete her dissertation. The stimulant effects that help her stay awake are primarily due to caffeine's _________ of central _________ receptors—a system involved in promoting sleepiness during extended periods of wakefulness.

   A. Agonism, adenosine
   B. Antagonism, dopamine
   C. Agonism, dopamine
   D. Antagonism, adenosine
   E. Partial agonism, mu-opioid

   Answer: D
   Explanation: Endogenous adenosine agonizes central A_1 and A_{2A} adenosine receptors, which leads to the experience of increased sleepiness. Caffeine's psychomotor-reinforcing effects and hyperarousal are the result of the antagonism of central A_1 and A_{2A} adenosine receptors.
2. A 25-year-old man with a history of intravenous cocaine use has entered a residential drug and alcohol treatment program. As part of his recovery plan, he participates in a structured intervention that provides incentives for submitting cocaine-negative urine samples and applies consequences for positive results. This evidence-based behavioral approach, which uses targeted reinforcement to encourage abstinence, is known as

   A. Contingency management (Voucher-Based Reinforcement Therapy)
   B. Acceptance and commitment therapy

C. Motivational enhancement therapy
D. Cognitive behavioral therapy
E. Mindfulness-based stress reduction

Answer: A

Explanation: Contingency management (or Voucher-Based Reinforcement Therapy) is an evidence-based behavioral therapy that has been shown to be effective in the treatment of various stimulant use disorders, but cocaine use disorder in particular. In this treatment, individuals are given the opportunity to receive behavioral incentives such as gift cards if they adhere to some predetermined and agreed upon desirable behavior (e.g., attendance at counseling sessions, providing a negative toxicology screen). Correspondingly, individuals receive sanctions (e.g., no gift card, reduction in number of take-home methadone doses provided) should they not adhere to the predetermined and agreed upon desirable behavior.

3. A 47-year-old male with severe opioid use disorder has maintained 4 years of abstinence while on sublingual buprenorphine-naloxone. During a social event, he tries methamphetamine for the first time. He later reports that the experience was more intensely pleasurable than any other drug he has used in the past, including cocaine. One pharmacological reason methamphetamine may have produced such a powerful reinforcing effect is

A. Methamphetamine not only blocks reuptake of dopamine in the synapse but also causes vesicular release of dopamine into the synaptic cleft. This results in a surge in dopamine that accounts for methamphetamine's intensely rewarding experience relative to most other drugs of abuse.
B. Methamphetamine potently stimulates serotonin receptors, whereas cocaine does not.
C. Methamphetamine blocks the effects of the most widespread inhibitory neurotransmitter in the brain, gamma-aminobutyric acid (GABA), leading to a potent stimulatory effect.
D. Cocaine's ability to block neuronal sodium channels lessens its pleasurable effect relative to methamphetamine which has no effect on neuronal sodium channels.
E. The patient must have also used a sedative medication or alcohol with the methamphetamine in order to produce an intensely pleasurable "speedball" effect, since methamphetamine alone is not very reinforcing or rewarding.

Answer: A

Explanation: Much of cocaine's psychostimulatory effects are mediated through its ability to increase synaptic dopamine levels by inhibiting dopamine reuptake. By contrast, methamphetamine (and amphetamine) produce their psychostimulatory effects by both blocking dopamine (and other catecholamine) reuptake, as well as disrupting monoamine vesicular storage causing an intracellular release of catecholamine stores with consequent increased release of synaptic catecholamines.

4. While speaking with her physician at a residential treatment center, a 25-year-old woman with a history of methamphetamine use expresses curiosity about treatment options. "People with heroin addiction can take medications like methadone or buprenorphine," she says. "Is there something like that for meth?" The physician, who is board-certified in addiction medicine, provides the most accurate response:

    A. "That's fantastic. There is a great new option of a methamphetamine vaccine that just got approved for use in the U.S."
    B. "Methadone and buprenorphine are just replacing one addiction for another, so I would not recommend thinking about any medications for your addiction, or any addiction for that matter."
    C. "I'll get you started today with a prescription for amphetamine that you can take instead of taking methamphetamine."
    D. "Several large-scale studies have demonstrated that topiramate is effective in treating methamphetamine addiction. I recommend that we start that today."
    E. "Researchers have tried many different kinds of medications to treat methamphetamine use disorder, and unfortunately none of them have shown a strong enough positive effect to warrant widespread use."

    Answer: E

    Explanation: Small studies have demonstrated some possible effect of mirtazapine and risperidone on the use of methamphetamine. However, larger studies have not demonstrated large enough beneficial effects for any medication in the treatment of methamphetamine use disorder to warrant widespread use in treatment.

References

1. American Psychiatric Association and American Psychiatric Association. DSM-5 Task Force. Diagnostic and statistical manual of mental disorders: DSM-5. 5th ed. Washington, DC: American Psychiatric Association; 2013, xliv, 947 p.
2. Anthony JC, Warner LA, Kessler RC. Comparative epidemiology of dependence on tobacco, alcohol, controlled substances, and inhalants: basic findings from the National Comorbidity Survey. Exp Clin Psychopharmacol. 1997;2(3):244–68.
3. Woody GE, Cottler LB, Cacciola J. Severity of dependence: data from the DSM-IV field trials. Addiction. 1993;88(11):1573–9.
4. Compton WM, Wargo EM, Volkow ND. Neuropsychiatric model of addiction simplified. Psychiatr Clin North Am. 2022;45(3):321–34.
5. Friedman J, Shover CL. Charting the fourth wave: geographic, temporal, race/ethnicity and demographic trends in polysubstance fentanyl overdose deaths in the United States, 2010–2021. Addiction. 2023;118(12):2477–85.
6. Quality CfBHSa. Key substance use and mental health indicators in the United States: results from the 2023 National Survey on Drug Use and Health. SAMHSA, editor. Rockville: Center for Behavioral Health Statistics and Quality, Substance Abuse and Mental Health Services Administration; 2024.

7. Shearer RD, et al. Racial and ethnic differences in heroin, methamphetamine, and cocaine use, treatment, and mortality trends in 3 national data sources-United States, 2010–2019. Med Care. 2024;62(3):151–60.
8. Administration SAaMHS. Lesbian, gay, and bisexual behavioral health: results from the 2021 and 2022 National Surveys on Drug Use and Health. SAaMHSA, editor. Rockville: Center for Behavioral Health Statistics and Quality; 2023.
9. Pippard NS, Bandoli G, Baer RJ. Trends and adverse pregnancy and birth outcomes associated with stimulant-related disorder diagnosis. Addiction. 2024;119(11):2006–14.
10. Mariano V, Berk J. "Coke in the dope": the underrecognized complications of a cocaine-adulterated fentanyl supply. J Addict Med. 2024;18(5):471–3.
11. Brust JC. Neurologic complications of illicit drug abuse. Continuum (Minneap Minn). 2014;20(3 Neurology of Systemic Disease):642–56.
12. Courtney KE, Ray LA. Methamphetamine: an update on epidemiology, pharmacology, clinical phenomenology, and treatment literature. Drug Alcohol Depend. 2014;143:11–21.
13. Sordo L, et al. Cocaine use and risk of stroke: a systematic review. Drug Alcohol Depend. 2014;142:1–13.
14. Kevil CG, et al. Methamphetamine use and cardiovascular disease. Arterioscler Thromb Vasc Biol. 2019;39(9):1739–46.
15. Glauser J, Queen JR. An overview of non-cardiac cocaine toxicity. J Emerg Med. 2007;32(2):181–6.
16. Foulds JA, et al. Methamphetamine use and violence: findings from a longitudinal birth cohort. Drug Alcohol Depend. 2020;207:107826.
17. McKetin R, et al. Does methamphetamine use increase violent behaviour? Evidence from a prospective longitudinal study. Addiction. 2014;109(5):798–806.
18. Brecht ML, Herbeck D. Methamphetamine use and violent behavior: user perceptions and predictors. J Drug Issues. 2013;43(4):468–82.
19. McKetin R. Methamphetamine psychosis: insights from the past. Addiction. 2018;113(8):1522–7.
20. Glasner-Edwards S, Mooney LJ. Methamphetamine psychosis: epidemiology and management. CNS Drugs. 2014;28(12):1115–26.
21. Hajebi A, et al. Twelve-month course and outcome of methamphetamine-induced psychosis compared with first episode primary psychotic disorders. Early Interv Psychiatry. 2018;12(5):928–34.
22. Gerra G, et al. Experimentally induced aggressive behavior in subjects with 3,4-methylened ioxy-methamphetamine ("Ecstasy") use history: psychobiological correlates. J Subst Abus. 2001;13(4):471–91.
23. Tyner EF, Fremouw WJ. The relation of methamphetamine use and violence: a critical review. Aggress Violent Behav. 2008;13(4):285–97.
24. Srisurapanont M, Kittiratanapaiboon P, Jarusuraisin N. Treatment for amphetamine psychosis. Cochrane Database Syst Rev. 2001;4:CD003026.
25. Ruha AM, Yarema MC. Pharmacologic treatment of acute pediatric methamphetamine toxicity. Pediatr Emerg Care. 2006;22(12):782–5.
26. Martel M, et al. Management of acute undifferentiated agitation in the emergency department: a randomized double-blind trial of droperidol, ziprasidone, and midazolam. Acad Emerg Med. 2005;12(12):1167–72.
27. Connors NJ, et al. Antipsychotics for the treatment of sympathomimetic toxicity: a systematic review. Am J Emerg Med. 2019;37(10):1880–90.
28. Clinical Guideline Committee M, et al. The ASAM/AAAP clinical practice guideline on the management of stimulant use Disorder. J Addict Med. 2024;18(1S Suppl 1):1–56.
29. Richards JR, et al. Treatment of toxicity from amphetamines, related derivatives, and analogues: a systematic clinical review. Drug Alcohol Depend. 2015;150:1–13.
30. Pham D, et al. Outcomes of beta blocker use in cocaine-associated chest pain: a meta-analysis. Emerg Med J. 2018;35(9):559–63.

31. Wilson T, Pitcher I, Bach P. Avoidance of beta-blockers in patients who use stimulants is not supported by good evidence. CMAJ. 2022;194(4):E127–8.
32. Kampman KM, et al. A double-blind, placebo-controlled trial of topiramate for the treatment of comorbid cocaine and alcohol dependence. Drug Alcohol Depend. 2013;133(1):94–9.
33. Kampman KM, et al. Cocaine withdrawal severity and urine toxicology results from treatment entry predict outcome in medication trials for cocaine dependence. Addict Behav. 2002;27(2):251–60.
34. Kampman KM, et al. Cocaine withdrawal symptoms and initial urine toxicology results predict treatment attrition in outpatient cocaine dependence treatment. Psychol Addict Behav. 2001;15(1):52–9.
35. Mulvaney FD, et al. Cocaine abstinence symptomatology and treatment attrition. J Subst Abus Treat. 1999;16(2):129–35.
36. Hjorthoj CR, Hjorthoj AR, Nordentoft M. Validity of timeline follow-back for self-reported use of cannabis and other illicit substances–systematic review and meta-analysis. Addict Behav. 2012;37(3):225–33.
37. McNeely J, et al. Performance of the tobacco, alcohol, prescription medication, and other substance use (TAPS) tool for substance use screening in primary care patients. Ann Intern Med. 2016;165(10):690–9.
38. Smith PC, et al. A single-question screening test for drug use in primary care. Arch Intern Med. 2010;170(13):1155–60.
39. Skinner HA. The drug abuse screening test. Addict Behav. 1982;7(4):363–71.
40. Tiet QQ, et al. Screen of drug use: diagnostic accuracy of a new brief tool for primary care. JAMA Intern Med. 2015;175(8):1371–7.
41. Chasnoff IJ, et al. Validation of the 4P's Plus screen for substance use in pregnancy validation of the 4P's Plus. J Perinatol. 2007;27(12):744–8.
42. Drake LR, Scott PJH. DARK classics in chemical neuroscience: cocaine. ACS Chem Neurosci. 2018;9(10):2358–72.
43. Jenkins AJ, Cone EJ. Pharmacokinetics: drug absorption, distribution, and elimination. In: Karch SB, editor. Drug abuse handbook. Boca Raton: CRC Press; 1998. p. 1138.
44. Pergolizzi J, et al. Cocaethylene: when cocaine and alcohol are taken together. Cureus. 2022;14(2):e22498.
45. Pennings EJ, Leccese AP, Wolff FA. Effects of concurrent use of alcohol and cocaine. Addiction. 2002;97(7):773–83.
46. Verstraete AG. Detection times of drugs of abuse in blood, urine, and oral fluid. Ther Drug Monit. 2004;26(2):200–5.
47. Studies OoA. Results from the 2013 national survey on drug use and health: summary of national findings. SAaMHS Administration, editor; 2014.
48. Rogers RD, Robbins TW. Investigating the neurocognitive deficits associated with chronic drug misuse. Curr Opin Neurobiol. 2001;11(2):250–7.
49. Marzuk PM, et al. Prevalence of cocaine use among residents of New York City who committed suicide during a one-year period. Am J Psychiatry. 1992;149(3):371–5.
50. Vijayakumar L, Kumar MS, Vijayakumar V. Substance use and suicide. Curr Opin Psychiatry. 2011;24(3):197–202.
51. Mantinieks D, et al. Stimulant use in suicides: a systematic review. Forensic Sci Int. 2022;338:111391.
52. Friedman H, Pross S, Klein TW. Addictive drugs and their relationship with infectious diseases. FEMS Immunol Med Microbiol. 2006;47(3):330–42.
53. van Harten PN, et al. Cocaine as a risk factor for neuroleptic-induced acute dystonia. J Clin Psychiatry. 1998;59(3):128–30.
54. Tseng W, Sutter ME, Albertson TE. Stimulants and the lung: review of literature. Clin Rev Allergy Immunol. 2014;46(1):82–100.
55. Kuczkowski KM. The effects of drug abuse on pregnancy. Curr Opin Obstet Gynecol. 2007;19(6):578–85.
56. Cocaine. In: Drugs and lactation database (LactMed(R)). Bethesda; 2006.

57. Levin FR, et al. Extended release mixed amphetamine salts and topiramate for cocaine dependence: a randomized clinical replication trial with frequent users. Drug Alcohol Depend. 2020;206:107700.
58. Kampman KM. The treatment of cocaine use disorder. Sci Adv. 2019;5(10):eaax1532.
59. Penberthy JK, et al. Review of treatment for cocaine dependence. Curr Drug Abuse Rev. 2010;3(1):49–62.
60. Dutra L, et al. A meta-analytic review of psychosocial interventions for substance use disorders. Am J Psychiatry. 2008;165(2):179–87.
61. Minozzi S, et al. Psychosocial interventions for stimulant use disorder. Cochrane Database Syst Rev. 2024;2(2):CD011866.
62. Palazon-Llecha A, et al. Predictors of cocaine use disorder treatment outcomes: a systematic review. Syst Rev. 2024;13(1):124.
63. Stotts AL, et al. Motivational interviewing with cocaine-dependent patients: a pilot study. J Consult Clin Psychol. 2001;69(5):858–62.
64. McKee SA, et al. Enhancing brief cognitive-behavioral therapy with motivational enhancement techniques in cocaine users. Drug Alcohol Depend. 2007;91(1):97–101.
65. Hedden SL, Kennet J, Lipari R, Medley G, Tice P. Key substance use and mental health indicators in the United States: results from the 2015 National Survey on Drug Use and Health. DoHaH Services, editor; 2016.
66. Coviello DM, et al. The effectiveness of two intensities of psychosocial treatment for cocaine dependence. Drug Alcohol Depend. 2001;61(2):145–54.
67. McLellan AT, et al. "Intensive" outpatient substance abuse treatment: comparisons with "traditional" outpatient treatment. J Addict Dis. 1997;16(2):57–84.
68. Stitzer ML, Petry NM, Peirce J. Motivational incentives research in the National Drug Abuse Treatment Clinical Trials Network. J Subst Abus Treat. 2010;38 Suppl 1(Suppl 1):S61–9.
69. Services CDoHC. The recovery incentives program: California's contingency management benefit. 2022 [cited 2025 January 21]. Available from: https://www.dhcs.ca.gov/CalAIM/Documents/CM-Fact-Sheet.pdf.
70. Hatch-Maillette M, et al. Predictors of 12-step attendance and participation for individuals with stimulant use disorders. J Subst Abus Treat. 2016;68:74–82.
71. Mattson ME. Emergency department visits involving attention deficit/hyperactivity disorder stimulant medications. In: The CBHSQ report. Rockville; 2013. p. 1–8.
72. McCabe SE, et al. Prescription stimulant medical and nonmedical use among US secondary school students, 2005 to 2020. JAMA Netw Open. 2023;6(4):e238707.
73. Heal DJ, et al. Amphetamine, past and present–a pharmacological and clinical perspective. J Psychopharmacol. 2013;27(6):479–96.
74. Ciccarone D. The rise of illicit fentanyls, stimulants and the fourth wave of the opioid overdose crisis. Curr Opin Psychiatry. 2021;34(4):344–50.
75. Kirkpatrick MG, et al. Comparison of intranasal methamphetamine and d-amphetamine self-administration by humans. Addiction. 2012;107(4):783–91.
76. Schep LJ, Slaughter RJ, Beasley DM. The clinical toxicology of metamfetamine. Clin Toxicol (Phila). 2010;48(7):675–94.
77. Baselt RC. Disposition of toxic drugs and chemicals in man. 7th ed. Foster City: Chemical Toxicology Institute; 2004.
78. Hemphill K, et al. A review of methamphetamine use and stroke in the young. Front Neurol. 2024;15:1397677.
79. Jayanthi S, Daiwile AP, Cadet JL. Neurotoxicity of methamphetamine: main effects and mechanisms. Exp Neurol. 2021;344:113795.
80. Sitte HH, Freissmuth M. Amphetamines, new psychoactive drugs and the monoamine transporter cycle. Trends Pharmacol Sci. 2015;36(1):41–50.
81. Sekine Y, et al. Brain serotonin transporter density and aggression in abstinent methamphetamine abusers. Arch Gen Psychiatry. 2006;63(1):90–100.
82. Papaseit E, et al. Clinical pharmacology of the synthetic cathinone mephedrone. Curr Top Behav Neurosci. 2017;32:313–31.

83. Baumann MH, et al. The designer methcathinone analogs, mephedrone and methylone, are substrates for monoamine transporters in brain tissue. Neuropsychopharmacology. 2012;37(5):1192–203.
84. Cox S, et al. Hospitalizations with amphetamine abuse among pregnant women. Obstet Gynecol. 2008;111(2 Pt 1):341–7.
85. Smid MC, Metz TD, Gordon AJ. Stimulant use in pregnancy: an under-recognized epidemic among pregnant women. Clin Obstet Gynecol. 2019;62(1):168–84.
86. Cohen JM, et al. Placental complications associated with psychostimulant use in pregnancy. Obstet Gynecol. 2017;130(6):1192–201.
87. Ornoy A. Pharmacological treatment of attention deficit hyperactivity disorder during pregnancy and lactation. Pharm Res. 2018;35(3):46.
88. Dinger J, et al. Methamphetamine consumption during pregnancy – effects on child health. Pharmacopsychiatry. 2017;50(3):107–13.
89. Committee Opinion No. 479: methamphetamine abuse in women of reproductive age (reaffirmed 2021). Obstet Gynecol. 2021;117(3):751–5.
90. Gorelick DA. Pharmacological treatment of stimulant use disorders. In: Miller SC, Fiellin DA, Rosenthal R, Saitz R, editors. The ASAM principles of addiction medicine. Wolters Kluwer: Philadelphia; 2019. p. 847–62.
91. Vocci FJ, Montoya ID. Psychological treatments for stimulant misuse, comparing and contrasting those for amphetamine dependence and those for cocaine dependence. Curr Opin Psychiatry. 2009;22(3):263–8.
92. Rawson RA, et al. A multi-site comparison of psychosocial approaches for the treatment of methamphetamine dependence. Addiction. 2004;99(6):708–17.
93. Khan S, et al. Caffeine intoxication treated with hemodialysis. Semin Dial. 2023;36(5):414–8.
94. Boeck CSDSR. Caffeine. In: Gupta R, editor. Reproductive and developmental toxicology. 3rd ed. Academic Press; 2022. p. 489–502.
95. Fischer TW, Hipler UC, Elsner P. Effect of caffeine and testosterone on the proliferation of human hair follicles in vitro. Int J Dermatol. 2007;46(1):27–35.
96. Volker JM, et al. Caffeine and its pharmacological benefits in the management of androgenetic alopecia: a review. Skin Pharmacol Physiol. 2020;33(3):93–109.
97. Mitchell DC, et al. Beverage caffeine intakes in the U.S. Food Chem Toxicol. 2014;63:136–42.
98. Mitchell DC, et al. An update on beverage consumption patterns and caffeine intakes in a representative sample of the US population. Food Chem Toxicol. 2025;196:115237.
99. Saraiva SM, et al. Overview of caffeine effects on human health and emerging delivery strategies. Pharmaceuticals (Basel). 2023;16(8):1067.
100. Carman AJ, et al. Current evidence for the use of coffee and caffeine to prevent age-related cognitive decline and Alzheimer's disease. J Nutr Health Aging. 2014;18(4):383–92.
101. Grosso G, et al. Coffee, tea, caffeine and risk of depression: a systematic review and dose-response meta-analysis of observational studies. Mol Nutr Food Res. 2016;60(1):223–34.
102. Saab S, et al. Impact of coffee on liver diseases: a systematic review. Liver Int. 2014;34(4):495–504.
103. Schmidt B, et al. Caffeine therapy for apnea of prematurity. N Engl J Med. 2006;354(20):2112–21.
104. Storm KK, et al. Caffeine therapy for apnea of prematurity: single center study on dosing practices and perceived effectiveness. Neonatology. 2024:1–20.
105. Derry CJ, Derry S, Moore RA. Caffeine as an analgesic adjuvant for acute pain in adults. Cochrane Database Syst Rev. 2014;2014(12):CD009281.
106. James JE. Critical review of dietary caffeine and blood pressure: a relationship that should be taken more seriously. Psychosom Med. 2004;66(1):63–71.
107. Devitt S. Growing popularity of energy drinks associated with an increase in pediatric cases reported to poison centers. 2024 [cited 2025 Jan 20]. Available from: https://poisoncenters.org/news-alerts/13414265.
108. Evatt DP, Juliano LM, Griffiths RR. A brief manualized treatment for problematic caffeine use: a randomized control trial. J Consult Clin Psychol. 2016;84(2):113–21.

109. Sweeney MM, et al. A randomized controlled trial of a manual-only treatment for reduction and cessation of problematic caffeine use. Drug Alcohol Depend. 2019;195:45–51.
110. Strain EC, et al. Caffeine dependence syndrome. Evidence from case histories and experimental evaluations. JAMA. 1994;272(13):1043–8.
111. Oliveto AH, et al. Effects of d-amphetamine and caffeine in humans under a cocaine discrimination procedure. Behav Pharmacol. 1998;9(3):207–17.
112. Hagg S, et al. Effect of caffeine on clozapine pharmacokinetics in healthy volunteers. Br J Clin Pharmacol. 2000;49(1):59–63.
113. Carrillo JA, Benitez J. Clinically significant pharmacokinetic interactions between dietary caffeine and medications. Clin Pharmacokinet. 2000;39(2):127–53.
114. Greenwood DC, et al. Caffeine intake during pregnancy and adverse birth outcomes: a systematic review and dose-response meta-analysis. Eur J Epidemiol. 2014;29(10):725–34.
115. Weng X, Odouli R, Li DK. Maternal caffeine consumption during pregnancy and the risk of miscarriage: a prospective cohort study. Am J Obstet Gynecol. 2008;198(3):279 e1–8.
116. Savitz DA, et al. Caffeine and miscarriage risk. Epidemiology. 2008;19(1):55–62.
117. Opinion TACoOaGC. Moderate caffeine consumption during pregnancy. 2020 [cited 2025 January 20]. Reaffirmation of Committee Opinion Number 462 from August 2010. Available from: https://www.acog.org/-/media/project/acog/acogorg/clinical/files/committee-opinion/articles/2010/08/moderate-caffeine-consumption-during-pregnancy.pdf?rev=005f71cc7fa04a8fa7deae4935f921a3&hash=F401F5697A61D867B87226F47A765A58.
118. ACOG Committee Opinion No. 462: moderate caffeine consumption during pregnancy. Obstet Gynecol. 2010;116(2 Pt 1):467–8.
119. Caffeine During Pregnancy. [cited 2025 January 20]. Available from: https://americanpregnancy.org/healthy-pregnancy/pregnancy-health-wellness/caffeine-intake-during-pregnancy/.
120. Aldridge A, Bailey J, Neims AH. The disposition of caffeine during and after pregnancy. Semin Perinatol. 1981;5(4):310–4.
121. McCreedy A, et al. Effects of maternal caffeine consumption on the breastfed child: a systematic review. Swiss Med Wkly. 2018;148:w14665.
122. Caffeine. In: Mother to baby | Fact sheets. Brentwood; 1994.
123. Prevention CfDCa. Maternal diet and breastfeeding. 2024 [cited 2025 January 20]. Available from: https://www.cdc.gov/breastfeeding-special-circumstances/hcp/diet-micronutrients/maternal-diet.html#:~:text=exposure%20and%20breastfeeding.-,Caffeine,Chocolate.

Steroids, Dissociatives, Club Drugs, Inhalants, and Hallucinogens

13

Mashal Khan, Abdo Semaan, and Anil Thomas

High-Yield Review Points

- Anabolic-androgenic steroid use is common among men, especially those with negative bodily perceptions, and their use comes along with adverse psychiatric and medical effects affecting multiple organ systems.
- Inhalants, used most commonly by adolescents, vary in their pharmacological properties, though most fall into one of several categories: volatile hydrocarbons, nitrous oxide, or nitrites.
- Hallucinogens are a pharmacologically diverse group of substances that cause an alteration in sensory perception, mood, and cognition and include, though are not limited to, lysergic acid diethylamide (LSD), psilocybin (mushrooms), N,N-dimethyltryptamine (DMT), mescaline, 5-dimethoxy-4-bromophenethylamine (2C-B), salvia, NBOMe Series, and DOx Series.
- Dissociative anesthetics exert their psychoactive effects by acting as antagonists at the NMDA receptor and produce a dissociative state with a greater degree of cognitive and neurological impairment than that produced by classic hallucinogens.

M. Khan (✉) · A. Semaan
Department of Psychiatry, NewYork-Presbyterian Weill Cornell Medical Center, New York, NY, USA
e-mail: mak9268@med.cornell.edu; aes9024@nyp.org

A. Thomas
Department of Psychiatry, NYU Grossman School of Medicine, New York, NY, USA
e-mail: anil.thomas@nyulangone.org

C. Marienfeld, M. Soltani (eds.), *AAAP Review of Addiction Psychiatry*,
https://doi.org/10.1007/978-3-032-24174-0_13

- Researchers are investigating some hallucinogens (psilocybin) and dissociative anesthetics (ketamine) for SUD treatment; clinicians must balance potential benefits with the risk of nonmedical use and addiction to these compounds.
- Falling under NIDA's classification of "club drugs," being able to recognize the intoxication and withdrawal symptoms, and the treatment, of both MDMA and GHB, are critical.

Anabolic-Androgenic Steroids (AAS)

Introduction

Anabolic-androgenic steroids (AAS) are a class of hormones that includes testosterone and its synthetic derivatives. Similar to testosterone, these compounds bind to the androgen receptor and produce varying degrees of anabolic (muscle-building) and androgenic (masculinizing) effects. These drugs are used therapeutically for various conditions, mainly utilizing the anabolic and/or androgen enhancement properties. These compounds have been used in higher than prescribed doses for physical or performance enhancement by weightlifters, bodybuilders, and other athletes, and they have been misused.

Epidemiology

In the United States, roughly 1% of the population (>three million) are estimated to have used AAS, and approximately one million men have experienced AAS dependence. Even though the use of AAS may start as early as teens, the average age of the onset of use appears to be in the early 20s, with the majority of users being men in their 20s–30s aiming to be lean and muscular, contrary to popular belief that use is relatively less prevalent among athletes [1]. Their use is more common among men than females (>50:1), and long-term users are predominantly men; up to one-third of users are thought to develop dependence [2]. Surveys of high school-attending teenagers suggest a decline in use; i.e., self-reported lifetime prevalence among 8th–12th graders declined from 3.3% (2001) to 1.1% (2023) [3]. AAS use is rare among girls and women, though some anonymous surveys with high selection bias have suggested that substantial number of teenage girls have used AASs [4].

Body dysmorphic disorder, especially its subset muscle dysmorphia, is notably present among users of AAS; in two studies, 10 of 23 men (44%) [5] and 11 of 24 men (46%) [6] with muscle dysmorphia reported lifetime use of anabolic-androgenic steroids (AASs). These individuals also show elevated rates of mood and anxiety disorders, obsessive and compulsive behaviors, substance use disorders, and impairment of social and occupational functioning.

Types of Anabolic Steroids and Sources

AASs are available in four forms: oral, intramuscular, topical (creams/gels), and patches. The oral and intramuscular are predominantly used outside of therapeutic indications. Typically, the oral form is a 17-alpha-alkylated androgen (such as stanozolol), which requires daily dosing and is associated with a higher incidence of hepatotoxicity. IM formulations include testosterone esters (depot testosterone) and testosterone enanthate. These are slower to absorb than their oral counterparts; their effects last 2–4 weeks. Once in the body, these compounds are metabolized by 5a-reductase to dihydrotestosterone (DHT) (which also contributes to male pattern baldness) and then by aromatase to estradiol (which contributes to gynecomastia) and neurosteroids (which are responsible for psychoactive effects).

Users most often obtain androgens from peers at their local gym or the Internet. Suppliers usually provide packages containing a variety of drugs: testosterone, synthetic androgens, aromatase inhibitors, human chorionic gonadotropin (hCG), clomiphene, and phosphodiesterase inhibitors. Some dietary supplements may also contain AASs.

Pharmacodynamics

Different types of AASs bind to androgen receptors with varying affinity. Androgen receptor complexes translocate to the cell nucleus, augmenting gene transcription, resulting in protein synthesis and increasing muscle mass. Psychoactive effects occur via AAS action at the membrane on the androgen receptor and via allosteric sites on the GABA receptor. Androgen metabolites, estradiol, and neurosteroids can also have psychoactive effects. The neurosteroid metabolite of testosterone (3-alpha-androstanediol) is a positive allosteric modulator of the GABA receptor and can potentiate GABA receptors.

Patterns of Use

Individuals use these drugs for their anabolic properties in three common concepts. Often, individuals titrate and taper off (pyramiding) utilizing either an individual or a combination of steroids (stacking). Androgen users often pyramid their doses in "cycles" of 6–12 weeks. Most users follow each "cycle" with an "off-cycle" phase for recovery. Stacks are intended to reduce unwanted side effects or for additive effects. Combinations used include both androgens and other drugs, such as growth hormone for additional anabolic effect, human chorionic gonadotropin (hCG) to counteract the reduction in testicular size resulting from high-dose androgen use, aromatase inhibitors to counteract gynecomastia, 5-alpha reductase inhibitors to prevent balding and acne, and diuretics to promote water loss or to mask steroid misuse.

Presentation and Adverse Medical Effects

Several typical situations bring AAS users to the attention of clinicians. These include the following:

1. AAS dependence syndromes
2. Hypomanic and manic syndromes during AAS exposure
3. Syndromes of depression and anxiety associated with AAS withdrawal
4. Body image disorders associated with AAS use
5. Co-occurring substance use disorders
6. Medical conditions associated with long-term AAS use
7. Forensic situations, such as cases of AAS-induced violence or criminality.

AAS users may experience the following adverse effects:

Cardiovascular: The use of supraphysiologic doses of AAS is associated with several adverse cardiovascular effects, including dyslipidemia via the induction of hepatic lipase (reducing HDL): dose-dependent increase in left ventricular mass and related diastolic dysfunction [2, 7]; hypertension; thrombosis, erythrocytosis, and polycythemia [8]; accelerated atherosclerosis related to dyslipidemias [2]; and increased risk of cardiac ischemia during peak exercise.

Endocrine: Exogenous androgens result in the suppression of gonadotropins and impact the hypothalamic-pituitary-gonadal axis, causing feminization of men and masculinization of women. This results in men possibly developing hypogonadism, reduced testicular size (reduced spermatogenesis and fertility) [9], erectile dysfunction, gynecomastia, and early-onset prostatic hypertrophy. Women may experience shrinkage of breast tissue, oligomenorrhea/amenorrhea, hirsutism, clitoromegaly, and an irreversible deepening of the voice.

Hepatic: Adverse effects concerning the liver are typically limited to oral AAS (i.e., 17a-alkylated agents) [2]. Hepatic peliosis (proliferation of sinusoidal hepatic capillaries that result in cystic blood-filled cavities), cholestatic jaundice, and hepatic neoplasms (rare) are related to cumulative dose and duration of use.

Neuro-psychiatric/behavioral: Supratherapeutic doses of AAS most commonly lead to the following adverse psychiatric symptoms: aggression, irritability, anxiety, reduced inhibitory control, impulsive behavior, hypomania, mania, and even psychotic reactions. Alterations in the GABAergic system are thought to mediate many of the behavioral effects of AAS [10]. AASs exert a dose-dependent effect on the brain, with high doses eliciting manic symptoms in normal men [11]. AAS withdrawal can present with mood swings, depression with suicidal behavior, and aggression with violent and assaultive behaviors, sometimes dramatic reductions in size and strength.

Musculoskeletal: AAS users who aim to increase skeletal muscle mass over short periods are at risk of tendon rupture [2, 12] due to tendons' slower rate of adaptation to rapidly increased muscle mass. Specific to adolescents and the use of aromatized AAS is the premature closure of the epiphyses in teenage users, which may result in reduced final height.

Skin: Frequently, individuals using AAS develop acne and oily skin; this is in part due to the overactivity of sebaceous glands and the related overproduction of skin surface lipids and the consequent increases in the population of cutaneous *Propionibacterium acnes* and *Staphylococcus aureus* bacteria [13]. Acne generally tends to resolve upon the cessation of AAS. Male pattern baldness may be seen in both male and female users, is related to the effects of excess circulating DHT, and tends to be irreversible.

Assessment and Management

In the DSM-5-TR [14], misuse of AASs does not have a category of its own and falls under *Other (or Unknown) Substance Disorders.* The criteria are similar to the *Substance Use Disorder* criteria in the DSM-5-TR; the severity of the use disorder is classified based on the number of criteria met. Within this category are subcategories of other substance use disorders, other substance intoxications, other substance withdrawals, other substance-induced disorders, and unspecified other substance-related disorders.

To improve clinical management, the history obtained should include information about use (i.e., stacks, pyramids, cycles, off-cycles), formulations and doses used, other pharmacological agents that they may have used to counter side effects (e.g., tamoxifen for gynecomastia, human chorionic gonadotropin for testicular atrophy, diuretics for edema, opioids for pain relief, and anxiolytics for anxiety), medical symptoms and their reversibility, and symptoms of mood, anxiety, substance use, and body image disorders.

A focused physical exam should include assessment for body composition (height, weight, body mass index, signs of rapid increase in lean body mass), skin (acne, male pattern baldness, needle marks, hirsutism, striae, or keloids), breasts (lactation, gynecomastia), genitourinary (testicular atrophy, clitoromegaly, enlarged prostate), and systemic signs of cardiac and liver disease.

Lab workup is based on presenting symptoms and possible organ systems affected, in addition to a hormonal panel (i.e., luteinizing hormone (LH), follicle-stimulating hormone (FSH), estradiol (E2), testosterone (T), free testosterone (free T), sex hormone-binding globulin (SHBG), and prolactin (PRL)); initial testing should include complete blood count (CBC), complete metabolic profile, creatine kinase (CK), lipid profile, prostate-specific antigen, urine drug screen, electrocardiogram (EKG), echocardiogram, and semen analysis. Tests may present with the following abnormalities: CBC (↑ RBC count, Hct and Hgb), liver function tests (↑ALT, AST, and LDH are often muscular in origin and may not indicate liver disease), muscle enzymes (↑CK, LDH, AST, and ALT may be elevated), lipid profile (may show ↓ HDL-C, ↑ LDL-C, ↑ or no change in total cholesterol and triglycerides), hormonal levels (↑testosterone and estradiol—with the use of testosterone esters, ↓testosterone—without the use of testosterone esters or during withdrawal, or ↓ LH and FSH), EKG (can show left ventricular hypertrophy), echocardiogram (can show decreased ventricular ejection fraction, impaired diastolic function), and semen analysis (↓sperm count and motility, abnormal morphology).

AAS detection is possible via mass spectrometry testing of urine samples. Misuse should be suspected with high testosterone in association with suppressed LH and FSH levels. A T/E ratio of greater than 4 can confirm testosterone misuse [2].

While addiction professionals can assist with treatments for the substance use disorder, management of AAS-induced adverse effects should be directed to specialists. Hypogonadism and gynecomastia should be addressed and managed by consulting with endocrine specialists. Heart and liver problems should also be directed to those respective specialists.

There are limited data and a lack of published clinical trials to support formal indications for treating AAS-related disorders; however, experts recommend utilizing cognitive behavioral therapies to address body image concerns, such as muscle dysmorphia, and to consider SSRI value in AAS users showing prominent and refractory obsessions related to body image. Depression is commonly seen in the withdrawal phase and treated with antidepressants, and, if resistant, ECT can be considered. Couples therapy is recommended for cases where the partner reports distress in living with the person.

Inhalants

Introduction

Inhalants are volatile substances that produce chemical vapor that can be breathed in to induce a mind-altering/psychoactive effect and are believed to have specific pharmacological properties and effects in common. See Table 13.1 for common types of inhalants. The DSM-5-TR [14] identified volatile hydrocarbons as "inhalants" in its diagnostic criteria of "inhalant-related disorder." Inhalants are found in various everyday products, such as paint, solvents, glue, aerosol propellants, and fuels. The DSM-5-TR classifies conditions related to either anesthetic gases, such as nitrous oxide, or nitrites, such as amyl, butyl, and isobutyl nitrites, under "other (or unknown) substance-related disorders." Nitrous oxide is used as a propellant in canisters of whipped cream, as a power booster in automobiles and motorcycles, and as an anesthetic agent for painful medical and dental procedures. Volatile hydrocarbons can be categorized based on structure as aromatic, aliphatic, and halogenated hydrocarbons.

An inhalant can be administered in multiple ways, which are explained in Table 13.2.

Table 13.1 Types of inhalants [15]

Inhalant type	Examples
Aromatic hydrocarbons	Petroleum products (gasoline and kerosene), propane, butane
Aliphatic hydrocarbons[a]	Toluene (used in paint thinner and model glue), xylene
Haloalkanes[a]	Hydrofluorocarbons, chlorofluorocarbons (including many aerosols and propellants)
Nitrites—amyl/butyl nitrites	"Poppers"
Nitrous oxide	Found in whipped cream canisters

[a]Volatile hydrocarbons

Table 13.2 Methods of administering inhalants [16]

Method of use	Description
Sniffing, snorting	Inhaling through the nose from the original container
Huffing	Inhaling through the mouth from the original container or inhaling from a chemically saturated rag held to the face or mouth
Bagging	Paper or plastic bag containing an inhalant being held over the mouth and nose or over the head
Dusting	Inhaling aerosol computer dusting spray via the mouth or nose
Glading	Inhaling air freshener

Epidemiology

Inhalant use is more common among adolescents and less common among adults. According to the 2023 National Survey on Drug Use and Health (NSDUH) [17], approximately 2.6 million Americans (0.9%) aged 12 years or older used inhalants in the past year; their use was most common in those aged 12–17 years. The most recent report by Monitoring the Future Study (MTF) [3] states that 9.0% of eighth graders, 6.5% of tenth graders, and 6.3% of 12th graders had ever used inhalants and that current inhalant use remains highest among eighth graders (i.e., 2.6% vs. 0.9% in tenth graders and 1.2% in 12th graders). Inhalant use has decreased over the last two decades; the prevalence of 30-day use for grades 8, 10, and 12 combined was 3.4%, 2.6%, and 1.5% in 1998, 2008, and 2023, respectively.

Adults at risk for use are those with ready access to chemicals or anesthetics, such as doctors, nurses, factory workers, dentists, shoemakers, hair stylists, painters, and dry-cleaning workers. Nitrite use is prevalent among men who have sex with other men (MSM) [18] and is utilized for its aphrodisiac properties.

Pharmacokinetics and Pharmacodynamics

Inhalants are highly lipid-soluble. Upon inhalation, they rapidly cross alveolar membranes and the blood-brain barrier to reach high concentrations in the brain while also bypassing first-pass hepatic metabolism. The onset of symptoms is within seconds of use, with peak plasma concentration 15–20 min after inhalation [15]. The mode of administration determines the inhaled concentration. Sniffing (inhaling through the nose from the original container) offers the lowest concentration, followed by huffing (inhaling by mouth from the original container or inhaling from a chemically saturated rag held to the face or mouth), and bagging (a paper or plastic bag containing an inhalant is held over the mouth and nose or over the head) offers the highest concentration. Most inhalants undergo elimination primarily through the lungs, usually unaltered by exhalation. However, some inhalants, such as aromatics, alkyl nitrites, and methylene chloride, undergo hepatic metabolism, producing damaging and toxic byproducts such as free nitrites and carbon monoxide.

Inhalants are varied in their pharmacological properties. There is some overlap between volatile hydrocarbons and nitrous oxide in that they act as CNS depressants, although the mechanism of action is not entirely understood for most inhalants. The mechanism of action for volatile hydrocarbons is theorized to be similar to the mechanism of action of ethanol, with the stimulation of gamma-aminobutyric acid (GABA) and glycine alpha-1 receptors and the inhibition of the N-methyl-D-aspartate (NMDA) receptor, leading to inhibition in the CNS [19]. Nitrous oxide is theorized to exert its effect by mediating the release of endogenous beta-endorphins and direct binding on mu, delta, and kappa opiate receptors. In addition, it acts as an NMDA receptor antagonist [15]. Alkyl nitrites release nitric oxide, a potent vasodilator that causes smooth muscle relaxation, a vital effect related to its use [20].

Clinical Features

Volatile Hydrocarbons

Immediate effects often include an initial stimulating "rush," followed by lightheadedness, disinhibition, and impulsivity. The effects of intoxication last minutes (typically 15–30 min) but can be extended by inhaling repeatedly. Euphoria is often followed by drowsiness, lethargy, headache, and sleep, especially with repeated cycles of inhalation use. Slurred speech, dizziness, diplopia, ataxia, and disorientation occur as the inhalant dose increases. With prolonged use, visual hallucinations and marked time distortion occur, which are cited as motivators for continued use. Low-frequency users report more pleasurable experiences, whereas chronic users have mixed pleasurable and unpleasant or noxious experiences [19].

Table 13.3 below details the toxic effects of inhalants on organ systems. In addition to the effects mentioned, mortality has been noted in the context of asphyxiation or suffocation, choking on vomit, and careless or dangerous behavior in potentially dangerous settings. "Sudden sniffing death" [22] can also occur, though the mechanism is unclear. It is theorized that inhalant-related increases in myocardial cell depolarization and reduced conductivity lead to arrhythmia paired with increased blood concentration of epinephrine [19].

Table 13.3 Toxic effects of inhalants by organ system [15, 19]

Organ System	Toxic effects
CVS	Sinus bradycardia, increased QT dispersion [21], hypoxia-induced heart block, myocardial fibrosis, sudden sniffing death syndrome
Hematologic	Bone marrow suppression, leukemia, aplastic anemia
Pulmonary	Cough, wheezing, dyspnea, emphysema, pneumonitis
Dermatologic	Perioral rash/eczema, contact dermatitis, burns, angioedema, frostbite injury
Neurologic	Change in speech, drowsiness, nystagmus, peripheral neuropathy, sensorimotor polyneuropathy, tremor, ataxia, white matter degeneration, cerebellar degeneration
Gastrointestinal	Nausea, vomiting, diarrhea, abdominal pain/cramps, hepatotoxicity
Renal	Hypokalemia, acid-base disturbance, acute renal failure, Fanconi's syndrome, renal tubular acidosis
Neuro-psych	Apathy, depression, insomnia, poor attention, memory loss, dementia, psychosis

Nitrites

The effects of nitrites are instantaneous, brief, and intense. Nitrites cause vasodilation, resulting in a sudden surge of blood to the heart and brain. Users often experience a "head rush," which is a combination of elated mood, light-headedness, heat flush, and heightened sensual awareness [23]. The effects wear off within 5 min of use. Nitrites are also used to enhance sexual pleasure by prolonging penile erection and promoting anal sphincter relaxation.

Negative effects include headache, nausea, and syncope, which are related to the vasodilatory effects of nitrites. Nasotracheal irritation, sinusitis, and dermatitis may occur. Users can also develop methemoglobinemia, and acute impairment of oxygen delivery to tissues can present as headache, fatigue, dyspnea, and lethargy [15]. At higher methemoglobin levels (e.g., greater than 70%), respiratory depression, altered consciousness, shock, seizures, and death may occur [24]. Taking sildenafil with nitrites can cause severe hypotension, leading to syncope and cerebral or myocardial ischemia.

Nitrous Oxide

The onset of action for nitrous oxide is 2–3 min, and the duration of effect is less than 5 min. Intoxication causes euphoria, dizziness, dulling of the senses, decreased pain sensation, and distorted audiovisual processes.

Nitrous oxide causes mild cardiac depression and indirect sympathetic stimulation [25]. Little change in blood pressure occurs because a mild increase in peripheral resistance offsets the mild cardiac depressant effect.

Users inhaling from a pressurized tank are at risk of pneumothorax [26]. Neurological and hematological effects are due to vitamin B12 inactivation by nitrous oxide; chronic use produces clinical effects similar to the subacute combined degeneration syndrome associated with pernicious anemia [27].

Assessment and Management

All persons suspected of inhalant use should have the following labs performed: complete blood count (CBC), pulse oximetry, EKG, basic metabolic profile (BMP), methemoglobin, and liver function tests (LFT). Urine toxicology does not identify inhalants; however, it may prove useful in screening for other substances. Specific findings that may indicate inhalant use include bone marrow suppression (associated with benzene); poor oxygen saturation, arrhythmias, hypokalemia, and hypophosphatemia (associated with toluene); methemoglobinemia (seen with nitrites); acidosis (seen with toluene); and liver and renal function abnormalities, particularly with halogenated hydrocarbons.

Management of acute inhalant intoxication is supportive care, primarily for cardiac and respiratory systems. Upon removing the source of intoxication, address any hypoxia with supplemental oxygen. Patients presenting in a coma with respiratory depression require endotracheal intubation and mechanical ventilation. Arrhythmias are corrected based on commonly accepted guidelines. Electrolyte abnormalities should be corrected. Patients with methemoglobinemia should receive high-dose oxygen and IV methylene blue that accelerates the enzymatic reduction of methemoglobin (contraindicated in persons with G6PD deficiency) [28]. Chelation therapy may be required for lead toxicity, but the treatment has limitations in only clearing inorganic lead and organolead (lead attached to carbon molecules) over time [29].

Hallucinogens

Introduction

The term "hallucinogen" is an umbrella term used to describe substances that primarily cause an alteration in sensory perception, mood, and cognition. They are a pharmacologically diverse group of compounds that range from plant- and animal-sourced compounds to synthetic drugs. Organically sourced hallucinogens (plant, mushroom, or animal) have been used in religious rituals and recreationally for thousands of years [30], and examples include the genus *Psilocybe*, ayahuasca, peyote, and *Salvia divinorum*. Lysergic acid diethylamide (LSD) was the first synthesized hallucinogen, created by Albert Hofmann in 1938; its psychoactive properties were discovered by accident 5 years later [31].

Also known as classical psychedelics, classical hallucinogens are organically sourced compounds and synthetic drugs that produce varying degrees of alterations in consciousness. They are divided into two chemical classes. Tryptamines, which are serotonin-like in structure, include LSD, psilocybin, and dimethyltryptamine (DMT). Phenylethylamines include the drug mescaline [32]. They mediate effects via 5-HT2A receptor agonism or partial agonism [32]. Their effects are similar (LSD-like); however, they differ principally in the time course (onset and duration of effects), which in turn depends on the substance, the dose, and the route of administration. Table 13.4 shows the pharmacologic features of classic hallucinogens.

Table 13.4 Pharmacological features of classic hallucinogens [16, 32–34]

Hallucinogen	Typical dose	Onset (min) (post ingestion)	Peak effects (h) (post ingestion)	Duration (h) (post ingestion)
LSD	Oral: 25–200 μg	30–90	3–5	6–12
Psilocybin	Oral: 10 mg (20–30 g fresh, mushrooms or 1–2 g dried)	20–30	1–2	6–8
DMT	Oral: 35–75 mg IV/smoked: 30–50 mg	20–60	1–2	2–8
Mescaline	Oral: 200–500 mg (6–12 dried buttons)	30–120	2–4	6–12
2C-B	Oral: 10–30 mg Insufflated: 5–20 mg	45–75 5–15	1–2	4–8 2–4
NBOMe Ex. 25I-NBOMe	Sublingual: 500–1000 μg Insufflated: 250–750 μg	15–45 5–15	1–3	6–10 4–6
DOx Ex. DOC	Oral: 1.5–3 mg Insufflated: 1–2 mg	60–120 20–60	4–8	12–24 8–16

Epidemiology

Hallucinogen use occurs worldwide, although the prevalence is generally considered to be low relative to other drugs misused. LSD remains the prototypical hallucinogen and the most extensively studied of such drugs. Hallucinogens account for approximately 7% of United States emergency department (ED) visits involving illicit drugs. According to the 2023 National Survey on Drug Use and Health [17], 3.1% of Americans aged 12 and older reported use in the past year of hallucinogens (0.6% LSD, <0.1% phencyclidine (PCP), 1.3% ketamine, 0.8% 3,4-methylenedioxy-methamphetamine (MDMA), 0.6% GHB). Individuals under 17-years-old have higher rates of use for serotonergic hallucinogens like LSD, whereas those over 26-years-old have higher rates of use for MDMA.

LSD

LSD is the most potent classic hallucinogen (effects starting at 25 μg). Despite its potency, there is a considerable safety margin. It is often distributed and sold on small squares of blotter paper, colloquially referred to as "tabs" or "hits," that often contain 50 μg of LSD; a moderate dose (75–150 μg) will significantly alter the state of consciousness [35].

The effects of LSD can vary widely, but typical perceptual changes include illusions, pseudo-hallucinations, and synesthesias, as well as alterations of thinking and time experience. Religious and mystical experiences may occur and can be produced reliably under controlled conditions [36]. Unwanted effects can occur, such as dysphoria, anxiety, fear of insanity, and feelings that one is dying. These are colloquially referred to as a "bad trip" and usually resolve during the time course of acute drug action [37]. There are no documented human deaths from LSD overdose

[35]. In some rare cases, acute psychotic episodes have occurred. Hallucinogen persisting perceptual disorder (HPPD) or "flashback," which is the intermittent reemergence of perceptual distortions weeks, months, or longer after the drug's effects have worn off, occurs in very low prevalence [38].

Psilocybin

Found in over 100 species of mushroom, including the members of the genus *Psilocybe*, psilocybin was first isolated in 1958. Typically referred to as "shrooms" or "magic mushrooms," they can be consumed fresh or dried. It is intermediate in potency between LSD and mescaline, with a dose of 10–15 mg being roughly equivalent to 100 μg of LSD. The effects of psilocybin are very similar to those of LSD but of shorter duration. Perceptual changes such as illusions, synesthesia, affective activation, alterations of thought, time sense, and body experience are especially noteworthy [39]. A mild headache is common for up to 24 h following psilocybin use.

DMT

DMT is a naturally occurring tryptamine found in various plants and is the active ingredient in ayahuasca, a traditional South American drink. Oral consumption of DMT leads to inactivation due to rapid metabolism by monoamine oxidase A (MAO-A) [40]. However, it can be rendered orally active by the administration of MAO inhibitors (MAO-I) before or along with DMT. Ayahuasca preparations utilize the same principle; the brew contains harmala alkaloids (MAO-Is), which prevent inactivation. DMT, on its own, is usually smoked or occasionally injected or insufflated. In smoked doses of around 40–50 mg, DMT produces a brief (<30 min) [40] and extremely intense experience that can involve complete loss of contact with reality, intense visual experiences, terrifying disorientation, incoordination, loss of ordinary sense of reality and self, mystical experience, and/or the experience of contact with other worlds or beings. The effects of ayahuasca are more prolonged (~4 h) and are generally similar to those of the classic hallucinogens described above [41]. Nausea and vomiting are common and considered to be related to the harmala alkaloids. Unlike frequent LSD use, tolerance to DMT does not seem to develop [40], but it is unusual for people to use it frequently due to the intense and sometimes overwhelming nature of the experience. Complications are infrequent, especially by the oral route, and may not appear in clinical settings because of the short duration of DMT's action. Individuals consuming ayahuasca or DMT along with an MAO-I are at increased risk of developing serotonin syndrome.

Mescaline

Mescaline (3,4,5-trimethoxyphenethylamine) is the active ingredient in peyote cactus, found in the Southwest US and Northern Mexico. The "dried button" (fleshy tops of the cactus) is ingested or crushed to a powder and prepared as a tea [42]. Mescaline is the least potent of the classic hallucinogens; a typical dose is between 6 and 12 buttons, and the effects are LSD-like. Individuals frequently experience nausea or vomiting after ingestion. Users have reported experiencing recurring visual patterns, including stripes, checkerboards, angular spikes, multicolored dots, and fractals [43]. At higher doses, users may experience hyperthermia, headache, vomiting, hypotension, ataxia, diaphoresis, and depressed cardiac and respiratory function. These effects may precede the hallucinogenic effects, which may last 8–12 h.

2C-B

2C-B (4-bromo-2,5-dimethoxyphenethylamine) is a synthetic phenethylamine hallucinogen often sold as a pink powder or pill. It is popularly nicknamed "pink cocaine," or "tusi." Notably, it is structurally unrelated to cocaine. Typical oral doses range 10–30 mg, while insufflated doses range 5–20 mg. It produces both a stimulant-like and hallucinogen-like effect, leading to euphoria, wakefulness, visual distortions, synesthesia, and altered time perception. Effects typically last 4–8 h for oral dosing and 2–4 h for insufflated dosing. Its pharmacology involves 5-HT2A receptor partial agonism, but the whole mechanism remains unclear [44]. Reported side effects include dysphoria, anxiety, increased heart rate, and elevated blood pressure [45].

Salvia

Salvinorin A, a diterpene alkaloid and kappa-opioid agonist, is the active ingredient in *Salvia divinorum*, a herb from the mint family that has been used in religious ceremonies for Mazatec Indians native to Oaxaca, Mexico. Salvia is pharmacologically distinct from classical hallucinogens in that it does not exert its psychoactive effect via serotonin; instead, it does so by stimulating the kappa-opioid receptor [46]. It is not a federally controlled substance and, as such, is sold in the form of leaves, which are available to recreational users at smoke shops and over the Internet. It can be chewed, smoked, vaporized, and ingested. The method of use can impact how long the effects last, with smoking or vaporizing having short effects (15–25 min), whereas chewing can have effects lasting 1–2 h. When chewed, the leaf mass and juice are maintained within the cheek area, with absorption occurring across the lining of the oral mucosa (buccal); it has poor absorption via the GI tract [46]. The sought-after subjective effects include elevation of mood, relaxation, feeling calm, introspection, mild dissociative effects, hallucinations, and synesthesia. At higher doses, users may experience dissociation, with intense hallucinatory effects and loosening contact with reality [47]. Larger doses are typically aversive.

NBOMes

The NBOMe compounds are synthetic phenethylamine hallucinogens in which an N-methoxybenzyl (NBOMe) group is attached to a 2C-series backbone. The most widely encountered of these compounds is 25I-NBOMe (2-(4-iodo-2,5-

dimethoxyphenyl)-N-[(2-methoxyphenyl)methyl]ethanamine). They are highly potent 5-HT2A receptor agonists, commonly sold on blotter paper (frequently misrepresented as LSD) or in powder, liquid, or tablet form [48]. Typical sublingual/buccal doses range 500–1000 μg, while insufflated doses range 250–750 μg. They produce intense hallucinogen-like effects, including euphoria, altered perception, and visual hallucinations, accompanied by marked sympathomimetic stimulation. Effects typically last 6–10 h for sublingual/buccal dosing and 4–6 h for insufflated dosing. Reported side effects include agitation, confusion, hypertension, tachycardia, hyperthermia, seizures, and rhabdomyolysis [49].

DOx

The DOx compounds (4-substituted-2,5-dimethoxyamphetamines) are synthetic phenethylamine hallucinogens in which an alpha-methyl group is added to the 2C-series backbone, producing potent and long-lasting psychoactive effects. One of the most widely encountered of these is DOC (2,5-dimethoxy-4-chloroamphetamine). They are potent 5-HT2A receptor agonists [50], typically sold as blotter paper frequently mg, while insufflated doses range 1–2 mg. They produce pronounced hallucinogen-like effects, including euphoria, visual hallucinations, altered perception, and a sympathomimetic response. Effects typically last 12–24 h for oral dosing and 8–16 h for insufflated dosing [51] seizures [52].

Clinical Features

Mood can vary from euphoria and feelings of spiritual insight to depression, anxiety, and terror. Perception usually is intensified and distorted, with alterations in the sense of time, space, and body boundaries; illusions (visual and auditory distortions of perception) are common; true hallucinations (perceptions that do not have any basis in reality) are rare, while synesthesia (a blending of the senses wherein colors are heard and sounds are seen) may often be experienced [32, 53]. Reality testing is usually intact; however, confusion and disorientation may occur.

A "bad trip" usually takes the form of an anxiety attack or panic reaction, with the user feeling out of control. An experience of depersonalization may precipitate the fear of losing one's mind permanently. While higher doses are associated with more intense experiences, adverse reactions are less a function of the dose than of context and environment. Of note, mental "set" (mental state/intention/preparation of the person) and "setting" (environment) are thought to strongly influence the psychological content and emotional tone of the individuals' experience.

The acute somatic effects are typically mild to moderate, including nausea (+/− vomiting), dry mouth, chills, tremors, paresthesia, blurred vision, mild tachycardia, and hypertension [53]. Hallucinogen ingestion may also result in an acute toxic delirium that is characterized by delusions, hallucinations, agitation, confusion, paranoia, and inadvertent suicide attempts (e.g., attempts to fly or perform other impossible activities).

Assessment and Management

Hallucinogen use disorder (other than PCP) can be diagnosed using the DSM-5-TR [14] criteria for *Other Hallucinogen Intoxication* or *Other Hallucinogen Use Disorder*; the criteria are similar to other substance intoxication and use disorder criteria in the DSM-5-TR; the severity of the use disorder is classified based on the number of criteria met. Hallucinogen withdrawal syndrome is not a recognized phenomenon in the DSM-5-TR; however, some users do report having withdrawal symptoms such as fatigue, irritability, and anhedonia. The DSM-5-TR describes hallucinogen persisting perception disorder (HPPD) as a disorder found in individuals with past exposure to hallucinogens experiencing flashbacks, vivid memories, or brief recurrences of sensory distortions reminiscent of intoxication during periods of sobriety.

Classical hallucinogen use rarely requires medical attention. Individuals seeking medical attention do so in the context of an overdose, acute anxiety or panic reactions, or accidental ingestion. Except in cases of delirium or overdose, the treatment of acute ingestion of a classic hallucinogen includes reassurance and a calm and safe environment. Reassuring patients that the drug is causing their anxiety and that the effects are transient should aid in partly mitigating symptoms. There is no role for medication in the treatment of uncomplicated hallucinogen withdrawal.

Severe reactions can include delirium or serotonin syndrome. In the case of agitation, dysphoria, and distress, benzodiazepines are the first line of treatment [54]; neuroleptics are a reasonable adjunct only if distress and concerning behaviors persist. Haldol may decrease the seizure threshold. Restraints are rarely necessary but recommended if there is an immediate danger of self-harm or assaultive behavior. Close observation of intoxicated patients and periodic monitoring of mental status are indicated due to rapid changes in mood and thought content during intoxication. Serotonin syndrome may occur in individuals who have ingested an ayahuasca brew or taken DMT with MAO-Is [55]. These individuals would present with increased autonomic activity (mydriasis, tachycardia, increased blood pressure), delirium, nausea, and vomiting and can be treated with the serotonin antagonist cyproheptadine. Following acute intoxication or severe reactions, short-term therapy is helpful for individuals who have had very intense, disturbing, or traumatic experiences; it can help them integrate their experience and identify/address any psychological sequelae.

At-risk individuals may experience recurrences of flashbacks with the initiation of selective serotonin reuptake inhibitors (esp. sertraline) [56]. Risperidone should be avoided; it has been noted to worsen visual disturbances and accompanying anxiety, presumably due to its alpha-2 presynaptic antagonism and noradrenaline release.

Benzodiazepines, clonidine, first-generation antipsychotics at low doses (esp. haloperidol), carbamazepine, and psychotherapy have been reported to have positive therapeutic effects, although the evidence to support their efficacy is limited [57].

Future Considerations

Several classic hallucinogens are currently under investigation for their potential therapeutic applications in substance use disorders (SUDs). For example, psilocybin administered in conjunction with structured psychotherapy has shown preliminary efficacy in reducing cravings and promoting abstinence in individuals with alcohol use disorder [58, 59] and cocaine use [60].

Ibogaine, an indole alkaloid derived from *Tabernanthe iboga*, has also shown promise in observational studies for reducing opioid withdrawal symptoms and craving [61]. However, its clinical development has been limited by safety concerns, including QT-interval prolongation, ventricular arrhythmias, and cardiac-related fatalities. Notably, some studies have utilized co-administration of magnesium with ibogaine to decrease the risk of cardiac side effects [62].

While these findings are promising, large-scale randomized controlled trials are needed to confirm efficacy, refine dosing paradigms, and ensure safety before these compounds can be integrated into evidence-based SUD treatment protocols. Notably, the growing availability and medical framing of hallucinogens could paradoxically contribute to increased rates of hallucinogen use disorder in vulnerable individuals [63], underscoring the need for careful screening, ongoing monitoring, and robust public health surveillance alongside clinical development.

Dissociative Anesthetics

Dissociative drugs cause a disconnection among thoughts, identity, consciousness, and memory. This heterogeneous group of chemicals can produce hallucinogenic effects. However, unlike the classic hallucinogens, they exert their psychoactive effects by acting as NMDA antagonists. Dissociatives include arylcyclohexylamines (phencyclidine (PCP) and ketamine), dextromethorphan (DXM), and nitrous oxide (discussed along with inhalants). These drugs produce a dissociative state with a greater degree of cognitive and neurological impairment than that produced by classic hallucinogens. At higher doses, symptoms become more severe and can result in delirium, coma, and seizures. Table 13.5 shows features of dissociative anesthetics.

PCP

Initially utilized as an anesthetic agent, it was soon discontinued due to prolonged delirium, psychosis, agitation, and dysphoria after surgery [64]. Manufactured illicitly, it is available in various forms and a wide range of doses. In its purest form,

Table 13.5 Pharmacologic features of typical dissociative [16, 32–34]

Dissociative	Typical dose	Onset (min) (post ingestion)	Peak effects (h) (post ingestion)	Duration (h) (post ingestion)
PCP	Oral: 2–6 mg IV/nasal/smoked: 1–3 mg	30–60 (swallowing) 2–5 (smoking)	1–4	4–8
Ketamine	Oral: 200–300 mg IN: 60–250 mg IM: 75–125 mg IV: 50–100 mg	15–20	0.5–1	1.5–2
DXM	Oral: 100–600 mg	15–30	2.5	4–6

phencyclidine (PCP) is a white crystalline powder that dissolves readily in water or alcohol; however, it is typically sprayed onto leafy material, such as cannabis, mint, oregano, tobacco, parsley, and ginger leaves and then smoked. It may also be insufflated and ingested orally. It is pharmacologically similar to ketamine, but it is more potent, longer acting, and more likely to produce seizures. A typical street dose is ~5 mg, with doses of 120 mg of PCP able to cause death.

PCP produces a range of intoxicated states that can be grouped into three stages [64, 65]: Stage I—conscious, with psychological effects and mild physiologic effects; Stage II—stuporous or in a light coma yet responsive to pain; and Stage III—comatose and unresponsive to pain. Intoxication at the mild Stage I is desired by users and is associated with few serious medical complications. Stage I would clinically present with euphoria, nystagmus (mostly horizontal but is one of a few drugs that can cause vertical), tachycardia, increased blood pressure, disorientation, agitation, ataxia, dysarthria, numbness, increased salivation, and hyperreflexia. Higher stages are associated with severe medical effects, including hypertensive crisis, hyperthermia, seizures, rhabdomyolysis, acute renal failure, stroke, cardiac failure, coma, and death [64].

Ketamine

Ketamine is widely used as a general anesthetic (in combination with other agents) in animals and humans, in addition to its newer utilization in the treatment of pain and treatment-resistant depression [66]. It is pharmacologically similar to PCP and similarly a noncompetitive NMDA receptor antagonist [67] but less potent as an anesthetic with a faster onset and shorter duration of action. Primarily diverted from veterinary clinics to the streets, ketamine is available as a liquid or a white powder and can be smoked, insufflated, injected, or taken orally.

The hallucinatory effects of ketamine last 1 h or less, but the user's senses, judgment, and coordination may be affected for up to 24 h. Euphoria and hallucinosis peak effects occur in roughly 2.5 h. Doses of ketamine as large as 900–1000 mg given intravenously or intramuscularly are lethal. Although ketamine is often self-administered by insufflation, some are injecting it, increasing the risk for hepatitis C, HIV, and other infectious diseases [68]. Ketamine-induced coma occurs in a dose-dependent manner.

The clinical effects of ketamine are similar to PCP. Of note, in the short term, ketamine causes problems with attention, learning, and memory. It also causes dreamlike states, hallucinations, sedation, confusion, speech problems, loss of memory, and movement problems progressing to immobility [69]. Elevated blood pressure, unconsciousness, and slowed breathing can occur. Large doses of ketamine may produce what users refer to as a "K-hole," which is a state reached when the user is on the brink of being fully sedated, often likened to an out-of-body or near-death experience. Although rare, overdose can cause death [70]. Ketamine can also cause kidney problems, stomach pain, and depression. Long-term ketamine use can cause damage to the bladder and urinary tract, which can result in a condition known as ketamine bladder syndrome [71]. The syndrome may cause ulcers in the bladder, blood in the urine, and incontinence.

DXM

Dextromethorphan (D-3-methoxy-N-methylmorphinan, DM, DXM) is the D-isomer of a codeine analog, methorphan. In contrast to the L-isomer, which is an opioid analgesic, DXM is not. In addition to NMDA antagonism, DXM has activity at the sigma receptor, which likely contributes to its therapeutic effects as a cough suppressant. DXM is available as an ingredient in more than 100 different over-the-counter cough and cold medicines. Terms such as "robotripping," "tussin," and "skittling" refer to illicit use. Antitussive dose ranges 15–30 mg, and recreational use can range 240–1500 mg; clinically significant psychological and behavioral effects of DXM begin to occur at approximately five times the therapeutic dose. Its psychoactive effect overlaps with the effects of classic hallucinogens, including perceptual distortions, changes in the sense of time and space, alterations in body awareness, and spiritual experiences [72]. Psychoactive effects may be noted within 1 h of ingestion; these are dose-related and are described by users as occurring in "plateaus" [73, 74]. At lower levels, i.e., 100–200 mg (1.5–2.5 mg/kg), users may experience euphoria and restlessness; 200–500 mg doses (2.5–7.5 mg/kg) result in exaggerated auditory and visual sensations and closed-eye hallucinations and imbalance; doses of 500–1000 mg (7.5–15 mg/kg) may result in altered consciousness, hallucinations, partial dissociation symptoms, and agitation; doses greater than 1000 mg (>15 mg/kg) can result in intense hallucinations, delusions, complete dissociation, and ataxia. Overdose can also cause respiratory depression, hyperthermia, and metabolic acidosis [73]. Additional ingredients in cough medicine (e.g., decongestants, antihistamines, acetaminophen, bromides) can cause other problems in overdose amounts.

Assessment and Management

In the DSM-5-TR [14], diagnosis related to phencyclidine use can fall under *Phencyclidine Intoxication*, *Phencyclidine Use Disorder*, or *Other Phencyclidine-Induced Disorders* (includes diagnostic criteria for PCP-induced psychosis, mania, depression, anxiety, and intoxication delirium under specific subcategories). The severity of the use disorder is classified based on the number of criteria met. Ketamine and dextromethorphan use can be diagnosed using the criteria of *Other Hallucinogen Use Disorder*.

Management of PCP intoxication should consider the level/stage of intoxication and aim at minimizing medical emergencies (seizures, hypertension, hyperthermia, and rhabdomyolysis) and behavioral consequences.

Initial assessment should follow the stabilization of breathing, circulation, and temperature. PCP is detectable in urine for up to 8 days after use; other hallucinogens are not included in routine tests. Mild Stage I intoxication is best treated without medication. Sensory input should be minimal; unlike classic hallucinogens, reassuring and reality-oriented communication (talking down) rarely works with agitated PCP intoxication. Violent behavior can be prevented with physical restraints but can also increase agitation and the probability of rhabdomyolysis. Benzodiazepines are primarily used to treat agitation and seizures [64]. If agitation does not respond adequately to benzodiazepines, antipsychotics may be used. Antipsychotics should be used in moderation since they can lower the seizure threshold, cause dystonia, and exacerbate hyperthermia and anticholinergic symptoms. Tachycardia and hypertension may be treated with beta-blockers, such as labetalol, or calcium channel blockers, such as verapamil, and in cases of severe hypertension can be treated with IV nitroprusside. Standard cooling measures may be applied to address hyperthermia. Rhabdomyolysis can be treated with IV fluids and diuretics.

Clinical support of distress associated with ketamine and DXM is similar to the methods used with classic hallucinogens. For DXM, which is often consumed orally, activated charcoal is effective for gastrointestinal decontamination [73]. Naloxone (an opioid antagonist) has been recommended for the treatment of respiratory depression in the context of DXM overdose [75]. DXM toxicity may result from the other ingredients found in cough or cold preparations (e.g., acetaminophen, pseudoephedrine, phenylephrine, guaifenesin, and antihistamines). The evaluation and treatment of patients with suspected DXM overdose must attend to the possibility of acetaminophen or other concomitant toxicity.

Future Considerations

Some dissociative anesthetics are being investigated for their potential therapeutic applications in the treatment of SUDs. Ketamine, administered in conjunction with motivational enhancement, has demonstrated preliminary efficacy in increasing rates of AUD abstinence [76–78].

While these findings are promising, translating ketamine and dextromethorphan into effective, evidence-based treatments for SUDs will require large-scale randomized controlled trials. As with classic hallucinogens, the increasing medical use and destigmatization of these compounds could paradoxically contribute to greater rates of nonmedical use and ketamine or dextromethorphan use disorders, particularly in vulnerable populations [79]. This underscores the importance of integrating careful supervised use alongside their continued therapeutic development.

Club Drugs

The term "club drugs" is inclusive of a range of compounds, including various hallucinogens, stimulants, sedatives, and other drugs that have been associated with use at bars, nightclubs, concerts, and parties. The term is slightly misleading since drugs predominantly utilized in clubs, such as tobacco and alcohol, are not included in this category. NIDA identifies the following substances as club drugs: GHB, Rohypnol (flunitrazepam), ketamine, MDMA, methamphetamine, and LSD. Rohypnol and methamphetamines are covered under benzodiazepines and stimulants, respectively.

MDMA

The substance 3,4-methylenedioxy-methamphetamine (MDMA), commonly known as ecstasy, is a synthetic drug that is structurally similar to amphetamine. Categorized as an entactogen or empathogen due to its ability to evoke a sense of emotional openness and connection [80], it also elicits a unique mix of mood enhancement and stimulant-like and hallucinogenic effects.

MDMA exerts its psychoactive effect by promoting the release of serotonin, norepinephrine, and dopamine, preventing the reuptake of serotonin, and inhibiting serotonin synthesis; its mechanism of action contributes to an acute depletion of central serotonin. A typical dose of MDMA (75–150 mg) may take 30–60 min for onset and may last up to 4–6 h. Users report experiencing euphoria, increased sense of closeness toward others and empathy, energy, and reduced appetite; at higher doses, users may experience psychedelic hallucinogenic effects. Individuals who use MDMA often experience a "hangover" the day after use, characterized by insomnia, fatigue, drowsiness, sore jaw muscles from teeth clenching, loss of balance, and headaches. Users may experience minor adverse reactions from use, such as bruxism (grinding teeth), diaphoresis, nausea, blurry vision, tachycardia, and hypertension. Hyperthermia can occur as a result of MDMA's effects on the CNS, prolonged physical exertion, and environmental conditions. Hyponatremia may also occur and is often related to both dehydration and individuals drinking an excess amount of water [81].

Assessment and Management

Diagnosis is made using the DSM-5-TR [14] criteria under the heading of *Other Hallucinogen Use Disorder*. As with other substances, the severity of the use disorder is classified based on the number of criteria met.

MDMA intoxication typically comes to attention in cases of overdose, with the majority of the cases presenting with serotonin syndrome. Such patients should be evaluated emergently, and an ICU admission may be required. Cardiac monitoring and frequent monitoring of vital signs and mental status aid in its management. Activated charcoal should be administered if recent ingestion is suspected. Cooling measures are indicated in cases of hyperthermia. Dantrolene is sometimes used to treat hyperthermia due to MDMA ingestion, but its efficacy is not proven. Seizures, hypertension, and agitation are treated with benzodiazepines. In cases of rhabdomyolysis, intravenous fluids, alkalization of the urine, and furosemide are recommended [81].

GHB

Gamma-hydroxybutyric acid (GHB, sodium oxybate) is a short-chain fatty acid that occurs naturally in the brain. First synthesized in the 1960s, it was used as an anesthetic. In the US, it is FDA-approved as a Schedule-III controlled substance for the treatment of cataplexy and excessive daytime sleepiness in persons with narcolepsy. In some European countries, it is used for the management of alcohol withdrawal and off-label to attenuate symptoms of opiate withdrawal. GHB has a wide range of formulations, use patterns, and associated health risks. It is used recreationally as a "club drug," as an aid to enhance muscle growth by bodybuilders, and by individuals for insomnia. The misuse potential of GHB is most likely the result of its anxiolytic, hypnotic, and euphoric effects. Recreationally, it is frequently used in combination with stimulants and/or alcohol.

Sources include supplements and industrial chemicals containing GHB analogs (GBL, BD), homemade GHB (recipes available on the Internet), and pharmaceutical formulations that can be prescribed and diverted from their intended use.

It is structurally similar to GABA and binds to endogenous GHB and GABA-B receptors. It modulates dopamine, opioid, serotonin, noradrenaline, and growth hormone release. Gamma-butyrolactone (GBL) and 1,4 butanediol (BD) are GHB precursors that, upon ingestion, are metabolized to GHB and have the same effect.

The effects of GHB intoxication are comparable to alcohol and MDMA. Users report feeling euphoric, relaxed, and disinhibited; elevated libido, energy, and stamina; and increased empathy and sensuality. Severe manifestations of GHB intoxication include CNS depression, hypoventilation, bradycardia, myoclonus, and seizures [82]. Users may also present with agitation and delayed delirium, as well as complications such as metabolic acidosis and Wernicke's encephalopathy.

Patterns of use vary significantly, from daily use among bodybuilders or nightly use among persons self-treating insomnia to binge use (every 30–60 min over consecutive days) among recreational users. Tolerance develops quickly. The withdrawal phenomenon is associated with frequent dosing and a daily dose greater than 10 g [83].

Assessment and Management

Diagnosis is made using the DSM-5-TR [14] criteria under the heading of *Sedative, Hypnotic, or Anxiolytic Use Disorder*. As with other substances, the severity of the use disorder is classified based on the number of criteria met.

The presentation of GHB withdrawal is like that of alcohol and benzodiazepines in that dependent individuals may present with tremors, tachycardia, hypertension, diaphoresis, anxiety, agitation, and confusion. However, there is often a more rapid and abrupt onset and more prominent delirium and psychosis (with paranoia, auditory hallucinations, and visual hallucinations); insomnia can be a notable feature.

Treatment of GHB toxicity and withdrawal consists of supportive care, including airway protection, cardiac and pulse oxygen monitoring, sedation for agitation, and treatment of complications. The first-line treatment for managing withdrawal symptoms is high-dose benzodiazepines (up to 120 mg of diazepam daily). Barbiturates and propofol may be utilized in cases of benzodiazepine-resistant individuals [83]. Individuals using more than 30 g of GHB (or >15 g of GBL) per day may benefit from inpatient management of their withdrawal. Severely depressed respirations indicate a need for intensive care treatment and mechanical ventilation. Once stabilized, oral benzodiazepines are commonly tapered off over 7–10 days.

Chapter Review Questions

1. A 30-year-old recreational weightlifter presents to his primary care physician with new onset acne and mood irritability. Physical exam reveals pronounced muscle hypertrophy. He reports recently starting "performance supplements." What is the most common reason individuals in the United States use anabolic-androgenic steroids (AAS)?

   A. Preparation for competitive bodybuilding
   B. Enhance physical appearance and strength
   C. Improve athletic performance
   D. Increase cardiovascular stamina
   E. Reduce body fat

   Correct Answer: B.

   Explanation: Over the past few decades, the trends in anabolic-androgenic steroid (AAS) use have changed. The majority of users are not athletes or bodybuilders; rather, they are individuals who desire to increase and improve their physical strength and appearance.

   Reference: Kanayama et al. [83].

2. A 22-year-old college student presents for his annual physical examination. He reports using anabolic-androgenic steroids for the past several months. Vital signs are within normal limits. Which of the following physical exam findings is most associated with anabolic-androgenic steroid use?

A. Gynecomastia
B. Androgenic Alopecia
C. Hepatomegaly
D. Testicular atrophy
E. Hypertension

Correct Answer: D.

Explanation: Exogenous AAS in high doses results in testicular shutdown of testosterone production and consequent atrophy. The other options listed are possible outcomes of AAS use as well; however, testicular atrophy is directly related to its use and is the most common outcome.

Reference: Rahnema et al. [84].

3. A 14-year-old boy is brought to the clinic by his parents for evaluation of a rash. They report that over the past few months, he has had decreased appetite, worsening school performance, and complaints from teachers about reduced attention and incomplete assignments. On examination, there are perioral papules. Which of the following substances is the most likely cause of his presentation?

A. Kratom
B. Ketamine
C. Volatile hydrocarbons
D. Alcohol
E. LSD

Correct Answer: C.

Explanation: Use of volatile hydrocarbons should be considered in persons showing intermittent changes compatible with inhalant use, together with an odor of organic solvents, inhalation paraphernalia, or the occasional presence of perioral or perinasal papular "glue-sniffers" rash. Other options listed can contribute to some aspects of this patient's presentation but do not cause a perioral papular rash.

Reference: Sadock et al. [85, p. 1335].

4. A 30-year-old woman reports using various hallucinogens several times per month for the past 10 years. She states that her experiences often enhance her sense of connection with nature. Friends have expressed concern about what they describe as unusual beliefs she has developed. Which of the following is the most likely long-term effect associated with chronic classic hallucinogen use?

A. Anxiety
B. Psychosis
C. Flashbacks
D. Depression
E. Mania

Correct Answer: C.

Explanation: The most commonly associated long-term risk of classic hallucinogen use is hallucinogen persisting perception disorder, frequently referred to as "flashbacks." A flashback typically involves unexpectedly reexperiencing the perceptual, emotional, or somatic effects of a previous hallucinogen experience.

Reference: Halpern and Pope [38].

5. A 40-year-old male patient with a history of frequent hallucinogen use reports that he now requires much larger doses than before to achieve the same effects, and sometimes notices little effect at all. Marked tolerance can develop with repeated use of most classical hallucinogens. Which of the following is an exception to this pattern?

   A. MDMA
   B. Psilocybin
   C. LSD
   D. DMT
   E. Mescaline

   Correct Answer: C.

   Explanation: Tolerance to LSD develops very rapidly, with significant decreases in the effect of subsequent doses after a single dose. Cross-tolerance exists among LSD, mescaline, and psilocybin, further evidence of their shared mechanism of action. This effect may be due to downregulation or internalization of 5HT2A receptors and is completely reversed within a week of abstinence. DMT may be an exception to this effect as marked tolerance is not observed. MDMA is not a classical hallucinogen.

   Reference: Sadock et al. [85, p. 1316].

6. A 19-year-old college student presents with recurrent, unpredictable episodes of visual distortions resembling his past LSD experiences, despite abstaining from drug use for the past year. Stress and anxiety have increased recently with upcoming exams. After ruling out other causes, he is diagnosed with hallucinogen persisting perception disorder (HPPD). Which of the following treatments is most likely to worsen his symptoms?

   A. Cognitive Behavioral Therapy
   B. Lorazepam
   C. Risperidone
   D. Haloperidol
   E. Clonidine

   Correct Answer: C.

   Explanation: Risperidone (and possibly the atypical antipsychotics in general) should be avoided as a treatment option in HPPD as there is evidence that risperidone worsens the HPPD symptoms. Other interventions mentioned have been shown to alleviate some of the symptoms of HPPD.

   Reference: Sadock et al. [85, pp. 1324–1325].

References

1. Kanayama G, Pope HG Jr. History and epidemiology of anabolic androgens in athletes and non-athletes. Mol Cell Endocrinol. 2018;464:4–13.
2. Pope HG Jr, Wood RI, Rogol A, Nyberg F, Bowers L, Bhasin S. Adverse health consequences of performance-enhancing drugs: an Endocrine Society scientific statement. Endocr Rev. 2013;35(3):341–75.
3. Monitoring the Future. National survey results of drug use. [Internet]. 2024 [cited 2024 October 30]. Available from: https://monitoringthefuture.org/wp-content/uploads/2024/01/mtfoverview2024.pdf.
4. Kanayama G, Boynes M, Hudson JI, Field AE, Pope HG. Anabolic steroid abuse among teenage girls: an illusory problem? Drug Alcohol Depend. 2007;88(2–3):156–62.
5. Cafri G, Olivardia R, Thompson JK. Symptom characteristics and psychiatric comorbidity among males with muscle dysmorphia. Compr Psychiatry. 2008;49(4):374–9.
6. Olivardia R, Pope J, Hudson JI. Muscle dysmorphia in male weightlifters: a case-control study. Am J Psychiatry. 2000;157(8):1291–6.
7. Herschman Z. Cardiac effects of anabolic steroids. Anesthesiology. 1990;72(4):772–3.
8. Coviello AD, Kaplan B, Lakshman KM, Chen T, Singh AB, Bhasin S. Effects of graded doses of testosterone on erythropoiesis in healthy young and older men. J Clin Endocrinol Metab. 2008;93(3):914–9.
9. Coward RM, Rajanahally S, Kovac JR, Smith RP, Pastuszak AW, Lipshultz LI. Anabolic steroid induced hypogonadism in young men. J Urol. 2013;190(6):2200–5.
10. Henderson LP, Penatti CA, Jones BL, Yang P, Clark AS. Anabolic androgenic steroids and forebrain GABAergic transmission. Neuroscience. 2006;138(3):793–9.
11. Pope HG, Katz DL. Psychiatric and medical effects of anabolic-androgenic steroid use: a controlled study of 160 athletes. Arch Gen Psychiatry. 1994;51(5):375–82.
12. Kanayama G, DeLuca J, Meehan WP III, Hudson JI, Isaacs S, Baggish A, Weiner R, Micheli L, Pope HG Jr. Ruptured tendons in anabolic-androgenic steroid users: a cross-sectional cohort study. Am J Sports Med. 2015;43(11):2638–44.
13. Zomorodian K, Rahimi MJ, Taheri M, Asad AG, Khani S, Ahrari I, Pakshir K, Khashei R. The cutaneous bacterial microflora of the bodybuilders using anabolic-androgenic steroids. Jundishapur J Microbiol. 2015;8(1):e12269.
14. American Psychiatric Association. Diagnostic and statistical manual of mental disorders. 5th ed., text rev. (DSM-5-TR®). American Psychiatric Pub; 2022.
15. Brouette T, Anton R. Clinical review of inhalants. Am J Addict. 2001;10(1):79–94.
16. The Vaults of Erowid. Available from: https://www.erowid.org/psychoactives/.
17. 2023 National Survey on Drug Use and Health (NSDUH). Published July 30, 2024. Accessed 30 Oct 2024. https://www.samhsa.gov/data/report/2023-nsduh-annual-national-report.
18. Dutta A, Uno H, Holman A, Lorenz DR, Wolinsky SM, Gabuzda D. Long-term nitrite inhalant exposure and cancer risk in MSM. AIDS. 2017;31(8):1169–80.
19. Tormoehlen LM, Tekulve KJ, Nañagas KA. Hydrocarbon toxicity: a review. Clin Toxicol. 2014;52(5):479–89.
20. Balster RL. Neural basis of inhalant abuse. Drug Alcohol Depend. 1998;51(1–2):207–14.
21. Alper AT, Akyol A, Hasdemir H, Nurkalem Z, Güler Ö, Güvenç TS, Erdinler I, Cakmak N, Eksik A, Gürkan K. Glue (toluene) abuse: increased QT dispersion and relation with unexplained syncope. Inhal Toxicol. 2008;20(1):37–41.
22. Bass M. Sudden sniffing death. JAMA. 1970;212(12):2075–9.
23. Haverkos HW, Dougherty J. Health hazards of nitrite inhalants. Am J Med. 1988;84(3):479–82.
24. Coleman MD, Coleman NA. Drug-induced methaemoglobinaemia. Drug Saf. 1996;14(6):394–405.
25. Becker DE, Rosenberg M. Nitrous oxide and the inhalation anesthetics. Anesth Prog. 2008;55(4):124–31.

26. Garbaz L, Mispelaere D, Boutemy M, Jounieaux V. Pneumothorax following recreational inhalation of nitrous oxide. Rev Mal Respir. 2007;24(5):622–4.
27. Sanders RD, Weimann J, Maze M. Biologic effects of nitrous oxidea mechanistic and toxicologic review. Anesthesiology. 2008;109(4):707–22.
28. Romanelli F, Smith KM, Thornton AC, Pomeroy C. Poppers: epidemiology and clinical management of inhaled nitrite abuse. Pharmacotherapy. 2004;24(1):69–78.
29. Tenenbein M. Leaded gasoline abuse: the role of tetraethyl lead. Hum Exp Toxicol. 1997;16(4):217–22.
30. Schultes RE, Hofmann A, Rätsch C. Plants of the gods: their sacred, healing, and hallucinogenic powers. Rochester, VT: Healing Arts Press; 2001.
31. Hofmann A. LSD: my problem child. New York: Oxford University Press; 2013.
32. Nichols DE. Hallucinogens. Pharmacol Ther. 2004;101(2):131–81.
33. Drug Enforcement Administration, US Department of Justice. Drugs and chemicals of concern. [Internet]. Available from: http://www.deadiversion.usdoj.gov/drug_chem_info/index.html.
34. Baselt RC. Disposition of toxic drugs in man. Foster City: Chemical Toxicology Institute; 2000.
35. Passie T, Halpern JH, Stichtenoth DO, Emrich HM, Hintzen A. The pharmacology of lysergic acid diethylamide: a review. CNS Neurosci Ther. 2008;14(4):295–314.
36. Liechti ME, Dolder PC, Schmid Y. Alterations of consciousness and mystical-type experiences after acute LSD in humans. Psychopharmacology. 2017;234(9–10):1499–510.
37. Strassman RJ. Adverse reactions to psychedelic drugs. A review of the literature. J Nerv Ment Dis. 1984;172(10):577–95.
38. Halpern JH, Pope HG Jr. Hallucinogen persisting perception disorder: what do we know after 50 years? Drug Alcohol Depend. 2003;69(2):109–19.
39. Passie T, Seifert J, Schneider U, Emrich HM. The pharmacology of psilocybin. Addict Biol. 2002;7(4):357–64.
40. Carbonaro TM, Gatch MB. Neuropharmacology of N, N-dimethyltryptamine. Brain Res Bull. 2016;126:74–88.
41. Hamill J, Hallak J, Dursun SM, Baker G. Ayahuasca: psychological and physiologic effects, pharmacology and potential uses in addiction and mental illness. Curr Neuropharmacol. 2019;17(2):108–28.
42. Cassels BK, Saez-Briones P. Dark classics in chemical neuroscience: mescaline. ACS Chem Neurosci. 2018;9(10):2448–58.
43. Klüver H. Mescal, and mechanisms of hallucinations. Chicago: University of Chicago Press; 1928.
44. Gil-Martins E, Barbosa D, Borges F, Remião F, Silva R. Toxicodynamic insights of 2C and NBOMe drugs – is there abuse potential? Toxicol Rep. 2025;14:101890.
45. Papaseit E, Farré M, Pérez-Mañá C, Torrens M, Ventura M, Pujadas M, de la Torre R, González D. Acute pharmacological effects of 2C-B in humans: an observational study. Front Pharmacol. 2018;9:206.
46. Roth BL, Baner K, Westkaemper R, Siebert D, Rice KC, Steinberg S, Ernsberger P, Rothman RB. Salvinorin a: a potent naturally occurring nonnitrogenous κ opioid selective agonist. Proc Natl Acad Sci. 2002;99(18):11934–9.
47. El-Khoury J, Sahakian N. The association of Salvia divinorum and psychotic disorders: a review of the literature and case series. J Psychoactive Drugs. 2015;47(4):286–92.
48. Zawilska JB, Kacela M, Adamowicz P. NBOMes – highly potent and toxic alternatives of LSD. Front Neurosci. 2020;14:78.
49. Suzuki J, Dekker MA, Valenti ES, Arbelo Cruz FA, Correa AM, Poklis JL, Poklis A. Toxicities associated with NBOMe ingestion—a novel class of potent hallucinogens: a review of the literature. Psychosomatics. 2015;56(2):129–39.
50. Canal CE, Morgan D. Head-twitch response in rodents induced by the hallucinogen 2,5-dim ethoxy-4-iodoamphetamine: a comprehensive history, a re-evaluation of mechanisms, and its utility as a model. Drug Test Anal. 2012;4(7–8):556–76.
51. Shulgin AT, Shulgin A. PiHKAL: a chemical love story. Berkeley: Transform Press; 1991.

52. Burish MJ, Thoren KL, Mangan AM, Bursua AJ, Owens SM, Gussow L. Hallucinogens causing seizures? A case report of the synthetic amphetamine 2,5-dimethoxy-4-chloroamphetamine. Neurol Clin Pract. 2015;5(1):84–7.
53. Hollister LE. Effects of hallucinogens in humans. In: Hallucinogens: neurochemical, behavioral, and clinical perspectives. New York: Raven; 1984. p. 19–33.
54. Taylor RL, Maurer JI, Tinklenberg JR. Management of bad trips in an evolving drug scene. JAMA. 1970;213(3):422–5.
55. Callaway JC, Grob CS. Ayahuasca preparations and serotonin reuptake inhibitors: a potential combination for severe adverse interactions. J Psychoactive Drugs. 1998;30(4):367–9.
56. Markel H, Lee A, Holmes RD, Domino EF. LSD flashback syndrome exacerbated by selective serotonin reuptake inhibitor antidepressants in adolescents. J Pediatr. 1994;125(5):817–9.
57. Martinotti G, Santacroce R, Pettorruso M, Montemitro C, Spano M, Lorusso M, di Giannantonio M, Lerner A. Hallucinogen persisting perception disorder: etiology, clinical features, and therapeutic perspectives. Brain Sci. 2018;8(3):47.
58. Bogenschutz MP, Forcehimes AA, Pommy JA, Wilcox CE, Barbosa P, Strassman RJ. Psilocybin-assisted treatment for alcohol dependence: a proof-of-concept study. J Psychopharmacol. 2015;29(3):289–99.
59. Johnson MW, Garcia-Romeu A, Griffiths RR. Long-term follow-up of psilocybin-facilitated smoking cessation. Am J Drug Alcohol Abuse. 2017;43(1):55–60.
60. Thomas G, Lucas P, Capler NR, Tupper KW, Martin G. Ayahuasca-assisted therapy for addiction: results from a preliminary observational study in Canada. Curr Drug Abuse Rev. 2013;6(1):30–42.
61. Noller GE, Frampton CM, Yazar-Klosinski B. Ibogaine treatment outcomes for opioid dependence from a twelve-month follow-up observational study. Am J Drug Alcohol Abuse. 2018;44(1):37–46.
62. Cherian KN, Keynan JN, Anker L, Faerman A, Brown RE, Shamma A, Keynan O, Coetzee JP, Batail JM, Phillips A, Bassano NJ. Magnesium–ibogaine therapy in veterans with traumatic brain injuries. Nat Med. 2024;30(2):373–81. Keyes KM, Patrick ME. Hallucinogen use among young adults ages 19–30 in the United States: changes from 2018 to 2021. Addiction. 2023;118(12):2449–54.
63. Bey T, Patel A. Phencyclidine intoxication and adverse effects: a clinical and pharmacological review of an illicit drug. Cal J Emerg Med. 2007;8(1):9.
64. Gorelick DA. Phencyclidine (PCP). In: Psychopharmacology, the fourth generation of progress. New York: Raven Press; 1995. p. 1767–76.
65. Gao M, Rejaei D, Liu H. Ketamine use in current clinical practice. Acta Pharmacol Sin. 2016;37(7):865.
66. Mion G, Villevieille T. Ketamine pharmacology: an update (pharmacodynamics and molecular aspects, recent findings). CNS Neurosci Ther. 2013;19(6):370–80.
67. Mathias R. Study suggests ketamine injection poses new disease risks for street youths. NIDA Notes. 2003;18(4):1–3.
68. Liu Y, Lin D, Wu B, Zhou W. Ketamine abuse potential and use disorder. Brain Res Bull. 2016;126:68–73.
69. Schifano F, Corkery J, Oyefeso A, Tonia T, Ghodse AH. Trapped in the "K-hole": overview of deaths associated with ketamine misuse in the UK (1993–2006). J Clin Psychopharmacol. 2008;28(1):114–6.
70. Srirangam S, Mercer J. Ketamine bladder syndrome: an important differential diagnosis when assessing a patient with persistent lower urinary tract symptoms. BMJ Case Rep. 2012;2012:bcr2012006447.
71. Reissig CJ, Carter LP, Johnson MW, Mintzer MZ, Klinedinst MA, Griffiths RR. High doses of dextromethorphan, an NMDA antagonist, produce effects similar to classic hallucinogens. Psychopharmacology. 2012;223(1):1–5.
72. Boyer EW. Dextromethorphan abuse. Pediatr Emerg Care. 2004;20(12):858–63.
73. Antoniou T, Juurlink DN. Dextromethorphan abuse. CMAJ. 2014;186(16):E631.

74. Chyka PA, Erdman AR, Manoguerra AS, Christianson G, Booze LL, Nelson LS, Woolf AD, Cobaugh DJ, Caravati EM, Scharman EJ, Troutman WG. Dextromethorphan poisoning: an evidence-based consensus guideline for out-of-hospital management. Clin Toxicol. 2007;45(6):662–77.
75. Dakwar E, et al. A single ketamine infusion combined with motivational enhancement therapy improved drinking outcomes in individuals with alcohol dependence. Am J Psychiatry. 2020;177(2):125–33.
76. Huang E-Y-K, Hung H-Y, Chen Y-H, Kao J-H, Tsai A-L, Chow L-H. Effects of dextromethorphan on nicotine-induced reward, behavioral sensitization, withdrawal signs, and drug-seeking–related behavior in rats. Nicotine Tob Res. 2023;25(7):1251–60.
77. Axsome Therapeutics Inc. A Phase II, randomized, double-blind study to evaluate the effects of dextromethorphan–bupropion (AXS-05) on smoking behavior (NCT03471767). ClinicalTrials.gov. Completed.
78. Marongiu S, van Eijk M, Gresnigt FMJ, Croes EA, Franssen EJF. Rising incidence of recreational ketamine use: clinical cases and management in emergency settings. Toxicol Rep. 2025;14:101940.
79. Nichols DE. Differences between the mechanism of action of MDMA, MBDB, and the classic hallucinogens. Identification of a new therapeutic class: entactogens. J Psychoactive Drugs. 1986;18(4):305–13.
80. Hall AP, Henry JA. Acute toxic effects of 'Ecstasy' (MDMA) and related compounds: overview of pathophysiology and clinical management. Br J Anaesth. 2006;96(6):678–85.
81. Busardò FP, Jones AW. GHB pharmacology and toxicology: acute intoxication, concentrations in blood and urine in forensic cases and treatment of the withdrawal syndrome. Curr Neuropharmacol. 2015;13(1):47–70.
82. Kamal RM, van Noorden MS, Wannet W, Beurmanjer H, Dijkstra BAG, Schellekens A. Pharmacological treatment in γ-hydroxybutyrate (GHB) and γ-butyrolactone (GBL) dependence: detoxification and relapse prevention. CNS Drugs. 2017;31(1):51–64.
83. Kanayama G, Hudson JI, Pope HG Jr. Illicit anabolic–androgenic steroid use. Horm Behav. 2010;58(1):111–21.
84. Rahnema CD, Lipshultz LI, Crosnoe LE, Kovac JR, Kim ED. Anabolic steroid-induced hypogonadism: diagnosis and treatment. Fertil Steril. 2014;101(5):1271–9.
85. Sadock BJ, Sadock VA, Ruiz P. Kaplan & Sadock's comprehensive textbook of psychiatry. 10th ed., 50th Anniversary ed. Philadelphia: Wolters Kluwer; 2017.

Behavioral Addictions

14

Hector A. Colon-Rivera and Kavita K. Fischer

High-Yield Review Points

- Behavioral addictions resemble substance use disorders in many domains, including natural history, phenomenology, genetic factors, and response to treatment.
- Family history and genetic information support heritability for behavioral addictions.
- External factors for ongoing participation such as aggressive marketing and incentivization need to be considered in gambling disorder.
- Behavioral addictions are characterized by changes in multiple brain areas and neurotransmitter systems.

H. A. Colon-Rivera (✉)
Asociación Puertorriqueños en Marcha, Inc (APM), Philadelphia, PA, USA

UPMC Jameson Partial Hospitalization Program | Intensive Outpatient Program, New Castle, PA, USA

Intrinsic Me TM Psychiatry, Bluebell, PA, USA
e-mail: colonriveraha@upmc.edu; Hector.colon-rivera@apmphila.org

K. K. Fischer
Community Care Behavioral Health, Pittsburgh, PA, USA

University of Pittsburgh School of Medicine, Pittsburgh, PA, USA
e-mail: Fischerk6@upmc.edu

C. Marienfeld, M. Soltani (eds.), *AAAP Review of Addiction Psychiatry*,
https://doi.org/10.1007/978-3-032-24174-0_14

Introduction

Defining components of behavioral addictions include a recurrent pattern of behavior despite adverse consequences, reduced self-control, excessive engagement, and an appetitive urge or craving state prior to engaging in the behavior. All behavioral addictions have a dysphoric state, analogous to withdrawal, and these usually involve irritability, restlessness, anxiety, and cravings. However, unlike in certain substance withdrawals, there are no life-threatening physical withdrawal symptoms from behavioral addictions.

The dysfunction in financial, educational, occupational, and marital relations is common in behavioral addictions. The repetitive maladaptive engagement in these behaviors results in clinically significant impairment and/or distress in a person's level of function, like substance use disorders [1].

Gambling Disorder (GD)

Gambling involves risking something of value in the hopes of obtaining something of greater value in the event of an uncertain outcome. Gambling has faced heavier commercialization internationally since the reinterpretation of previous rulings banning this activity. Gambling activities include those in brick-and-mortar casinos, public lotteries, and video terminals and now have quickly expanded to online and offline sports betting and online casinos. Other forms to consider that may have blurred lines to gambling but can become problematic include investment platforms that allow for day trading, "social casino" applications, and video games that involve opening "loot bags" or "packs." Loot boxes are digital containers [2, 3] that players can buy to potentially reveal a game feature that enhances a character's looks or gives a player a competitive advantage but is not guaranteed. Some of these activities are of particular concern among adolescents and have shown to act as grooming behaviors to develop problematic gambling behaviors over time [4].

Growing evidence of shared neurobiological and genetic substrates with substance-related disorders has led to revisions in diagnostic classification. Starting with DSM-5, the previous diagnosis of "pathological gambling" was replaced with "gambling disorder." Additionally, Gambling Disorder (GD) was moved from the "impulse control disorders not classified elsewhere" category to "substance-related and addictive disorders." DSM-5-TR reports GD as featuring repetitive, maladaptive gambling behavior, leading to severe adverse impact on the individual, familial, and social levels [5]. Of note, ICD-11 has further categorized GD into predominantly online and predominantly offline [5].

The lifetime prevalence of GD is thought to be increasing amid the rapid expansion of online gambling and legalized sports betting following reinterpretation of prior rulings that had restricted such activity in many states [2, 3]. Previous estimates for adults vary in the range 1–2%, around the same rates as bipolar disorder and schizophrenia, with higher rates among high-risk populations such as adolescents (up to 12%) [6]. More recently, rates of problem gambling (subthreshold GD) have been shown to be much higher with a 2024 global metanalysis showing considerable variance in adults depending on the gambling product: the pooled estimated prevalence of problematic gambling among those using online casinos (15.8%), casino gambling (10.0%), online gambling (8.6%), and sports betting (8.9%) was considerably higher than for other forms [7].

GD may have the highest rate of suicide among addictive behaviors, and although comorbidities may contribute to this high rate, a 2022 review demonstrated that the two main processes that connect gambling and suicidal behavior include indebtedness and shame [8]. Roughly one in two individuals with GD have been reported to contemplate suicide, with one in five completing suicide [9]. In clinical populations and those involved in treatment services, estimates ranging 22–81% of individuals have been found to have suicidal ideations, while those ranging 7–30% of individuals have had suicide attempts [8]. Historically, however, only 10% of gamblers have been shown to present for treatment which may lead to an underestimation of these rates [10]. Barriers to treatment include poverty, lack of social support, childcare, and access to appropriate treatment.

Populations that may be more vulnerable to gambling disorder include adolescents, college students, older adults, homeless individuals, indigenous people, active military members and veterans, members of certain ethnic and racial groups including black and Hispanic individuals, and prisoners, each with their own unique risk factors. Risk factors for developing GD include genetic predisposition, male gender (although gender differences may be narrowing since the explosion of online gambling), co-occurring disorders, and environmental factors such as widespread commercialization and increased access [11–13].

Women may be at greater risk for GD than previously recognized. Contributing factors include increased access to gambling, the expansion of online platforms, and higher rates of trauma exposure. Women are more likely to engage in chance-based games, which may function as a means of escape or emotional regulation, whereas men more often prefer sports betting and other competitive forms of gambling associated with excitement-seeking. In some women, GD also appears to follow a "telescoping" course, with lower initial intensity or frequency followed by more rapid escalation [14].

Screening

Screening is extremely important given the high risk of suicide with GD and due to historically low rates of those with GD seeking treatment [15, 16]. Open-ended questions may also be useful as part of a clinical interview (see example questions in the last row of Table 14.1).

Public Health/Advocacy: Improved screening and prevention measures, including a comprehensive public health approach, are needed to mitigate the harm faced by the public [8, 17, 18]. Several self-reported statistics by casinos and studies have shown that the top addicted gamblers account for up to 90% of the income from a casino [19]. A study done prior to widespread commercialization showed that a casino within 10 miles of one's home is associated with a 90% increase in the odds of having problem gambling or a GD [20]. Now with gambling platforms available at one's fingertips always via mobile devices and incentives such as VIP hosts, data tracking, bonuses, and prizes that encourage starting and continuing with gambling activities, prevalence is expected to steadily increase without new regulatory policies.

Table 14.1 Screening tools for gambling disorder

Lie-Bet Questionnaire	This two-question screening tool derives from DSM-IV criteria for pathological gambling. These two questions were selected for their substantial predictive value. The tool helps identify individuals who may benefit from a more comprehensive screening or further clinical assessment
Gamblers Anonymous 20 Question survey	This self-assessment tool helps individuals determine whether they have a problem with gambling. The survey consists of 20 yes/no questions that explore various aspects of gambling behavior, including financial issues, loss of control, dishonesty, and the impact on personal relationships. A standard guideline is that answering "yes" to seven or more questions suggests the individual may be experiencing a compulsive gambling problem and could benefit from support such as Gamblers Anonymous meetings or professional treatment
Brief Biosocial Gambling Screen (BBGS)	This three-item screening tool identifies individuals at risk of gambling disorder. It is based on the DSM-IV diagnostic criteria for pathological gambling
Problem Gambling Severity Index (PGSI)	This 9-item screening tool assesses the severity of gambling problems in the past year. Each item is scored on a 4-point scale, evaluating behaviors such as chasing losses, financial strain, and feelings of guilt. Based on the total score, individuals are categorized from non-problem to problem gamblers. The PGSI is widely used in both clinical and research settings to identify individuals at risk and guide intervention strategies
The Early Intervention Gambling Health Test (EIGHT)	This brief, 8-question screening tool identifies individuals who may be experiencing gambling-related harm. It focuses on emotional, behavioral, and financial indicators such as guilt, concealment, and chasing losses. A score of four or more "yes" responses suggests a potential gambling problem and indicates the need for further assessment. The EIGHT is designed for use in general healthcare and counseling settings to facilitate early detection and intervention
The Case-finding and Help Assessment Tool (CHAT)	This brief screening tool serves primary care settings to identify lifestyle and mental health issues, including gambling. It consists of a series of questions covering domains such as substance use, mental health, and behavioral concerns. CHAT helps clinicians quickly identify areas where patients may need support, facilitate early intervention and referral to appropriate services
Brief Problem Gambling Screen (BPGS)	While not fully validated, this tool is the only one to accurately identify all levels of problem gambling in individuals seeking mental health treatment
Open-ended questions/ commands	Open-ended questions or statements are prompts that encourage individuals to share detailed, thoughtful responses rather than simple yes/ no answers. Common in therapeutic and clinical settings, they help individuals explore their experiences, emotions, and motivations. Examples include the following: Please let me know if you participate in any gambling activities. Please tell me about your relationship with gambling? How have you gambled using any form of money or currency? What apps have you used on an electronic device that requires payment to continue using them? (This may also capture some blurred forms of gambling that children and adolescents may easily partake in.) How is gambling part of your lifestyle? How do you spend your entertainment budget? How would you describe your current financial health?

Treatment

Treatment for GD can be examined through a "biopsychosocial" lens and categorized as biological, psychotherapeutic, and psychosocial modalities.

Biological Treatment

Currently there are no FDA-approved medications for GD. Treating any co-occurring mental health/substance use disorder should be the initial focus. Opioid antagonists, monoaminergic drugs, and glutamatergic agents have been most frequently studied, and the literature is summarized in Table 14.2. While more research is needed, pharmacotherapy may be considered part of a comprehensive treatment approach after weighing risks, side effects, benefits, and alternatives for each individual.

One should keep in mind that medications with dopamine agonism, including partial agonism, such as those used to treat Parkinson's disease, restless leg syndrome, psychosis, and some mood disorders, may have a rare side effect that results in compulsive behaviors. The pathological over-activation of the dopaminergic reward and reinforcement system is one hypothesized mechanism for these drugs to increase gambling behavior [21].

Psychotherapeutic Treatments

Several forms of psychotherapy may be equally useful in treating GDs with positive predictors including length of time in treatment, commitment to doing the recovery work, and involvement of natural support in treatment [22, 23]. Good evidence exists for both motivational Interviewing (MI) and Cognitive Behavioral Therapy (CBT) with the combination (sometimes called brief motivational treatment) shown to have support. Psychodynamic and supportive therapy have also been used. Mindfulness strategies, contingency management, and cognitive-based remediation may also be incorporated. Rehabilitation in a drug and alcohol setting specializing in gambling within inpatient settings or intensive outpatient settings may also be helpful, but they are not highly prevalent in the United States [6]. One meta-analysis suggested that Internet-based treatments for problematic gambling may be helpful, especially if a patient prefers virtual treatment or if face-to-face treatment options are unavailable [24].

Psychosocial Treatments

Despite no available peer-reviewed studies on efficacy, Gamblers Anonymous is a 12-step program that reports to be helpful, especially those individuals who attend consistently [25]. Another resource shown to be helpful is Gambler, Friends, and Family in Recovery which arose during the COVID-19 pandemic to support those no longer able to attend face-to-face meetings. This is an international noticeboard to find online group meetings worldwide and support families and patients [26]. Self-exclusion is an option offered by some state gaming boards that involve individuals voluntarily banning themselves from different forms of gambling [27].

Table 14.2 Classes of medications studied for gambling disorder

Opioid antagonists:	Naltrexone: Commonly used for alcohol and opioid use disorders, naltrexone has shown promise in reducing gambling urges and behaviors by modulating the brain's reward pathways. Mixed but robust evidence suggests that naltrexone appears to be more effective than placebo, and some studies indicate that higher doses may be necessary. May be more effective in those with more severe urges. Consider more so if comorbid alcohol use disorder Nalmefene: Like naltrexone, nalmefene has been studied for its potential to decrease the reinforcing effects of gambling
Glutamate modulators: N-acetylcysteine (NAC)	NAC: Available as an over-the-counter supplement, NAC influences glutamate levels and has shown some efficacy in reducing gambling behaviors in preliminary studies. Studies show promise; low side-effect profile; more research needed
Selective Serotonin Reuptake Inhibitors (SSRIs)	Fluvoxamine, paroxetine, sertraline, citalopram, escitalopram: These antidepressants have been explored for their ability to alleviate gambling behaviors, particularly in individuals with co-occurring mood or anxiety disorders
Atypical Antipsychotics	Olanzapine: An antipsychotic, it has been examined for its potential to reduce gambling urges, though findings are mixed, and further research is needed. It does not demonstrate superiority over placebo in two studies. Haloperidol: Has been found to increase gambling urges in GD
Mood Stabilizers	Lithium: Primarily used for bipolar disorder, lithium has been investigated for its potential benefits in individuals with GD, especially those exhibiting mood instability. Valproate: An anticonvulsant and mood stabilizer, valproate has been studied for its effects on impulsivity and compulsive behaviors associated with gambling
Others	Topiramate: An anticonvulsant that has been studied for its potential to reduce gambling urges and improve impulse control. Bupropion: An antidepressant with dopaminergic and noradrenergic activity, bupropion has been explored for its effects on gambling behaviors, particularly in individuals with comorbid depression. Modafinil: A wakefulness-promoting agent, modafinil has been studied its potential to reduce gambling urges, though evidence is limited. Guanfacine: An alpha-2A adrenergic receptor agonist, guanfacine has been explored for its effects on impulsivity and decision-making in GD

Public Health/Advocacy

Some other treatment approaches include asking patients to track screen time and app usage and incorporating supports such as parents or a significant other to block apps or reduce time on apps through various built-in smart phone restrictions. Gambling blocking software can also be downloaded, such as "Betblocker" and

"Gamban" to prevent individuals from using online betting apps. Using a mobile device incompatible with apps may also be considered. A mobile device that does not include apps may also be considered. The National Council for Problem Gambling provides the helpline 1-800-Gambler. This is widely advertised, but caution must be used as funding is received from members and donors, many of which are part of the gambling or sports industry. Conflicts with self-regulation should be considered.

Technological Addictions

The Internet has become increasingly integrated in the activities of people's lives, but the degree to which we use the Internet or play video games determines if these behaviors are problematic or addictive. The defining characteristics include the dysregulation of arousal, impulsivity, and compulsivity. Multiple studies indicate that social isolation plays a critical role in the development of Internet addiction, a pattern than became particularly evident during the COVID-19 pandemic, when individuals experiencing loneliness were more likely to turn to online activities in an effort to mitigate social disconnection. Addiction specialists generally agree on seven major technological addictions that involve the Internet: Internet gaming disorder, Internet gambling disorder, online shopping disorder, cybersex, Internet surfing and infobesity (information overload), texting/email addiction, and social media addiction [28, 29]. In this section, we will focus on Internet gaming disorders.

Internet Gaming Disorder (IGD)/Gaming Disorder

Internet Gaming Disorder (IGD) was added as a tentative disorder as a condition for further study starting with DSM 5. The DSM 5-TR defines IGD as the persistent and recurrent use of the Internet to engage in games, often with other players, leading to clinically significant impairment or distress [5]. In 2019, the ICD-11 officially recognized Gaming Disorder as a persistent and compulsive pattern of game use lasting for longer than 12 months that includes impaired control and increasing priority of, and continued involvement in, gaming, despite the negative consequences. Digital and video gaming (which may be online or offline) were specified in the ICD-11 criteria [30].

Gaming Disorder appears to be most prevalent among adolescent and young adult males aged 12–20 years. The pooled global prevalence of IGD among adolescents and young adults was shown to be 9.9% in a 2022 metanalysis which also showed the following as risk factors of IGD in this group: stress, long average game time, family dysfunction, poor academic performance, being bullied, bullying, interpersonal problems, hyperactivity/inattention, anxiety, depression, emotional distress, and low self-esteem [31].

Specific Internet game genres have been shown to have varying levels of addiction risk and players may exhibit different clinical characteristics depending on genres which include role-playing games (RPGs), strategy (STR) games, action shooter (ACS) games, and brain and skill (BRS) games. For example, higher neuroticism and lower conscientiousness were recently shown to be related to STR, ACS, and RPG groups. RPG and STR players were also found to be more vulnerable to developing IGD compared to ACS and BRS players [32].

Effective treatments that have all been shown to decrease severity of gaming disorder include group therapy, Craving Behavioral Intervention (CBI), Acceptance and Cognitive Restructuring Intervention Program (ACRIP), and short-term Cognitive Behavioral Therapy (CBT). Multidimensional family therapy has also been shown to reduce problematic gaming in adolescents [33].

Compulsive Buying Disorder or Shopping Addiction

This disorder is a condition in which people are preoccupied with shopping and suffer from recurrent buying impulses (or episodes) and lose control over their buying behavior [34]. Individuals with this disorder may acquire objects in an effort to alleviate distress arising from unmet belonging needs and frequently report associated negative consequences, including social, occupational, familial, and financial impairment. The prevalence ranges 5.8–8.0%. Neurocognitive data suggest impairments in response inhibition, risk adjustment during decision-making, and spatial working memory [35]. Problems in these distinct cognitive domains support the similarities between compulsive buying and other behavioral and substance addictions. Pharmacological studies with selective serotonin re-uptake inhibitors (SSRIs) or topiramate did not indicate superiority over placebo [36]. The Yale-Brown Obsessive-Compulsive Scale-Shopping Version is a measure of compulsive buying disorder treatment response and can be used to help with the clinical diagnosis of compulsive buying disorder.

Sex Addiction and Hypersexual Behaviors

This behavioral disorder involves persistent preoccupation with sexual activities, failed attempts to exert control, and engagement in sexual behaviors despite clear negative consequences. These patterns must be present for at least 6–12 months, depending on diagnostic guidelines, and must cause significant distress or functional impairment in domains such as relationships, finances, work, and social life [37, 38]. The prevalence of sex addiction disorders is estimated to be 3–6% of the general population. The addictive sexual behaviors are more common in men, with onset usually in late adolescence [37, 39].

Cue reactivity, the degree of sexual arousal elicited by erotic stimuli, is the single most powerful predictor of pornography-driven sexual addiction, symptom severity, and functional impairment, surpassing metrics such as total hours spent.

Terms like sex addiction, sexual addiction, addictive sexual behavior, compulsive sexual behavior, hypersexual disorder, sexual compulsivity, and sexual impulsivity generally describe the *same core phenomenon*: persistent, often uncontrolled sexual thoughts or behaviors that result in adverse consequences and distress [38].

Other related terms include the following:

1. Paraphilias: In DSM-5-TR, paraphilic disorders are classified as atypical sexual interests that cause distress or harm to the individual or others. They are characterized by recurrent, intense fantasies, urges, or behaviors involving nonconsenting partners, non-human objects, or non-genital body parts that cause significant distress or impairment. The DSM-5-TR distinguishes between paraphilias (atypical sexual interests) and paraphilic disorders (those causing distress or harm) [5].
2. Nonparaphilic: These include sexual acts that do not meet criteria for a paraphilia or paraphilic disorder and include compulsive sexual acts with multiple partners, compulsive masturbation, frequent use of pornography, and compulsive sex acts within a consensual relationship [5].

Eating Addictions

The correlations between eating addictions and substance use disorder are linked to the reward-responsive phenotype of eating with, and without, obesity [40–42]. Eating addiction behaviors have a high negative urgency, high reward dependence, and lack of premeditation. Compared with controls, individuals with eating addiction demonstrate heightened dopaminergic signaling response, particularly within reward-related neural circuits [40, 41]. Food addiction commonly co-occurs with binge-eating disorder, which is characterized by recurrent episodes of consuming large amounts of food accompanied by a sense of loss of control. The combination of these conditions has been related to higher psychiatric comorbidities, weight concerns, and psychological distress.

Binge-eating disorder is an eating disorder characterized by heightened reward responsiveness, especially in the ventral striatum, during anticipatory phases resulting in overpowering urges to eat and consequent binge episodes. Neurohormonal circuits mediate these reward-driven behaviors. Leptin deficiency removes inhibitory control over hypothalamic–mesolimbic pathways, increasing susceptibility to pathological eating. Conversely, ghrelin activates the mesolimbic dopamine system, especially the VTA to nucleus accumbens pathway, to enhance reward-seeking and binge behaviors when administered directly into the VTA [42, 43].

The Yale Food Addiction Scale (YFAS) was the first validated instrument designed to measure addictive-like eating behaviors. Comprised of 25 items, it adapts the DSM-IV substance dependence criteria (tolerance, withdrawal, loss of control) to food consumption patterns, producing both a symptom count and a diagnostic threshold requiring ≥3 symptoms plus impairment or distress.

Lisdexamfetamine dimesylate is currently the only FDA-approved medication for treating moderate-to-severe binge-eating disorder (BED) in adults, demonstrating efficacy in decreasing frequency of binge episodes and boosting remission rates through dopaminergic and noradrenergic mechanisms [44]. Atomoxetine, another drug approved for ADHD, significantly outperformed placebo in reducing binge eating and achieving remission in a small, randomized trial; however, its use in BED remains off-label.

Neurobiology and Genetics

Behavioral addictions share genetic and environmental contributions in twin studies, and demonstrate similarities, as well as differences, at neurobiological levels. See Table 14.3.

Table 14.3 Behavioral addiction and key genetic and neurobiological points [40, 45–53]

Behavioral addiction	Key results
Gambling	Genetic heritability is substantial, with twin studies estimating 50–60% heritable influence and no significant sex differences in the genetic contribution: Earlier US twin research had similar findings, with heritability ranging 46–54% in men and 49% overall, with negligible influence from the shared family environment and equivalent genetic contributions across sexes. Dopamine D2 receptor gene (DRD2, Taq IA): Several initial studies linked the A1 allele to a higher risk for pathological gambling. Serotonin transporter (5-HTTLPR) and MAO-A polymorphisms: Among males with gambling addiction, specific variants in these genes are associated with increased impulsivity and riskier choices. Neurotrophin-related genes: Recent genetic association studies have identified polymorphisms in NTF3 and the BDNF receptor gene NTRK2 as linked to an increased risk of GD, underscoring the potential role of neurotrophic signaling in behavioral addictions. Individuals with GD show higher concordance with ADHD and attention-deficit traits, suggesting shared genetic vulnerability rooted in dopamine–prefrontal circuitry—supported by family and twin-study comorbidity data

(continued)

Table 14.3 (continued)

Behavioral addiction	Key results
Internet addictions	Linked to altered reward sensitivity and compulsive behaviors. The DRD2 Taq1A1 allele is associated with reduced receptor density and heightened vulnerability to addictive behaviors. SS variant associated with impulsivity and emotional dysregulation in male patients with Internet Addiction Disorder (IAD). Specific polymorphisms are associated with heightened impulsivity and aggression, which may elevate the risk of IAD. Reduced D2-like receptor availability in the dorsal striatum in individuals with IAD: No significant changes were observed in the ventral striatum. Suggests impairment in habit formation and executive control circuits. Lower dopamine transporter (DAT) density in the striatum. Indicates a hypodopaminergic state, like other behavioral and substance addictions. Over 72 single-nucleotide polymorphisms (SNPs) are linked to IAD. Many SNPs are in genes related to dopaminergic, serotonergic, and MAO pathways. Overlap found with genetic risks for ADHD and mood disorders [49–58]
Videogame playing (change to gaming disorder/Internet gaming disorder?)	TDRD2 A1 and low-activity COMT alleles are linked to vulnerability toward compulsive gaming behaviors. PET studies reveal metabolic imbalances, including hyperactive reward centers (orbitofrontal and caudate) and diminished activity in motor and prefrontal regions. These findings suggest IGD shares biomarker features with other addictions, characterized by reinforcement sensitivity and diminished cognitive control [59]
Shopping	Familial Patterns: Compulsive shoppers are more likely to have first-degree relatives with psychiatric conditions. Associated disorders in family members include mood disorders, anxiety, and substance use disorders. Suggests a heritable or familial vulnerability to compulsive shopping behavior. 5-HTTLPR Polymorphisms: Studies show no significant difference in the frequency of 5-HTT gene polymorphisms (short vs. long alleles) between compulsive buyers and controls. Indicates a limited role of serotonin transporter gene variation in the direct development of compulsive shopping. SSRI Treatment Response: SSRIs, such as fluvoxamine and escitalopram, have shown inconsistent outcomes in reducing compulsive shopping behaviors. Some patients report improvement, while placebo-controlled trials show no consistent benefit. The response to SSRIs is not clearly influenced by 5-HTT genotype.

(continued)

Table 14.3 (continued)

Behavioral addiction	Key results
Sex	First-degree relatives are more likely to have SUDs: Limited positive clinical results suggest a possible role for serotonergic activity. Family link: First-degree relatives of compulsive shoppers often have other psychiatric disorders. 5-HTT genetics: No significant allelic difference in 5-HTTLPR polymorphisms found. SSRI efficacy: Evidence for SSRI effectiveness in compulsive shopping/sex addiction remains inconsistent and inconclusive
Eating	Low central serotonin availability may promote intense cravings for high-sugar and high-fat foods by impairing satiety regulation. Polymorphisms in serotonin receptor subtypes—especially 5-HT_2C—have been associated with altered appetite and susceptibility to binge-eating behaviors. Functional variants in 5-HT_3A/B genes have been linked to eating disorder risk, influencing satiety and consumption behavior. Though widely studied, the evidence remains mixed regarding its association with binge-eating disorder (BED) [60–63]

Psychosocial Treatments of Gambling Disorder and Other Behavioral Addictions

The research continues psychodynamic therapy, motivational interviewing, and cognitive behavioral therapy effectiveness as treatments and their neurobiological underpinnings on behavioral addictions continue to develop. Many of these studies have small sample sizes and other limitations. Much of the current evidence-based treatments focused on cognitive behavioral therapy (CBT).

CBT is the most common psychological intervention for treating and reducing symptoms of behavioral addictions generally, and it is the most effective psychological intervention for treating and reducing problem-gambling behavior specifically [34]. Studies have shown how CBT interventions increased insula activation from gaming-related cues and decreased connectivity between the orbitofrontal cortex and hippocampus, as well as between the posterior cingulate and motor-related brain regions [32]. These findings suggest that CBT is associated with reduced connectivity strength during cue exposure within neural circuits implicated in cue-induced craving across addictive behaviors [64]. CBT is combined with motivational enhancement therapy (MET) to move patients from ambivalence to engagement concerning behavioral change (Table 14.4).

Group Psychotherapy

Group psychotherapy that uses a CBT model reduces the distress associated with compulsive and maladaptive behaviors. Impulse control training is a core component of behavioral addiction group therapy. Mutual help group models are available

Table 14.4 Psychosocial treatments of gambling disorder [33, 65–72]

Treatment	Description	Evidence Base
Cognitive Behavioral Therapy (CBT)	Identifies and restructures gambling-related cognitive distortions and behaviors. Includes exposure and relapse prevention	Strongest empirical support with multiple RCTs and meta-analysis confirming efficacy
Motivational Interviewing (MI)	Client-centered approach aimed at enhancing motivation and resolving ambivalence. Often combined with CBT	Effective in improving engagement and outcomes, especially when paired with CBT
Group Therapy	Peer-supported sessions guided by therapists may follow CBT, psychoeducational, or supportive formats	Effective for building accountability and support; used widely in treatment settings
12-Step Programs (e.g., GA)	Peer-led recovery groups emphasize abstinence, spirituality, and community support	Mixed evidence; helpful for some but often best as a supplement to therapy
Acceptance and Commitment Therapy (ACT)	Mindfulness-based therapy helps clients accept cravings and act based on values	Promising results in preliminary studies; growing but still emerging evidence base
Craving Behavioral Intervention (CBI)	Targets craving triggers using behavioral and cognitive coping strategies	Demonstrated reductions in craving intensity and emotional regulation improvement
Acceptance and Cognitive Restructuring Intervention Program (ACRIP)	Combines acceptance-based and cognitive restructuring strategies to reduce gambling urges	Effective in reducing symptom severity in short-term trials
Psychodynamic Psychotherapy	Explores unconscious drives, emotional conflicts, and developmental patterns related to gambling	Limited but emerging evidence; more commonly used in complex or resistant cases
Mindfulness-Based Interventions (MBIs)	Develops nonjudgmental awareness of urges, thoughts, and emotional triggers	Early studies suggest a reduction in frequency and urge intensity

worldwide and are linked to favorable outcomes, particularly in conjunction with professional treatment for addictive behaviors [34].

Craving Behavioral Intervention

Based on cognitive neuroscience, the craving behavioral intervention was developed for patients with IGD to reduce cravings and enhance coping skills [32, 64]. It is conducted weekly in a group format with eight to nine participants. Topics for each weekly session include the following:

(a) Perceiving subjective craving
(b) Recognizing and testing irrational beliefs regarding the desires of doing the behavior

(c) Detecting craving and relieving craving-related negative emotions
(d) Coping with cravings and altering participant fulfillment of psychologic needs
(e) Learning time management and skill training for dealing with cravings
(f) Reviewing, practicing, and implementing skills
(g) Mindfulness training.

Pharmacologic Treatments

Opioid Receptor Antagonists

Two randomized, double-blind, placebo-controlled trials have demonstrated that naltrexone and nalmefene can significantly reduce symptoms in behavioral addictions, including binge-eating disorder, compulsive sexual behavior, and gambling disorder. While naltrexone is FDA-approved for the treatment of substance use disorders in the U.S., nalmefene is not currently approved for use in the U.S. but has demonstrated promising efficacy as compared to placebo in European trials [36, 37]. The opioid antagonists demonstrated a small but significant benefit and are the only evidence-based pharmacological treatments for some of the addictive behaviors [36, 37]. The medications appear to help reduce urges/cravings in the treatment of addictive behaviors.

N-Acetylcysteine (NAC)

N-acetylcysteine (NAC) is an amino acid that is an over-the-counter dietary supplement. It has been reported to influence glutamatergic systems, particularly mGluR2 and mGluR3 receptors [39]. In an open-label study active, NAC was superior to placebo in maintaining diminished problem-gambling severity [39].

Glutamate and N-Methyl-D-Aspartate (NMDA) Receptor Modulators

Glutamate plays a pivotal role in behavioral addictions, and the N-methyl-D-aspartate (NMDA) glutamate receptor subtype serves as a molecular target for behavioral addictions [40, 73]. The release of glutamate by nerve cells leads to the rapid activation of these receptors and the depolarization of the neurons, creating a behavior-related stimuli, producing related memories that will enable cues to drive addiction behaviors. The NMDA receptors are believed to mediate depolarization and/or induction of plasticity in individuals suffering from behavioral addictions [40, 73, 74].

Conclusion

Progress in understanding the genetic, clinical, and neuro-hormonal mechanisms is ongoing. Neuroimaging and neuropsychological research have shown changes in brain structure, allowing psychological and pharmacological therapies to be developed. Research has improved clinical management and understanding of the similarities and differences between character traits like impulsivity, compulsivity, and substance use disorders. However, access continues to be limited to evidence-based treatments, and people with behavioral addictions continue to suffer isolation, stigma, and shame. Understanding the characteristics of the disease and differences among patients suffering from behavioral addictions can help guide clinician decision-making. Targeted multimodal, multidisciplinary treatment both individually and in a group, medication management (if necessary) could help patients recover from behavioral addictions.

Chapter Review Questions

1. A 47-year-old female presents due to increased symptoms of anxiety in the last 2 weeks. She is having financial difficulties and reports increasing time spent day trading stocks over the past 3 months, replacing her prior casino gambling with her ex-husband, from whom she divorced last year. Her trading has escalated significantly in the past month. Based on what we know about gambling behaviors, which of the following is most likely true?

   A. Day trading is not considered a form of gambling because it involves financial markets.
   B. Behavioral addictions like gambling rarely co-occur with mood or anxiety disorders.
   C. Day trading can function as a form of gambling when it becomes repetitive, risky, and driven by a reward-seeking behavior.
   D. Women who gamble tend to prefer strategic forms of gambling, such as sports betting or poker.
   E. Anxiety symptoms are usually protective against the development of gambling disorders.

   Correct Answer: C.

   Explanation: While investing is not inherently pathological, day trading can become a form of gambling when it is characterized by repetitive, high-risk behavior driven by the desire for quick rewards, often with a loss of control. This patient's escalation, financial problems, and emotional distress raise concern for gambling disorder. Gambling disorder frequently co-occurs with mood and anxiety disorders, and women more often engage in non-strategic gambling (slot machines or lottery). However, there are exceptions, as in this case. Day trading, while socially sanctioned, may fulfill the criteria for gambling when it meets patterns of compulsion and negative consequences.

2. A 39-year-old female presents to the office for a mental health evaluation before bariatric surgery. She reports daily struggles over the past 14 months with loss of control when eating foods high in carbohydrates, fat, and salt. She often feels guilty after eating certain foods yet finds herself eating them again soon after. Which patient statement best demonstrates the expected emotional response to binge eating?

   A. "After a binge, I feel well for a little while."
   B. "I know this is bad sometimes; I will stop soon."
   C. "Everyone in my gym class is on a diet."
   D. "It will pass after I fix my social stressors."
   E. "I hate myself after I eat like that, but I can't stop."

   Correct Answer: A.

   Explanation: Eating behaviors exhibit high negative urgency, high reward dependence, and a lack of premeditation. Food addiction usually presents concomitantly with binge-eating disorder, when the person eats a large quantity of food in one session and feels unable to stop. After binging food, the person usually feels better and sometimes happy due to the release of neurotransmitters in the brain, followed by feelings of guilt or failure after binging are common.

3. A 42-year-old man presents for psychiatric evaluation after being referred by his primary care physician. He reports on difficulty controlling his gambling, which has escalated from occasional lottery tickets to frequent online poker over the past year. He spends several hours per day gambling and has accumulated significant debt. He describes intense cravings for gambling and emotional relief when doing so. He denies substance use but reports a history of depression. You consider starting pharmacologic treatment to help reduce his gambling urges. Which of the following medications has shown the most consistent evidence for reducing gambling urges and behaviors?

   A. Fluoxetine
   B. Naltrexone
   C. Risperidone
   D. Topiramate
   E. Modafinil

   Correct Answer: B.

   Explanation: Naltrexone, an opioid receptor antagonist, has demonstrated efficacy in reducing cravings and the rewarding effects of gambling by modulating the brain's reward system. It is one of the most studied and supported pharmacologic options for gambling disorder.

4. A 35-year-old man presents to the clinic reporting symptoms of anxiety, low mood, and difficulty sleeping for the past several months. He also reveals that he has been struggling with compulsive online sports betting, which has caused financial stress and tension with his partner. He expresses guilt and regret after gambling but finds it hard to stop. He denies any history of substance use but has a past diagnosis of generalized anxiety disorder. After discussing treatment options, you consider pharmacologic support in addition to therapy. Which of the following statements is most accurate regarding SSRIs in the treatment of gambling disorder?

A. SSRIs are first-line FDA-approved medications for gambling disorder.
B. SSRIs consistently reduce gambling urges in all patients.
C. SSRIs may be beneficial in patients with gambling disorder and co-occurring anxiety or depression.
D. SSRIs are known to increase the risk of gambling behavior.
E. SSRIs are contraindicated in gambling disorder.

Correct Answer: C.

Explanation: Although SSRIs are not FDA-approved specifically for gambling disorder and their efficacy in reducing gambling urges alone is inconsistent, they can be helpful in individuals with co-occurring mood or anxiety disorders. Treating these underlying conditions can reduce emotional triggers that contribute to gambling behaviors.

5. A 29-year-old man is referred to your clinic by his primary care provider due to concerns about possible gambling problems. He reports spending several hours each day betting on sports and recently borrowed money from family members to cover losses. He denies substance use and has no prior psychiatric history. You want to quickly screen him for gambling disorder before conducting a complete diagnostic assessment. Which of the following screening tools is most appropriate for identifying individuals at risk for gambling disorder in a brief clinical encounter?

A. DSM-5 Gambling Disorder Criteria Checklist
B. Alcohol Use Disorders Identification Test (AUDIT)
C. Brief Biosocial Gambling Screen (BBGS)
D. Patient Health Questionnaire-9 (PHQ-9)
E. Clinical Institute Withdrawal Assessment for Alcohol (CIWA-Ar)

Correct Answer: C.

Explanation: The BBGS is a validated 3-item screening tool specifically designed to quickly identify individuals who may be at risk for gambling disorder. It is brief, easy to administer, and effective in primary care and mental health settings. The DSM-5 checklist is more comprehensive but not as efficient for initial screening. AUDIT and PHQ-9 assess alcohol use and depression, respectively, and CIWA-Ar is used for alcohol withdrawal.

References

1. Brand M, Antons S, Bőthe B, Demetrovics Z, Fineberg NA, Jimenez-Murcia S, et al. Current advances in behavioral addictions: from fundamental research to clinical practice. Am J Psychiatry. 2025;182(2):155–63.
2. Office of Legal Counsel. U.S. Department of Justice. Whether the Wire Act applies to non-sports gambling, 35 Op. O.L.C. 134. 2011. https://www.justice.gov/olc/file/1121531/download.
3. Murphy v. National Collegiate Athletic Association. 584 U.S. 2018. https://www.supremecourt.gov/opinions/17pdf/16-476_dbfi.pdf.
4. Wardle H, Degenhardt L, Marionneau V, Reith G, Livingstone C, Sparrow M, et al. The Lancet Public Health Commission on gambling. Lancet Public Health. 2024;9(11):e950–94.

5. American Psychiatric Association. Diagnostic and statistical manual of mental disorders. Arlington: American Psychiatric Association Publishing; 2022.
6. Stefanovics EA, Potenza MN. Update on gambling disorder. Psychiatr Clin N Am. 2022;45(3):483–502.
7. Tran LT, Wardle H, Colledge-Frisby S, Taylor S, Lynch M, Rehm J, et al. The prevalence of gambling and problematic gambling: a systematic review and meta-analysis. Lancet Public Health. 2024;9(8):e594–613.
8. Marionneau V, Nikkinen J. Gambling-related suicides and suicidality: a systematic review of qualitative evidence. Front Psych. 2022;13:980303.
9. Moghaddam JF, Yoon G, Dickerson DL, Kim SW, Westermeyer J. Suicidal ideation and suicide attempts in five groups with different severities of gambling: findings from the National Epidemiologic Survey on Alcohol and Related Conditions. Am J Addict. 2015;24(4):292–8.
10. Calado F, Griffiths MD. Problem gambling worldwide: an update and systematic review of empirical research (2000–2015). J Behav Addict. 2016;5(4):592–613.
11. Davis CN, Slutske WS, Martin NG, Agrawal A, Lynskey MT. Genetic and environmental influences on gambling disorder liability: a replication and combined analysis of two twin studies. Psychol Med. 2019;49(10):1705–12.
12. Błoch M, Misiak B. Understanding the emergence of comorbidity between problematic online gaming and gambling: a network analysis approach. Brain Sci. 2024;14(9):929.
13. Moreira D, Azeredo A, Dias P. Risk factors for gambling disorder: a systematic review. J Gambl Stud. 2023;39(2):483–511.
14. Miller L, Mide M, Arvidson E, Söderpalm Gordh A. Clinical differences between men and women in a Swedish treatment-seeking population with gambling disorder. Front Psych. 2023;13:1054236.
15. Lee K, Kim H, Kim Y. Gambling disorder symptoms, suicidal ideation, and suicide attempts. Psychiatry Investig. 2021;18(1):88–93.
16. National Council on Problem Gambling. Gambling assessment manual [Internet]. Washington, DC: NCPG; 2025. Available from: https://www.ncpgambling.org.
17. World Health Organization. ICD-11 beta draft. 2016. Retrieved from http://apps.who.int/classifications/icd11/browse/l-m/en.
18. Ukhova D, Marionneau V, Volberg R, Wardle H. The expansion of gambling across the Americas poses risks to mental health and wellbeing. Lancet Reg Health Am. 2024;37:100855.
19. Deng X, Lesch T, Clark L. Pareto distributions in online casino gambling: sensitivity to timeframe and associations with self exclusion. Addict Behav. 2021;120:106968.
20. Welte JW, Wieczorek WF, Barnes GM, Tidwell MC, Hoffman JH. The relationship of ecological and geographic factors to gambling behavior and pathology. J Gambl Stud. 2004;20(4):405–23.
21. Wolfschlag M, Håkansson A. Drug-induced gambling disorder: epidemiology, neurobiology, and management. Pharmaceut Med. 2023;37(1):37–52.
22. Rash CJ, Petry NM. Psychological treatments for gambling disorder. Psychol Res Behav Manag. 2014;7:285–95.
23. Bergeron PY, Giroux I, Chrétien M, Jacques C, Goulet A. Exposure therapy for gambling disorder: systematic review and meta-analysis. Curr Addict Rep. 2022;9(2):179–94.
24. Sagoe D, Griffiths Mark D, Erevik EK, Høyland T, Leino T, Lande IA, et al. Internet-based treatment of gambling problems: a systematic review and meta-analysis of randomized controlled trials. J Behav Addict. 2021;10(3):546–65.
25. Gamblers Anonymous. Home. Available from: https://www.gamblersanonymous.org/ga/. Accessed 5 Jun 2025.
26. Gamblers, family and friends in recovery. Gamblers in recovery [Internet]. 2025 [cited 2025 Jun 5]. Available from: https://gamblersinrecovery.com/.
27. Motka F, Grüne B, Sleczka P, Braun B, Örnberg JC, Kraus L. Who uses self-exclusion to regulate problem gambling? A systematic literature review. J Behav Addict. 2018;7(4):903–16.
28. Levounis P. Technological addictions: the new frontier of addiction psychiatry. Austen Riggs Center & American Psychiatric Association; 2022.

29. Association AP. Special report: be prepared to address technological addictions in practice. Psychiatr News. 2022;57(2):1, 23–26.
30. World Health Organization. ICD-11 for mortality and morbidity statistics [Internet]. Geneva: World Health Organization; 2022.
31. Gao YX, Wang JY, Dong GH. The prevalence and possible risk factors of internet gaming disorder among adolescents and young adults: systematic reviews and meta-analyses. J Psychiatr Res. 2022;154:35–43.
32. Liao Z, Chen X, Huang S, Huang Q, Lin S, Li Y, et al. Exploring the associated characteristics of Internet gaming disorder from the perspective of various game genres. Front Psych. 2023;13:1103816.
33. Chen L, Lu Z, Wang X, Gao Y. Effective interventions for gaming disorder: a systematic review of randomized controlled trials. J Behav Addict. 2023;14:1098922.
34. Ridgway NM, Kukar-Kinney M, Monroe KB. An expanded conceptualization and a new measure of compulsive buying. J Consum Res. 2008;35(4):622–39.
35. Derbyshire KL, Chamberlain SR, Odlaug BL, Schreiber LNR, Grant JE. Neurocognitive functioning in compulsive buying disorder. Ann Clin Psychiatry. 2014;26(1):57–63.
36. Müller A, Laskowski NM, Thomas TA, Antons S, Tahmassebi N, Steins-Loeber S. Update on treatment studies for compulsive buying-shopping disorder: a systematic review. J Behav Addict. 2023;12(3):631–51.
37. Kraus SW, Krueger RB, Briken P, First MB, Stein DJ, Kaplan MS, et al. Compulsive sexual behaviour disorder in the ICD-11. World Psychiatry. 2018;17(1):109–10.
38. Karila L, Wéry A, Weinstein A, Cottencin O, Petit A, Reynaud M, et al. Sexual addiction or hypersexual disorder: different terms for the same problem? A review of the literature. Curr Pharm Des. 2014;20(25):4012–20.
39. Carnes PJ, Green BA, Merlo LJ, Polles A, Carnes S, Gold MS. PATHOS: a brief screening application for assessing sexual addiction. J Addict Med. 2012;6(1):29–34.
40. Davis C. Compulsive overeating as an addictive behavior: overlap between food addiction and binge eating disorder. Curr Obes Rep. 2013;2(2):171–8.
41. Wolz I, Hilker I, Granero R, Jiménez-Murcia S, Gearhardt AN, Dieguez C, et al. "Food addiction" in patients with eating disorders is associated with negative urgency and difficulties to focus on long-term goals. Front Psychol. 2016;7:61.
42. Haynos AF, Camchong J, Pearson CM, Lavender JM, Mueller BA, Peterson CB, et al. Resting state hypoconnectivity of reward networks in binge eating disorder. Cereb Cortex. 2021;31(5):2494–504.
43. Naef L, Pitman KA, Borgland SL. Mesolimbic dopamine and its neuromodulators in obesity and binge eating. CNS Spectr. 2015;20(6):574–83.
44. Guerdjikova AI, Mori N, Casuto LS, McElroy SL. Novel pharmacologic treatment in acute binge eating disorder – role of lisdexamfetamine. Neuropsychiatr Dis Treat. 2016;12:833–41.
45. Haghighatfard A, Ghaderi AH, Mostajabi P, Kashfi SS, Mohabati Somehsarayee H, Shahrani M, et al. The first genome-wide association study of internet addiction; revealed substantial shared risk factors with neurodevelopmental psychiatric disorders. Res Dev Disabil. 2023;133:104393.
46. Solé-Morata N, Baenas I, Etxandi M, Granero R, Gené M, Barrot C, et al. Underlying mechanisms involved in gambling disorder severity: a pathway analysis considering genetic, psychosocial, and clinical variables. Nutrients. 2023;15(2):418.
47. Rehn M, Nilsson KW, Hultman C, Vadlin S, Åslund C. Differential susceptibility effects of the 5-HTTLPR and MAOA genotypes on decision making under risk in the Iowa gambling task. Front Psych. 2025;16:1456490.
48. Leeman RF, Potenza MN. A targeted review of the neurobiology and genetics of behavioural addictions: an emerging area of research. Can J Psychiatr. 2013;58(5):260–73.
49. Hahn T, Notebaert K, Dresler T, Kowarsch L, Reif A, Fallgatter AJ. Serotonin transporter gene variation impacts innate fear processing: a functional magnetic resonance imaging study. Biol Psychiatry. 2014;75(5):373–9.
50. Hou H, Jia S, Hu S, Fan R, Sun W, Sun T, et al. Reduced striatal dopamine transporters in people with Internet addiction disorder. J Biomed Biotechnol. 2012;2012:854524.

51. Kim SH, Baik SH, Park CS, Kim SJ, Choi SW, Kim SE, et al. Reduced striatal dopamine D2 receptors in people with Internet addiction. Neuroreport. 2011;22(8):407–11.
52. Kim SJ, Lee H, Kim SH, Jung YC, Lee JY. Genetic influences on Internet addiction: a review of the literature. Psychiatry Investig. 2006;3(2):67–72.
53. Lee YS, Han DH, Yang KC, Daniels MA, Na C, Kee BS, et al. Depression-like characteristics of 5HTTLPR polymorphism and temperament in excessive Internet users. J Affect Disord. 2008;109(1–2):165–9.
54. Montag C, Kirsch P, Sauer C, Markett S, Reuter M. The role of the CHRNA4 gene in Internet addiction: a case–control study. J Addict Med. 2012;6(3):191–5.
55. Park S, Kim SH, Bang SA, Yoon Y, Cho SS. MAO-A polymorphism and aggression in male Internet addiction. Neurosci Lett. 2013;548:65–9.
56. Park M, Lee JE, Namkoong K. Genetic markers and genome-wide associations in Internet and gaming addiction: emerging targets and shared vulnerabilities. Front Psych. 2023;14:1189223.
57. Weinstein A, Lejoyeux M. New developments on the neurobiological and pharmaco-genetic mechanisms underlying Internet and videogame addiction. Am J Addict. 2015;24(2):117–25.
58. Zai CC, Maes MS, Fuselli S, Tiwari AK, Kennedy JL. The genetics of impulsivity: a review of the role of catechol-O-methyltransferase and the dopamine receptor D4 gene. J Psychiatry Neurosci. 2014;39(5):296–307.
59. Kim E, Lee D, Do K, Kim J. Interaction effects of DRD2 genetic polymorphism and interpersonal stress on problematic gaming in college students. Genes (Basel). 2022;13(3):449.
60. Carroll ME, Smethells JR. Sex differences in behavioral dyscontrol: role in drug addiction and novel treatments. Front Psych. 2016;6:175.
61. Groleau P, Potenza MN. Serotonin 2C receptor gene variants and disordered eating: a systematic review. Int J Eat Disord. 2019;52(7):753–66.
62. Hinney A, Volckmar AL, Scherag A. Genetics of eating disorders. Curr Psychiatry Rep. 2013;15(12):423.
63. Hainerová I, Snejková V, Hainer V. Genetic variants in serotonin receptors 5-HT2A, 5-HT2C, and 5-HT3 and their associations with eating behavior: a review. Nutrients. 2021;13(4):1201.
64. Nielsen P, Christensen M, Henderson C, Liddle HA, Croquette-Krokar M, Favez N. Multidimensional family therapy reduces problematic gaming in adolescents: a randomised controlled trial. J Behav Addict. 2021;10(2):234–43.
65. Cowlishaw S, Merkouris S, Dowling N, Anderson C, Jackson A, Thomas S. Psychological therapies for pathological and problem gambling. Cochrane Database Syst Rev. 2012;11(11):CD008937.
66. Gooding P, Tarrier N. A systematic review and meta-analysis of cognitive-behavioural interventions to reduce problem gambling. Behav Res Ther. 2009;47(7):592–607.
67. Hodgins DC, Currie SR, el-Guebaly N, Diskin KM. Does motivational interviewing predict relapse in problem gambling? Addict Behav. 2007;32(4):1096–102.
68. Yakovenko I, Quigley L, Hemmelgarn BR, Hodgins DC, Ronksley PE, Rush B. The efficacy of motivational interviewing for disordered gambling: a meta-analysis. Addiction. 2020;115(5):809–23.
69. Leichsenring F, Klein S. Evidence for psychodynamic psychotherapy in specific mental disorders: a systematic review. Psychol Bull. 2014;140(2):318–37.
70. Garland EL, Hanley AW, Nakamura Y, Froeliger B. Mindfulness-oriented recovery enhancement for addiction, stress, and pain. Washington, DC: American Psychological Association; 2017.
71. Luquiens A. Acceptance and commitment therapy for problem gambling: a pilot study. J Gambl Stud. 2016;32(3):1025–40.
72. Petry N. Group therapy for gambling disorder: a cognitive-behavioral approach. J Consult Clin Psychol. 2006;74(3):555–67.
73. Wolz I, Hilker I, Granero R, Jiménez-Murcia S, Gearhardt AN, Dieguez C. Food addiction: patients with eating disorders is associated with negative urgency and difficulties to focus on long-term goals. Front Psychol. 2016;7:61.
74. Barry D, Clarke M, Petry NM. Obesity and its relationship to addictions: is overeating a form of addictive behavior? Am J Addict. 2009;18(6):439–51.

Part III

Populations

Adolescents and Students

15

Jose Vito, Justin Morales, and Irshan Shaik

High-Yield Review Points

- The use of e-cigarettes has risen significantly compared with regular cigarette use, making it the most commonly misused substance in adolescents.
- Alcohol is the second most misused substance in adolescents; cannabis closely follows. Studies indicate that the perceived risk of cannabis has decreased with legalization, the advertisement of supposed medical uses, and perceived availability.
- Screening tools, such as HEADSS, SBIRT, S2BI, and BSTAD, have been shown to be effective for adolescents.
- Personality traits and childhood temperaments are often cited as key risk factors to adolescent engagement in risky behaviors, including substance use.
- Treatment should include behavioral approaches, family engagement, and medication interventions. Current FDA-approved treatments for adults are not necessarily approved by the FDA for adolescents.

J. Vito (✉) · J. Morales
NYU School of Medicine, New York, NY, USA
e-mail: jose.vito@nyulangone.org; justin.morales@nyulangone.org

I. Shaik
BronxCare Health System, New York, NY, USA

C. Marienfeld, M. Soltani (eds.), *AAAP Review of Addiction Psychiatry*,
https://doi.org/10.1007/978-3-032-24174-0_15

Introduction

Neurobiological, psychological, developmental, social, and environmental considerations contribute to adolescent substance use. Understanding the development of substance use in the child and adolescent population and utilizing appropriate early intervention and treatment decrease the risk of developing an adult substance use disorder (SUD) [1]. Assessing substance use in children and adolescents requires a different approach than in adults, considering factors such as the most commonly used substances and the limitations of screening and treatment options. While there are roughly 105,000 child and adolescent psychiatrists in the United States, the child and adolescent population is over 72 million, requiring adult psychiatrists and primary care providers like pediatricians to appropriately screen, diagnose, and treat this vulnerable population [2–4]. Substance use before 14, compared to later exposure, has been associated with numerous short- and long-term consequences. These include, but are not limited to, poor academic performance, including higher rates of dropout; SUDs in adulthood; unintentional overdose; suicide; accidents, including risk of a traumatic brain injury; increased risk of HIV and some forms of hepatitis; and memory disturbances [5].

Epidemiology

There has been a downward trend of substance use for most substances by American 8th, 10th, and 12th graders since the 1990s, according to the Monitoring the Future Study [6]. Now, the average age of substance use initiation in North America has increased to 15–17 years of age [7, 8]. Despite the improving trends, in 2024 there were over 11 million adolescents who were estimated to have met diagnostic criteria for a SUD (2.0 million ages 12–17 and 9.1 million ages 18–25), with the majority remaining untreated [9]. Interestingly, there are also consistent themes that suggest that single substance use is rare in adolescence, and multiple substance use is more common [10]. There are also racial differences in use with White youth outpacing Black and Latinx youth in almost all substance use [11].

Alcohol is the second most commonly used substance among adolescents, with approximately 1.7 million (6.6%) reporting monthly alcohol consumption and 900,000 engaging in binge-drinking at least once a month, and it is the second most common substance for which adolescents seek treatment [9, 12]. There is also a recent trend that females aged 12–20 are reporting higher rates of past-month alcohol consumption and binge-drinking than their male peers, although they are relatively equal on heavy alcohol consumption [13]. Apart from cannabis and e-cigarettes, most substance use is declining; though their prevalence shows many adolescents use substances (Table 15.1).

Cannabis is the third most commonly used substance by adolescents with approximately 1.6 million reporting monthly use, but cannabis is the most common illicit substance, due to federal designation despite many states having legalized cannabis-related products, for which adolescents seek treatment [12]. Studies indicate that the perceived risk of cannabis has decreased with legalization, the

Table 15.1 Prevalence estimates of substance use [9]

Substance	Number and percentage of adolescents (ages 12–17)
Past Month	
Tobacco and Vape Nicotine products	1.9 million (7.2%)
Alcohol	1.7 million (6.6%)
Cannabis	1.6 million (6%)
Past Year	
Cannabis	2.7 million (10.4%)
Inhalants	967,000 (3.7%)
Prescribed pain relievers	425,000 (1.6%)
Hallucinogens	405,000 (1.6%)
Opioids	400,000 (1.5%)
Prescription Stimulants	203,000 (0.8%)
Tranquilizers and Sedatives	172,000 (0.7%)
Cocaine	72,000 (0.3%)
Methamphetamines	57,000 (0.2%)
Heroin	10,000 (less than 0.1%)

advertisement of purported medicinal uses, and perceived availability, which has led to use no longer decreasing after decades of decline [14]. While nicotine use has decreased among 8th–12th graders, the use of e-cigarettes has risen significantly compared with regular cigarette use, making it the most used substance in adolescents [9, 15].

Earlier use of illicit substances is associated with a higher risk of developing any SUD, as there is an inverse correlation between the age of first use and the likelihood of developing a SUD. Individuals who begin using substances in early adolescence are 3–5 times more likely to develop a SUD compared to those who start in early adulthood [16–18]. The majority of those who have a SUD started using before age 18 and developed their disorder by age 20.

Neurobiological Considerations

Understanding the basic principles regarding the neurobiological development of the brain will help clinicians conceptualize why children and adolescents are at elevated risk for substance use. There is a general theory that an adolescent's risk behavior is due to a dual system model and the asynchronous maturation of the emotional limbic regions of the brain, which peaks during adolescence, and the regulatory prefrontal cortex, which occurs last in young adulthood [1]. The prefrontal cortex is the portion of the brain that is involved with executive function, which includes decision-making, planning, response inhibition, and working memory [19]. Gray matter volume in the prefrontal cortex peaks between the ages of 11 and 13, leading to synaptic pruning, a process in which synaptic connections that are underutilized are "pruned" away. This process occurs much later in development as other portions of the brain undergo synaptic pruning before the prefrontal cortex [20]. In contrast, the striatum and the emotional limbic system, responsible for emotional responsiveness and reward, go through their respective maturation process during adolescence [21]. Another aspect of neuronal development includes alterations in myelination where insulation of the neurons leads to faster cell signaling and processing. Similar to synaptic pruning, myelination of the remaining and connected neurons occurs later in development, particularly in young adulthood [22]. Since synaptic pruning and myelination do not complete until later in young adulthood (late twenties), the consequence of an immature prefrontal cortex against a mature striatum and emotional limbic system includes poor impulse control, increased risk-taking behavior due to lack of response inhibition, and difficulty with planning. The hyperactivity of the striatum and the reward system are also linked to an "impulsivity theory" further suggesting vulnerability to substance use [23, 24].

The tonic and phasic firing of dopamine also contributes to substance use in children and adolescents. Tonic dopamine firing, or low frequency but sustained release of dopamine, leads to incentive motivation or the act of pursuing a stimulus that will provide an external reward [5]. In adolescents, the tonic firing of dopamine occurs at a faster rate than that of adults, and they have more dopamine receptors than adults, leading to a heightened response to substances [25, 26]. This leads to adolescents being more likely to pursue illicit substance use if they believe there is an external reward associated with that substance. These external rewards would include peer approval, excitement for getting high, or taking away emotional pain. The unfortunate consideration is that since the adolescent brain is not fully developed and mature, it is more vulnerable to the lasting effects of substances, increasing the risk of neurocognitive deficits that may alter further development of the regulatory reward and inhibitory neural system, leading to increased risk for addiction [27–29].

Psychological and Developmental Considerations

The exact mechanism by which adolescents develop SUDs is not well understood and appears to be a complex function of biological, psychological, developmental, societal, and environmental considerations [30]. From a psychological and developmental perspective, adolescence is a period of experimentation and identity formation. It is during this period that children attempt to refine their sense of autonomy from their parents and simultaneously gain acceptance from their peers [22]. It has been theorized that some adolescents use substances to seek this sense of independence from family members and social elevation from peers [22]. Similarly, adolescents' desire to conform to "normal" behaviors leads to behavioral changes influenced by social media, celebrities, and advertisements. Therefore, those that have friends who use substances are 1.5–2 times more likely to begin using substances themselves [31–34].

Individual Risk Factors and Protective Factors

Personality traits and childhood temperaments are often cited as key risk factors to adolescent engagement in risky behaviors, including substance use. Individuals who are prone to *sensation seeking* and *impulsivity* have been associated with an increased risk of adolescent alcohol use and an increased risk of substance use, respectively [35]. Other psychological risk factors include decreased ability to self-regulate when compared to peers and a difficult temperament [5, 35].

While research is limited and the exact way these factors influence risk is complex, some factors that have been identified as protective are increased competence, positive or easy temperament, and self-control [5, 30]. One hypothesis is that children's personality and temperamental factors influence the parenting that they receive and therefore the attachment and bonds that are later made [35]. Another recommendation is to include youth in their treatment planning so they can express their own opinions and develop their independence in a positive way [36].

Environmental (Familial, Peer, Community, School) and Societal Considerations

Firstly, with the transition out of primary school, there is a greater exposure to different peers and a new potential for acceptance into or rejection from new peer groups. Secondly, in later school years, there is usually more autonomy and less direct supervision from school authorities as classroom sizes tend to be larger, and students are shared among a larger number of teachers [30]. Furthermore, amid all these changes, there is a shift away from time spent with family members in favor of increased time spent with peers [26]. While adolescents are spending more time with peers, familial relationships, and dynamics also play a significant role in the risk of adolescent substance use [30].

Societal factors that contribute to adolescent substance use include but are not limited to laws, policies, and popular media portrayal [30]. These considerations are further discussed below regarding risk factors and protective factors for adolescent substance use.

Social Risk Factors and Protective Factors

Families play a key part in the risk of adolescent substance use. Genetics have been shown to explain more than half of the total variance in adolescent substance use. The roles that families play can best be broken down into familial use, attitudes, and parenting styles [35]. Higher rates of alcohol use have been described in adolescents with parents who use alcohol [30]. Additionally, parental attitudes toward substance use seem to have both a risk and a protective role [26]. Adolescents with parents who have negative views on substance use or a more authoritarian role have lower rates of use, and conversely those who perceive their parents as having more permissive or even positive views of substance use have increased rates of use [35, 37]. Furthermore, parental styles and the parent–child relationship are key components. A favorable parent–child relationship where the child feels cared for and accepted and receives adequate supervision and rules has been associated with lower rates of adolescent alcohol use [30]. Conversely, adverse childhood events, such as inconsistent parenting, abuse, neglect, and high parent–child conflicts, have all been associated with increased risk [26, 35]. Abuse from any perpetrator (familial or not) is associated with an increased risk of substance use [35]. This is also highlighted in the estimated 437,000 children and adolescents in foster care during 2018, who are up to 5 times more likely to be diagnosed with a SUD than those living with their parents [38]. Similarly, LGBTQ youth face additional challenges such as stigma and estrangement from family, which contribute to higher rates of SUDs [39].

Adolescents who are associated with peers who use substances and engage in other risky behaviors are more likely to use substances themselves, whereas adolescents who have peer groups that do not use substances or have negative views on substance use are less likely to use substances [30]. Likewise, having coaches, mentors, counselors, and clinicians share the repetitive stance that substances are bad gives adolescents a foundation to diminish their potential for use [36]. A thought-provoking argument though is that student-athletes have a higher rate of alcohol use than nonathletic peers, but are less likely to use tobacco, cannabis, or other illicit drugs [40, 41]. Also, social popularity plays a role in risk, with students who self-identify as popular having a higher risk of substance use. One theory for this is that these students may feel more pressured to use substances to gain a more positive view from their peers to maintain their popularity [22, 30].

Students with poor academic performance and who attend schools where drugs are readily available are at a higher risk for substance use, whereas students who identify as having a prominent level of school connectedness and academic competence are at a reduced risk [30]. From a community standpoint, lower socioeconomic status has been associated with a higher risk, although the exact mechanism is unknown [5, 35].

Societal views and norms also contribute to substance use risk. If an adolescent believes that substances are lethal or looked down upon largely by society, they are at lower risk of substance use [30]. Of the 31 million adolescents involved in the criminal justice system in 2018, up to 67% had prior substance use [42]. This view can be developed via news and popular media portrayal of substance use, as well as laws surrounding the legalization and criminalization of substance use. One concrete example of this is that increased taxes on alcohol are associated with a decreased drinking rate among adolescents, but lower legal drinking age is associated with a higher drinking rate [35].

Risk and protective factors are further summarized in Table 15.2.

Table 15.2 Key risk and protective factors for adolescent substance use

	Risk factors	Protective factors
Individual	Impulsivity Sensation seeking ADHD Depression	Self-control Competence Easy temperament
Family	Child abuse and neglect Inconsistent parenting Permissive parenting style Parental substance use Elevated level of parental–child conflict	Positive parent–child relations Clear parental expectations Negative perceived parental view of substance use Positive parental–child relationships
Peer	Maladaptive peer relationships Perception of popularity Gang affiliation	Friends who abstain from substances Belief that peers have negative view of substance use
School/community	Poor academic performance Poverty Lower socioeconomic status Drug availability	School connectedness Academic competence Community attachment Illegal status/laws

Co-occurring Psychiatric Conditions

When evaluating children and adolescents for SUDs, it is also important to address mental health comorbidities, such as mood and anxiety disorders, attention deficit/hyperactivity disorder (ADHD), and post-traumatic stress disorder (PTSD), which may place the youth at risk of developing or further increasing their substance use. Theories regarding the association between substance use and mental health comorbidities focus on three main mechanisms: (1) shared risk factors or biological predispositions, (2) substance use as a form of "self-medication" in an attempt to relieve mental health symptoms, and (3) substance use as a cause of or contributor to worsening mental illness [43, 44]. Research suggests that anywhere ranging 37–80% of adolescents with SUD have at least one other mental health disorder, and the relationship is bidirectional [11]. When unrecognized or untreated, psychiatric comorbidities can significantly interfere with abstinence or harm reduction interventions addressing substance use.

ADHD

Adolescents diagnosed with ADHD are significantly more likely to try a range of substances during their lifetime compared to their non-ADHD diagnosed peers [45]. Evidence supports that youths with ADHD symptoms who are treated with stimulants have lower risks of developing a SUD [46]. In addition, the younger the initiation of medications to address symptoms interfering with functioning, the greater the protective effect against developing a SUD [47]. However, some other studies showed no benefit of medication in addition to CBT with motivational interviewing on the remission of SUD, as measured by self-reported days of use and urine drug screen [48, 49]. A small naturalistic chart review study showed that bupropion reduced substance use, depression, and ADHD symptoms [50]. Pharmacotherapy for co-occurring ADHD and SUDs can be beneficial but must be considered on a case-by-case basis, weighing the risks of stimulant use, including diversion and misuse.

Conduct Disorder

Established therapy and behavioral treatments, not medications, have been shown to work well to reduce substance use in patients with conduct disorder. Multisystemic therapy (MST) is a well-established treatment for conduct disorder and criminal activity with evidence supporting its use in comorbid SUDs and conduct disorder. In addition, multidimensional family therapy (MDFT) has been shown to be effective for high acuity SUDs, as well as improved educational outcomes and decreased arrests.

Major Depressive and Bipolar Disorder

Pharmacotherapy in adolescents with depression has mixed evidence. A meta-analysis of randomized placebo-controlled studies showed that antidepressants had a significant effect on depression but minimal to no effect on substance use [51]. Studies highlight the importance of high-quality behavioral therapy (such as CBT and MI) and accurate diagnosis rather than specific antidepressants. Signs of changes in behavior and mood should also prompt consideration for a major depressive episode or social/environmental factors such as bullying at school or difficulties in the family.

Few studies have focused on treatments for co-occurring bipolar disorder and substance use, partly because of the low prevalence of this disorder in younger age groups. Very few studies have focused on pharmacotherapy, with a small randomized controlled trial showing Lithium benefits in patients with bipolar disorder and substance use [51].

Anxiety

There is little research in comorbid anxiety and substance use treatment in adolescents. Studies show promising results for behavioral family system therapy (BFST), as well as CBT with MI and mindfulness.

PTSD

Adolescents with PTSD and substance use are more likely to be female and of an ethnic minority status, highlighting the interrelated connections between social and environmental inequalities and mental health [52]. A randomized trial of Seeking

Safety for adolescent girls with PTSD and substance use showed benefits. Mixed trauma-focused CBT and MST also have preliminary evidence in a small trial of sexually assaulted adolescents. Adolescents may seek substances to address symptoms of hypervigilance and hyperarousal when not utilizing other coping skills.

Screening

Discussing substance use with adolescents and youths is a skill that requires taking a nonjudgmental attitude, showing genuine interest, and forming a therapeutic alliance. Guidelines recommend asking about substance use at age 11 during primary care and mental health visits, as primary care providers (PCPs) typically have long-term relationships with the child or adolescent and have a keen sense of the family history, home environment, and behavioral concerns at school [22, 36, 53]. The unfortunate element is that less than 50% of adolescents get annual well-child visits and are never screened; so, training other caring adults such as coaches, teachers, mentors, caseworks, and others to screen is critical [36, 54]. Being clear about expectations and limits of confidentiality at the beginning of the interview, especially with respect to parental disclosures, will be important in forming trust.

The HEADSS mnemonic (Home Education Activities Drug use Sexuality and Suicidality/mood) developed for primary care settings is a useful tool to explore topics that may be difficult to discuss. Clinicians should ask open-ended questions related to each of these domains, including Home, Education, Activities, Drug use, Sexuality, and Suicidality/mood. Other screening measures include the Screening, Brief Intervention, and Referral to Treatment (SBIRT) [55]; the Screening to Brief Intervention model (S2BI) [56], which is endorsed by the American Academy of Pediatrics; the Car, Relax, Alone, Friends/Family, Forget, Trouble questionnaire (CRAFFT) [57]; the National Institute of Alcohol Abuse and Alcoholism (NIAA) set for alcoholism; and the Brief Screener for Tobacco, Alcohol, and Other Drugs (BSTAD) [58]. These tools have been shown to be effective for adolescents, however, with varying sensitivity and specificity depending on age groups.

Treatment Considerations

Consent, Confidentiality, and Decision-Making

Laws differ by state, and, in most states, adolescents younger than the age of 18 can consent for their own substance use treatment. Even in states that require parental approval, teens over the age of 13 should be provided with the space for a private interview, and the providers should seek assent from the patient while working as a mediator for the discussion with parents. Providers should openly discuss with adolescents the limits of confidentiality prior to gathering any information. Sensitive information that does not pertain to safety should not be disclosed to parents without the patient's consent. Adolescents should be made aware that if they are on their parent's health insurance, insurers may send an explanation of benefits or a bill containing the details of any potential diagnoses. However, treatment-related conversations are most effective when parents are also involved and have better treatment outcomes [59]. The patient's support network is crucial to treatments that require frequent appointments, medication administrations, and harm reduction approaches.

Behavioral Approaches

Therapy and behavioral approaches have the most robust evidence in this population, compared with research on pharmacological treatment. Cognitive behavioral therapy (CBT) has been shown to be effective for reducing tobacco, alcohol, and cannabis use in adolescents [60]. CBT courses tailored for youth according to their developmental stage are especially effective. Motivational enhancement therapy, the manualized version of MI, can be combined with CBT and involves short, problem-focused sessions aimed at resolving ambivalence and promoting internal motivation and empowerment. This technique is good for youth with limited attention capacity. The adolescent community reinforcement approach (A-CRA) uses cognitive and behavioral techniques to encourage prosocial activities toward recovery. Contingency management is a treatment that uses systems of incentives and rewards to encourage healthy behaviors, which can be combined with other behavioral treatments. Adjuncts to traditional clinical treatment, such as 12-step programs, residential programs, and youth community groups, offer peer support and facilitate identity formation separate from parents.

Family engagement is key to treatment success. Multidimensional family therapy (MDFT) is a technique developed for adolescent substance use that has benefits even years later based on research-derived evidence about adolescent and family development. MDFT is a manualized weekly family therapy that occurs over 5–6 months. It aims to change parenting behaviors and family interactions. Other family interventions shown to be effective for substance use include multifamily educational intervention (MEI), which involves more structure and psychoeducation compared to MDFT [61].

For more novel initiatives, KEEP SAFE is a 16-week support and educational program to improve the caregiving environment and the youth–caregiver relationship, teaches parenting techniques, and coaches communication skills, with evidence to support significantly less substance use [62]. Additional preventive interventions can be seen in Table 15.3, with the understanding that they aim to increase prosocial behaviors, peer relationships, academic functioning, provide adequate duration of treatment, include follow-up care, and simultaneously address comorbid psychiatric disorders through psychosocial therapies and/or medications [63]. For most addiction treatments, a 3-month timeline is often considered the

Table 15.3 Novel preventive interventions for substance use

Prevention level	Name of the program	Age (years)	Comments
Primary	Good Behavior Game	6–10	Teaches self-control, delayed gratification, teamwork, and problem-solving
	Alcohol from SAMHSA	10–12	Games explore brain science and allow practice responding to difficult social situations involving alcohol
	PlayForward: smokeSCREEN	10–16	Encourages decision-making and risk analysis of e-cigarette and vaping
	Line Up Live Up	13–18	A "sports-based life skills training curriculum" aiming to reduce violence, crime, and drug use among at-risk and marginalized youth
Secondary	SBIRTOregon.org Screening App	10+	Guides the patient through self-administered substance and depression screening using validated tools based on their age, summarizes the results for the provider, and provides handouts and guidance for a brief intervention
	iHELP	16–20	A smartphone-based motivational interviewing intervention to reduce substance use among foster youth transitioning to independent living
Tertiary	This is quitting	13—24	Text-to-quit vaping service with real-time messaging for managing cravings and triggers
	reSET and reSET-O	18+	CBT-based app to be used in combination with treatment for nonopioid or opioid-SUD. FDA-approved prescription only

minimum duration of care, while recognizing that for adolescents, 2 of the 3 pillars of treatment (medical/psychiatric care, counseling, and peer support) will likely go on indefinitely, to help assist with the various transitions that will occur on their path to adulthood (i.e., relationships, housing transitions, college or academic changes, and employment) [36, 63].

Pharmacotherapy Approaches

Treatment of adolescents with SUDs ought to include multiple approaches, addressing psychosocial issues, family dynamics, individual therapy, and 12-step programs, in addition to considering pharmacological interventions. Due to the limited number of child and adolescent addiction specialists, PCPs are encouraged to treat SUDs with the support of programs like Project Echo and the Prescriber's Clinical Support System (PCSS) Mentoring Program that can help expand PCPs' scope of practice via specialist outreach directly to pediatric addiction specialists [36].

Outside of the need for acute intoxication or withdrawal management, currently, medications are generally not recommended for youth, except for buprenorphine, which has evidence supporting its use for opioid use disorder, due to limited research and lack of US FDA approval for other treatments. This is understandable when you consider that developmental differences exist in adolescents' neurobiology, maturation of neurotransmitters, pharmacodynamics, and pharmacokinetics, including age-related changes in body fat, extracellular water, hepatic and renal function altering bioavailability, metabolism, and clearance of drugs [64–66]. Medications currently play a limited role beyond improving withdrawal and short-term intoxication, but there should be an examination for their use, especially when considering multiple substance use.

Alcohol

Current FDA-approved treatments for adults are not formally approved in adolescents and youth. However, following a recent literature review, naltrexone, disulfiram, and topiramate were suggested to be safe, well-tolerated, and showed promising results as an adjunctive treatment for AUD in youth [67]. Separately, acamprosate has limited data, but one double-blind placebo-controlled study revealed significantly more abstinence among adolescents taking acamprosate after 90 days [68]. Regarding treatments for acute intoxication and withdrawal, there are no adolescent or youth-specific guidelines, and treatment is similar to adults. For all these medications, use in adolescents regarding dosing and laboratory monitoring is the same as for adults.

Tobacco and Nicotine

For tobacco addiction, psychosocial treatments are the first line for adolescents. Unlike adults, pharmacotherapy has shown limited results with youth and adolescents. There are currently no FDA-approved medications or nicotine replacement therapies (NRT) for adolescents under age 18; however, NRT and bupropion are the most used in conjunction with psychosocial treatments in adolescents. Of NRT, research exists only for the patch and the gum in adolescents, which have some mixed results, but many show decreased withdrawal and decreased rates of cigarette use [69]. Further discussion should be given to varenicline, as it performed like bupropion, but there is hesitation due to previously documented psychiatric side effects [67].

However, cigarette smoking prevalence is at its lowest level ever recorded in high school-age students (14–18 years old) following the expansion of electronic cigarettes, also called e-cigarettes or vapes, and nicotine pouches [70]. Vapes are battery-powered devices that heat a liquid, usually containing nicotine and flavorings, and produce an aerosol that users inhale. They have become the most commonly used commercial tobacco and nicotine product in youth. Nicotine pouches are small, prefilled, spit-free microfiber pouches designed to deliver nicotine through the oral mucosa that contain nicotine powder rather than tobacco leaf, typically found in smokeless tobacco. Despite only having 34 e-cigarette marketing authorizations from the FDA in July 2024, there are an abundance of illicit brands flooding the market, while there are at least 24 new nicotine pouch brands that are "coming soon." While e-cigarettes and nicotine pouches can and likely will help cigarette smokes transition to less risky products, their lack of FDA authorizations and monitoring come with their own risks [70]. There is emerging data that varenicline can be helpful in increasing vaping abstinence for those who vape and do not smoke tobacco [71].

Benzodiazepines

Misuse of prescription medications such as benzodiazepines is increasingly common among youth. Overdose and withdrawal can be life-threatening, and currently there are no youth- or adolescent-specific guidelines. Prescription drug monitoring programs have been shown to decrease prescription dispensing in adolescents but caused no change in benzodiazepine-related overdoses [72]. Treatment for withdrawal should follow general medical principles used in the management of adults. Currently, there is little research on youth-specific treatment for maintenance or long-term treatment. Management usually involves tapering the dose of the misused agent with psychosocial support, group, and individual therapy.

Cannabis

Despite being one of the third most used substances in adolescence, and having a similar pattern in adults, there are no FDA treatments of Cannabis Use Disorder in adults or adolescents. There have been open-label pilot studies and controlled pharmacotherapy trials, and two studies suggest N-acetylcysteine (NAC) may be helpful in reducing cannabis use in adolescents, aged 15–21, by more than doubling the likelihood of abstinence at 12 weeks [67]. Future clinical practice guidelines should come out of future NIDA CTN studies.

Opioids

Opioid Use Disorder is one of the only SUDs that does have an FDA-approved pharmacological treatment in pediatric patients. This comes with a caveat because despite the evidence suggesting that buprenorphine is better than clonidine in treating withdrawal symptoms and can be effective in active treatment, alongside methadone, there are hesitations in its use [67]. The concern is that using an agonist-based therapy in an adolescent leads to impacts on their developing brain, endocrine system, and long-term effects of prolonged physical dependence in youth. Interestingly, buprenorphine-naloxone and counseling are more effective than detoxification followed by behavioral counseling, but once medications are discontinued, adolescents typically relapse, and 12-month outcomes are the same [67]. Under specific situations, requiring documentation of two treatment failures of drug-free detoxication followed by a psychosocial intervention, adolescents can be referred to a licensed and regulated specialty clinic and prescribed methadone [67]. With all these considerations, clinicians may opt to use Naltrexone XR, although this should not be considered first line given documented poor adherence and data, in addition to ensuring intranasal naloxone is given for the potential overdose [73].

The hesitation to prescribe agonist medication is shown in 2020 data, where pediatricians, where most children under 18 get their care, had only prescribed 1% of the buprenorphine dispensed; multistate Medicaid data indicates that less than a 25% of adolescents and young adults with OUD, and only 1-in-21 youth aged under 18 years old, received MOUD within 3 months of diagnosis; and 1.9% of youth were prescribed any medications within 30 days of a nonfatal overdose [74]. Despite the delay in care, there are several studies showing adolescents starting on anywhere ranging 2–8 mg within a buprenorphine induction, with additional doses in the same range, and maximum doses usually ranging 8–16 mg, and rare instances of the total daily dose reaching 32 mg [75, 76]. Additional studies assessed "low-dose" methadone maintenance with doses ranging 10–60 mg, with an average of 20 mg, during a 14-week maintenance period followed by a 14-week taper off [76]. Comparatively, data demonstrates that buprenorphine has lower retention rates compared to methadone, but both equally suppress illicit opioid use in youths [76].

Chapter Review Questions

1. A meta-analysis investigating the relationship between adolescent cannabis use and later anxiety outcomes found a significant association between frequent cannabis use during adolescence and an increased risk of anxiety disorders or symptoms in adulthood. Which of the following actions would be most appropriate based on these findings?

   A. A Encourage cannabis use during adolescence to prevent anxiety disorders.
   B. Focus public health efforts on reducing adolescent cannabis use to lower future anxiety risks.
   C. Ignore the relationship between cannabis use and anxiety disorders, as it is insignificant.
   D. Prioritize addressing anxiety disorders in adolescence over reducing cannabis use to lower future mental health risks.
   E. Limit discussions about cannabis risks to adults, as adolescent substance use is unlikely to persist into adulthood.

   Correct Answer: B.

   Explanation: The findings highlight a clear link between adolescent cannabis use and an increased risk of developing anxiety disorders later in life. Public health interventions should focus on reducing cannabis use in adolescents to minimize these future mental health risks.

   Reference: Lowe et al. [77].

2. Which of the following statements best describes the effects of e-cigarettes on children and adolescents?

   A. E-cigarette use in adolescents is associated with a reduced likelihood of using other psychoactive substances later in life.
   B. E-cigarette use in adolescents has no significant impact on mental health or future substance use.
   C. E-cigarette use in adolescents increases the risk of future use of psychoactive substances, including cannabis and alcohol.
   D. E-cigarette use in adolescents is only harmful if nicotine is present in the e-liquid.
   E. E-cigarettes are a healthy alternative to cigarettes.

   Correct Answer: C.

   Explanation: Research has shown that e-cigarette use in adolescents is linked to a higher likelihood of using other substances, such as cannabis and alcohol, later in life. This highlights the importance of preventive measures in this age group.

   Reference: Lau et al. [78].

3. Which of the following best describes primary, secondary, and tertiary prevention in treating cannabis-induced psychosis (CIP) with antipsychotics?

   A. *Primary prevention* educates people on the risks of cannabis use, *secondary prevention* involves early detection and intervention, and *tertiary prevention* focuses on using antipsychotics to treat established psychosis.
   B. *Primary prevention* involves giving antipsychotics to all cannabis users, *secondary prevention* treats only severe cases, and *tertiary prevention* requires long-term care without medication.
   C. *Primary prevention* starts after psychosis has already occurred, *secondary prevention* involves avoiding medication, and *tertiary prevention* encourages discontinuing cannabis use.
   D. *Primary prevention* stops cannabis use, *secondary prevention* only uses antipsychotics once psychosis is fully established, and *tertiary prevention* avoids all future treatment.
   E. *Primary prevention* screening for cannabis use disorder, *secondary prevention* attending cannabis anonymous groups, and *tertiary prevention* encourages discontinuing cannabis use.

   Correct Answer: A.

   Explanation: Primary prevention efforts aim to prevent disease or injury. For example, health education programs on substance use prevention in schools. Secondary prevention efforts aim to detect and address disease or injury in its early states before significant symptoms or complications occur: for example, screening adolescents for substance use to intervene before dependency develops. Finally, tertiary prevention efforts aim to manage and reduce the impact of established disease or injury, improving quality of life and preventing further complications: for instance, support groups and counseling individuals with chronic health conditions. In this instance answer choice *A* meets these criteria: *Primary prevention* educates people on the risks of cannabis use, *secondary prevention* involves early detection and intervention, and *tertiary prevention* focuses on using antipsychotics to treat established psychosis.

Reference: Chuenchom et al. [79].

4. Unintentional injuries are the leading cause of death in teens and most often are associated with substance use. Which of the following is an example of universal prevention for reducing unintentional injuries related to substance use in adolescents?

   A. Screening adolescents with a history of substance use for early signs of addiction.
   B. Implementing school-based programs that educate all students about the risks of alcohol and drug use while driving.
   C. Providing counseling services for teens who have already been involved in drug-related accidents.
   D. Offering rehabilitation programs for teens with a substance use disorder.
   E. Offering an educational workshop to parents with teens who have substance use disorders.

   Correct Answer: B.

   Explanation: This answer represents *universal prevention*, which targets the entire population (all adolescents) to prevent risky behaviors like driving under the influence of substances, aiming to reduce unintentional injuries before they occur.

   Reference: Cunningham et al. [80].

5. Which of the following medications is FDA-approved for treating opioid use disorder in adolescents aged 16 and older?

   A. Methadone
   B. Buprenorphine
   C. Naltrexone
   D. Naloxone
   E. Vivitrol

   Correct Answer: B.

   Explanation: Buprenorphine is the only FDA-approved medication for opioid use disorder in adolescents aged 16 and older. While methadone is approved for adults, it is not FDA-approved for adolescents under 18. Naltrexone can be used in certain cases but is not specifically FDA-approved for adolescents.

   Reference: AACAP et al. [81].

References

1. Casey BJ, Jones RM. Neurobiology of the adolescent brain and behavior: implications for substance use disorders. J Am Acad Child Adolesc Psychiatry. 2010;49(12):1189–201.
2. Shatkin JP. Child & adolescent mental health: a practical, all-in-one guide. New York: W. W. Norton & Company; 2015. Print.
3. The American Academy of Child and Adolescent Psychiatry. Severe shortage of child and adolescent psychiatrists illustrated in AACAP workforce maps [Internet]. [cited 2025 Aug 17]. Available from: https://www.aacap.org/AACAP/zLatest_News/Severe_Shortage_Child_Adolescent_Psychiatrists_Illustrated_AACAP_Workforce_Maps.aspx#:~:text=There%20are%20approximately%2010%2C500%20practicing,adolescent%20psychiatrists%20is%2052%20years.
4. U.S. Census Bureau Quickfacts: United States [Internet]. [cited 2025 Aug 17]. Available from: https://www.census.gov/quickfacts/fact/table/US/AGE295223#AGE295223.
5. Cleveland MJ, Feinberg ME, Bontempo DE, Greenberg MT. The role of risk and protective factors in substance use across adolescence. J Adolesc Health. 2008;43(2):157–64.
6. Johnston LD, Miech RA, Bachman JG, et al. Monitoring the future national survey results on drug use, 1975–2016: overview, key findings on adolescent drug use. Ann Arbor: University of Michigan Institute for Social Research; 2017.
7. Boak A, Elton-Marshall T, Mann RE, Hamilton HA. Drug use among Ontario students, 1977–2019: detailed findings from the Ontario Student Drug Use and Health Survey (OSDUHS). Toronto: Centre for Addiction and Mental Health; 2020.
8. Richmond-Rakerd LS, Slutske WS, Wood PK. Age of initiation and substance use progression: a multivariate latent growth analysis. Psychol Addict Behav. 2017;31(6):664.
9. Results from the 2024 National Survey on Drug Use and … [Internet]. 2025 [cited 2025 Dec 20]. Available from: https://www.samhsa.gov/data/sites/default/files/reports/rpt56287/2024-nsduh-annual-national-report.pdf.
10. Halladay J, Woock R, El-Khechen H, Munn C, MacKillop J, Amlung M, Ogrodnik M, Favotto L, Aryal K, Noori A, Kiflen M. Patterns of substance use among adolescents: a systematic review. Drug Alcohol Depend. 2020;216:108222.
11. Simon KM, Levy SJ, Bukstein OG. Adolescent substance use disorders. NEJM Evid. 2022;1(6):EVIDra2200051.
12. Abuse S. Treatment episode data set (TEDS): 2002–2012. National admissions to substance abuse treatment services. In: BHSIS Series S-71, HHS Publication No.(SMA) 14-4850. Rockville: Substance Abuse and Mental Health Services Administration; 2014.
13. Lipari RN, Park-Lee E. Key substance use and mental health indicators in the United States: results from the 2019 National Survey on Drug Use and Health. Rockville: Center for Behavioral Health Statistics and Quality, Substance Abuse and Mental Health Services Administration; 2020. HHS publication no. PEP20-07-01-001, NSDUH Series H-55.
14. Johnson SB, Blum RW, Giedd JN. Adolescent maturity and the brain: the promise and pitfalls of neuroscience research in adolescent health policy. J Adolesc Health. 2009;45:216–21. https://doi.org/10.1016/j.jadohealth.2009.05.016.
15. Sowell ER, Thompson PM, Holmes CJ, Jernigan TL, Toga AW. In vivo evidence for post-adolescent brain maturation in frontal and striatal regions. Nat Neurosci. 1999;2(10):859–61.
16. Hingson RW, Zha W. Age of drinking onset, alcohol use disorders, frequent heavy drinking, and unintentionally injuring oneself and others after drinking. Pediatrics. 2009;123(6):1477–84.
17. Le Strat Y, Dubertret C, Le Foll B. Impact of age at onset of cannabis use on cannabis dependence and driving under the influence in the United States. Accid Anal Prev. 2015;76:1–5.
18. McCabe SE, West BT, Morales M, Cranford JA, Boyd CJ. Does early onset of non-medical use of prescription drugs predict subsequent prescription drug abuse and dependence? Results from a national study. Addiction. 2007;102(12):1920–30.
19. Willuhn I, Wanat MJ, Clark JJ, Phillips PE. Dopamine signaling in the nucleus accumbens of animals self-administering drugs of abuse. Curr Top Behav Neurosci. 2010;3:29–71.

20. Ernst M, Luciana M. Neuroimaging of the dopamine/reward system in adolescent drug use. CNS Spectr. 2015;20(4):427–41.
21. Jordan CJ, Andersen SL. Sensitive periods of substance abuse: early risk for the transition to dependence. Dev Cogn Neurosci. 2017;25:29–44.
22. NIDA. Principles of adolescent substance use disorder treatment: a research-based guide. National Institute on Drug Abuse website; 2014. https://www.drugabuse.gov/publications/principles-adolescent-substance-use-disorder-treatment-research-based-guide. Accessed 18 Oct 2018.
23. Bjork JM, Chen G, Smith AR, Hommer DW. Incentive-elicited mesolimbic activation and externalizing symptomatology in adolescents. J Child Psychol Psychiatry. 2010;51(7):827–37.
24. Bjork JM, Smith AR, Chen G, Hommer DW. Mesolimbic recruitment by nondrug rewards in detoxified alcoholics: effort anticipation, reward anticipation, and reward delivery. Hum Brain Mapp. 2012;33(9):2174–88.
25. Dwyer JB, McQuown SC, Leslie FM. The dynamic effects of nicotine on the developing brain. Pharmacol Ther. 2009;122(2):125–39.
26. Schoenfelder EN, Faraone SV, Kollins SH. Stimulant treatment of ADHD and cigarette smoking: a meta-analysis. Pediatrics. 2014;133(6):1070–80.
27. Squeglia LM, Jacobus J, Tapert SF. The influence of substance use on adolescent brain development. Clin EEG Neurosci. 2009;40(1):31–8.
28. Wade NE, Bagot KS, Tapert SF, Gruber SA, Filbey FM, Lisdahl KM. Cognitive functioning related to binge alcohol and cannabis co-use in abstinent adolescents and young adults. J Stud Alcohol Drugs. 2020;81(4):479–83.
29. Cawkwell PB, Hong DS, Leikauf JE. Neurodevelopmental effects of cannabis use in adolescents and emerging adults with ADHD: a systematic review. Harv Rev Psychiatry. 2021;29(4):251–61.
30. National Research Council (U.S.), O'Connell M, Boat T, Warner K, Boat T, Warner KE, et al. Preventing mental, emotional, and behavioral disorders among young people: progress and possibilities. Washington, DC: National Academies Press; 2009.
31. Cruz JE, Emery RE, Turkheimer E. Peer network drinking predicts increased alcohol use from adolescence to early adulthood after controlling for genetic and shared environmental selection. Dev Psychol. 2012;48(5):1390.
32. Liu J, Zhao S, Chen X, Falk E, Albarracín D. The influence of peer behavior as a function of social and cultural closeness: a meta-analysis of normative influence on adolescent smoking initiation and continuation. Psychol Bull. 2017;143(10):1082.
33. Davis JP, Pedersen ER, Tucker JS, Dunbar MS, Seelam R, Shih R, D'Amico EJ. Long-term associations between substance use-related media exposure, descriptive norms, and alcohol use from adolescence to young adulthood. J Youth Adolesc. 2019;48:1311–26.
34. Weitzman M, Lee L. Similarities between alcohol and tobacco advertising exposure and adolescent use of each of these substances. J Stud Alcohol Drugs Suppl. 2020;19:97–105.
35. Hawkins JD, Catalano RF, Miller JY. Risk and protective factors for alcohol and other drug problems in adolescence and early adulthood: implications for substance abuse prevention. Psychol Bull. 1992;112(1):64.
36. Nelson LF, Weitzman ER, Levy S. Prevention of substance use disorders. Med Clin. 2022;106(1):153–68.
37. Calafat A, Garcia F, Juan M, et al. Which parenting style is more protective against adolescent substance use? Evidence within the European context. Drug Alcohol Depend. 2014;138:185–92.
38. Pilowsky DJ, Wu LT. Psychiatric symptoms and substance use disorders in a nationally representative sample of American adolescents involved with foster care. J Adolesc Health. 2006;38(4):351–8.
39. Goldbach JT, Tanner-Smith EE, Bagwell M, et al. Minority stress and substance use in sexual minority adolescents: a meta-analysis. Prev Sci. 2014;15(3):350–63.
40. Lisha NE, Sussman S. Relationship of high school and college sports participation with alcohol, tobacco, and illicit drug use: a review. Addict Behav. 2010;35(5):399–407.

41. Mays D, DePadilla L, Thompson NJ, Kushner HI, Windle M. Sports participation and problem alcohol use: a multi-wave national sample of adolescents. Am J Prev Med. 2010;38(5):491–8.
42. Chassin L. Juvenile justice and substance use. Futur Child. 2008;18(2):165–83.
43. Bolton JM, Robinson J, Sareen J. Self-medication of mood disorders with alcohol and drugs in the National Epidemiologic Survey on Alcohol and Related Conditions. J Affect Disord. 2009;115(3):367–75.
44. Fergusson DM, Boden JM, Horwood LJ. Structural models of the comorbidity of internalizing disorders and substance use disorders in a longitudinal birth cohort. Soc Psychiatry Psychiatr Epidemiol. 2011;46:933–42.
45. Köck P, Meyer M, Elsner J, Dürsteler KM, Vogel M, Walter M. Co-occurring mental disorders in transitional aged youth with substance use disorders–a narrative review. Front Psych. 2022;13:827658.
46. Quinn PD, Chang Z, Hur K, Gibbons RD, Lahey BB, Rickert ME, Sjölander A, Lichtenstein P, Larsson H, D'Onofrio BM. ADHD medication and substance-related problems. Am J Psychiatry. 2017;174(9):877–85.
47. Özgen H, Spijkerman R, Noack M, Holtmann M, Schellekens A, Dalsgaard S, van den Brink W, Hendriks V. Treatment of adolescents with concurrent substance use disorder and attention-deficit/hyperactivity disorder: a systematic review. J Clin Med. 2021;10(17):3908.
48. Dalsgaard S, Mortensen PB, Frydenberg M, et al. ADHD, stimulant treatment in childhood and subsequent substance abuse in adulthood—a naturalistic long term follow-up study. Addict Behav. 2014;39(1):325–8.
49. Bukstein OG, Horner MS. Management of the adolescent with substance use disorders and comorbid psychopathology. Child Adolesc Psychiatr Clin N Am. 2010;19(3):609–23.
50. Spas J, et al. All might have won, but not all have the prize: optimal treatment for substance abuse among adolescents with conduct problems. Subst Abuse. 2012;6:141–55.
51. Scott K, Becker SJ, Helseth SA, Saldanha IJ, Balk EM, Adam GP, Konnyu KJ, Steele DW. Pharmacotherapy interventions for adolescent co-occurring substance use and mental health disorders: a systematic review. Fam Pract. 2022;39(2):301–10.
52. Chasser YM. Profiles of youths with PTSD and addiction. J Child Adolesc Subst Abuse. 2016;25(5):448–54. https://doi.org/10.1080/1067828X.2015.1081115.
53. Burkstein O. Substance use disorder in adolescents: epidemiology, pathogenesis, clinical manifestations and consequences, course, assessment, and diagnosis. UpToDate. 2020. https://www.uptodate.com/contents/.
54. Adams SH, Park MJ, Twietmeyer L, Brindis CD, Irwin CE. Association between adolescent preventive care and the role of the Affordable Care Act. JAMA Pediatr. 2018;172(1):43–8.
55. Screening, brief intervention, and referral to treatment (SBIRT) [Internet]. 2024 [cited 2025 Aug 7]. Available from: https://www.samhsa.gov/substance-use/treatment/sbirt.
56. Screening to brief intervention (S2BI) [Internet]. [cited 2025 Aug 1]. Available from: https://www.samhsa.gov/resource/ebp/screening-brief-intervention-s2bi.
57. The Center for Adolescent Behavioral Health Research [Internet]. 2018 [cited 2025 Aug 7]. Available from: https://crafft.org/.
58. Teens screening tool: brief screener for tobacco, alcohol, and other drugs [Internet]. U.S. Department of Health and Human Services; [cited 2025 Aug 7]. Available from: https://nida.nih.gov/bstad/.
59. Hogue A, Henderson CE, Becker SJ, Knight DK. Evidence base on outpatient behavioral treatments for adolescent substance use, 2014–2017: outcomes, treatment delivery, and promising horizons. J Clin Child Adolesc Psychol. 2018;47(4):499–526.
60. Waldron HB, Kaminer Y. On the learning curve: the emerging evidence supporting cognitive-behavioral therapies for adolescent substance abuse. Addiction. 2004;99 Suppl 2(Suppl 2):93–105. https://doi.org/10.1111/j.1360-0443.2004.00857.x. PMID: 15488108; PMCID: PMC1781376.
61. Filges T, Rasmussen PS, Andersen D, Jørgensen AM. Multidimensional family therapy (MDFT) for young people in treatment for non-opioid drug abuse: a systematic review. Campbell Syst Rev. 2015;11(1):1–24.

62. Kim HK, Buchanan R, Price JM. Pathways to preventing substance use among youth in foster care. Prev Sci. 2017;18:567–76.
63. Spencer AE, Valentine SE, Sikov J, Yule AM, Hsu H, Hallett E, Xuan Z, Silverstein M, Fortuna L. Principles of care for young adults with co-occurring psychiatric and substance use disorders. Pediatrics. 2021;147(Supplement 2):229–39.
64. Fernandez E, Perez R, Hernandez A, Tejada P, Arteta M, Ramos JT. Factors and mechanisms for pharmacokinetic differences between pediatric population and adults. Pharmaceutics. 2011;3(1):53–72.
65. Vitiello B. Developmental aspects of pediatric psychopharmacology. In: Findling RL, editor. Clinical manual of child & adolescent psychopharmacology. Arlington, VA: American Psychiatric Association; 2008. p. 1–31.
66. van den Anker JN, Schwab M, Kearns GL. Developmental pharmacokinetics. Pediatr Clin Pharmacol. 2011;205:51–75.
67. Hammond CJ. The role of pharmacotherapy in the treatment of adolescent substance use disorders. Child Adolesc Psychiatr Clin. 2016;25(4):685–711.
68. Niederhofer H, Staffen W. Acamprosate and its efficacy in treating alcohol dependent adolescents. Eur Child Adolesc Psychiatry. 2003;12(3):144–8.
69. Karpinski JP, Timpe EM, Lubsch L. Smoking cessation treatment for adolescents. J Pediatr Pharmacol Ther. 2010;15(4):249–63.
70. Delnevo CD, Hrywna M. Lessons learned from E-cigarettes should affect FDA regulation of nicotine pouches. JAMA. 2025;333(5):373–4.
71. Evins AE, Cather C, Reeder HT, Evohr B, Potter K, Pachas GN, Gray KM, Levy S, Rigotti NA, Iroegbulem V, Dufour J, Casottana K, Costello MA, Gilman JM, Schuster RM. Varenicline for youth nicotine vaping cessation: a randomized clinical trial. JAMA. 2025;333(21):1876–86. https://doi.org/10.1001/jama.2025.3810. PMID: 40266580; PMCID: PMC12019676.
72. Toce MS, Michelson KA, Hudgins JD, Olson KL, Monuteaux MC, Bourgeois FT. Association of prescription drug monitoring programs with benzodiazepine prescription dispensation and overdose in adolescents and young adults. Clin Toxicol. 2023;61(4):234–40.
73. Mitchell SG, Monico LB, Gryczynski J, Fishman MJ, O'Grady KE, Schwartz RP. Extended-release naltrexone for youth with opioid use disorder. J Subst Abus Treat. 2021;130:108407.
74. Terranella A, Guy GP Jr, Mikosz C. Buprenorphine dispensing among youth aged ≤19 years in the United States: 2015–2020. Pediatrics. 2023;151(2):e2022058755.
75. Borodovsky JT, Levy S, Fishman M, Marsch LA. Buprenorphine treatment for adolescents and young adults with opioid use disorders: a narrative review. J Addict Med. 2018;12(3):170–83.
76. Robinson CA, Wilson JD. Management of opioid misuse and opioid use disorders among youth. Pediatrics. 2020;145(Supplement_2):S153–64.
77. Lowe DJE, Sorkhou M, George TP. Cannabis use in adolescents and anxiety symptoms and disorders: a systematic review and meta-analysis. Am J Drug Alcohol Abuse. 2024;50(2):150–61. https://doi.org/10.1080/00952990.2023.2299922. Epub 2024 Jan 29. PMID: 38285048.
78. Lau L, Conti AA, Hemmati Z, Baldacchino A. The prospective association between the use of E-cigarettes and other psychoactive substances in young people: a systematic review and meta-analysis. Neurosci Biobehav Rev. 2023;153:105392. https://doi.org/10.1016/j.neubiorev.2023.105392. Epub 2023 Sep 14. PMID: 37714228.
79. Chuenchom O, Suansanae T, Lukanapichonchut L, Suwanmajo S, Suthisisang C. Real world clinical outcomes of treatment of cannabis-induced psychosis and prevalence of cannabis-related primary psychosis: a retrospective study. BMC Psychiatry. 2024;24(1):626.
80. Cunningham RM, Walton MA, Carter PM. The major causes of death in children and adolescents in the United States. N Engl J Med. 2018;379(25):2468–75. https://doi.org/10.1056/NEJMsr1804754.
81. AACAP. Opioid use disorder treatment for Youth [Internet]. [cited 2025 Aug 19]. Available from: https://www.aacap.org/AACAP/Policy_Statements/2020/Opioid_Use_Disorder_Treatment_Youth.aspx#:~:text=Buprenorphine%2Fnaloxone%20is%20a%20medication,to%20increase%20abstinence%20in%20youth%20.

Women and Pregnancy

16

Natasia S. Courchesne-Krak
and Stephanie A. Meyers-Pantele

High-Yield Review Points

- Women who use substances may progress more quickly from first use to substance use disorder, may experience more intense withdrawal symptoms, and may respond differently to pharmacological treatments.
- Women face greater barriers to entering substance use treatment, including greater substance-use-related stigma, family responsibilities, fear of child protective service involvement, and a greater likelihood of comorbid mood and anxiety disorders.
- Clinicians should adopt sex- and gender-responsive and trauma-informed approaches when treating women who use substances, including motivational interviewing techniques, contingency management, community reinforcement approaches, and medications as appropriate.

Introduction

Historically, substance misuse has been primarily conceptualized as a male problem, and, as such, most substance use treatment research has focused on male populations. In more recent years, however, the scientific community has recognized that there are significant sex and gender differences in substance use processes,

N. S. Courchesne-Krak (✉)
Department of Psychiatry, University of California San Diego, La Jolla, CA, USA
e-mail: ncourchesne@health.ucsd.edu

S. A. Meyers-Pantele
Division of Infectious Diseases and Global Public Health, University of California San Diego, La Jolla, CA, USA
e-mail: s3meyers@health.ucsd.edu

C. Marienfeld, M. Soltani (eds.), *AAAP Review of Addiction Psychiatry*,
https://doi.org/10.1007/978-3-032-24174-0_16

trajectories, and related harms. It is important to acknowledge that significant gender differences also exist in these processes and trajectories for transgender, nonbinary, and gender-diverse populations (see Chap. 17). This chapter, however, focuses specifically on the processes and harms affecting cisgender women—those whose gender identity aligns with the sex they were assigned at birth. Throughout this chapter, the term "women" or "men" will predominantly refer to cisgender women and men, while recognizing that gender diversity exists, and some aspects may also apply to a broader range of gender identities. A thorough discussion of the epidemiology, consequences of use, screening and diagnostic tools, and treatment considerations for women who use substances, including during pregnancy, follows.

Epidemiology

Substance Use Among Women

Substance use rates vary significantly between women and men, influenced by both biological and social factors. Sex-based differences in brain function, hormonal regulation, and social environments shape how individuals experience and engage with substances. Compared to women, men are more likely to use almost every type of substance (including cannabis and prescription medication misuse) [1], and their use is more likely to result in emergency department visits or overdose deaths [1]. Additionally, though women tend to have higher rates of the psychotherapeutic use of substances with potential for misuse (e.g., pain relievers, tranquilizers, stimulants, or sedatives, not including over-the-counter drugs), men have higher rates of misuse of these substances [2]. Although men are more likely to engage in substance use, and therefore their rates of substance dependence are higher, women are *as* likely to develop a substance use disorder (SUD) as men [3], and they use smaller amounts of certain drugs for less time before they develop an SUD [2]. Women who misuse substances such as stimulants may do so for reasons related to gendered social roles and responsibilities, such as managing work and family duties, which may contribute to patterns of use and dependence that differ from those observed in men [4]. Research suggests that women may be more susceptible to cravings and relapse when compared to men, which are important components of the SUD cycle [2]. However, men are more vulnerable to overdose deaths caused by opioid and stimulant drugs, even when factoring in differing state-level environmental conditions and drug misuse levels [5]. These differences may stem from culturally influenced differences between women and men, particularly their tendency toward risky behaviors, which go beyond the inherent risks of opioid or stimulant misuse. Examples include injecting drugs while alone, taking excessively large doses, or using unreliable suppliers. Treatment engagement is relatively similar between sexes, with males and females aged 12 years or older receiving treatment at similar rates (~2%; Table 16.1). However, despite substantial treatment need, national reports have shown that SUD treatment utilization remains low overall, with only 10.6% of adults with a past-year SUD receiving treatment [6]. Collectively, these findings underscore the importance of considering sex and gender differences, as well as shared patters in substance use trajectories, treatment engagement, and clinical outcomes.

Table 16.1 Substance use disorder and treatment in past year among those 12 or older, by **sex**: numbers in the thousands, 2023

	Total, *n* (%)	Males, *n* (%)	Females, *n* (%)
Substance use disorder			
Any substance use disorder	48,464 (17.1)	27,735 (20.0)	20,729 (14.3)
Alcohol use disorder	28,859 (10.2)	16,838 (12.1)	12,022 (8.3)
Marijuana use disorder	19,164 (6.8)	11,380 (8.2)	7784 (5.4)
Opioid use disorder	5679 (2.0)	2697 (1.9)	2982 (2.1)
Stimulant use disorder	4322 (1.5)	2502 (1.8)	1820 (1.3)
Drug use disorder	27,153 (9.6)	15,375 (11.1)	11,778 (8.1)
Treatment for substance use disorder			
Alcohol use treatment	4519 (1.6)	2549 (1.8)	1970 (1.4)
Drug use treatment	6073 (2.1)	2939 (2.1)	3134 (2.2)
Both alcohol and drug use treatment	1669 (0.6)	1024 (0.7)	645 (0.5)

Source: SAMHSA, Center for Behavioral Health Statistics and Quality, National Survey on Drug Use and Health, 2023. Tobacco use disorder was not reported in the 2023 report. Information on tobacco product use or nicotine vaping can be found here: https://www.samhsa.gov/data/release/2023-national-survey-drug-use-and-health-nsduh-releases#detailed-tables

Substance Use among Pregnant Women

Among pregnant women, legal substances (e.g., nicotine, alcohol) are the most problematic in terms of effect and magnitude. Estimates from the Centers for Disease Control (CDC) indicate that maternal smoking still poses a significant risk for infant health complications, contributing to around 23% of sudden infant death syndrome (SIDS) cases annually [7]. The detrimental effects of alcohol consumption during pregnancy, such as miscarriage, stillbirth, and fetal alcohol spectrum disorder (FASD), continue to make it the leading preventable cause of birth defects in the United States [8]. According to data from the 2023 National Survey on Drug Use and Health (NSDUH), 9.4% reported tobacco use or vaping and 8.4% of pregnant women reported alcohol use in the past month [9]. Pregnant women's use of other substances, though less common compared to nicotine and alcohol use, is still significant. Cannabis use, in particular, has increased in states where it is legalized, though past-month cannabis use among pregnant women was found to have decreased from 9.6% in 2022 to 4.9% in 2023 [9]. Additionally, opioid misuse during pregnancy has remained a significant concern, with about 6.6 per 1000 women giving birth diagnosed with an opioid use disorder (OUD) in 2020 [10]. The opioid epidemic has led to a marked rise in neonatal opioid withdrawal syndrome (NOWS), with figures showing that rates increased from 7 per 1000 births in 2016 to 8.8 per 1000 in 2020 [11]. Opioid-related complications in pregnancy have quadrupled since 1999, continuing to exert pressure on maternal and infant healthcare systems [10]. See the treatment section of this chapter for more detailed risks associated with each substance type (e.g., nicotine, alcohol, cannabis, stimulants, opioids).

Considerations of Use in Women and Pregnancies

Physiological Considerations

Women who misuse substances or have an SUD experience unique and severe physiological consequences, including higher risks for cardiovascular disease, liver damage, reproductive health issues, and immune system suppression [12]. They are more prone to conditions such as osteoporosis and cognitive decline and have an increased likelihood of co-occurring mental and physical health disorders [13–16]. These effects, compounded by sex differences in metabolism and hormonal regulation, result in heightened vulnerability to adverse health outcomes, including overdose and mortality.

Substance use during pregnancy poses concerns for maternal, fetal, and neonate health and wellness. Maternal morbidity outcomes related to substance use include preterm birth, placental complications such as placental abruption, hypertensive disorders such as pre-eclampsia, infections, and cardiac complications [17–21].

Many substances could potentially harm a fetus and increase the risk of long-term and fatal effects, such as congenital malformations, low birth weight for gestational age due to intrauterine growth restriction (IUGR), prematurity, microcephaly (small head circumference), prenatally acquired infections, complications of delivery, SIDS, and miscarriage [22]. Among women who use substances during pregnancy, the risk of stillbirth is two to three times greater compared to women who do not use these substances while pregnant [23]. Symptoms of NOWS can develop immediately or up to 14 days (about 2 weeks) post birth and may include diarrhea, excessive or high-pitched crying, irritability, increased heart rate, blotchy skin, seizures, rapid breathing, trembling, vomiting, or slow weight gain [24].

Social Considerations

Women who use substances also face several unique social consequences due to their substance dependence when compared to men. For example, women who use substances have been found to be more likely to have come from families in which one or more members are substance-dependent, to have experienced more disruption in their families, to be in relationships with substance-dependent partners, to cite relationship problems as a significant contributor to their own substance use, and to be diagnosed with a mood or anxiety disorder [25]. In addition, women who inject drugs (WWID) have been found to be more likely to have been initiated into injection drug use by a male intimate partner, to be injected after their initiator, and to share injection equipment. These practices place women at increased risk of blood-borne infections such as human immunodeficiency virus (HIV) and hepatitis C (HCV), bacterial infections, abscesses, and physical harm from being injected by someone who is intoxicated [26]. Further, women who use substances, including racially and ethnically diverse women, experience high rates of violence and intersectional stigma [26, 27], both of which have been linked to HIV transmission risk and healthcare service avoidance [26, 28].

Legal Considerations

In addition to the aforementioned risks, and due to the criminalization of many substances, women who use substances are at significant risk of involvement with law enforcement agencies and could face separation from their children if they are detained or incarcerated [26]. The number of women in jails and prisons in the United States remains at or near a historic high, with the majority incarcerated for nonviolent and drug-related offenses [29]. Importantly, although overall rates of incarceration have decreased in recent years, the decrease has been less pronounced for women than men [29]. These trends are particularly concerning given research indicating that women in prisons have higher prevalence of blood-borne infections and sexually transmitted infections, as well as more health problems overall, when compared to their male counterparts [26].

There are also several state laws and legal concerns that pertain to pregnant women who use substances, specifically. Over the past two decades, more states have adopted punitive rather than supportive policies related to substance use during pregnancy, in stark contrast with guidance from professional societies and federal agencies (e.g., the American College of Obstetricians and Gynecologists [ACOG], the American Academy of Pediatrics [AAP], and the Substance Abuse and Mental Health Services Administration [SAMHSA]) [30]. According to the most recent data available, there were 23 states and the District of Columbia that, under civil child welfare statutes, considered substance use during pregnancy to be child abuse or neglect in 2019 [31]. Research has consistently demonstrated that these punitive state-level policies do not serve to reduce neonatal abstinence syndromes (NAS), including NOWS, or maternal narcotic exposure at birth [32]. These policies do, however, deter women from seeking substance use treatment and prenatal care [32]. Due to the rapidly evolving policy landscape surrounding women's sexual and reproductive health, and the ever-changing nature of state laws, it is recommended that professionals refer to the Guttmacher Institute's website for up-to-date information on the specific state laws pertaining to pregnant women who use substances: https://www.guttmacher.org/state-policy/explore/substance-use-during-pregnancy.

Another important social consequence of substance dependence for women is involvement with Child Protective Services (CPS). Women who use drugs and WWID face a significant risk that disclosure of their drug use will lead to the notification of child protection authorities and that their children will be removed from their care [33]. Furthermore, once a report has been substantiated, the children of parents with substance issues are more likely to be placed in out-of-home care and to stay in care longer than other children [33]. The impact of child custody loss has been found to be akin to trauma for mothers who use substances, with many women reporting persistent post-traumatic stress disorder (PTSD) symptoms and increased substance use to cope with the separation [34]. These social consequences are important for clinicians to understand as they have implications for understanding the barriers to care that these women face and should guide approaches to treatment for this population.

Barriers to Care for Women Who Use Substances

Women have been found to be more likely than men to encounter barriers that prevent them from seeking or completing treatment [35]. For example, women are more likely to report having difficulty regularly attending treatment sessions due to family responsibilities and feelings of stigma, shame, and embarrassment because of being in substance use treatment [35]. Further, women remain underrepresented in SUD treatment, and many SUD treatment options are male-dominated spaces. This can further deter women who may feel unsafe in those spaces and/or feel like those spaces are not meant for them [36]. Additionally, women are disproportionately affected by mood and anxiety disorders, violence, and multiple, intersecting social stigmas (e.g., gender-, substance use-, race-related stigma), all of which have been demonstrated to act as significant barriers to accessing substance use treatment and other critically needed healthcare services [35]. Providing comprehensive services such as housing, transportation, education, and income support has been found to significantly reduce substance use after treatment for both women and men, but a greater proportion of women need these services [35]. Other barriers to care that have been cited by women include substance use itself, a lack of transportation, a lack of health insurance, financial barriers, and being unhoused [37]. Pregnant women who use substances have also reported additional barriers to seeking prenatal care, including delays in discovering their pregnancy, a lack of doctors willing to initiate treatment with women in their third trimester, fear of involvement with CPS, and/or incarceration [37]. Women who use substances, including pregnant women, may also have multiple, intersecting barriers that need to be addressed.

Screening and Diagnosis

Many women presenting for primary care visits and/or prenatal care will not self-identify as being at risk for SUDs [38]. Due to the stigma and barriers that women who use substances face, clinicians serving women should ensure that they are creating an environment where women are comfortable discussing their substance use histories [38]. Screening tools, often developed for men, may under-identify SUDs in women due to differing patterns of use, co-occurring disorders (e.g., trauma, depression), and underreporting. For example, women are less likely to report frequent binge drinking but may engage in lower, chronic levels of alcohol use, which some tools may not detect as problematic. Women-specific recommendations, such as those from the ACOG and United States Preventive Services Task Force (USPSTF), emphasize the need for integrated screenings in primary and prenatal care to better capture these differences.

ACOG recommends that all women who seek gynecological or maternity care be screened for substance use, especially alcohol, annually [39]. These screenings should be applied uniformly, regardless of age, sex, race, ethnicity, or socioeconomic status. For women with high-risk substance use, brief interventions or motivational interviewing (MI) techniques are recommended [38]. Screening Brief Intervention and Treatment (SBIRT), a comprehensive and integrated public health model for delivering early intervention services, has been recommended for addressing at-risk substance use in primary care settings for women [38]. The USPSTF endorses screening instruments for SBIRT, including the Alcohol Use Disorders Identification Test (AUDIT), validated for women [38], and the Drug Abuse Screening Test (DAST), which is useful across diverse populations, including women in the criminal justice system [40].

Early identification of SUDs in pregnant women is critical for minimizing harm to both mother and neonate. For example, ACOG recommends carefully phrased questions during prenatal visits, including inquiries about prescription opioids and other potential misused medications [41]. Screening should start at the initial prenatal visit and continue throughout pregnancy, with annual alcohol screenings recommended for all women and within the first trimester for pregnant women [39]. Though no universal tool exists to screen pregnant women for substance use, non-judgmental, open-ended questions during interviews or structured self-report tools like the 4Ps Plus can elicit valid substance use information and assess adverse pregnancy outcomes [42].

For screening alcohol use, validated tools include T-ACE [43], TWEAK [44], and AUDIT-C [41], which show high sensitivity for identifying risky prenatal drinking in systematic reviews [45]. For pregnant adolescents and young adults, the CRAFFT questionnaire is validated and includes questions related to substance use behaviors and risks [46]. The ALPHA tool, using CAGE-style questions, assesses maternal substance use and identifies psychosocial risk factors such as family violence and postpartum depression [47].

Co-occurring depression is common among women with SUDs, particularly during and after pregnancy [48]. Depression screenings should be conducted during intake and between four and six weeks postpartum [49]. Additionally, assessing trauma, such as childhood physical or sexual abuse, is vital and can be measured with tools such as the Trauma Symptom Inventory [50].

Approaches to Improve Outcomes and Treatment Considerations

Gender-Responsive and Trauma-Informed Harm Reduction and Treatment

Despite the wealth of research demonstrating that women have unique substance use-related trajectories, outcomes, and consequences, harm reduction and treatment options tailored directly toward women are still scarce. Gender responsive treatments (GRTs), however, have shown preliminary effectiveness in improving substance use and mental health treatment outcomes [51]. GRTs have been defined, more specifically, as treatment modalities that consider the unique gender-specific needs and concerns of people who use substances. While we recognize that transgender and non-binary persons have gender-specific needs within substance use treatment (see Chap. 17), this chapter is focused on the gender-specific needs of women within treatment settings (e.g., family responsibilities, increased levels of substance use-related stigma, higher prevalence of mood and anxiety disorders) and the use of GRT with this population [51]. Correspondingly, a systematic review of 24 studies employing GRT-based interventions has demonstrated that GRT is a promising approach that yields significantly better substance use and mental health outcomes for women over time relative to comparison groups [51].

Other gender-focused suggestions for substance use treatment have included providing transportation and daycare options for women looking to access substance use-related services. Additionally, treatment options that are tailored for specific populations of women, such as those that have co-occurring SUDs and other psychiatric disorders (e.g., mood or anxiety disorders), have been recommended [51]. Others have also suggested that family-centered treatment services, such as inpatient treatment options for mothers where their children can stay with them, be implemented [33]. Further, those calling for GRT options for women with SUDs have underscored the need for trauma-informed care-based approaches, given the high rates of violence this population experiences, and the negative impacts violence and trauma has on treatment engagement and retention [51]. Lastly, approaches that can address and reduce stigma for women who use drugs are critically needed considering the multiple, intersecting social stigmas (e.g., gender-, substance use-, and race-related stigma) this group experiences, and the barriers to care stigma creates [27]. More information on treatment for women with SUDs is included in the following section.

Treatment for Substance Use Disorders Among Women and Pregnant Women

Treatment for SUDs may progress differently in women than for men. For example, women have reported a shorter duration of substance use prior to entering treatment, indicating that women's substance use tends to progress more quickly from first use to SUD [52]. Research has also shown that women tend to respond better to treatments that address psychosocial stressors, trauma, and mental health comorbidities (such as anxiety and depression) [12].

For pregnant women, the optimal treatments for SUDs have been assessed in several randomized trials and observational studies, showing that treatment engagement and prenatal care improve maternal and neonatal outcomes [53]. Recent studies emphasize the effectiveness of treatment models that integrate medical care with behavioral health interventions [54]. Motivational Interviewing (MI), with or without behavioral incentives, has been shown to reduce maternal substance use and improve engagement in prenatal care [55]. Cognitive Behavioral Therapy (CBT), in conjunction with MI, demonstrated a significant reduction in substance use by approximately 50% in pregnant women during pilot studies [55]. Contingency Management (CM) remains the most supported approach for improving treatment attendance and substance abstinence, with consistent success in pregnant populations [56]. The community reinforcement approach (CRA) has also demonstrated effectiveness in some trials, particularly when combined with other interventions [53]. In a comprehensive care setting for pregnant women with SUDs, those treated with a combination of MI, CM, and CRA exhibited greater treatment utilization, higher abstinence rates, and reduced neonatal hospital stays compared to those receiving standard care [57]. In recent years, harm reduction approaches tailored to pregnant women have received increased attention. These models—grounded in nonjudgmental, trauma-informed care and strong therapeutic alliances—prioritize engagement over immediate abstinence, supporting safer use or reduced use while connecting individuals to social services, prenatal care, and behavioral health. Evidence shows such approaches improve retention in care, reduce substance use, enhance birth outcomes, and reduce healthcare costs [58–61]. Core to their success is building trust and self-efficacy through unconditional positive regard and motivational interviewing, which helps reduce stigma and fears around treatment disengagement, legal repercussions, or involvement with child welfare [62–64]. These strategies help pregnant women remain engaged in services that benefit both maternal and neonatal health [65–68]. Women- and pregnancy-focused treatment recommendations for specific substances are included in the sections below.

Alcohol

Women metabolize alcohol differently from men, leading to higher blood alcohol concentrations even with the same alcohol intake due to factors such as lower body water content, slower gastric emptying, and differences in liver enzyme activity. This increases their risk for alcohol-related conditions such as liver disease and cardiovascular complications at lower consumption levels [69]. Treatment for women with alcohol use disorders (AUD) typically begins with psychotherapeutic interventions (e.g., CBT, MI, mutual-help groups). If these approaches are insufficient, medications such as naltrexone, acamprosate, and disulfiram may be used to reduce cravings and prevent relapse. Care plans should also address psychosocial and medical needs, particularly if co-occurring conditions are present. While pharmacological treatments such as naltrexone are equally effective for both women and men in managing cravings and relapse, side effects such as nausea may be more common in women [70].

In pregnancy, brief psychotherapeutic interventions, particularly MI, are the preferred approach to reducing alcohol use. While some studies report positive reductions in alcohol use among pregnant women, others indicate minimal change, depending on factors such as the intensity of the intervention, baseline drinking behaviors, and individual characteristics of the participants [71]. The effectiveness of MI may also be influenced by how interventions are implemented, with outcomes differing based on the delivery method (e.g., online) and participant engagement

[72]. Most medications used to treat AUD, such as naltrexone, acamprosate, and disulfiram, are either teratogenic or have unknown safety profiles for the fetus, making them unsuitable for use during pregnancy.

Tobacco

Nicotine replacement therapy (NRT) (e.g., patch, gum, lozenges, nasal spray) does not work as well for women as for men [73]. Nicotine withdrawal symptoms are also generally more intense for women, possibly due to hormonal fluctuations influencing nicotine metabolism [74]. Among pregnant women, brief psychotherapeutic interventions (e.g., CBT, MI, CM) are preferred in targeting smoking cessation and preventing relapse, though success rates remain modest. Specifically, reduced smoking through MI has shown limited efficacy in reducing smoking among methadone-maintained [75] and low-income pregnant women [76]. CM using financial incentives has been more successful, showing improved rates of smoking cessation and better birth outcomes in this population [77]. Data on the safety and efficacy of pharmacological treatments such as varenicline and bupropion for smoking cessation during pregnancy remain limited [78].

Cannabis

Cannabis use tends to differ between women and men, with men using cannabis more frequently and in higher quantities. However, women are more likely to use cannabis to cope with stress, anxiety, and mood disorders, which can lead to a faster progression to dependence [79]. During pregnancy, cannabis use is of particular concern due to potential adverse outcomes for both the mother and fetus, including low birth weight, preterm birth, and developmental issues [80]. With cannabis legalization, its use during pregnancy has been increasing, further highlighting the need for effective treatment interventions. Reducing cannabis use among women and pregnant women through psychotherapeutic interventions and therapies has shown some success [81]. Currently, there are no FDA-approved medications specifically for treating cannabis use disorder (CUD).

Stimulants

Stimulant use, including cocaine and methamphetamines, often presents differently in women and men. While men typically engage in higher levels of stimulant use, women are more vulnerable to developing dependence more quickly and are more likely to use stimulants as a coping mechanism for stress, trauma, or mental health issues. During pregnancy, stimulant use is particularly concerning due to its association with adverse outcomes such as preterm birth, low birth weight, and neurodevelopmental issues in infants [82].

Psychotherapeutic interventions (e.g., MI, CM, CRA) are reliable evidence-based treatments for cocaine use in pregnant women [83]. CM has demonstrated the greatest potential, with randomized clinical trials showing that CM is associated with longer durations of abstinence, more negative urine tests, and higher proportions of abstinent participants compared to CRA or 12-step programs [84]. Evidence-based pharmacological treatments for prenatal cocaine use are currently not available. For other stimulants such as methamphetamines, treatment options remain limited. Reinforcement-based therapy (RBT), modeled after CRA and combined with women-focused interventions, has shown promise in reducing methamphetamine use among pregnant women. Interestingly, studies have observed reductions in methamphetamine use in both intervention and control groups, which suggests that even non-specific interventions may have beneficial effects for stimulant users in certain contexts [85].

Sedatives/Depressants

Women are more often prescribed sedatives and depressants, such as benzodiazepines and barbiturates, and may experience heightened sensitivity to these medications leading to a greater risk of dependence and side effects even at lower doses [86]. Anxiety, insomnia, and mood disorders have a higher prevalence in women, which contributes to the disparity in prescription and misuse rates. Treatment approaches for women with sedative or depressant use disorders often start with psychotherapeutic interventions, such as CBT. When necessary, tapering strategies and pharmacological interventions, including medications such as flumazenil for sedative use disorder, are used to manage dependence.

In pregnancy, brief psychotherapeutic interventions (e.g., CBT, MI) are the preferred first-line treatments for sedative or depressant use disorders. While MI shows potential in promoting behavioral changes, its effectiveness varies depending on factors such as intervention intensity, baseline substance use, and participant engagement. Pharmacological treatments, such as flumazenil or benzodiazepine antagonists, are generally avoided due to potential fetal risks, reinforcing the preference for non-pharmacological approaches during pregnancy [87].

Opioids

Women tend to progress more rapidly from the onset of opioid use to entering treatment compared to men [88, 89]. They often present with more severe medical and psychiatric comorbidities and face additional social challenges, such as being younger, unemployed, or engaging in risky behaviors. Rates of women seeking treatment for OUD have increased over the last few decades and now are nearly equal to men [90]. Medications for opioid use disorder (MOUD; e.g., methadone, buprenorphine) alongside supportive clinical follow-up are considered the standard of care for persons, including women, with OUD [91]. Treatment outcomes for women and men with OUD are generally similar. However, recent studies suggest women in buprenorphine treatment may experience better outcomes than men, although the reasons for this difference remain unclear [92].

Access to treatment during pregnancy is critical. Methadone has been a standard treatment for pregnant women with OUD since the 1970s, improving prenatal care and reducing fetal mortality and morbidity. Recent data continue to support methadone's effectiveness in reducing opioid use and maintaining abstinence compared to medical withdrawal and psychosocial interventions. However, methadone's metabolism changes significantly during pregnancy, requiring dose adjustments to maintain therapeutic levels [93]. The half-life of methadone in pregnant women averages around 8.1 h, much shorter than the 22–24 h in non-pregnant women [94]. This difference is attributed to an accelerated metabolism due to increased expression of the CYP3A4 enzyme in organs such as the liver, intestines, and placenta [95]. As pregnancy progresses, methadone clearance increases, and many women require higher or split doses to achieve optimal therapeutic effects. Buprenorphine, a partial agonist, has also shown positive outcomes, with research suggesting reduced NOWS severity and shorter hospital stays compared to methadone (MOTHER trial) [96]. However, higher dropout rates with buprenorphine have been reported, possibly due to underdosing or patient dissatisfaction with the drug's effects.

Methadone is typically administered through certified opioid treatment programs (OTPs), while buprenorphine may be prescribed in office-based settings. Both treatments are safe and effective, and the choice often depends on clinical severity, treatment availability, and patient preference. These medications remain the primary treatments for OUD during pregnancy and can be continued safely into the postpartum period to reduce the risk of relapse. This is particularly important, as women are especially vulnerable to opioid misuse and treatment discontinuation during the postpartum phase. Long-acting injectable naltrexone is not recommended during pregnancy due to limited safety data and the need for complete detoxification prior to initiation.

Substance Use and Breastfeeding

Mothers and infants impacted by SUD have a significant potential benefit in breastfeeding. Breastfeeding is encouraged for mothers who have discontinued non-prescribed substance use at the time of delivery and who remain engaged in postpartum care, including lactation support and SUD treatment. The Academy of Breastfeeding Medicine (https://www.bfmed.org/protocols) has developed protocols to guide safe breastfeeding practices for mothers with SUDs, emphasizing the need for standardized approaches across healthcare settings to mitigate bias and ensure equitable care [97]. Given the complexities associated with breastfeeding in this population, individualized care plans should be developed with input from a multidisciplinary team, including addiction specialists, lactation consultants, and pediatricians, to provide appropriate guidance and follow-up.

Although limited data are available on the concentrations of specific drugs in breast milk and their effects on breastfeeding infants, studies have demonstrated that breastfeeding can reduce the severity of NOWS among infants born to mothers receiving methadone or buprenorphine treatment [98]. Further research is needed to better understand the impacts of various substances on breastfeeding infants and to optimize breastfeeding recommendations for this population.

Conclusion

Substance use among women and in pregnancy continues to be a significant public health concern. Women who use substances have been found to have significantly different physiological, legal, and social consequences because of substance use when compared to men. It is recommended that clinicians utilize substance use screening measures that have been validated for women and/or pregnant women when assessing female patients that may have SUDs. In addition, it is recommended that clinicians create nonjudgmental environments and engage in gender-responsive and trauma-informed treatment approaches for women who use substances to reduce potential stigma and barriers to treatment access, engagement, and retention.

Chapter Review Questions

1. A 26-year-old woman presents for psychiatric services. Upon intake, she discloses that she has a history of intimate partner violence and has developed a substance use disorder. Given that women who use drugs are disproportionately impacted by certain psychiatric disorders, what should the clinician also screen for?

   A. Attention deficit hyperactivity disorder
   B. Antisocial personality disorders
   C. Mood and anxiety disorders
   D. Schizophrenia and schizoaffective disorders
   E. Neurodevelopmental disorders

   Correct Answer: C.

   Explanation: Women who use substances are disproportionately impacted by mood and anxiety disorders when compared to their male counterparts. Additionally, men who use substances are disproportionately impacted by antisocial personality disorder. No sex or gender differences in attention deficit hyperactivity disorder or schizoaffective disorder comorbidity have been documented among people who use substances.
2. A 25-year-old pregnant woman at 14 weeks gestation presents to your clinic seeking assistance with nicotine cessation. She has a history of anxiety and depression, both well-managed without medications for the past year. She vapes daily, using a nicotine concentration of approximately 12 mg/mL and estimates using about 2 mL of e-liquid per day. She expresses a strong desire to quit, but she is concerned about the safety of using cessation medications during pregnancy. She has no other significant medical conditions and reports no alcohol or substance use.

   Which of the following is the most appropriate initial treatment plan to address her tobacco use?

A. Psychotherapeutic counseling combined with nicotine replacement therapy (NRT) if necessary.
B. Prescribe varenicline for smoking cessation, as it has the highest efficacy in non-pregnant populations.
C. Advise quitting smoking without pharmacotherapy, as all smoking cessation medications are harmful to the fetus.
D. Start bupropion (Zyban) as the first-line treatment, as it also helps with anxiety and depression.
E. Recommend continuing vaping as a safer alternative to traditional cigarettes during pregnancy.

Correct Answer: A. The first-line treatment for nicotine cessation during pregnancy is psychotherapeutic counseling.

Explanation: Option A is correct because psychotherapeutic counseling is the first-line treatment for smoking cessation in pregnant women, which should be offered to all pregnant women who use nicotine. If psychotherapeutic interventions alone are insufficient, NRT can be considered. Although nicotine exposure itself carries risks, NRT is safer than continued vaping or smoking and can help reduce the amount of nicotine the fetus is exposed to. Option B is incorrect because varenicline has not been adequately studied during pregnancy and may carry unknown risks. Option C is incorrect as relying solely on quitting without pharmacotherapy may result in continued smoking if counseling fails. Option D is incorrect because bupropion is not a first-line treatment and should only be used when other options fail. Option E is incorrect because vaping is not proven to be safe during pregnancy and may still expose the fetus to harmful substances.

3. A 33-year-old woman presents for a psychiatric evaluation to determine the best course of treatment and to assess whether referrals to other services are necessary. Though the evaluation has determined the woman has an opioid use disorder and post-traumatic stress disorder from a past history of trauma, she is resistant to beginning treatment. She has expressed that, as the sole caregiver of her two children, she is worried about child protective service involvement and the stigma associated with being seen accessing substance use disorder treatment services.

   Which of the following standard of care and stigma reduction approaches should be applied to help reduce potential barriers to being retained in care?

   A. Motivational interviewing alone
   B. Exposure therapy
   C. Medications for opioid use disorder alone
   D. Motivational interviewing, gender-responsive and trauma-informed care, and medications for opioid use disorder
   E. Contingency management

   Correct Answer: D.

   Explanation: The standard of care for treating opioid use disorders can involve medications (MOUDs), like buprenorphine, and motivational interviewing techniques. In addition, women who use substances are disproportionately impacted by violence and experience unique barriers to accessing care including stigma, family and childcare responsibilities, and fear of child protective service involvement. Preliminary research has demonstrated that gender-responsive and trauma-informed approaches can help retain women in care and improve treatment outcomes.

4. A 28-year-old pregnant woman at 16 weeks gestation presents to your clinic seeking help for alcohol use disorder. She reports drinking approximately 4–5 alcoholic beverages daily and has unsuccessfully tried to reduce her consumption since learning of her pregnancy. She has a history of depression, which was managed well prior to pregnancy, but she has been experiencing increased stress and anxiety. She is concerned about the impact of alcohol on her baby but is unsure how to stop drinking alcohol. She denies the use of other substances and is not on any psychiatric medications. Her prenatal course was otherwise uncomplicated.

   Which of the following is the most appropriate initial management for this patient's alcohol use disorder during pregnancy?

   A. Recommend gradual alcohol tapering without medical intervention to avoid withdrawal symptoms.
   B. Start disulfiram to help her abstain from alcohol.
   C. Refer her for inpatient detoxification and initiate a benzodiazepine taper to manage alcohol withdrawal symptoms, followed by behavioral counseling.
   D. Prescribe naltrexone as a first-line treatment to reduce cravings and prevent relapse.
   E. Begin outpatient behavioral counseling and refer her to a 12-step support group, with close monitoring for alcohol withdrawal symptoms.

   Correct Answer: C.

   Explanation: In pregnant women with alcohol use disorder, the priority is to prevent the harm that alcohol withdrawal can cause to both the mother and the fetus. In cases of moderate-to-severe alcohol dependence, inpatient detoxification with medical management of withdrawal, including the use of benzodiazepines (which are safer than alcohol during withdrawal), is often indicated. After detoxification, behavioral counseling and long-term support should be provided to help her maintain sobriety.

5. A 32-year-old pregnant woman at 20 weeks gestation presents to your clinic seeking help for prescription opioid use disorder. She reports using oxycodone daily for the past year due to chronic back pain and now takes up to 80 mg per day without a prescription. She has tried to cut back but experiences withdrawal symptoms such as nausea, sweating, and anxiety, which make it difficult to stop. She is concerned about the impact of her opioid use on her pregnancy but is afraid of experiencing withdrawal. Her prenatal course has been uneventful, and she has no significant psychiatric or medical history aside from her opioid use. She expresses a strong desire to quit and wants to know the safest treatment options during pregnancy.

Which of the following is the most appropriate treatment plan for this patient's prescription opioid use disorder during pregnancy?

A. Advise her to gradually taper off oxycodone on her own to avoid withdrawal, with regular prenatal monitoring.
B. Initiate methadone or buprenorphine to manage opioid dependence and provide ongoing prenatal care.
C. Refer her for inpatient detoxification and manage her withdrawal symptoms without medications for opioid use disorder.
D. Delay treatment until after delivery to avoid neonatal withdrawal.
E. Encourage abrupt cessation of oxycodone and provide outpatient follow-up for withdrawal management.

Correct Answer: B.

Explanation: The standard of care for pregnant individuals with OUD is treatment with MOUD specifically methadone or buprenorphine, either as monotherapy or as a combination product with naloxone (e.g., Suboxone). Recent data and practice guidelines (e.g., ACOG, SAMHSA) support the use of buprenorphine, with or without naloxone, during pregnancy, particularly when the patient is already stabilized on it or when office-based access is more feasible than treatment through an OTP. Both medications are associated with improved maternal and fetal outcomes and should be continued postpartum to reduce the risk of relapse.

Tapering, abrupt cessation, or detoxification without MOUD is associated with high relapse risk and is not recommended during pregnancy. Delaying treatment increases the risk of adverse outcomes for both the mother and fetus.

References

1. Center for Behavioral Health Statistics and Quality. 2017 National Survey on drug use and health: detailed tables. Rockville: Substance Abuse and Mental Health Services Administration; 2018.
2. National Institute on Drug Abuse, National Institutes of Health, U.S. Department of Health and Human Services. Substance Use in Women Research Report. 2020.
3. Anthony JC, Warner LA, Kessler RC. Comparative epidemiology of dependence on tobacco, alcohol, controlled substances, and inhalants: basic findings from the national comorbidity survey. 1997.
4. Motyka MA, Al-Imam A, Haligowska A, Michalak M. Helping women suffering from drug addiction: needs, barriers, and challenges. Int J Environ Res Public Health. 2022;19(21):14039.
5. Butelman ER, Huang Y, Epstein DH, Shaham Y, Goldstein RZ, Volkow ND, et al. Overdose mortality rates for opioids and stimulant drugs are substantially higher in men than in women: state-level analysis. Neuropsychopharmacology. 2023;48(11):1639–47.
6. Martin CE, Parlier-Ahmad AB, Beck L, Scialli A, Terplan M. Need for and receipt of substance use disorder treatment among adults, by gender, in the United States. Public Health Rep. 2022;137(5):955–63.
7. Centers for Disease Control and Prevention. Health effects of cigarettes: reproductive health 2024 [updated May 15]. Available from: https://www.cdc.gov/tobacco/about/cigarettes-and-reproductive-health.html.

8. Centers for Disease Control and Prevention. About alcohol use during pregnancy 2024 [updated May 15]. Available from: https://www.cdc.gov/alcohol-pregnancy/about/index.html.
9. Substance Use and Mental Health Services Administration. 2023 National Survey on Drug Use and Health (NSDUH): detailed tables and findings. 2024.
10. Haight SC. Opioid use disorder documented at delivery hospitalization—United States, 1999–2014. MMWR Morbidity and mortality weekly report; 2018. p. 67.
11. Healthcare Cost Utilization Project. Neonatal abstinence syndrome (NAS) among newborn hospitalizations, agency for healthcare research and quality. 2021.
12. Greenfield SF, Brooks AJ, Gordon SM, Green CA, Korthuis PT, Bernstein J. Substance use disorders in women: epidemiology, course, & gender-specific treatment approaches. Psychiatr Clin N Am. 2022;45(2):339–56.
13. Bourgault Z, Rubin-Kahana DS, Hassan AN, Sanches M, Le Foll B. Multiple substance use disorders and self-reported cognitive function in US adults: associations and sex-differences in a nationally representative sample. Front Psychiatry. 2022;12:797578.
14. Substance Abuse and Mental Health Services Administration. Co-occurring disorders and other health conditions. 2022.
15. Xie C, Wang C, Luo H. Increased risk of osteoporosis in patients with cognitive impairment: a systematic review and meta-analysis. BMC Geriatr. 2023;23(1):797.
16. Gomez KU, McBride O, Roberts E, Angus C, Keyes K, Drummond C, et al. The clustering of physical health conditions and associations with co-occurring mental health problems and problematic alcohol use: a cross-sectional study. BMC Psychiatry. 2023;23(1):89.
17. Chen D, Gao X, Yang T, Xin X, Wang G, Wang H, Liu M. Independent risk factors for placental abruption: a systematic review and meta-analysis. BMC Pregnancy Childbirth. 2025;25(1):351.
18. Courchesne NS, Smith LR, Zúñiga ML, Chambers CD, Reed MB, Ballas J, Marienfeld CB. Association of alcohol and other substance-related diagnoses with severe maternal morbidity. Alcohol Clin Exp Res. 2021;45(9):1829–39.
19. Courchesne-Krak NS, Zúñiga ML, Chambers C, Reed MB, Smith LR, Ballas J, Marienfeld C. Substance-related diagnosis type predicts the likelihood and co-occurrence of preterm and cesarean delivery. J Addict Dis. 2023;41(2):137–48.
20. Evans K, Wu P, Mamas MA, Irwin C, Kang P, Perlow JH, Foley M, Gulati M. Substance use in pregnancy and its association with cardiovascular events. JACC Adv. 2023;2(8):100619.
21. Keller JM, Al-Hammadi N, Bass S, Chavan NR. Substance use disorder and severe maternal morbidity: is there a differential impact? Am J Obstetr Gynecol MFM. 2025;7(1):101544.
22. Viteri OA, Soto EE, Bahado-Singh RO, Christensen CW, Chauhan SP, Sibai BM. Fetal anomalies and long-term effects associated with substance abuse in pregnancy: a literature review. Am J Perinatol. 2015;32(05):405–16.
23. Eunice Kennedy Shriver National Institute of Child Health and Human Development. Tobacco, drug use in pregnancy can double risk of stillbirth 2013 [updated December 11]. Available from: https://www.nih.gov/news-events/news-releases/tobacco-drug-use-pregnancy-can-double-risk-stillbirth#:~:text=Smoking%20tobacco%20or%20marijuana%2C%20taking,thetaking,the%20National%20Institutes%20of%20Health.
24. Jilani SM, Jones HE, Grossman M, et al. Standardizing the clinical definition of opioid withdrawal in the neonate. J Pediatr. 2022;243:33–9. PMID: 34942181. pubmed.ncbi.nlm.nih.gov/34942181/
25. Tuchman E. Women and addiction: the importance of gender issues in substance abuse research. J Addict Dis. 2010;29(2):127–38.
26. Iversen J, Page K, Madden A, Maher L. HIV, HCV, and health-related harms among women who inject drugs: implications for prevention and treatment. JAIDS J Acquir Immune Defic Syndr. 2015;69:S176–S81.
27. Meyers S, Earnshaw V, D'Ambrosio B, Courchesne N, Werb D, Smith L. The intersection of gender and drug use-related stigma: a mixed methods systematic review and synthesis of the literature. Drug Alcohol Depend. 2021;223:108706.

28. Meyer JP, Springer SA, Altice FL. Substance abuse, violence, and HIV in women: a literature review of the syndemic. J Women's Health. 2011;20(7):991–1006.
29. Heimer K, Malone SE, De Coster S. Trends in women's incarceration rates in US prisons and jails: a tale of inequalities. Ann Rev Criminol. 2023;6(1):85–106.
30. Carroll JJ, El-Sabawi T, Ostrach B. The harms of punishing substance use during pregnancy. Int J Drug Policy. 2021;98:103433.
31. Guttmacher Institute. Substance use during pregnancy 2019. Available from: https://www.guttmacher.org/state-policy/explore/substance-use-during-pregnancy
32. Faherty LJ, Kranz AM, Russell-Fritch J, Patrick SW, Cantor J, Stein BD. Association of punitive and reporting state policies related to substance use in pregnancy with rates of neonatal abstinence syndrome. JAMA Netw Open. 2019;2(11):e1914078-e.
33. Child Welfare Information Gateway. Parental substance use and the child welfare system 2021. Available from: https://cwig-prod-prod-drupal-s3fs-us-east-1.s3.amazonaws.com/public/documents/parentalsubuse.pdf?VersionId=v4euBVU4yf8bb2QQEKblAClxFy3phGJK
34. Kenny KS, Barrington C, Green SL. "I felt for a long time like everything beautiful in me had been taken out": women's suffering, remembering, and survival following the loss of child custody. Int J Drug Policy. 2015;26(11):1158–66.
35. Green CA. Gender and use of substance abuse treatment services. Alcohol Res Health. 2006;29(1):55.
36. Harris MT, Laks J, Hurstak E, Jain JP, Lambert AM, Maschke AD, et al. "If you're strung out and female, they will take advantage of you": a qualitative study exploring drug use and substance use service experiences among women in Boston and San Francisco. J Subst Use Addict Treat. 2024;157:209190.
37. Roberts SC, Pies C. Complex calculations: how drug use during pregnancy becomes a barrier to prenatal care. Matern Child Health J. 2011;15:333–41.
38. Shogren MD, Harsell C, Heitkamp T. Screening women for at-risk alcohol use: an introduction to screening, brief intervention, and referral to treatment (SBIRT) in women's health. J Midwifery Women's Health. 2017;62(6):746–54.
39. American College of Obstetricians and Gynecologists. Committee opinion no. 496: at-risk drinking and alcohol dependence: obstetric and gynecologic implications. Obstet Gynecol. 2011;118(2 Pt 1):383–8.
40. Yudko E, Lozhkina O, Fouts A. A comprehensive review of the psychometric properties of the Drug Abuse Screening Test. J Subst Abus Treat. 2007;32(2):189–98.
41. American College of Obstetricians and Gynecologists. Committee Opinion No. 711: opioid use and opioid use disorder in pregnancy. Obstet Gynecol. 2017;130(2):e81–94.
42. Chasnoff I, Wells A, McGourty R, Bailey L. Validation of the 4P's Plus© screen for substance use in pregnancy validation of the 4P's Plus. J Perinatol. 2007;27(12):744–8.
43. Sokol RJ, Martier SS, Ager JW. The T-ACE questions: practical prenatal detection of risk-drinking. Am J Obstet Gynecol. 1989;160(4):863–70.
44. Chang G, Wilkins-Haug L, Berman S, Goetz M. The TWEAK: application in a prenatal setting. J Stud Alcohol. 1999;60(3):306–9.
45. Burns E, Gray R, Smith LA. Brief screening questionnaires to identify problem drinking during pregnancy: a systematic review. Addiction. 2010;105(4):601–14.
46. Chang G, Orav EJ, Jones JA, Buynitsky T, Gonzalez S, Wilkins-Haug L. Self-reported alcohol and drug use in pregnant young women: a pilot study of associated factors and identification. J Addict Med. 2011;5(3):221–6.
47. Carroll JC, Reid AJ, Biringer A, Midmer D, Glazier RH, Wilson L, et al. Effectiveness of the Antenatal Psychosocial Health Assessment (ALPHA) form in detecting psychosocial concerns: Aa randomized controlled trial. CMAJ. 2005;173(3):253–9.
48. Martin PR, Arria AM, Fischer G, Kaltenbach K, Heil SH, Stine SM, et al. Psychopharmacologic management of opioid-dependent women during pregnancy. Am J Addict. 2009;18(2):148–56.
49. Jones HE, Kaltenbach K. Treating women with substance use disorders during pregnancy: a comprehensive approach to caring for mother and child. Oxford University Press; 2013.

50. Briere J, Elliott DM, Harris K, Cotman A. Trauma Symptom Inventory: psychometrics and association with childhood and adult victimization in clinical samples. J Interpers Violence. 1995;10(4):387–401.
51. Johnstone S, Dela Cruz GA, Kalb N, Tyagi SV, Potenza MN, George TP, et al. A systematic review of gender-responsive and integrated substance use disorder treatment programs for women with co-occurring disorders. Am J Drug Alcohol Abuse. 2023;49(1):21–42.
52. National Institute of Drug Abuse. Sex, gender, and drug use 2024 [updated June 3]. Available from: https://nida.nih.gov/research-topics/sex-gender-and-drug-use
53. Jones HE, Kaltenbach K, Heil SH. Community reinforcement approach for substance use disorders during pregnancy: evidence and future directions. J Subst Abus. 2022;27(3):277–86.
54. Terplan M, Martin CE, Premkumar A, Krans EE. Caring for pregnant and parenting women with opioid use disorder. Treating Opioid Use Disorder in General Medical Settings; 2021. p. 203–21.
55. Herron AJ, Amaro H, Matta B. Motivational interviewing and cognitive behavioral therapy in the treatment of pregnant women with substance use disorders. Addict Sci Clin Pract. 2022;17(1):19–27.
56. Higgins ST, Washio Y, Heil SH. Contingency management in the treatment of pregnant women with substance use disorders: review of clinical trials and implications for practice. J Subst Abus Treat. 2022;138
57. Mckinney JR, Russell M, Avellaneda-Ojeda A, Gannon C, Zambare S, Hansford M, et al. A comprehensive care approach for pregnant persons with substance use disorders. Int J Ment Heal Addict. 2023;21(5):2865–76.
58. Eibl JK, Gauthier G, Pellegrini D, Daiter J, Varenbut M, Hogenbirk JC, Marsh DC. The effectiveness of telemedicine-delivered opioid agonist therapy in a supervised clinical setting. Drug Alcohol Depend. 2017;176:133–8.
59. Jones HE, Andringa K, Carroll S, Johnson E, Horton E, O'Grady K, Thorp J. Comprehensive treatment for pregnant and parenting women with substance use disorders and their children: the UNC Horizons story. Matern Child Health J. 2024;28(3):409–25.
60. Klaman SL, Isaacs K, Leopold A, Perpich J, Hayashi S, Vender J, Jones HE. Treating women who are pregnant and parenting for opioid use disorder and the concurrent care of their infants and children: literature review to support national guidance. J Addict Med. 2017;11(3):178–90.
61. Ordean A, Kahan M, Graves L, Abrahams R, Kim T. Obstetrical and neonatal outcomes of methadone-maintained pregnant women: a Canadian multisite cohort study. J Obstet Gynaecol Can. 2015;37(3):252–7.
62. Puccio J. They will never forget how you made them feel: implementing harm reduction in the perinatal setting. Matern Child Health J. 2023;27(Suppl 1):122–7.
63. Roberts DL. Reframing the response to the opioid crisis: the critical role of resilience in public health. Open Health. 2024;5(1):20230006.
64. Stone R. Pregnant women and substance use: fear, stigma, and barriers to care. Health Justice. 2015;3:1–15.
65. Terplan M, Kennedy-Hendricks A, Chisolm MS. Article commentary: prenatal substance use: exploring assumptions of maternal unfitness. Subst Abuse Res Treat. 2015;9:SART-S23328.
66. Weber A, Miskle B, Lynch A, Arndt S, Acion L. Substance use in pregnancy: identifying stigma and improving care. Subst Abus Rehabil. 2021:105–21.
67. Wolfson L, Schmidt RA, Stinson J, Poole N. Examining barriers to harm reduction and child welfare services for pregnant women and mothers who use substances using a stigma action framework. Health Soc Care Commun. 2021;29(3):589–601.
68. Wright TE, Schuetter R, Fombonne E, Stephenson J, Haning WF. Implementation and evaluation of a harm-reduction model for clinical care of substance using pregnant women. Harm Reduct J. 2012;9:1–10.
69. White AM. Gender differences in the epidemiology of alcohol use and related harms in the United States. Alcohol Res Curr Rev. 2020;40(2)

70. Bahji A, Bach P, Danilewitz M, Crockford D, Devoe DJ, El-Guebaly N, et al. Pharmacotherapies for adults with alcohol use disorders: a systematic review and network meta-analysis. J Addict Med. 2022;16(6):630–8.
71. Popova S, Dozet D, Pandya E, Sanches M, Brower K, Segura L, et al. Effectiveness of brief alcohol interventions for pregnant women: a systematic literature review and meta-analysis. BMC Pregnancy Childbirth. 2023;23(1):61.
72. Ondersma SJ, Beatty JR, Svikis DS, Strickler RC, Tzilos GK, Chang G, et al. Computer-delivered screening and brief intervention for alcohol use in pregnancy: a pilot randomized trial. Alcohol Clin Exp Res. 2015;39(7):1219–26.
73. Smith PH, Bessette AJ, Weinberger AH, Sheffer CE, McKee SA. Sex/gender differences in smoking cessation: a review. Prev Med. 2016;92:135–40.
74. Jones ASK. Nicotine withdrawal and hormonal fluctuations: impact on smoking cessation in women. Tob Control. 2022;31(1):85–91.
75. Haug NA, Svikis DS, DiClemente C. Motivational enhancement therapy for nicotine dependence in methadone-maintained pregnant women. Psychol Addict Behav. 2004;18(3):289.
76. Heckman CJ, Egleston BL, Hofmann MT. Efficacy of motivational interviewing for smoking cessation: a systematic review and meta-analysis. Tob Control. 2010;19(5):410–6.
77. Wilson SM, Newins AR, Medenblik AM, Kimbrel NA, Dedert EA, Hicks TA, et al. Contingency management versus psychotherapy for prenatal smoking cessation: a meta-analysis of randomized controlled trials. Womens Health Issues. 2018;28(6):514–23.
78. Turner E, Jones M, Vaz LR, Coleman T. Systematic review and meta-analysis to assess the safety of bupropion and varenicline in pregnancy. Nicotine Tob Res. 2019;21(8):1001–10.
79. Cooper ZD, Craft RM. Sex-dependent effects of cannabis and cannabinoids: a translational perspective. Neuropsychopharmacology. 2018;43(1):34–51.
80. Volkow ND, Han B, Compton WM, McCance-Katz EF. Self-reported medical and nonmedical cannabis use among pregnant women in the United States. JAMA. 2019;322(2):167–9.
81. Ghafouri M, Correa da Costa S, Zare Dehnavi A, Gold MS, Rummans TA. Treatments for cannabis use disorder across the lifespan: a systematic review. Brain Sci. 2024;14(3):227.
82. Smid MC, Metz TD, Gordon AJ. Stimulant use in pregnancy: an under-recognized epidemic among pregnant women. Clin Obstet Gynecol. 2019;62(1):168–84.
83. Terplan M, Ramanadhan S, Locke A, Longinaker N, Lui S. Psychosocial interventions for pregnant women in outpatient illicit drug treatment programs compared to other interventions. Cochrane Database Syst Rev. 2015;4
84. Schottenfeld RS, Moore B, Pantalon MV. Contingency management with community reinforcement approach or twelve-step facilitation drug counseling for cocaine dependent pregnant women or women with young children. Drug Alcohol Depend. 2011;118(1):48–55.
85. Jones HE, Myers B, O'Grady KE, Gebhardt S, Theron GB, Wechsberg WM. Initial feasibility and acceptability of a comprehensive intervention for methamphetamine-using pregnant women in South Africa. Psychiatry J. 2014;2014(1):929767.
86. Edinoff AN, Nix CA, Hollier J, Sagrera CE, Delacroix BM, Abubakar T, et al. Benzodiazepines: uses, dangers, and clinical considerations. Neurol Int. 2021;13(4):594–607.
87. Blanco C, Wesson DR, Smith DE. Disorders due to substance use: sedatives, hypnotics, and anxiolytics. Tasman's psychiatry. Springer; 2024. p. 2825–41.
88. Straub L, Bateman BT, Hernández-Díaz S, Zhu Y, Suarez EA, Vine SM, Huybrechts KF. Comparative safety of in utero exposure to buprenorphine combined with naloxone vs buprenorphine alone. JAMA. 2024;332(10):805–16.
89. Link HM, Jones H, Miller L, Kaltenbach K, Seligman N. Buprenorphine-naloxone use in pregnancy: a systematic review and meta-analysis. Am J Obstetr Gynecol MFM. 2020;2(3):100179.
90. Huhn AS, Dunn KE. Challenges for women entering treatment for opioid use disorder. Curr Psychiatry Rep. 2020;22:1–10.
91. Suarez EA, Huybrechts KF, Straub L, Hernández-Díaz S, Jones HE, Connery HS, et al. Buprenorphine versus methadone for opioid use disorder in pregnancy. N Engl J Med. 2022;387(22):2033–44.

92. Campbell AN, Barbosa-Leiker C, Hatch-Maillette M, Mennenga SE, Pavlicova M, Scodes J, et al. Gender differences in demographic and clinical characteristics of patients with opioid use disorder entering a comparative effectiveness medication trial. Am J Addict. 2018;27(6):465–70.
93. Kinsella M, Halliday LO, Shaw M, Capel Y, Nelson SM, Kearns RJ. Buprenorphine compared with methadone in pregnancy: a systematic review and meta-analysis. Subst Use Misuse. 2022;57(9):1400–16.
94. Swift RM, Dudley M, DePetrillo P, Camara P, Griffiths W. Altered methadone pharmacokinetics in pregnancy: implications for dosing. J Subst Abus. 1989;1(4):453–60.
95. Tracy TS, Venkataramanan R, Glover DD, Caritis SN. Temporal changes in drug metabolism (CYP1A2, CYP2D6 and CYP3A Activity) during pregnancy. Am J Obstet Gynecol. 2005;192(2):633–9.
96. Jones HE, Fischer G, Heil SH, Kaltenbach K, Martin PR, Coyle MG, Arria AM. Maternal Opioid Treatment: Human Experimental Research (MOTHER) – approach, issues and lessons learned. Addiction. 2012;107:28–35.
97. Harris M, Schiff DM, Saia K, Muftu S, Standish KR, Wachman EM. Academy of Breastfeeding Medicine Clinical Protocol# 21: breastfeeding in the setting of substance use and substance use disorder (revised 2023). Breastfeed Med. 2023;18(10):715.
98. Doerzbacher M, Chang Y-P. Supporting breastfeeding for women on opioid maintenance therapy: a systematic review. J Perinatol. 2019;39(9):1159–64.

LGBTQIA+: Lesbian, Gay, Bisexual, Transgender, Queer or Questioning, Intersex, Asexual, and More

17

Matthew P. Abrams

High-Yield Review Points

- Use warmth, respect, and curiosity to create an open dialogue with LGBTQIA+ persons about substance use, gender identity, and sexual orientation.
- Use of "party drugs" such as crystal methamphetamine, ecstasy, GHB, 2C, and ketamine is higher in many LGBTQIA+ populations and disproportionately so among gay men.
- LGBTQIA+ people may use psychoactive substances to relieve increased stress stemming from experiences of discrimination, stigma, and shame or to enhance sexual pleasure during sex (i.e., chemsex).
- Providing supportive LGBTQIA+ affirming care that is trauma-informed is vital to reducing SUD treatment barriers and promoting positive health outcomes.
- Addressing experiences of discrimination, violence, and anti-transgender stigma together with SUD treatment improves clinical outcomes for transgender patients.

Introduction

Understanding, appreciating, and celebrating the lives of LGBTQIA+ people (lesbian, gay, bisexual, transgender, queer or questioning, intersex, and asexual, or LGBTQ+ for short) and the cultures of their communities help mental health and addiction treatment practitioners provide optimal care to their patients. Part of

M. P. Abrams (✉)
Department of Psychiatry, University of California San Diego, La Jolla, CA, USA
e-mail: maabrams@health.ucsd.edu

C. Marienfeld, M. Soltani (eds.), *AAAP Review of Addiction Psychiatry*,
https://doi.org/10.1007/978-3-032-24174-0_17

understanding and treating LGBTQ+ people effectively is recognizing the higher rates of substance use in this group. In the LGBTQ+ population, 20–30% struggle with addiction, compared with approximately 17% of the general population [1–3]. Higher rates of SUD can be best understood in the context of the many challenges that LGBTQ+ communities face daily, including stigma, marginalization, and shame [4]. Some multiply marginalized or intersectional groups, like Black transgender individuals, also experience higher rates of substance use [5, 6]. Supportive, trauma-informed, and affirming LGBTQ+ care is vital to reducing treatment barriers and promoting positive health outcomes [7].

While many underserved communities face similar problems, some challenges are unique to LGBTQ+ communities. LGBTQ+ people face a disproportionate amount of shame from family and friends due to discrimination, stigma, abuse, threats, hate crimes, public humiliation, and, frequently, internalized homophobia and transphobia [4, 6]. Likewise, LGBTQ+ people have historically had fewer social spaces to find community apart from bars and night clubs, which functioned as critical social infrastructure in the absence of broader societal acceptance, but also facilitated substance use [8]. In the face of these psychosocial stressors and social conditions, use of illicit drugs, alcohol, and other substances became common among LGBTQ+ communities.

Substance use among LGBTQ+ people may serve as a maladaptive coping mechanism used to try to avoid negative mental health or trauma-related symptoms or ameliorate psychiatric conditions such as generalized anxiety disorder, major depressive disorder, eating disorders, post-traumatic stress disorder, and other disorders (or subclinical problems) that occur in the context of widespread stigmatization. While the need for general psychiatric care is increased in LGBTQ+ populations due to the differential prevalence of mental health disorders, many healthcare providers feel uncomfortable providing culturally informed care—or even express outright hostility toward LGBTQ+ populations—thus inhibiting care-seeking and limiting their access to health care [9, 10]. Many members of LGBTQ+ communities have learned to distrust a traditionally stigmatizing and inhospitable healthcare system and may not seek help even when it is needed. With this cycle, mental health and substance use problems go untreated, and suicide rates in the LGBTQ+ community remain high [1, 11–14].

Language and the LGBTQ+ Patient

Not asking about sexual orientation and gender identity as an attempt to avoid incorrect language usage is misguided and sub-optimal care, and it may inadvertently alienate patients and compromise their care. Many well-meaning and otherwise supportive health providers feel uncomfortable when meeting a patient that belongs to a sexual or gender minority group for the first time due to a general lack of knowledge about these minority communities and the terminology used to describe LGBTQ+ individuals and their practices. This section will define some of the most common terms that one should know to appropriately engage with LGBTQ+

patients. This section is not an exhaustive list that encapsulates all the nuanced terminology used to describe these groups. As mentioned above, LGBTQ+ refers to people who identify as lesbian, gay, bisexual, transgender, intersex, queer or questioning, intersex, and asexual. Many of these terms are not mutually exclusive. For example, transgender is used to identify people belonging to a gender group, and these people may continue to use terms such as lesbian, gay, and bisexual to describe their sexual orientation. Likewise, someone who identifies as queer may be referring to their gender or their sexual orientation not aligning with their cisgender or heterosexual counterparts, and that same person may or may not also identify as gay when sexually attracted to the same gender. In short, the term LGBTQ+ is meant to encompass a wide variety of people whose gender identity, gender expression, biological sex, and sexual orientation are outside of heteronormativity, and who are seeking to best self-identify consistent with their preferred terminology.

Gender and sexual orientation are separate concepts [15]. The former is mostly contained within an individual, while the latter refers to how the individual relates sexually or romantically with others (or not). Gender is further understood as gender identity, gender expression, and biological sex. Similarly, sexual orientation is further understood as sexual orientation identity, sexual behavior, and sexual attraction. These are essential elements of our humanity and have distinct meanings [15]. Table 17.1 summarizes some of these concepts. It is especially important not to conflate gender and sexuality when interfacing with LGBTQ+ patients.

Most of these terms are not binary and can be best appreciated as a spectrum. Firstly, gender identity refers to how a person conceives themselves, in their own minds, regarding their gender role. The spectrum of gender identity goes from "man-ness" on one end to nongendered in the center to "woman-ness" on the other end. Next, gender expression is fundamentally different from gender identity. Whereas gender identity refers to one's inner conception of their gender, gender expression is an outward portrayal of gender. On the spectrum of gender expression, there is "feminine" on one side, androgynous in the center, and "masculine" on the other side. Gender expression can encompass dress, how one presents themselves, and other outward signifiers of gender. Biological sex is assigned at birth and refers to the measurable organs, hormones, and chromosomes that one possesses. Biological sex, while mostly binary with "female" and "male" genetic makeups, also includes intersex people, including those with rare conditions such as androgen insensitivity syndrome and congenital adrenal hyperplasia and changes in the sex chromosomes from the more common XX (female sex) and XY (male sex) to

Table 17.1 Gender and sexual orientation

Sexual orientation	Gender
Identity	*Identity*
Examples: gay, lesbian, bisexual, straight, asexual, queer	Examples: woman, gender fluid, man
Behavior	*Expression*
Examples: same-gender partners, opposite-gender partners, both, neither	Examples: feminine, androgynous, masculine

include variations such as XO (one X chromosome) or XXY (having an extra sex chromosome).

Sexual orientation encompasses many identities. Sexual identity is how one chooses to describe themselves with terms such as "straight," "gay," "lesbian," "bisexual," "pansexual," and so on. Sexual behavior may or may not be tied to sexual identity and refers to the sexual encounters that one is choosing to partake in. These encounters can be with same-gender partners, opposite-gender partners, neither, or both. Lastly, there is sexual attraction. This refers to whether one prefers sex with or is sexually attracted to men, women, neither, or people from multiple gender categories. Sometimes one's sexual attraction does not align with their romantic attraction. Various scales of attraction have been proposed, but the most commonly cited is the Kinsey scale, which describes attraction in terms of gradations of orientation rather than simply "straight" or "gay." This scale runs from 0, meaning exclusively heterosexual, to 6, meaning exclusively homosexual. A person who falls on a 3 on the Kinsey scale is equally attracted to both the same and opposite genders. The scale also includes an X, which denotes those who indicate that they have no sexual encounters.

Table 17.2 provides a list of helpful and commonly used terms to describe those in the LGBTQ+ community or other common terms important for understanding substance use in these communities. This list and definitions were adapted from the list generated by the authors at the LGBTQ+ Resource Center at UC Davis [16] and the World Professional Association for Transgender Health (WPATH) guidelines for Standards of Care for the Health of Transgender and Gender Diverse People [17].

Table 17.2 Glossary

Bisexual	A person whose sexual orientation is toward people of more than one gender (for example, being interested in both men and women)
Cisgender	A gender identity that aligns with the person's assigned sex at birth
Chemsex	Substance use before or during sex (e.g., sexualized drug use)
Gay	A sexual orientation toward people of the same gender identity
Gender-expansive youth	Young people whose gender identity, expression, or experience does not align with the sex they were assigned at birth or with traditional gender roles. This broad term can include individuals who identify as transgender, nonbinary, gender fluid, or other identities outside the typical gender binary
Gender expression	How one expresses oneself in terms of dress and/or behaviors; it may be described as "masculine," "feminine," or "androgynous"
Gender identity	Sense of one's self as woman, man, trans, or some other identity, which may or may not correspond with the sex and gender that one is assigned at birth
Gender queer	A person whose gender identity and/or gender expression falls outside of the dominant societal norm for their assigned sex
Gender minority	A gender minority refers to individuals whose gender identity, expression, or experience differs from the dominant societal norms of their culture, typically those who do not identify strictly as cisgender
Harm reduction	An approach to care that aims to reduce the negative consequences of substance use and to promote a person's quality of life and self-determination. It is a non-judgmental, person-centered approach that does not require substance abstinence

(continued)

Table 17.2 (continued)

Heteronormativity	A set of lifestyle norms, practices, and institutions that assume heterosexuality as a fundamental and natural norm
Homosexuality	A term to describe a sexual orientation in which a person feels physically and emotionally attracted to people of the same gender
Intersex	The experience of naturally developing primary or secondary sex characteristics that do not fit neatly into society's definitions of male or female
Lesbian	A woman whose primary sexual and affectional orientation is toward people of the same gender
MSM	An abbreviation for men who have sex with men; they may or may not identify as gay
Orientation	One's attraction or non-attraction to other people; it may be fluid or consistent and can change throughout the course of one's life
Pansexual	Pansexual refers to a sexual orientation characterized by attraction to people regardless of their gender or gender identity. Pansexual individuals may be attracted to men, women, nonbinary people, and those of other gender identities
Pronouns	Linguistic tools used to refer to someone in the third person; examples are they/them/theirs, ze/hir/hirs, she/her/hers, he/him/his
Queer	A historical epithet used against people whose gender and/or sexuality does not conform to dominant expectations; some people have reclaimed the word to describe sexual orientations and gender identities that do not conform to dominant heteronormative and cisnormative standards
Sex	A medically constructed categorization; sex chromosomes X and Y; though, sex is often assigned based on the appearance of the genitalia, either via ultrasound or at birth
Straight	A word commonly used to describe a heterosexual person
Transgender	Adjective used most often as an umbrella term and frequently abbreviated to "trans"; this adjective describes a wide range of identities, including the two terms below to describe members of the many varied communities that exist globally of people with gender identities or expressions that differ from the gender socially attributed to the sex assigned to them at birth
Trans man	An identifier of someone who was assigned female sex at birth that identifies as a man; some trans men may also use the term FTM for "female to male"
Trans woman	An identifier of someone who was assigned male sex at birth that identifies a woman; some trans women may also use MTF for "male to female"
Transphobia	The fear, hatred, disbelief, or discrimination against transgender and gender nonconforming people

Providing Optimal Care to LGBTQ+ Populations

Healthcare providers who have not treated many openly LGBTQ+ people may have a certain level of trepidation or uncertainty when first approaching their patients. LGBTQ+ patients face stigma daily. In general, the best way to approach LGBTQ+ patients is with a sense of acceptance and a non-judgmental attitude, much like any other patient. Creating a welcoming environment without judgment is a top priority.

Simple things that providers take for granted are often fraught subjects for those in the LGBTQ+ community, such as public restrooms, equal protections in the workplace, and marriage equality. Patients may hide certain struggles that they are facing unless the provider communicates a genuinely open and accepting stance. Providers may want to differentiate between the real, imagined, and potential risks that LGBTQ+ patients face. For example, a commonly circulated false myth is that same-gender parents face unique challenges when it comes to raising children, and the children of LGBTQ+ adults experience higher incidences of mental illness [18, 19]. Meanwhile, there are health risks that disproportionately effect LGBTQ+ people [20]. For example, the risk of HIV and HCV in LGBTQ+ populations who use substances has been shown to be relatively higher than those of their heterosexual and cisgender counterparts [14, 21]. Knowing these potential risks can guide the clinical interview and ensure patient safety.

When discussing substance use with LGBTQ+ persons, using motivational interviewing (MI) remains key to fostering a supportive environment that facilitates openness about their substance use. Use of MI has been shown to play an important role in healthcare providers' ability to assess LGBTQ+ persons' readiness for change and to promote positive behavior changes [22–24]. For example, in one study, participants in an MI group were 18% less likely to use drugs and 24% less likely to engage in unprotected anal intercourse compared to those in the education group over 12 months follow-up [22].

While a practitioner may not know which pronoun a patient uses, or where exactly they fit in the broad and rich tapestry that comprises LGBTQ+ communities, almost any missteps a provider makes can often be forgiven so long as a current of curiosity and acceptance flows through the encounter. The following example shows how even a provider who makes an incorrect assumption about the patient can be very effective when warmth and curiosity are at the forefront of one's non-judgmental approach. The example also highlights how important it is that providers take ownership for any missteps during the patient encounter, just as they should when committing medical errors:

- *Provider: Hello Mr. Elbe, my name is Dr. Masters, and I'd like to discuss the process of the initial intake and what you can expect as we continue to work together.*
- *Patient: Hello Dr. Masters. I appreciate that, but I'd like you to know that I am in the process of transitioning and would prefer it if you refer to me as Ms. Elbe from now on.*
- *Provider: My sincere apologies Ms. Elbe, I'll make a note and be sure to do so going forward. While we are on the subject, which pronouns do you use? I use "he" and "him."*
- *Patient: It's not a problem. I use the pronouns "she" and "her." I appreciate that you asked me.*
- *Provider: Thank you. If you feel comfortable, I'd like to ask where you are in terms of your transition. I ask this because certain patients making the transition are on medications, such as hormones, which may interact with certain medications I prescribe.*

- *Patient: I have begun seeing an endocrinologist but have not begun taking any medications yet.*
- *Provider: Thank you. Let's return to the initial intake…*

Taking a Sexual History as Part of a SUD History

Taking a sexual history as it relates to addiction is often overlooked when establishing care with an LGBTQ+ patient. The following are a few takeaway points to ensure that a sexual history is obtained in a respectful manner:

1. Avoid assumptions of heteronormativity. Ask neutral questions like "Do you have a partner or partners?" As appropriate, consider terms such as married, divorced, and widowed.
2. Remind yourself that marriage or being in a relationship and monogamy are not synonymous. People you treat in a medical setting may be in open relationships or have non-traditional relationship structures that should be addressed from a place of curiosity and non-judgment.
3. Ask whether the patient prefers sex with men, women, both, or neither, regardless of the patient's gender identity.
4. Ask about sexual health and relationship styles in an open and accepting manner that avoids shame for the patient.
5. After building a respectful foundation of understanding, inquire as to any substance use during sex and which drugs the person may use during sex.
6. Ask whether the person's sexual encounters are consensual and whether they are protected from sexual violence. If there is doubt in this regard, preface questions by saying that the provider has a duty to ensure safety, as well as maintain confidentiality.

The following example demonstrates how to use these takeaway points when taking a sexual history:

- *Provider: I know from our earlier discussions that you use methamphetamine weekly and that you mostly prefer sex with men. Do you ever use crystal meth right before or during sex?*
- *Patient: It's a little embarrassing to admit, but yeah, especially in clubs, it's just the way things work. And the sex is much better, honestly.*
- *Provider: You told me that you try to use condoms when possible since you typically sleep with multiple and sometimes unknown partners each week. When you are using methamphetamine, do you use a condom?*
- *Patient: Honestly, not really. I know I should, but it just doesn't always happen that way.*
- *Provider: So, while methamphetamine improves your experience during sex, your use also might contribute to some risks, as condomless sex exposes you to HIV and other diseases. I'd like to discuss those risks so that you can make the most informed decisions going forward. Have you heard of PrEP?*

Epidemiology of Substance Use in LGBTQ+ Populations

LGBTQ+ individuals are 2 to 3 times more likely to use illicit substances than heterosexuals [25]. Likewise, national prevalence data on substance use among lesbian, gay, and bisexual high school students indicate that LGB students use substances at significantly higher rates than their heterosexual peers [26]. Cocaine, heroin, hallucinogens, inhalants, methamphetamines, and prescription drug misuse are higher in the LGBTQ+ adult population [25, 27]. The biggest discrepancies appear to occur with cocaine, hallucinogens (including ecstasy), inhalants (e.g., "poppers"), and methamphetamines, where use among gay men is at least three times that of their heterosexual counterparts [25]. These increased rates of drug use cross the boundaries of sex and age within the LGBTQ+ community [25, 28, 29]. The increased use of these substances is partially linked to unique societal pressures and systems of oppression faced by the LGBTQ+ population [4].

It follows that more people in the LGBTQ+ community need treatment for substance use problems than their counterparts [2, 30]. For example, about one third of bisexual males, bisexual females, and gay males have a SUD, with rates 1.5 to 2 times higher than comparable straight populations [25, 28, 29]. Compared with the general population, those in the LGBTQ+ community are somewhat more likely to seek and receive treatment for substance use [25]. However, there is still much to be done to ensure that those in underserved communities can access the substance use treatments they need.

Gay and Bisexual Men

Gay men are only slightly more likely to use tobacco products than their heterosexual counterparts overall and only have a slightly higher prevalence of nicotine dependence [31]. Some studies suggest that men who report only having sex with men are far less likely to develop alcohol use disorders as compared with men who report only having sex with women [32]. However, other studies suggest rates of AUD are significantly higher among gay and bisexual men. For example, the prevalence of AUD is 31.5% among gay and bisexual men, compared to 20.8% among heterosexual men, with the highest prevalence observed in gay and bisexual men aged 18–45 [33]. Gay and bisexual men also experience significantly higher rates of hazardous alcohol use than heterosexual men. Moreover, gay men who do develop alcohol use disorders find it more difficult to quit. Relapse rates for alcohol are higher in gay men than lesbian or bisexual women in the same socioeconomic groups [32].

When considering substance use among gay men, one must also discuss a class of illicit substances that some refer to as "party drugs" that can include drugs with several different mechanisms of action. Party drugs can include methamphetamine, methylene-dioxy-methamphetamine (MDMA) (ecstasy), gamma-hydroxy-butyrate (GHB), psychedelic phenethylamines (2C), ketamine (Special K), and inhaled alkyl nitrites (poppers). While these substances are used throughout the general population, their use by gay and bisexual men is substantially higher than within other populations [25, 27]. Party drugs can enhance pleasure during sex and are routinely used by a subset of gay men [34]. This practice is sometimes referred to as "chemsex" [35]. It is also known as "party and play," or "PNP" a code phrase for using drugs (party) and having sex (play) [34].

GHB and its precursor GBL (gamma-butyrolactone) are among the most frequently used substances in night clubs by gay men [36]. GHB may be referred to as "liquid X" or "liquid ecstasy" as it is typically consumed orally and is available as an odorless, colorless liquid. GHB is a central nervous system (CNS) depressant that may lead to euphoria, increased sex drive, and tranquility, which can enhance sexual experiences. GHB has a narrow therapeutic window making it easy to overdose, especially when combined with other CNS depressants. This is why GHB should never be combined with alcohol, ketamine, or other CNS depressants like benzodiazepines. If someone combines GHB with alcohol, the depressant effects of both substances will act synergistically. Overdose symptoms can include unconsciousness, respiratory depression, and, in severe cases, death. It also has a short half-life, so it requires repeat dosing to maintain the desired effects, increasing the risk that someone could overdose inadvertently. This is colloquially referred to as "g-ing out." Withdrawal symptoms may be severe and include insomnia, anxiety, tremors, and, in some cases, hallucinations or delirium. Repeated use can result in memory blackouts, impaired judgment, and reduced ability to consent, increasing the risk of non-consensual sexual encounters. Harm-reduction strategies for GHB/GBL use among LGBTQ+ people include providing education and supplies for dosing and sexual risk mitigation. Users should be informed about the importance of accurate dosing, using milliliter syringes or pipettes, and understanding the potency of different batches and why it is important not to mix batches or combine with other substances.

Methamphetamine has affected the gay population disproportionately [37, 38]. The drug may be referred to as "crystal," "Tina" ("crystal" becomes "Christina," which then becomes "Tina"), or simply "meth." Methamphetamine is often used in "runs," involving continuous use for 24–72 h or longer with little or no sleep, or it can be used daily. It can be snorted, smoked, or injected ("slammed"). Injection carries added risks such as blood-borne infections. Many studies have documented the rise of amphetamine use in gay populations across the United States, with rates 4 times higher among gay men [25]. Crystal methamphetamine is sometimes found in gay clubs and also use by certain sexual minority groups to enhance pleasure during intercourse. Furthermore, even those who use the drug sporadically are at higher risk for sexually transmitted diseases such as HIV [37, 39, 40]. GHB and methamphetamine are frequently co-used during chemsex sessions, increasing the risk of dangerous cardiovascular and neurological events.

MDMA (ecstasy) use has reached high rates among gay and bisexual men populations, with over half reporting use at some point in their lifetime [25, 27]. An analog of methamphetamine, MDMA is psychoactive and can increase energy, empathy, and pleasure. It is also known as "X" or "Scooby snacks" and typically comes in brightly colored, small, and therefore easy to swallow tablets. Risks from ecstasy use include dehydration, overheating (hyperthermia), serotonin syndrome (especially when combined with other serotonergic drugs), anxiety, depression, and difficulty regulating emotions after use ("comedown"). Variability in MDMA purity poses a risk of overdose or toxic reactions; users may accidentally consume ecstasy contaminated with other dangerous substances.

While not as prevalent in the gay population overall, ketamine use among gay and bisexual men who go to clubs is high [37]. Ketamine is sometimes used by LGBTQ+ people to enhance dissociation, reduce inhibitions, and create altered sensory experiences at bars, clubs, or during sex. Like GHB, ketamine may come in a powdered or liquid form and may be consumed in drinks, snorted, or injected. At bars and clubs, ketamine is typically consumed via snorting. Unlike GHB, ketamine imparts a salty and distinct taste when it is dissolved in drinks. Its effects and use as a "party drug" are similar to those of GHB. However, the two drugs are very different in terms of their lethality. As mentioned above, GHB has a very narrow therapeutic window (i.e., a narrow dose range to achieve clinical effect), with the dose that will result in a desirable high being only modestly lower than a lethal dose, resulting in a very significant risk of respiratory collapse and death. It is more difficult to overdose on ketamine since it has a wider therapeutic window.

Lesbian and Bisexual Women

Like men with same gender attraction, lesbian and bisexual women experience disproportionately higher rates of substance use compared to their heterosexual counterparts [20, 41, 42]. Similarly, lesbians are more likely to meet diagnostic criteria for substance use disorders (SUDs), particularly alcohol use disorder and cannabis use disorder, compared to heterosexual women [30, 42].

Lesbian women are more likely to start smoking earlier and continue to use tobacco at higher rates than heterosexual women throughout adult life [31]. Furthermore, tobacco use disorder rates are higher among lesbians than their heterosexual counterpart regardless of the type of tobacco used [31].

As with tobacco, alcohol plays a large social role in the lesbian community. Lesbians are more than three times as likely to develop alcohol use disorders compared with their heterosexual counterparts [32, 42]. Binge drinking and heavy episodic drinking are also elevated among lesbians [20]. Lesbians are also more likely to report negative social and financial consequences due to alcohol use [32]. However, both lesbian and heterosexual women in recovery find it easier to abstain—or are more successful in abstaining—from alcohol as women have fewer relapses overall compared to men [32].

Lesbians have higher lifetime rates of MDMA, cocaine, methamphetamine, and lysergic acid diethylamide (LSD) use compared with heterosexual women [20, 41, 42]. Forty-nine percent of lesbian or bisexual women report using MDMA at least once in their lifetime compared with 40% of age-matched heterosexual women [43]. The same applies for ketamine (19% versus 15%), GHB

(9% versus 7%), and cocaine (47% versus 37%) [43]. More statistically relevant differences are seen with methamphetamine use (17% versus 9%) and LSD (33% versus 23%) [43]. When compared with substance use among gay men, lesbians have a more pronounced "age gap" with younger lesbian and bisexual women being much more likely to experiment with illicit substances compared with their older counterparts [43]. Stigma, discrimination, and internalized homophobia underlie these healthcare disparities among lesbian and bisexual women.

Transgender People and Gender Minorities

Transgender persons experience significantly higher rates of substance use disorders compared to their cisgender counterparts [44]; these disparities are influenced by factors such as discrimination and victimization [45, 46].

Transgender youth are 2.5 to 4 times more likely to use substances—including alcohol, cigarettes, marijuana, and other illicit drugs—than non-transgender peers, with higher rates of heavy episodic drinking and polysubstance use [47]. Furthermore, transgender youth tend to initiate substance use at earlier ages compared to non-transgender youth, leading to increased risk of chronic substance use issues [47]. Prescription drug misuse is particularly concerning, as transgender students are more than twice as likely to misuse prescription medications, including painkillers, and are significantly more likely to use substances like cocaine, methamphetamine, and inhalants [41].

Among transgender adults, nearly one-third (31.1%) report high-frequency substance use in the past year, with 11.8% meeting criteria for a substance use disorder and 11.6% having received treatment for substance use [45]. Nicotine use disorder (16.6% vs. 5.4%), alcohol use disorder (2.6% vs. 0.9%), and drug use disorder (4.3% vs. 1.2%) are all more prevalent among transgender adults compared to their cisgender peers [20, 44]. These disparities are greatest among transfeminine individuals, who exhibit higher rates of polysubstance use and specific substance use disorders compared to transmasculine individuals [2]. Also, 31.2% of transgender individuals report problematic drug use and 28.2% report hazardous drinking, rates notably higher than those observed among cisgender adults [48]. Correlates of substance use include experiences of discrimination and unemployment [45, 49].

Evidence supports the use of trauma-informed, gender-affirming approaches when treating substance use disorders among transgender individuals. It is crucial that transgender patients receive treatment for their substance use disorders especially when substance use would interfere with receiving care like gender-affirming medical procedures part of their treatment plan [17]. It is important clinicians provide gender-affirming approaches when screening, diagnosing, and treating SUDs in transgender patients to reduce these disparities. Addressing experiences of discrimination, violence, and stigma alongside addiction treatment improves health outcomes [6].

Chapter Review Questions

1. Alex, a 29-year-old woman with a self-reported history of anxiety and depression, comes to you, a physician, for help. As the initial interview progresses, Alex confirms she uses the pronouns "she" and "her" when referring to herself. Later, she tells you that her partner, Pat, a woman, occasionally encourages her to use methamphetamine during sex. A little embarrassed, you realize you have been referring to Pat as "he." Alex is now upset. You have made an erroneous assumption about __________.

   A. Gender identity
   B. Gender expression
   C. Biological sex
   D. Sexual Orientation
   E. Affectation

   Correct Answer: D.

   Explanation: Gender identity, gender expression, and biological sex are the three dimensions of gender. Gender identity refers to how one conceives of themselves regarding "man-ness" or "woman-ness." Gender expression refers to how one displays femininity or masculinity to the outside world. Biological sex refers to the sex that someone is assigned at birth. Sexual orientation is independent of the previous three factors and refers to the type(s) of person(s) that one relates to sexually. Identity, behavior, and attraction are the three elements that describe sexual orientation.

   In the vignette, the physician assumed heteronormativity, thinking that a patient whose gender identity leans toward "woman-ness" must be attracted to men. Furthermore, the physician may have assumed that transgender women (Alex, for example) must be heterosexual or would have been happy staying with their gender assigned at birth (male for Alex). This is not true.

2. Robert, a 24-year-old man who uses he/him pronouns, comes to you for help. He identifies as "straight" but reluctantly reports having sexual experiences with other men "once in a blue moon." Last night, he was at a club, used a "party drug," and he is now worried about any lasting effects that the mystery drug may have. He says, "I was careful only to use a little, since I saw a guy take a little too much and pass out on the dance floor." Robert answers your question about alcohol stating that "last night I made sure to only drink non-alcoholic sodas to stay hydrated." He notes afterward he felt "incredibly relaxed, sexed up, and sexy." Which of the following substances the patient most likely ingested? He denied experiencing hallucinations and dissociative properties from the drug.

   A. Methylene-dioxy-methamphetamine (MDMA or "ecstasy")
   B. Gamma-hydroxy-methamphetamine (GHB)
   C. Lysergic acid diethylamide (LSD)

D. Ketamine
E. Delta-9-tetra-hydro-cannabinol (THC)

Correct Answer: B.

Explanation: GHB may be referred to as "liquid X" or "liquid ecstasy" and is a central nervous system depressant that leads to euphoria, increased sex drive, and tranquility. It is available as an odorless, colorless drug. GHB should never be combined with alcohol, so those who use it recreationally typically will only drink non-alcoholic drinks when at the bars and clubs. Similarly, ketamine or "special K" may come in a powdered or liquid form and may be consumed in drinks, snorted, or injected. GHB has an acidic taste and is sometimes described as burning. Ketamine has a more pungent taste and smell that some users describe as "salty." Both could lead to the effects described by the patient, but only GHB is odorless. GHB is far more likely than ketamine to result in overdose and death.

LSD would have had more potent hallucinogenic effects. Ecstasy is a sensual rather than sexual drug and is most commonly taken as a pill. Cannabinoids such as THC and cannabidiol (CBD) are typically smoked or consumed with food.

3. A 35-year-old cisgender gay man presents to your clinic seeking help for managing his use of methamphetamine during sexual encounters [commonly referred to as "chemsex"]. He reports engaging in prolonged sexual sessions with multiple partners, facilitated through online dating apps. Which of the following factors could be contributing to his engagement in chemsex?

A. Desire to enhance sexual performance due to underlying erectile dysfunction
B. Cultural practices unrelated to sexual orientation
C. Minority stress stemming from societal attitudes toward LGBTQ+ individuals
D. Lack of access to recreational substances in his community
E. Peer pressure from heterosexual friends

Correct Answer: C.

Explanation: Chemsex is intricately linked to factors such as societal attitudes toward LGBTQ+ individuals, the trauma from the HIV/AIDS epidemic, chronic bullying, and peer pressure within gay communities to consume psychoactive substances during sex. These elements contribute to minority stress, which can lead individuals to engage in chemsex as a coping mechanism.

4. A 26-year-old transgender woman reports frequent use of substances like GHB and ketamine, especially when going out with her friends and sometimes during sex. She expresses concerns about the impact on her mental health and seeks guidance. Which of the following harm-reduction strategies would be most appropriate to recommend?

A. Immediate cessation of all substance use without support
B. Referral to a general addiction support group without LGBTQ+ focus
C. Engagement with LGBTQ+-affirming services that provide education on safer substance use and sexual practices
D. Prescription of lorazepam to manage withdrawal symptoms without further intervention

E. Advise her to avoid bad influences and isolate from all her friends and social contacts to prevent substance use triggers

Correct Answer: C.

Explanation: Harm-reduction approaches for LGBTQ+ patients are most effective when they are not only non-judgmental but also affirming of LGBTQ+ identities. Providing education on safer substance use, understanding the context of chemsex, and offering support through LGBTQ+-focused services are crucial components of effective harm-reduction strategies.

5. A 32-year-old lesbian woman presents for an initial psychiatric evaluation. She reports frequent binge drinking and recent use of cannabis to cope with work- and relationship-related stressors. She has no prior psychiatric diagnoses. Based on current epidemiologic data, which of the following statements best reflects substance use trends among lesbian individuals?

A. Lesbian women are less likely than heterosexual women to engage in hazardous drinking.
B. Lesbian women have similar rates of substance use disorder diagnoses as heterosexual women.
C. Lesbian women are more likely to engage in heavy episodic drinking and cannabis use than heterosexual women.
D. Discrimination and stigma have not been shown to influence substance use patterns in lesbian populations.

Correct Answer: C.

Explanation: Research consistently shows that lesbian women have higher rates of heavy episodic drinking, cannabis use, and other substance use compared to heterosexual women. These disparities are partially driven by minority stress factors such as stigma, discrimination, and internalized homophobia. Culturally responsive, affirming care is essential in addressing these issues.

6. Ali, an ally to LGBTQ+ communities, presents to the emergency department after experiencing an overdose related to GHB use during a party. In developing a harm-reduction plan, which of the following educational points is most critical to emphasize regarding GHB use?

A. GHB overdoses are best managed at home without medical supervision.
B. Mixing GHB with alcohol significantly increases the risk of respiratory depression.
C. GHB has a wide margin of safety and can be used freely during sexual encounters.
D. GHB withdrawal is mild and does not require medical attention.
E. The effects of GHB last more than 24 h, minimizing the need for dosing awareness.

Correct Answer: B.

Explanation: GHB use poses serious health risks, particularly when combined with other depressants like alcohol, which can lead to life-threatening respiratory depression. Educating patients about the dangers of polydrug use is a key harm-reduction strategy in this scenario.

7. Which of the following best describes an evidence-based approach for providing effective addiction care for transgender patients?

   A. Focus only on substance use treatment and avoid discussing gender identity to prevent discomfort.
   B. Integrate trauma-informed and gender-affirming care to address both substance use and psychosocial stressors.
   C. Recommend a "one-size-fits-all" treatment model, as evidence suggests similar needs across all patient populations with SUDs.
   D. Prioritize abstinence-only SUD treatment programs without considering gender-specific experiences.

   Correct Answer: B.

   Explanation: Evidence supports the use of trauma-informed, gender-affirming approaches when treating substance use disorders among transgender individuals. Addressing experiences of discrimination, violence, and anti-transgender stigma together with SUD treatment improves clinical outcomes.

References

1. National Academy of Medicine. The health of lesbian, gay, bisexual, and transgender people: building a foundation for better understanding. National Academies Press; 2011. p. 13128. https://doi.org/10.17226/13128.
2. Hughto JMW, Quinn EK, Dunbar MS, Rose AJ, Shireman TI, Jasuja GK. Prevalence and co-occurrence of alcohol, nicotine, and other substance use disorder diagnoses among us transgender and cisgender adults. JAMA Netw Open. 2021;4(2):e2036512. https://doi.org/10.1001/jamanetworkopen.2020.36512.
3. Gonzales G, Henning-Smith C. Health disparities by sexual orientation: results and implications from the behavioral risk factor surveillance system. J Commun Health. 2017;42(6):1163–72. https://doi.org/10.1007/s10900-017-0366-z.
4. Casey LS, Reisner SL, Findling MG, et al. Discrimination in the United States: experiences of lesbian, gay, bisexual, transgender, and queer Americans. Health Serv Res. 2019;54(Suppl 2):1454–66. https://doi.org/10.1111/1475-6773.13229.
5. Lett E, Abrams MP, Moberg E, Benson GP, Perlson JE. Syndemic relationship of depressive symptoms, substance use, and suicidality in transgender youth: a cross-sectional study using the U.S. youth risk behavior surveillance system. Soc Psychiatry Psychiatr Epidemiol. 2022;57(11):2293–304. https://doi.org/10.1007/s00127-022-02348-1.
6. Operario D, King W, Gamarel K, Iwamoto M, Tan S, Nemoto T. Stigma and substance use among transgender and Nonbinary young adults: results from the phoenix study. Transgend Health. 2024;9(4):317–25. https://doi.org/10.1089/trgh.2022.0144.
7. Paschen-Wolff MM, DeSousa A, Paine EA, Hughes TL, Campbell ANC. Experiences of and recommendations for LGBTQ+-affirming substance use services: an exploratory qualitative descriptive study with LGBTQ+ people who use opioids and other drugs. Subst Abuse Treat Prev Policy. 2024;19(1):2. https://doi.org/10.1186/s13011-023-00581-8.
8. Mattson G. The changing mix of gay bar subtypes after COVID-19 restrictions in the United States, 2017 to 2023. Socius Sociol Res Dyn World. 2023;9:23780231231181902. https://doi.org/10.1177/23780231231181902.

9. Nair JM, Waad A, Byam S, Maher M. Barriers to care and root cause analysis of LGBTQ+ patients' experiences: a qualitative study. Nurs Res. 2021;70(6):417–24. https://doi.org/10.1097/NNR.0000000000000541.
10. Paschen-Wolff MM, Velasquez R, Aydinoglo N, Campbell ANC. Simulating the experience of searching for LGBTQ-specific opioid use disorder treatment in the United States. J Subst Abuse Treat. 2022;140:108828. https://doi.org/10.1016/j.jsat.2022.108828.
11. Johns MM, Lowry R, Haderxhanaj LT, et al. Trends in violence victimization and suicide risk by sexual identity among high school students – youth risk behavior survey, United States, 2015–2019. MMWR Suppl. 2020;69(1):19–27. https://doi.org/10.15585/mmwr.su6901a3.
12. Johns MM, Lowry R, Andrzejewski J, et al. Transgender identity and experiences of violence victimization, substance use, suicide risk, and sexual risk behaviors among high school students – 19 states and large urban school districts, 2017. MMWR Morb Mortal Wkly Rep. 2019;68(3):67–71. https://doi.org/10.15585/mmwr.mm6803a3.
13. Marchi M, Arcolin E, Fiore G, et al. Self-harm and suicidality among LGBTIQ people: a systematic review and meta-analysis. Int Rev Psychiatry Abingdon Engl. 2022;34(3-4):240–56. https://doi.org/10.1080/09540261.2022.2053070.
14. Zachry CE, O'Brien RP, Clark KA, Ding ML, Blosnich JR. Mortality among sexual and gender minority populations: a systematic review. PLoS One. 2025;20(2):e0307688. https://doi.org/10.1371/journal.pone.0307688.
15. Killermann S. Breaking through the binary: gender explained using continuums. It's pronounced metrosexual. https://www.itspronouncedmetrosexual.com/2011/11/breaking-through-the-binary-gender-explained-using-continuums/. Accessed 24 Sept 2025
16. The Regents of the University of California, Davis Campus. LGBTQIA resource center – LGBTQIA resource center glossary. May 5, 2015. https://lgbtqia.ucdavis.edu/educated/glossary. Accessed 25 Aug 2025
17. Coleman E, Radix AE, Bouman WP, et al. Standards of care for the health of transgender and gender diverse people, Version 8. Int J Transgender Health. 2022;23(sup1):S1–S259. https://doi.org/10.1080/26895269.2022.2100644.
18. Miller S. Same-sex marriage ruling: 3 years later, bills threaten LGBT families. USA Today. April 6, 2018. https://www.usatoday.com/story/news/nation/2018/06/04/same-sex-marriage-ruling-undermined-gay-parents/650112002/. Accessed 24 Sept 2025
19. Thrasher SW. For gay and lesbian parents, equality is a myth when it comes to custody cases. The Guardian. 2014; https://www.theguardian.com/australia-news/2017/oct/23/children-raised-by-same-sex-parents-do-as-well-as-their-peers-study-shows. Accessed 25 Nov 2024
20. Gonzales G, Przedworski J, Henning-Smith C. Comparison of health and health risk factors between lesbian, gay, and bisexual adults and heterosexual adults in the united states: results from the national health interview survey. JAMA Intern Med. 2016;176(9):1344–51. https://doi.org/10.1001/jamainternmed.2016.3432.
21. Crepaz N, Hess KL, Purcell DW, Hall HI. Estimating national rates of HIV infection among MSM, persons who inject drugs, and heterosexuals in the United States. AIDS. 2019;33(4):701–8. https://doi.org/10.1097/QAD.0000000000002111.
22. Parsons JT, Lelutiu-Weinberger C, Botsko M, Golub SA. A randomized controlled trial utilizing motivational interviewing to reduce HIV risk and drug use in young gay and bisexual men. J Consult Clin Psychol. 2014;82(1):9–18. https://doi.org/10.1037/a0035311.
23. Kahler CW, Pantalone DW, Mastroleo NR, et al. Motivational interviewing with personalized feedback to reduce alcohol use in HIV-infected men who have sex with men: a randomized controlled trial. J Consult Clin Psychol. 2018;86(8):645–56. https://doi.org/10.1037/ccp0000322.
24. Taylor E, Patel D, Marconi V, et al. Pilot trial of a smartphone-based intervention to reduce alcohol consumption among veterans with HIV. Mil Behav Health. 2023;11(1-2):66–77. https://doi.org/10.1080/21635781.2023.2221465.
25. Richesson D, Magas I, Brown S. Lesbian, gay, and bisexual behavioral health: results from the 2021 and 2022 national surveys on drug use and health. Substance Abuse and Mental Health Services Administration (SAMHSA); 2023.

26. Jones CM, Clayton HB, Deputy NP, et al. Prescription opioid misuse and use of alcohol and other substances among high school students – youth risk behavior survey, United States, 2019. MMWR Suppl. 2020;69(1):38–46. https://doi.org/10.15585/mmwr.su6901a5.
27. Noel JK, Tudela SE, Rosenthal SR. Sexual minority status, illicit drug use, and depressive symptoms. J LGBT Youth. 2024;21(3):490–506. https://doi.org/10.1080/19361653.2023.2187918.
28. Grigsby TJ, Hoopsick R, Barker D, Devier E, Amis A, Yockey RA. Substance use and sexual orientation among adolescents: differences by age group and sex in the 2023 National Survey of Drug Use and Health. Am J Addict. 2025:ajad.70087. https://doi.org/10.1111/ajad.70087.
29. Schuler MS, Stein BD, Collins RL. Differences in substance use disparities across age groups in a national cross-sectional survey of lesbian, gay, and bisexual adults. LGBT Health. 2019;6(2):68–76. https://doi.org/10.1089/lgbt.2018.0125.
30. McCabe SE, West BT, Hughes TL, Boyd CJ. Sexual orientation and substance abuse treatment utilization in the United States: results from a national survey. J Subst Abuse Treat. 2013;44(1):4–12. https://doi.org/10.1016/j.jsat.2012.01.007.
31. Ganz O, Schulz JA, Ehlke SJ, King Jensen JL, Villanti AC. Cigarette smoking behaviors and nicotine dependence at the intersection of sexual identity and sex in the United States: findings from the national survey on drug use and health. Prev Med Rep. 2024;38:102593. https://doi.org/10.1016/j.pmedr.2024.102593.
32. Hughes TL, Wilsnack SC, Kantor LW. The influence of gender and sexual orientation on alcohol use and alcohol-related problems: toward a global perspective. Alcohol Res Curr Rev. 2016;38(1):121–32.
33. Fish JN, Exten C. Sexual orientation differences in alcohol use disorder across the adult life course. Am J Prev Med. 2020;59(3):428–36. https://doi.org/10.1016/j.amepre.2020.04.012.
34. Coronado-Muñoz M, García-Cabrera E, Quintero-Flórez A, Román E, Vilches-Arenas Á. Sexualized drug use and Chemsex among men who have sex with men in Europe: a systematic review and meta-analysis. J Clin Med. 2024;13(6):1812. https://doi.org/10.3390/jcm13061812.
35. Poulios A, Apostolidou A, Triantafyllidou S, et al. The distinction between Chemsex and sexualized drug use among men who have sex with men. Sex Cult. 2024;28(3):1276–88. https://doi.org/10.1007/s12119-023-10179-8.
36. Georgiadis N, Katsimpris A, Vatmanidou MA, Vassilakou T, Beloukas A, Sergentanis TN. Prevalence of chemsex and sexualized drug use among men who have sex with men: a systematic review and meta-analysis. Drug Alcohol Depend. 2025;275:112800. https://doi.org/10.1016/j.drugalcdep.2025.112800.
37. Pappas MK, Halkitis PN. Sexual risk taking and club drug use across three age cohorts of HIV-positive gay and bisexual men in New York City. AIDS Care. 2011;23(11):1410–6. https://doi.org/10.1080/09540121.2011.565027.
38. Halkitis PN, Parsons JT, Stirratt MJ. A double epidemic: crystal methamphetamine drug use in relation to HIV transmission. J Homosex. 2001;41(2):17–35. https://doi.org/10.1300/J082v41n02_02.
39. Halkitis PN, Mukherjee PP, Palamar JJ. Longitudinal modeling of methamphetamine use and sexual risk behaviors in gay and bisexual men. AIDS Behav. 2009;13(4):783–91. https://doi.org/10.1007/s10461-008-9432-y.
40. Halkitis PN, Green KA, Carragher DJ. Methamphetamine use, sexual behavior, and HIV seroconversion. J Gay Lesbian Psychother. 2006;10(3-4):95–109. https://doi.org/10.1300/J236v10n03_09.
41. Coulter RWS, Bersamin M, Russell ST, Mair C. The effects of gender- and sexuality-based harassment on lesbian, gay, bisexual, and transgender substance use disparities. J Adolesc Health Off Publ Soc Adolesc Med. 2018;62(6):688–700. https://doi.org/10.1016/j.jadohealth.2017.10.004.

42. Hughes TL, Veldhuis CB, Drabble LA, Wilsnack SC. Research on alcohol and other drug (AOD) use among sexual minority women: a global scoping review. Kabir R, ed. PLoS One. 2020;15(3):e0229869. https://doi.org/10.1371/journal.pone.0229869.
43. Parsons JT, Kelly BC, Wells BE. Differences in club drug use between heterosexual and lesbian/bisexual females. Addict Behav. 2006;31(12):2344–9. https://doi.org/10.1016/j.addbeh.2006.03.006.
44. Tordoff DM, Wanta JW, Collin A, Stepney C, Inwards-Breland DJ, Ahrens K. Mental health outcomes in transgender and nonbinary youths receiving gender-affirming care. JAMA Netw Open. 2022;5(2):e220978. https://doi.org/10.1001/jamanetworkopen.2022.0978.
45. Wolfe HL, Biello KB, Reisner SL, Mimiaga MJ, Cahill SR, Hughto JMW. Transgender-related discrimination and substance use, substance use disorder diagnosis and treatment history among transgender adults. Drug Alcohol Depend. 2021;223:108711. https://doi.org/10.1016/j.drugalcdep.2021.108711.
46. Wolford-Clevenger C, Flores LY, Bierma S, Cropsey KL, Stuart GL. Minority stress and drug use among transgender and gender diverse adults: a daily diary study. Drug Alcohol Depend. 2021;220:108508. https://doi.org/10.1016/j.drugalcdep.2021.108508.
47. Day JK, Fish JN, Perez-Brumer A, Hatzenbuehler ML, Russell ST. Transgender youth substance use disparities: results from a population-based sample. J Adolesc Health Off Publ Soc Adolesc Med. 2017;61(6):729–35. https://doi.org/10.1016/j.jadohealth.2017.06.024.
48. Kidd JD, Tettamanti NA, Kaczmarkiewicz R, et al. Prevalence of substance use and mental health problems among transgender and cisgender U.S. adults: results from a national probability sample. Psychiatry Res. 2023;326:115339. https://doi.org/10.1016/j.psychres.2023.115339.
49. Connolly D, Gilchrist G. Prevalence and correlates of substance use among transgender adults: a systematic review. Addict Behav. 2020;111:106544. https://doi.org/10.1016/j.addbeh.2020.106544.

Substance Use Disorders in Underserved and Historically Excluded Populations

18

Theddeus Iheanacho, Ayana Jordan, and Charles Dike

High-Yield Review Points

- People experiencing homelessness have significantly higher rates of substance use disorders (SUD) and worse health and psychosocial outcomes related to substance use.
- Racial and ethnic minoritized (REM) communities are disproportionately affected by substance use. This is driven by lower treatment initiation and engagement, an overwhelming mistrust of the healthcare system, and vulnerabilities related to structural determinants of health.
- While more than half of the people involved in the legal system have a SUD, treatment penetration for this population remains low.
- Structurally and culturally competent care by clinicians and providers can reduce disparities in SUD health outcomes.
- Improved care coordination across different agencies in the legal system can enhance linkage to care for individuals involved in the system who have SUD.
- Integrating and adapting SUD care in non-traditional and community settings has potential to increase access to treatment for underserved populations.

T. Iheanacho (✉) · C. Dike
Department of Psychiatry, Yale University School of Medicine, New Haven, CT, USA
e-mail: theddeus.iheanacho@yale.edu; charles.dike@yale.edu

A. Jordan
Department of Psychiatry, New York University Grossman School of Medicine, New York, NY, USA
e-mail: ayana.jordan@nyulangone.org

C. Marienfeld, M. Soltani (eds.), *AAAP Review of Addiction Psychiatry*,
https://doi.org/10.1007/978-3-032-24174-0_18

Homelessness and Substance Use Disorder (SUD)

Substance use disorders (SUD) are a major health-related cause of homelessness in the United States [1, 2]. Using data from Wave 3 of the National Epidemiologic Survey on Alcohol and Related Conditions (2012–2013), results showed that substance use disorders independently increased prospective risk for lifetime and 1-year prevalence of homelessness, after adjustment for ecological variables [3]. Analysis of data from the National Comorbidity Survey Replication (NCSR) in the United States showed that one of the strongest independent risk factors for past homelessness was lifetime substance use disorder and being identified as Black [4]. In the United Kingdom, data from the Adult Psychiatric Morbidity Surveys showed that the largest attributable risk factors for homelessness were SUD. A study on homelessness among United States military veterans found that the strongest risk factors for homelessness, other than extreme poverty, were SUD, especially alcohol and other SUD [4, 5]. Specifically, opioid use disorder (OUD) increases the risk of homelessness. A national study of Veteran Health Affairs (VHA) service users found the prevalence of homelessness among veterans with OUD to be 34.6%, 28.7 times that of veterans without OUD. This suggests that OUD is a major risk factor for homelessness and is substantially greater than for homelessness associated with unspecified SUD among veterans [6]. Furthermore, for people who exit homelessness into permanent supported housing, SUD raised the odds of eviction by about 150%, while those with alcohol use disorder (AUD) specifically were 50% more likely to be evicted [7].

Epidemiology of SUD Among Homeless Individuals

The major epidemiological surveys in the United States related to alcohol and other substance use—namely the National Epidemiological Survey on Alcohol and Related Conditions (NESARC) and the National Survey on Drug Use and Health (NSDUH)—do not include homeless individuals [8, 9]. The NESARC items do include questions on past year and lifetime homelessness. Consequently, available data on prevalence and correlates of SUD among people experiencing homelessness come from epidemiological studies of sub-groups of homeless populations and homeless research focused on cities, states, or the Veteran Affairs (VA) healthcare system.

Alcohol Use Disorder (AUD) In a study of homeless women (n = 780) seeking primary care services at Health Care for the Homeless clinics across 11 sites in the US, 19% reported a past year AUD [10]. Another study among sheltered homeless adults found that 17% of women (n = 211) and 26% of men (n = 370) were diagnosed with AUD [11]. These rates are significantly higher than the rates of AUD for women and men in the general population based on NESARC data (women=10%; n = 20,447 and men=18%; n = 15,862). In a national study of homeless veterans admitted to the VA-supported housing program (n = 29,143), 16.6% had an AUD

[12]. A study of 146 homeless street youth in 3 U.S. cities (Los Angeles, California; Austin, Texas; St. Louis, Missouri) found that 46.3% met criteria for AUD [13]. Additionally, among young people, the experience of homelessness prior to 12th grade is significantly associated with the development in young adulthood of the most severe forms of AUD [14].

Opioid Use Disorder Data on the prevalence of OUD among homeless adults is limited. A national study of homeless veterans receiving services in the VA healthcare system in 2012 ($n = 191,391$) showed that almost 18% had a diagnosis of OUD [6]. A survey of homeless-experienced persons engaged in primary care at five federally funded programs in the United States ($n = 601$) showed that 7.5% had used illicit opioids in the three months prior to the survey [15]. In a study of patients presenting to an urban hospital emergency department with questions about housing, substance use, and other health and social factors among patients who did or did not report current literal (streets/shelter) homelessness, patients who were currently homeless ($n = 316$, 13.7%) versus non-homeless ($n = 1993$, 86.3%) had higher rates of past year heroin use (16.7% vs. 3.8%) and prescription opioid use (12.5% vs. 4.4%) [16]. A review of national trends in SUD treatment showed that among all adults with OUD entering specialty treatment from 2013 to 2017, 12.5% reported experiencing homelessness [17]. These findings, although limited, indicate that OUD rate among homeless adults could be 15 to 20 times the 1% prevalence rate of opioid use disorder in the general adult US population [18].

Nicotine Use Disorder In a nationally representative cross-sectional survey of homeless and non-homeless individuals using federally funded community health centers in 2009, individuals with a history of homelessness had a substantially higher prevalence of current smoking than never homeless people (57.3 vs. 26.7%) while 74% of respondents with a history of homelessness were ever smokers, compared to 43.5% among those without a history of homelessness. A systematic review of 53 studies of adult individuals experiencing homelessness in the United States published in 2020 showed smoking prevalence of 57% to 82% [19]. These rates are almost four times the national average and in keeping with other studies of smoking among homeless adults in the United States [20–22].

Co-morbidities and Mortality

By far, the most prevalent infections among homeless adults in the United States are hepatitis c virus (HCV) with rates ranging from 9.8% to 52.5% and human immunodeficiency virus (HIV) with rates of 6.4% to 40%. SUD are common primary risk factors for HCV and HIV infections. Additionally, unsafe sexual practices, prior incarceration, and chronic psychiatric disorders and history of intimate partner violence, all of which are related to SUD, were also associated with a heightened risk of HCV and HIV infections [6, 23].

Homeless adults are more likely to die of overdose and have poorer health and social outcomes compared to matched cohorts in the general population [24–26]. One study of homeless adults in Boston showed that opioid overdose accounted for over 80% of drug overdose-related deaths among homeless adults [27]. Another study showed that drug overdose accounted for 1 in 4 deaths among people experiencing homelessness with mortality patterns over time showing a substantial increase in synthetic opioid overdose mortality and increasing involvement of opioids in polysubstance overdose deaths [28].

Barriers to Treatment

Although there is a great need for SUD services for people experiencing homelessness, many do not use or receive these services. Only about 25% of homeless adults with SUD who are seeking treatment receive it. The most frequently cited barriers to treatment relate to insurance coverage, high copayments for services, lack of safe housing and place to stay to begin treatment, difficulty in accessing information about programs, not having personal contacts that could facilitate getting services, and maintaining contact with providers. At individual levels, frequently cited reasons by homeless adults for not accessing treatment include their own denial, the shame and guilt of relapsing, and not knowing how to stop even when they have decided to do so. For homeless women, particular barriers to treatment are having a child who is a minor and chronic homelessness and having "a more street-based social network" [25, 29]. For these reasons, compared to domiciled adults with SUD, homeless adults with SUD are less likely to initiate care, less likely to follow up with treatment, and less likely to access inpatient care [24, 25, 30]. This leads to poorer treatment outcomes.

Utilizing Existing Service Frameworks

With the high prevalence, morbidity and mortality burden of SUD and the treatment gap that exist for the homeless populations, innovative, tailored, effective, sustainable, and acceptable approaches are needed to increase their utilization of SUD treatment. One approach is using the integrated care model [31, 32] to include SUD treatment in the care package for the homeless by leveraging existing service frameworks and available resources including peer support and counseling, medications for addiction treatment (MAT), and mobile services. In fact, the National Healthcare for the Homeless Council specifically recommends "flexibility," "tailored treatment," and bringing "treatment to places where homeless people are, including shelters" [33]. For example, emergency department-based buprenorphine initiation is supported by a significant body of literature demonstrating a marked reduction in mortality in addition to increased engagement in care among people experiencing homelessness [34, 35]. Clinical case management programs for homeless adults anchored in community health centers, short-term housing agencies, and traditional shelters provide housing support, employment, and social services [36–38]. This is an example of a sustained and robust framework of screening, assessment, monitoring, and connection to treatment with potential for integrating specific SUD treatment modalities.

Treatment Interventions That Improve Outcomes for the Homeless Population

Over the past decade, "Housing first" models have showed some initial promise in reducing the burden of homelessness [39], and homeless services should screen for identify and provide access to care for SUD and common co-morbid conditions among their service users. Mobile treatment units offering "on-demand," flexible, and accessible MAT for opioid use disorder with medical and case management services is an example of a patient-centered approach to care delivery that can increase SUD treatment utilization among the homeless population. A program in New Jersey sought to reduce barriers to treatment by providing free, opioid agonist treatment (OAT) (i.e., methadone or buprenorphine) via mobile medication units (MMUs). The MMUs enrolled a greater proportion of homeless individuals than the fixed-site methadone clinics [40]. Earlier examples include the "methadone bus" project in Amsterdam [41] and the "mobile medical van" in New Haven [42].

Substance Use Disorders in Racial and Ethnic Minoritized Groups

Overview of Racial and Ethnic Disparities in Addiction

The overall prevalence of mental health conditions is similar across racial and ethnic groups in the United States. However, there continues to be a disproportionate burden of illness experienced among racial and ethnic minoritized (REM) populations [26]. A recent systematic review of randomized controlled trials (RCTs) that included Black or Latinx adults with any non-nicotine SUD that reported rates of treatment initiation, engagement, or substance use outcome by race or ethnicity showed that Black and Latinx participants had poorer treatment retention rates when compared with White participants [43]. The following sections summarize the major take-home points of the existing racial and ethnic disparities in addiction, specifically those related to treatment and health outcomes for SUD.

Tobacco The few studies that have looked at smoking by race have different results. Some have found there was no difference found in cigarette smoking prevalence by race and ethnicity [27], while others [28] found that American Indian/Alaskan Natives (AI/AN) and White people were found to use tobacco more than other REM groups. In general, Black and Latinx people are less likely to be daily smokers, use smokeless tobacco, or e-cigarettes, and had more reports of past-year quit attempts and higher use of menthol cigarettes compared to White people. Interestingly, more Black people were found to engage in smoking cessation treatment on the inpatient setting as compared with White people, who were less likely to be interested in cessation services during treatment [29]. This highlights the importance of culturally informed care, based on different racial preferences.

Alcohol Prevalence rates of alcohol use are higher among White people, compared with REM populations, including Black, Hispanic/Latino, AI/AN, Native Hawaiian/Pacific Islander (NH/PI), and Asians [25]. However Black and Latinx people have more adverse health consequences because of their alcohol use [30]. Latinx people are over-represented in DUI-related fatalities [30], and AI/AN have the greatest self-reported rates of DUIs. Further, Black and Latinx people are more likely to be involved in the legal system because of their alcohol use compared to White people [31]. This underscores the need for more advocacy at the local, state, and national levels to address biased policies that inherently result in the over-representation of Black and Hispanics/Latinos with AUDs in the legal system, as opposed to obtaining substance use treatment.

Cocaine People racialized as Black are more likely to use cocaine compared with White and Black people and Hispanics/Latinos have been shown to have higher rates of cocaine-related overdose deaths, compared with White people [32], but less likely to engage in treatment and more likely to be involved in the legal system as a result of their substance use [33]. A clearer understanding of the factors that underlie these health disparities is crucial in preventing further drug-related overdose deaths in REM populations.

Cannabis Studies on cannabis use by race and ethnicity have showed mixed results. There were indications that non-medical cannabis use had been decreasing among all racial and ethnic populations, with non-uniform rate of decrease among the different groups [44]. For example, among adolescents in tenth grade, Black youth were more likely to show an increase in cannabis use compared with White youth. Yet, all racial and ethnic groups in twelfth grade, except non-Hispanic/Latino White youth, demonstrate a linear increase in prevalence of cannabis across time [44]. Data from the National Survey on Drug Use and Health for 2003–2015 [45] revealed that among adult cannabis users, the odds of cannabis misuse and dependence were greater among Black, AI/AN, and Latinx people compared to White people. These REM groups are less likely to initiate substance use treatment compared with White people despite higher cannabis use [45]. A study examining changes in cannabis use following spate of legalizations in multiple states showed that living in a state after enactment of recreational cannabis laws was associated with increases in the odds of cannabis use within the past year and past month among Hispanic and non-Hispanic White individuals (as well as individuals identifying as Native American, Pacific Islander, Asian, or more than 1 race) compared with the period before the passage of recreational use laws; there were no increases among non-Hispanic Black individuals [46].

Opioids Misuse of opioids is the largest drug epidemic in the history of the U.S., affecting all racial and ethnic groups [47]. Initially, White people had the highest rate of opioid-related overdoses [47]. However, there has been a decline in deaths among this population, whereas rates of death among people racialized as Black, Latinx, and AI/AN individuals continue to increase [48, 49]. Despite these increased death rates, these REM groups have been excluded from greater sociopolitical discourse, with Black and Latinx people being far more likely to be arrested for their opioid use, rather than provided treatment [47].

Reasons Accounting for These Disparities

The exact reasons accounting for racial and ethnic disparities in addiction are not well understood. However, there have been several theories cited for lower treatment engagement among REM populations, including societal and cultural stigma associated with accessing substance use treatment, mistrust of the medical system due to historic maltreatment, lack of healthcare coverage, circuitous pathways to care, lower socioeconomic status, and the absence of culturally informed treatment options [37].

Furthermore, due to the interpersonal nature of medicine, a clinician's assumptions about a patient based upon their race or ethnicity can indeed impact interactions with, diagnosis of, and implementation of a treatment plan for the patient [31]. Race, both that of the patient and provider, can influence the care received, with several examples demonstrating substandard care of REM patients with SUD when compared to White people [31]. We must therefore acknowledge that stereotypes of racial and other groups do exist and can impact the perceptions, expectations, and interactions a person may have with the healthcare system, particularly if they belong to or are assigned to a REM group [31]. There has been more understanding and awareness about the role of *implicit bias*, the subconscious association of a stereotypical attribute with a particular racial group [38], in the care of minoritized populations with SUD [39].

Another key concept in understanding the disparities that exist among racial and ethnic minorities must include an understanding of the conditions in which people live, learn, work, and play, collectively known as the *Social Determinants of Health* (SDOH) [40], which can affect a wide range of health risks and outcomes. Unfortunately, racial and ethnic minorities are more likely to have poorer SDOH, including higher unemployment rates, unstable housing, low income, unsafe neighborhoods, and substandard education [40]. Taken together, not having stable SDOH can contribute to worsened health outcomes from substance use [40], and further decrease the likelihood of REM populations to initiate, engage, or complete substance use treatment [41].

Various Models of Care Hold Future Promise

There are many models of care to address disparities in addiction among REM people. Some examples of novel interventions that are culturally informed, meaning those that incorporate specific cultural norms into treatment considerations, which may prove useful can broadly be characterized as (1) integrated care models, (2) faith-based, and (3) models that address the SDOH [42].

Integrated health models that provide comprehensive, multi-disciplinary care are shown to be effective in the treatment of mental health disorders [43]. Primary care is often the entry point of care for many people, so co-localizing addiction treatment within primary care and utilizing peer recovery coaches (those with lived experience in SUD) or community resource workers may prove essential in addressing the complex needs of many REM populations. Further, the integration of cultural and linguistic preferences in care has also been shown to be effective in decreasing rates of attrition among REM populations [43]. An example of a cultural preference of care is the integration of faith into treatment models for addiction [44]. Given the importance and value of spirituality among many REM populations, the Substance Abuse and Mental Health Administration (SAMHSA) has specifically developed several faith-based programs to address substance use at the national, state, and local levels [44]. An example of a specific program that addresses SDOH includes the Center for Disease Control's Racial and Ethnic Approaches to Community Health (REACH), a national program geared at reducing racial and ethnic disparities in health, including tobacco use [42].

Substance Use Disorders and the Legal System

The association between substance use disorders (SUD) and criminal justice involvement is both robust and consistently demonstrated across studies. Individuals with SUD are significantly more likely to have extensive legal histories, with approximately 50% having received three or more sentences prior to probation or incarceration, compared to one-third of individuals without SUD [50]. This pattern is also evident in juvenile populations, where nearly half of adolescent boys and a comparable proportion of adolescent girls in detention facilities meet diagnostic criteria for a substance use disorder [51].

Co-morbid mental illness and SUD predominate in the offender population. A recent study found the worldwide prevalence of co-morbid SUD with non-affective psychosis, major depression, or axis I disorders was currently present in 3.5%, 9.1%, and 20.7% of the prison population, respectively. Approximately half of the prison population with serious mental illnesses had co-morbid substance use disorders [52]. Furthermore, released prisoners who were diagnosed with a substance use disorder (without a mental illness) while incarcerated had the highest rate of rearrest upon release, followed by those diagnosed with both mental illness and substance use disorder together, those with neither a substance use disorder nor a mental illness, and lastly by individuals diagnosed with mental illness alone [53]. For Black people, the "war on drugs" firmly established the connection between SUD and the legal system; punishment rather than treatment was emphasized [54]. This led to a dramatic increase in the incarceration of Black people, 5–7 times higher than White people in 2011, and to Black people accounting for almost half of all prisoners incarcerated with a sentence of more than one year for a drug-related offense [55].

High numbers of people with SUD in the legal system reflect, in part, the gap in treatment resources available in the community. For example, less than 12% of newly arrested individuals had been in outpatient or residential treatment for substance misuse in the preceding 12 months [56]. Research suggests that existing drug treatment programs have a capacity to serve only around 10% of offenders [57, 58].

Potential Interventions at Various Stages of the Legal System

Treatment interventions can be delivered from the point of arrest, through courts, during pre-incarceration, during incarceration, and at re-entry into the community.

Pre-incarceration Interventions In many jurisdictions, the police have a wide latitude in interacting with offenders who are under the influence of substances. They could, for example, divert the offender in lieu of arrest to the emergency room of an acute care hospital under statutes that allow them to transport persons whom the police assess as being a threat to themselves or others, or gravely disabled due to mental illness or intoxication. In these cases, police jurisdiction and involvement end when the person is admitted to the ED. Police have more options when they work with mobile crisis teams (MCTs). MCTs facilitate diversion of patients into one of various substance use treatments on the condition that the person agrees to voluntarily enter or engage in the treatment.

Alternatively, individuals taken into custody by the police can be diverted post booking with a promise to appear on the condition that they seek treatment. Such diversion occurs under the direction of the court and is then evaluated by the court at arraignment. Court diversion staff, from the department of mental health or similar agency assigned to the courts, advocate on behalf of patients, and following court approval of diversion, facilitate transfer to an available treatment facility. Treatment occurs independent of the court, although the court monitors success in terms of compliance with the treatment programs and avoidance of arrest.

Drug courts (an example of so-called specialty courts), present in many jurisdictions, but not in all states, work differently. They can assign criminal defendants and offenders (adults and juveniles) who have alcohol and drug problems to community-based substance use treatment and rehabilitation services with monitoring and supervision by the court [59]. A major difference between court diversion under the auspices of departments of mental health, and drug courts, is the requirement by the latter that the individual plead guilty, usually to misdemeanor charges. With successful completion of the program, the charges are usually expunged. In another example of a specialty court, offenders who have pleaded guilty to a felonious offense are sentenced for up to 2 years to a residential therapeutic community treatment system. The program, Drug Treatment Alternative To Prison (DTATP), significantly reduced recidivism and drug use and saved money over the cost of incarceration [60].

Pre-incarceration initiatives for managing SUD reflect the evolving recognition that punishment alone does not work for managing a chronic brain disease. They are more effective at reducing recidivism and significantly less expensive than incarceration in financial [61] and human costs [62]. There is less fracturing of family and neighborhood connections which is important for African American communities where many are under legal control on any given day.

Treatment in Jails (Shorter Term, Local) or Prisons (Longer Term, State or Federal) Jails provide an important step in interrupting problematic substance use and beginning treatment, especially because more than 15% of jail death and 7% of all deaths in state prisons in 2019 were attributed to drug and alcohol intoxication (overdose) [63]. However, given the short length of stay and rapid turnover, jails are more suited for screening and identification of SUD, initiation of brief interventions, and referral to community treatment programs [64]. Nevertheless, only 63% of jails in the US screen for OUD at intake, 24% continue MAT for those incarcerated in jails, and only 9% initiate MAT for those not on treatment. The picture is bleaker in prisons; in 2019, only 1% of individuals with SUD in federal or state prison received MAT, and in 2020 only 29% prisons had MAT available despite the fact that provision of MAT in corrections significantly reduces the likelihood of overdose, overdose deaths, and medical complications associated with SUD [65, 66]. Notably, although a majority of federal and state prisons provide other substance use treatments like withdrawal management, group or individual counseling, rehabilitation, self-help groups, and educational program, only 10% of incarcerated individuals received any form of treatment [65].

Post-incarceration Treatment The period immediately following release from incarceration is particularly dangerous for ex-prisoners. Former prisoners are at an increased risk of mortality compared to the non-incarcerated population, particularly from drug- and opioid-related overdose, especially in the 2 weeks following release from prison, compared to the general population [67]. Accidental drug overdose was the leading cause of death, followed by cardiovascular disease, cancer, homicide, suicide, and motor vehicle accidents [68]. Improved outcomes result from connection with identified protective factors against adverse outcome before or immediately following release from incarceration. These include structured SUD treatment programs, spirituality/religion, community-based resources (including self-help groups), and family [69].

The high rates of opioid overdose following release from incarceration provides a rationale for urgent intervention with medication treatment with buprenorphine or methadone [70]. In one study, prescription of MAT during incarceration and continuation on release from incarceration through coordination with outpatient services was associated with a 12.3% decrease in opioid-related overdose deaths compared to the preceding year [71]. 1115 Waiver: This waiver permits Medicaid to pay for SUD treatment for incarcerated individuals within 90 days (about 3 months) of their release from prison and subsequently connect them to outpatient services on release from prison.

For outpatient treatment to be successful, however, it is imperative that outpatient providers be comfortable working with patients with criminal history, and that they work closely with former incarcerated persons to access housing, transportation, health care, and vocational training/employment, and other life skills.

Conclusion

SUD are chronic, relapsing brain diseases associated with significant morbidity and mortality especially for vulnerable and underserved populations including the homeless, REM populations, and those involved in the legal system. Factors that increase the risk of worse SUD outcomes include poor socioeconomic status, impoverished environments, lack of or decreased access to medical and psychiatric care, challenges with housing and employment, and personally mediated and institutionalized racism. Individuals from disadvantaged, REM populations and those involved in the legal system are more likely to experience these barriers to recovery and to be exposed to the devastating consequences of addiction to substances. For treatments and interventions to be effective, they must address these issues in a coordinated, culturally and structurally relevant fashion.

Chapter Review Questions

1. A 58-year-old male U.S. military veteran presents to the clinic for a routine check-up. He reports being unemployed for the past year and admits to daily alcohol use. He also has a history of major depressive disorder and chronic back pain from an old training injury. His vital signs are stable, and physical examination is unremarkable. The clinician is discussing resources to help him maintain stable housing.

   Which of the following is the strongest independent risk factor for homelessness among U.S. military veterans?

   A. Unemployment
   B. Mental illness
   C. Substance use disorder
   D. Chronic pain
   E. Combat exposure

   Correct Answer: C.

   Explanation: While unemployment, mental illness, and chronic pain are significant contributing factors to homelessness among U.S. military veterans, substance use disorder (SUD) has consistently been identified as the strongest independent risk factor. Veterans with SUDs often face immense challenges in maintaining stable housing due to the pervasive impact of addiction on their financial stability, employment prospects, and social support systems. Addressing SUD is a critical component in preventing and resolving homelessness within this population.

References: Northern VA Medical Center [72], National Coalition for Homeless Veterans [73], US Department of Veterans Affairs [74].

2. A public health researcher is designing a national survey to assess the prevalence of substance use disorders (SUDs) across various demographic groups in the United States. The researcher is particularly interested in ensuring that all segments of the population are adequately represented to provide a comprehensive understanding of SUD epidemiology. Which of the following populations is most underrepresented in national surveys on substance use disorders (SUDs)?

   A. College students
   B. Elderly individuals
   C. Individuals experiencing homelessness
   D. Women
   E. Rural populations

   Correct Answer: C.

   Explanation: Individuals experiencing homelessness are consistently among the most significantly underrepresented populations in national surveys on substance use disorders. This underrepresentation is due to numerous factors, including difficulty in sampling this transient population, lack of stable addresses, distrust of institutions, and challenges in survey administration in non-traditional settings. Consequently, the true prevalence of SUDs in this vulnerable group is often underestimated in broader epidemiological studies. While other groups like the elderly, college students, women, or rural populations may face some challenges in survey participation, the barriers are generally less pronounced and pervasive than those encountered when surveying individuals experiencing homelessness.

   Reference: National Academies of Sciences, Engineering, and Medicine [75].

3. A 34-year-old Black man with a history of alcohol use disorder presents to the emergency department with a fractured arm after a fall. He reports he had been drinking heavily at the time of the fall. During his admission, the healthcare team focuses primarily on his acute injury and refers him to an outpatient alcohol treatment program upon discharge. He misses several follow-up appointments and experiences a relapse. Which of the following is one major reason Black and Latinx populations may experience worse outcomes from alcohol use, despite lower prevalence rates compared to White populations?

   A. Higher genetic susceptibility
   B. Preference for low-quality alcohol
   C. Greater legal system involvement and structural barriers
   D. Lower alcohol tolerance
   E. Less access to social support networks

   Correct Answer: C.

   Explanation: Black and Latinx populations often face greater involvement with the legal system and structural barriers, such as discrimination and lack of culturally competent care, which can significantly worsen outcomes related to alcohol use disorder. These factors can lead to delayed or inadequate treatment, perpetuating a cycle of poorer health outcomes despite potentially lower overall prevalence rates compared to White populations. Genetic susceptibility and alcohol tolerance are not consistently shown to be primary drivers of these disparities. While social support can be a factor, structural barriers often present more pervasive challenges.

Reference: Volkow et al. [76].

4. A 34-year-old man with a history of opioid use disorder is incarcerated in a local jail. He is not currently receiving any medication for opioid use disorder (MOUD). The jail's medical staff is evaluating him for treatment options. Which of the following percentages represents the approximate proportion of jails in the U.S. that initiate medications for addiction treatment (MAT) for new patients with Substance Use Disorder (SUD) who are not already on treatment?

   A. 63%
   B. 24%
   C. 9%
   D. 1%
   E. 45%

   Correct Answer: C.

   Explanation: The question asks for the percentage of jails that *initiate* MAT for new patients not already on treatment. Based on available data, only a small percentage of jails in the U.S. provide this service. The correct answer of 9% reflects the limited availability of MAT initiation in correctional facilities for new patients. Many facilities may continue treatment for those already on MAT, but initiation of new treatment is far less common.

   Reference: Brinkley-Rubinstein et al. [77].

5. A 35-year-old man with a history of opioid use disorder is being released from a correctional facility. During his incarceration, he participated in a medication for opioid use disorder (MOUD) program. As part of his discharge planning, the healthcare team is discussing strategies to prevent opioid overdose mortality post release. Which of the following interventions is most effective for reducing post-incarceration opioid overdose mortality?

   A. Mandatory drug testing
   B. Faith-based peer groups
   C. Continued MOUD from prison to outpatient care
   D. Isolated detox units
   E. Naloxone distribution at release only

   Correct Answer: C.

   Explanation: Opioid overdose mortality is significantly elevated in the post-incarceration period, particularly in the immediate weeks following release, due to decreased opioid tolerance. Continuity of care, specifically the continuation of medication for opioid use disorder (MOUD) from the correctional facility into outpatient settings, is the most effective intervention to reduce this risk. MOUD, which often includes buprenorphine or methadone, reduces opioid cravings and withdrawal symptoms, thereby decreasing the likelihood of relapse and fatal overdose.

- A. Mandatory drug testing:
  While drug testing can be a component of a comprehensive treatment plan, it alone is not as effective as continued MOUD in preventing overdose mortality, as it does not address the underlying physiological dependence or cravings.
- B. Faith-based peer groups:
  Peer support groups can be beneficial for recovery, but they are not a substitute for evidence-based medical treatment like MOUD in preventing overdose deaths, especially given the high physiological risk immediately post release.
- D. Isolated detox units:
  Withdrawal management alone, without subsequent MOUD, can be dangerous for individuals with opioid use disorder, as it rapidly reduces tolerance, increasing the risk of overdose if relapse occurs. Isolated units may not provide the necessary linkage to ongoing care.
- E. Naloxone distribution at release only:
  While naloxone distribution is a critical component of harm reduction and should be provided to all individuals at risk of opioid overdose, it is an overdose reversal medication and does not address the core issue of preventing opioid use or relapse itself. It should be used in conjunction with, not as a replacement for, effective treatment strategies like MOUD.

References: Binswanger et al. [78], Wakeman et al. [79].

Old Chapter Review Questions

1. Mr. Smith is a 56-year-old, employed, White male with history of diabetes, hypertension, and opioid use disorder. He lives in the rural areas of Ohio and recently became divorced from his wife of 20 years. Which of the following factors in Mr. Smith's history most likely puts him at risk of homelessness?

   A. Living in a rural area
   B. Being White
   C. Having a diagnosis of opioid use disorder
   D. Being recently divorced

   Correct Answer: C.

   Explanation: Data shows that a diagnosis of substance use disorder, especially opioid use disorder, is a strong risk factor for homelessness. Living in a rural area is in fact protective. Being Black is a risk factor for homelessness. Being divorced is not a known risk factor for homelessness.

2. Ms. Brown is a 45-year-old single, unemployed homeless female with history of substance use disorder, depression, and childhood sexual abuse. She drinks a pint of vodka daily and smokes crack cocaine a few times a week.

   Which of the following is more likely a comorbidity?

   A. Human Papillomavirus
   B. Human Immunodeficiency Virus
   C. Hepatitis C
   D. Hepatitis A

   Correct Answer: C.

   Explanation: Hepatitis C infection is the most common infection among homeless adults with up to 52% prevalence rate, and HIV is second with up to 40% prevalence. No strong evidence suggests that HPV and Hepatitis A viruses are highly prevalent among the homeless population.

3. An anthropology researcher examining the impact of social determinants of health in the United States will find that which of the following factors have been shown to potentially reduce disparities among racial and ethnic minorities with substance use disorder?

   A. Social and cultural stigma
   B. Racially concordant health providers
   C. Mistrust of the medical system
   D. Lack of healthcare coverage
   E. Lower socioeconomic status

   Correct Answer: B.

   Explanation: For racial and ethnic minoritized people (REM), having a provider of the same racial group is not implicated in health disparity and in fact can potentially enhance health outcomes for REM individuals. There have been several theories cited for lower treatment engagement among REM populations, including societal and cultural stigma associated with accessing substance use treatment, mistrust of the medical system due to historic maltreatment, lack of healthcare coverage, circuitous pathways to care, lower socioeconomic status, and the absence of culturally informed treatment options. In addition to these factors, the role of racism on various levels cannot be ignored.

4. During a court-ordered psychiatric evaluation of a jailed 22-year-old Black man awaiting trial on drug possession charges, the psychiatrist found one of the following to be correct regarding substance use in the legal system:

   A. 90% of all inmates reported drug use in the month before their offense
   B. Only 10% of adolescent boys in Juvenile detention have a diagnosis of substance use disorder
   C. Prisons are now aggressively treating identified inmates before their release back into the community

D. Drug courts, a specialty court that deals with individuals involved in the legal system with alcohol and other substance use problems, are not available in all US states

Correct Answer: D.

Explanation: The Bureau of Justice statistics report that over half of all inmates reported drug use in the month before their offense. In the juvenile population, approximately half of adolescent boys in Juvenile detention have a diagnosis of substance use disorder. Despite the recent escalation of deaths via opioid overdose, prescription of medication-assisted treatment for Opioid Use Disorders is sorely lacking. The majority of prisons provide drug treatment in the form of withdrawal management, counseling, and rehabilitation.

Drug courts, a specialty court that deals with individuals involved in the legal system with alcohol and other substance use problems, are not available in all US states. In some states with drug courts, they are not uniformly distributed throughout the state; they are not available in all counties of the state.

5. A post-doctoral research fellow, reviewing available data on substance use disorders among racial and ethnic groups in the legal system, would find which of the following to be correct?

A. The war on drugs targeted all racial and ethnic groups equally if cocaine was involved
B. Black and Latinx people involved in the legal system misused substances at rates higher than White people
C. It is now more likely that Black and Latinx people misusing substances will be committed to treatment in the community than to prison
D. Ready access to structured treatment programs, religious and self-help community groups, and family support have been shown to influence relapse and re-offending rates in Black people

Correct Answer: D.

Explanation: The war on drugs specifically targeted people racialized as Black and led to a dramatic increase in incarceration of Black people, 5–7 times more than White people. White people misused opioids more than Black and Latinx people. Black and Latinx people who misuse substances are still more likely to be incarcerated than sent to treatment; structured treatment programs and the other supportive structures listed in answer d are protective factors against re-offending.

References

1. Stablein GW, Hill BS, Keshavarz S, Llorente MD. Homelessness and substance use disorders. Clinical management of the homeless patient: social, psychiatric, and medical issues. Springer; 2021. p. 179–94.
2. Moxley VB, Hoj TH, Novilla MLB. Predicting homelessness among individuals diagnosed with substance use disorders using local treatment records. Addict Behav. 2020;102:106160.

3. Thompson RG Jr, Wall MM, Greenstein E, Grant BF, Hasin DS. Substance-use disorders and poverty as prospective predictors of first-time homelessness in the United States. Am J Public Health. 2013;103(S2):S282–S8.
4. Greenberg GA, Rosenheck RA. Mental health correlates of past homelessness in the National Comorbidity Study Replication. J Health Care Poor Underserved. 2010;21(4):1234–49.
5. Tsai J, Rosenheck RA. Risk factors for homelessness among US veterans. Epidemiol Rev. 2015:mxu004.
6. Iheanacho T, Stefanovics E, Rosenheck R. Opioid use disorder and homelessness in the Veterans Health Administration: the challenge of multimorbidity. J Opioid Manag. 2018;14(3):171–82.
7. Montgomery AE, Cusack M, Szymkowiak D, Fargo J, O'Toole T. Factors contributing to eviction from permanent supportive housing: lessons from HUD-VASH. Eval Progr Plan. 2017;61:55–63.
8. Hasin DS, Grant BF. The National Epidemiologic Survey on Alcohol and Related Conditions (NESARC) Waves 1 and 2: review and summary of findings. Soc Psychiatry Psychiatr Epidemiol. 2015;50(11):1609–40.
9. Abuse S, Administration MHS. 2015 National survey on drug use and health. 2016.
10. Upshur CC, Jenkins D, Weinreb L, Gelberg L, Orvek EA. Prevalence and predictors of substance use disorders among homeless women seeking primary care: an 11 site survey. Am J Addict. 2017;26(7):680–8.
11. Neisler J, Shree S, Reitzel LR, Chen T-A, Kendzor DE, Obasi EM, et al. Characterizing alcohol use behaviors among homeless men and women. Am J Health Behav. 2019;43(1):37–49.
12. Tsai J, Kasprow WJ, Rosenheck RA. Alcohol and drug use disorders among homeless veterans: prevalence and association with supported housing outcomes. Addict Behav. 2014;39(2):455–60.
13. Ferguson KM, Jun J, Bender K, Thompson S, Pollio D. A comparison of addiction and transience among street youth: Los Angeles, California, Austin, Texas, and St. Louis, Missouri. Community Ment Health J. 2010;46(3):296–307.
14. Moss HB, Ge S, Trager E, Saavedra M, Yau M, Ijeaku I, et al. Risk for Substance Use Disorders in young adulthood: associations with developmental experiences of homelessness, foster care, and adverse childhood experiences. Compr Psychiatry. 2020;100:152175.
15. Stringfellow EJ, Kim TW, Gordon AJ, Pollio DE, Grucza RA, Austin EL, et al. Substance use among persons with homeless experience in primary care. Subst Abus. 2016;37(4):534–41.
16. Doran KM, Rahai N, McCormack RP, Milian J, Shelley D, Rotrosen J, et al. Substance use and homelessness among emergency department patients. Drug Alcohol Depend. 2018;188:328–33.
17. Han BH, Doran KM, Krawczyk N. National trends in substance use treatment admissions for opioid use disorder among adults experiencing homelessness. J Subst Abus Treat. 2022;132:108504.
18. Saha TD, Kerridge BT, Goldstein RB, Chou SP, Zhang H, Jung J, et al. Nonmedical prescription opioid use and DSM-5 nonmedical prescription opioid use disorder in the United States. J Clin Psychiatry. 2016;77(6):772.
19. Soar K, Dawkins L, Robson D, Cox S. Smoking amongst adults experiencing homelessness: a systematic review of prevalence rates, interventions and the barriers and facilitators to quitting and staying quit. J Smok Cessat. 2020;15(2):94–108.
20. Baggett TP, Lebrun-Harris LA, Rigotti NA. Homelessness, cigarette smoking and desire to quit: results from a US national study. Addiction. 2013;108(11):2009–18.
21. Baggett TP, Rigotti NA. Cigarette smoking and advice to quit in a national sample of homeless adults. Am J Prev Med. 2010;39(2):164–72.
22. Tsai J, Rosenheck RA. Smoking among chronically homeless adults: prevalence and correlates. Psychiatr Serv. 2012;63(6):569–76.
23. Williams SP, Bryant KL. Sexually transmitted infection prevalence among homeless adults in the United States: a systematic literature review. Sex Transm Dis. 2018;45(7):494–504.

24. Wenzel SL, Burnam MA, Koegel P, Morton SC, Miu A, Jinnett KJ, et al. Access to inpatient or residential substance abuse treatment among homeless adults with alcohol or other drug use disorders. Med Care. 2001;39(11):1158–69.
25. Tucker JS, Wenzel SL, Golinelli D, Zhou A, Green HD. Predictors of substance abuse treatment need and receipt among homeless women. J Subst Abus Treat. 2011;40(3):287–94.
26. Lebrun-Harris LA, Baggett TP, Jenkins DM, Sripipatana A, Sharma R, Hayashi AS, et al. Health status and health care experiences among homeless patients in federally supported health centers: findings from the 2009 patient survey. Health Serv Res. 2013;48(3):992–1017.
27. Baggett TP, Hwang SW, O'Connell JJ, Porneala BC, Stringfellow EJ, Orav EJ, et al. Mortality among homeless adults in Boston: shifts in causes of death over a 15-year period. JAMA Intern Med. 2013;173(3):189–95.
28. Fine DR, Dickins KA, Adams LD, De Las Nueces D, Weinstock K, Wright J, et al. Drug overdose mortality among people experiencing homelessness, 2003 to 2018. JAMA Netw Open. 2022;5(1):e2142676-e.
29. Brubaker MD, Amatea EA, Torres-Rivera E, Miller MD, Nabors L. Barriers and supports to substance abuse service use among homeless adults. J Addict Offender Couns. 2013;34(2):81–98.
30. Priester MA, Browne T, Iachini A, Clone S, DeHart D, Seay KD. Treatment access barriers and disparities among individuals with co-occurring mental health and substance use disorders: an integrative literature review. J Subst Abus Treat. 2016;61:47–59.
31. Falloon IR, Fadden G. Integrated mental health care: a comprehensive, community-based approach. Cambridge University Press; 1995.
32. Shidhaye R, Lund C, Chisholm D. Closing the treatment gap for mental, neurological and substance use disorders by strengthening existing health care platforms: strategies for delivery and integration of evidence-based interventions. Int J Ment Heal Syst. 2015;9(1):40.
33. Matt Warfield BD. National Health Care for the Homeless Council (May 2016). Medication assisted treatment: buprenorphine in the HCH Community. 2016.
34. Hughes T, Nasser N, Mitra A. Overview of best practices for buprenorphine initiation in the emergency department. Int J Emerg Med. 2024;17(1):23.
35. Childers R, Castillo EM, Cronin AO, Swee S, Lasoff D. Emergency department-initiated buprenorphine treatment in a population with a high rate of homelessness: an observational study. J Emerg Med. 2023;64(2):129–35.
36. Hwang SW, Burns T. Health interventions for people who are homeless. Lancet. 2014;384(9953):1541–7.
37. de Vet R, van Luijtelaar MJ, Brilleslijper-Kater SN, Vanderplasschen W, Beijersbergen MD, Wolf JR. Effectiveness of case management for homeless persons: a systematic review. Am J Public Health. 2013;103(10):e13–26.
38. Winn JL, Shealy SE, Kropp GJ, Felkins-Dohm D, Gonzales-Nolas C, Francis E. Housing assistance and case management: improving access to substance use disorder treatment for homeless veterans. Psychol Serv. 2013;10(2):233.
39. Tsemberis S. Housing first: the pathways model to end homelessness for people with mental illness and addiction manual. Eur J Homelessness. 2011;5(2)
40. Hall G, Neighbors CJ, Iheoma J, Dauber S, Adams M, Culleton R, et al. Mobile opioid agonist treatment and public funding expands treatment for disenfranchised opioid-dependent individuals. J Subst Abus Treat. 2014;46(4):511–5.
41. Buning EC, van Brussel GH, van Santen G. The 'methadone by bus' project in Amsterdam. Br J Addict. 1990;85(10):1247–50.
42. Liebman J, Pat Lamberti M, Altice F. Effectiveness of a mobile medical van in providing screening services for STDs and HIV. Public Health Nurs. 2002;19(5):345–53.
43. Jordan A, Quainoo S, Nich C, Babuscio TA, Funaro MC, Carroll KM. Racial and ethnic differences in alcohol, cannabis, and illicit substance use treatment: a systematic review and narrative synthesis of studies done in the USA. Lancet Psychiatry. 2022;9(8):660–75.
44. Pacek LR, Malcolm RJ, Martins SS. Race/ethnicity differences between alcohol, marijuana, and co-occurring alcohol and marijuana use disorders and their association with public health and social problems using a national sample. Am J Addict. 2012;21(5):435–44.

45. James K, Jordan A. The opioid crisis in Black communities. J Law Med Ethics. 2018;46(2):404–21.
46. Martins SS, Segura LE, Levy NS, Mauro PM, Mauro CM, Philbin MM, et al. Racial and ethnic differences in cannabis use following legalization in US states with medical cannabis laws. JAMA Netw Open. 2021;4(9):e2127002-e.
47. Medlock MM, Shtasel D, Trinh N-HT, Williams DR. Racism and psychiatry: contemporary issues and interventions. Springer; 2018.
48. Gondré-Lewis MC, Abijo T, Gondré-Lewis TA. The opioid epidemic: a crisis disproportionately impacting Black Americans and urban communities. J Racial Ethn Health Disparities. 2023;10(4):2039–53.
49. Romero R, Friedman JR, Goodman-Meza D, Shover CL. US drug overdose mortality rose faster among hispanics than non-hispanics from 2010 to 2021. Drug Alcohol Depend. 2023;246:109859.
50. NCDAS. 2025 [02/08/2025]. Available from: https://drugabusestatistics.org/drug-related-crime-statistics/#:~:text=Drug%20arrests%20including%20marijuana%20make,11%25%20of%20total%20nationwide%20arrests
51. Teplin LA, Abram KM, McClelland GM, Dulcan MK, Mericle AA. Psychiatric disorders in youth in juvenile detention. Arch Gen Psychiatry. 2002;59(12):1133–43.
52. Baranyi G, Fazel S, Langerfeldt SD, Mundt AP. The prevalence of comorbid serious mental illnesses and substance use disorders in prison populations: a systematic review and meta-analysis. Lancet Public Health. 2022;7(6):e557–e68.
53. Zgoba KM, Reeves R, Tamburello A, Debilio L. Criminal recidivism in inmates with mental illness and substance use disorders. J Am Acad Psychiatry Law. 2020;48(2):209–15.
54. Rosenberg A, Groves AK, Blankenship KM. Comparing Black and White drug offenders: implications for racial disparities in criminal justice and reentry policy and programming. J Drug Issues. 2017;47(1):132–42.
55. Carson EA, Anderson E. Prisoners in 2014. 2015.
56. Golub A, Brownstein H, Dunlap E. Document title: Monitoring drug epidemics and the markets that sustain them using ADAM II: final technical report. 2012.
57. Taxman FS. Supervision-exploring the dimensions of effectiveness. Fed Probat. 2002;66:14.
58. Clark KJ, Vechinski J, Molfenter T, Taxman FS. Cascade of care in the legal system: best practices and goals for agencies providing care to patients concurrently navigating substance use disorders and criminal legal involvement. J Drug Issues. 2025;55(1):64–88.
59. Huddleston III CW, Freeman-Wilson JK, Marlowe DB, Roussell A. A national report card on drug courts and other problem solving court programs in the United States. US Department of Justice. 2008; 2(1)
60. Addiction NCo, University SAaC. Crossing the bridge: an evaluation of the Drug Treatment Alternative-to-Prison (DTAP) program. Author, New York; 2003.
61. Zarkin GA, Cowell AJ, Hicks KA, Mills MJ, Belenko S, Dunlap LJ, et al. Lifetime benefits and costs of diverting substance-abusing offenders from state prison. Crime Delinq. 2015;61(6):829–50.
62. McVay D, Schiraldi V, Ziedenberg J. Treatment or incarceration?: National and state findings on the efficacy and cost savings of drug treatment versus imprisonment. Justice Policy Institute; 2004.
63. Wang L, Widra E. An overview of health and access to healthcare for people in state prisons. In: Handbook on contemporary issues in health, crime, and punishment; 2024. p. 121–47.
64. Chandler RK, Fletcher BW, Volkow ND. Treating drug abuse and addiction in the criminal justice system: improving public health and safety. JAMA. 2009;301(2):183–90.
65. Widra E. Addicted to punishment: jails and prisons punish drug use far more than they treat it. 2024 01/30/2024.
66. Sufrin C, Kramer C, Terplan M, Fiscella K, Olson S, Voegtline K, et al. Availability of medications for opioid use disorder in US jails. J Gen Intern Med. 2023;38(6):1573–5.
67. O'Connor AW, Sears JM, Fulton-Kehoe D. Overdose and substance-related mortality after release from prison in Washington State: 2014–2019. Drug Alcohol Depend. 2022;241:109655.

68. Binswanger IA, Blatchford PJ, Mueller SR, Stern MF. Mortality after prison release: opioid overdose and other causes of death, risk factors, and time trends from 1999 to 2009. Ann Intern Med. 2013;159(9):592–600.
69. Binswanger IA, Nowels C, Corsi KF, Glanz J, Long J, Booth RE, et al. Return to drug use and overdose after release from prison: a qualitative study of risk and protective factors. Addict Sci Clin Pract. 2012;7(1):1–9.
70. Graves BD, Fendrich M. Community-based substance use treatment programs for reentering justice-involved adults: a scoping review. Drug Alcohol Depend Rep. 2024:100221.
71. Green TC, Clarke J, Brinkley-Rubinstein L, Marshall BD, Alexander-Scott N, Boss R, et al. Postincarceration fatal overdoses after implementing medications for addiction treatment in a statewide correctional system. JAMA Psychiatry. 2018;75(4):405–7.
72. Northern VA Medical Center. Homelessness among veterans: causes, risk factors, and solutions. https://www.va.gov/HOMES/docs/Homeless_Vet_Booklet_Web.pdf
73. National Coalition for Homeless Veterans. Homeless veterans: a hidden crisis. https://nchv.org/homeless-veterans/resources/
74. US Department of Veterans Affairs. The VA homeless programs; 2019. https://www.va.gov/HOMELESS/docs/Homeless_Programs_Fact_Sheet_FY19.pdf
75. National Academies of Sciences, Engineering, and Medicine. Homelessness, health, and human needs. The National Academies Press; 2018.
76. Volkow ND, et al. Alcohol and health disparities: a commentary. Alcohol Res Curr Rev. 2019;40(1):01.
77. Brinkley-Rubinstein L, Zaller N, Kuo I, et al. HIV and Hepatitis C virus infection among jail inmates: a systematic review. AIDS Behav. 2013;17(3):939–50.
78. Binswanger IA, Blatchford MR, Mueller SR. Mortality after release from prison and jail: an updated systematic review and meta-analysis. Ann Intern Med. 2022;175(2):226–36.
79. Wakeman SE, Bowman SE, Cunningham CO, Rich JD. Medication-assisted treatment for opioid use disorder in criminal justice settings: a review of the evidence and a call for action. J Subst Abuse Treat. 2020;116:108039.

Older Adults

19

Roberto D. Sanchez and Louis Trevisan

High-Yield Review Points

- As Baby Boomers retire, the proportion of older adults with substance use disorders has increased compared to earlier generations.
- The older adult population is less likely to be screened for substance use disorders and diagnoses may often be missed.
- Although not all seniors have serious medical problems, seniors who misuse substances generally face greater levels of medical comorbidity and functional impairment than their non-substance misusing peers.
- Physical illness and functional impairment can complicate addiction and the physical response to substances.
- Heavy and long-standing substance use has been shown to contribute to neurocognitive impairment.
- While many principles of addiction treatment remain constant across the age spectrum, good clinical care of the older adult requires an understanding of the aging process and how it alters the dynamics of treatment.
- Medications for substance use disorders can be effective in older adults but there should be special consideration of the age-related changes in drug metabolism and distribution that occur in late life.

R. D. Sanchez (✉)
Baylor College of Medicine, Houston, TX, USA
e-mail: Roberto.Sanchez@bcm.edu

L. Trevisan
Yale University School of Medicine, New Haven, CT, USA
e-mail: Louis.Trevisan@yale.edu

C. Marienfeld, M. Soltani (eds.), *AAAP Review of Addiction Psychiatry*,
https://doi.org/10.1007/978-3-032-24174-0_19

Introduction

Alcohol and drug use disorders are among the leading causes of disability worldwide. As the population of older adults increases, the magnitude of mental health and substance disorders will increase, and the public health impact of these disorders will increase. Additionally, the prevalence of addiction among older adults is predicted to increase due to cohort changes. Notably, the "Baby Boomer" generation is a group who were raised during the 1950s and 1960s and participated in the increased use of illicit drugs (e.g., heroin, cocaine), tobacco, and alcohol in the 1960s–1980s. This cohort is susceptible to both a history of and continued substance misuse, which will have physical and mental health consequences as it ages. However, relatively little research has been done examining the treatment and consequences of substance use disorders in older adults [1].

Substance use disorders are associated with social and health problems in seniors, including increased risk of hospitalization, nursing home placement, and death. Ninety percent of older adults use medications (both prescribed and over the counter) and many of these medications have potential adverse interactions with alcohol or illicit drugs. Additionally, older adults who are experiencing emotional and social issues such as bereavement, loneliness, and social isolation and medical problems such as chronic pain, insomnia, dementia, depression, or anxiety have an increased risk for substance misuse. These same problems may also be aggravated by substance use disorders [2].

However, substance use disorders in older adults are often not adequately diagnosed nor treated, as health professionals tend to overlook substance use disorders in the geriatric population, often attributing the symptoms to dementia, depression, or other problems instead. Additionally, older adults are more likely to hide their substance use problems and less likely to ask for help than younger adults. Although older adults respond well to age-specific, supportive and nonconfrontational group treatment targeted to their unique experience with substance use, only 7% of substance treatment centers reported having a program designed specifically for seniors in 2006 [2].

Demographics of Substance Use Disorders in Older Adults

The prevalence rates of substance use disorders have remained high among the Baby Boomers as they age, contrary to any generation preceding it. Substance use disorder rates among adults 50–64/≥65 years old increased from 2.8 million between 2002 and 2006 to 7.1 million between 2021 and 2022. This increase accounts for 9.1% of older adults. Of the 7.1 million, 5.6% had an alcohol use disorder, and 4.1% had a drug use disorder [2, 3].

Prevalence of Substance Use Among Older Adults

Alcohol

Although the geriatric population has increasing rates of illicit and prescription drug misuse, alcohol remains the most used substance among older adults. Alcohol is also the most common substance involved in older adults seeking substance use treatment [4]. Therefore, much of the research studying substance use among older adults has centered on alcohol use disorders.

Data from the 2022 National Survey on Drug Use and Health (NSDUH) shows that the estimated 12-month prevalence in the general population for alcohol use disorder as defined by the fifth edition of the Diagnostic and Statistical Manual of Mental Health Disorders is 5.6% for adults aged 60 and older. In this age group, the prevalence for binge alcohol use (defined by the use of 5 or more drinks for men or 4 or more drinks for women on the same occasion on at least 1 day in the past 30 days) is 12.8%, and the prevalence for heavy use (defined as binge drinking on the same occasion on each of 5 or more days in the past 30 days) is 3.2% [3]. This data confirms findings from a study examining primary care clinics across the United States, in which a majority (22%) of older alcohol users were moderate drinkers (defined as 1–7 drinks per week), while episodes of binge drinking were common among all drinkers (24%), whether they were categorized as moderate, at-risk, or heavy drinkers. In this sample, it was found that frequent binge drinkers who were also heavy drinkers were more likely to report fair or poor health. These findings are of critical significance due to older adults' increased susceptibility to the toxic effects of alcohol and the potential interactions of binging, medications, and co-occurring illnesses [5].

Risk factors for alcohol misuse in late life include male gender, affluence, Caucasian race, and being young-old (in the early stages of late life). Therefore, having more financial resources and longer financial horizons is a predictor of increased drinking in older age [6]. Moreover, many older adults have chronic medical conditions associated with pain. Those older adults who have drinking problems report more severe pain, more disruption of functioning due to pain, and more use of alcohol to manage pain than older nonproblem drinkers. Hence, it is important to monitor the drinking behavior of older patients who have pain complaints, especially those who have preexisting problems with alcohol [7].

Illicit Drugs

Older adults in the United States have one of the highest rates of illicit drug use compared to older adults in other countries [6]. The 2022 NSDUH data reveals that the 12-month prevalence rate of illicit drug use for adults aged 60 years and older was 12.1%, a jump from 5.7% in 2017 [3]. The Baby Boomer generation is unique as they have much higher rates of illicit drug use compared to their earlier cohorts, and they are a significantly larger group than previous cohorts. Baby Boomers, therefore, tend to have stark differences in attitudes toward recreational and illicit drugs compared to other generations.

Cannabis is the most common substance used after alcohol and tobacco by adults over the age of 50 in the United States and United Kingdom [8]. Although rates of illicit drug use among seniors have been relatively low historically, the prevalence of cannabis use among older adults is increasing in the United States. One study showed that the prevalence of past-year cannabis use among adults aged 65 years and older increased from 0.4% in 2006/2007 to 2.4% in 2015 and more recently 4.2% in 2018, a 75% relative increase [9]. Data from the 2022 NSDUH shows that for adults over the age of 60 years old, 7.7 million used cannabis in the last year with the primary mode of use being inhalation via smoking. Use was more common in older men (12.5%) than older women (7.5%) [3].

This trend of increased cannabis use in the older adult population is not unanticipated, given the high rates of substance use among Baby Boomers compared to previous generations. Additionally, this is occurring in the setting of shifting attitudes and legalization and decriminalization of cannabis use in a growing number of states for recreational and medicinal purposes. As cannabis use increases, it will be important to examine the health consequences of its use in older adults, as little to no research has focused on this. Although studies are emerging regarding the benefits of cannabis for medicinal use, such as for chronic pain, the risks for older adults have not been well-defined. It is therefore important to screen patients of all ages for substance misuse and to consider the unique vulnerabilities of older adults to the physiological effects of legal and illegal substances.

Prescription, Nonprescription, and OTC Medication Use

The United States is currently experiencing an opioid epidemic, with deaths from overdose of prescription opioids increasing from 3422 in 1999 to 14,716 in 2022 and overdose from any opioids increasing from 49,860 in 2019 to 81,806 in 2022. Based on data from the 2022 National Survey on Drug Use and Health (NSDUH), older adults were shown to have a 12-month prevalence of prescription opioid misuse of 2.3% in comparison with 3.2% in those between 18 and 25 years old.

A 2006 study found that 25% of older adults use prescription medications that have misuse potential (e.g., opioids and benzodiazepines) [10]. These medications can cause some of the most serious problems for seniors who use them. Most of these drugs are obtained legally, and misuse is usually unintentional. Older adults with the following characteristics may be more likely to have problems with psychoactive medications: being female, being socially isolated, and having a history of substance misuse or mental health disorder. Additionally, long-term use of psychoactive medications, like benzodiazepines, is associated with cognitive deficits, confusion, falls, and depression in older adults. The rate of hospital admissions for drug-related conditions among older adults is increasing exponentially. Combining alcohol and psychoactive medications has even more potential for bad outcomes. Older adults experiencing pain, anxiety, or sleep disturbances are especially at risk for substance misuse [11].

Diagnosis and Screening of Substance Use Disorders in the Older Adult

The criteria for the formal diagnosis of substance use disorders as laid out by the *DSM-5* may be less relevant for older adults. In a study exploring age-related biases among the criteria for alcohol use disorders, findings revealed that older adults were half as likely as middle-aged adults to endorse the criteria related to tolerance, activities to obtain alcohol, social/interpersonal problems, and physically hazardous situations. Older adults were also less likely to endorse recurrent physical/psychological problems than younger cohorts [12].

These findings may be explained by the unique biologic and social factors present in late life. For example, older adults generally experience a reduction in tolerance to substances due to the age-associated physiologic changes that increase the effects of alcohol and other substances. This interferes with one of the criteria of substance use disorders: increased tolerance. Additionally, interference with social or occupational areas of life or other consequences of substance use may be less likely to occur or less noticeable in old age due to a natural departure from these roles (i.e., through retirement or social isolation due to loss of peers). Furthermore, it may be that older adults blame the physical/psychological effects of alcohol on other areas in their life, such as the aging process itself, and in turn practitioners may be less likely to detect these issues as related to alcohol [6, 12].

As a result of these diagnostic issues, many who study substance use in the geriatric population deemphasize the reliance on *DSM* criteria to identify problematic substance use requiring treatment. They instead use a two-tier categorical classification: at risk and problem use. At-risk substance use refers to those who use substances above the recommended or prescribed levels but who experience few or no consequential physical, mental, emotional, or social problems. These individuals merit thorough screening and secondary prevention due to their high risk for developing such problems. Problem substance use, on the other hand, is characterized by those individuals who are already having problems in physical, mental, emotional, or social areas of life because of substance use. In contrast to at-risk substance users, identification of individuals with problem use does not depend on the quantity and frequency of use, but on the context in which substances are used. For example, older adults may have medical problems, such as gout or pancreatitis, even with minimal levels of alcohol consumption.

Older adults are less likely to be screened for substance use. Although awareness is increasing for the need for routine screening among older adults for substances, there are still several factors that inhibit adequate screening and identification of substance use disorders in older adults. For example, the potential stigma and discomfort related to the assessment of addiction and the similarities of a substance use disorder with both symptoms of normal aging and other illnesses common in later life can impede detection of substance use disorders. Additionally, older adults often have difficulty identifying their own risky behavior regarding substance use, making the identification of this behavior by the clinician even more difficult.

Moreover, many older adults and even their family members may view alcohol use as being their "one last pleasure," which creates a complex picture of substance use in late life. When assessing older adults for substance use, it is important to remember that older adults respond more to a supportive, nonconfrontational approach and that they are more likely to be forthcoming about potentially stigmatizing behaviors if they think the clinician is genuinely interested in their overall health.

Screening tools for the geriatric population include the CAGE questionnaire, which has been extensively studied and validated for use in older adults, or the MAST-G, which is a tool that was specifically designed to identify drinking problems in the geriatric population by modifying the Michigan alcohol screening test. The MAST-G is more relevant to alcohol use in later life as it focuses more on potential stressors and behaviors, rather than questions about family, vocational, and legal consequences of use. This tool is easy to administer, low cost, more specific than the CAGE in identifying problematic use, and useful to detect lifetime problematic use; however, it lacks information about frequency, quantity, and current problems.

The alcohol use disorders identification test (AUDIT) is also validated in older adults to assess current alcohol problems. Additionally, the comorbidity-alcohol risk evaluation tool (CARET) is useful for identifying older adults at risk of alcohol misuse as it assesses for quantity and frequency of alcohol consumption, presence of co-morbid diseases, high-risk behaviors, and concomitant use of medications that may interact adversely with alcohol. It too has shown validity with older adults and can detect a wider spectrum of hazardous use as it assesses criteria apart from just quantity and frequency of drinking that could present dangers more common in later life. The CARET is therefore more sensitive than the AUDIT and the MAST-G. Most older adults found to be at-risk drinkers by the CARET are identified as such due to their use of medications in combination with alcohol.

Physiology of Aging and Medical and Functional Complications of Substance Use for Geriatric Patients

Alcohol: As the percentage of lean body mass and total body water decreases with age, the ability of the liver to process alcohol is also decreased, while the permeability of the blood-brain barrier and neuronal receptor sensitivity to alcohol increase. As a result, older adults have higher blood alcohol concentrations and increased impairment than their younger counterparts in response to alcohol use at equivalent consumption levels. Older adults also have less awareness of their impairment, leading them to be more vulnerable to the effects of alcohol even in moderate amounts. Older at-risk drinkers are more likely to experience alcohol-related problems and functional impairment, such as impaired instrumental activities of daily living. This creates a unique and complicated picture of vulnerabilities for seniors, as they have increased rate of comorbid medical and psychiatric conditions. Even those older adults who had healthy drinking levels in young and middle age and then sustained these habits through older age may have increased risk for health problems [3]. The impact of alcohol use on the geriatric population has led the National Institute on Alcohol Abuse and Alcoholism (NIAAA) to lower recommended drinking thresholds. For adults ≥65, NIAA advises ≤1 standard drink/day and ≤7/week, and ≤3 on any single occasion; lower or zero for those with interacting meds/comorbidities [4].

Hazardous levels of drinking increase the risk of hypertension, diabetes, and other medical conditions in older adults. Alcohol misuse also significantly affects mood, sleep, and general health functioning. Depression in turn has been linked to relapses in drinking and increased alcohol intake. Low-risk drinkers, on the other hand, score better on general health, physical functioning, pain, mental health, and emotional functioning than both people who are hazardous drinkers and those who abstain from alcohol [11].

Some studies have shown that moderate alcohol consumption (no more than one standard drink per day) is associated with decreased morbidity and mortality among older adults. For example, older adult drinkers have been shown to have fewer falls, greater mobility, and improved physical functioning compared to non-drinkers. Despite these findings, it is important to note that there may be trade-offs of moderate alcohol use for older adults. Moderate drinking may decrease the risk of ischemic stroke and increase the risk of hemorrhagic stroke, for example. Alcohol also has many potential interactions with medications. Therefore, it is essential to weigh the benefits of alcohol for older adults with everyone's unique context, including age, comorbid illnesses, gender, and genetics [6].

Medications, tobacco, and illicit drugs: The same physiological differences that render older adults more vulnerable to effects of alcohol compared to other age groups also render them more vulnerable to drug effects and interactions. For example, older adults have less lean muscle mass and more body fat. Therefore, benzodiazepines, which are fat-soluble, have a longer duration of action in older adults and can cause excessive sedation. Benzodiazepines with long half-lives should be prescribed with caution. Additionally, older adults often see multiple providers, each of whom may prescribe medications that may interact with one other and/or with alcohol or other substances. Alcohol and cannabis, for example, increase the sedative effects of barbiturates, benzodiazepines, and opiates. Unintentional misuse may occur when older adults take more prescribed medications than intended, confuse pills, or borrow a medication from another person (e.g., use a dose of someone else's lorazepam or zolpidem for sleep).

Tobacco use in older adults is associated with several health consequences, including greater mortality, coronary events and cardiac deaths, cancer, COPD and pulmonary function decline, osteoporosis, hip fractures, loss of mobility, and poorer physical functioning. Tobacco also may decrease the efficacy of treatments for these conditions. It is not yet clear which of these health risks for tobacco use are also true for cannabis use [6].

Cannabis has been increasingly accepted both medicinally and recreationally. The risks of cannabis use have not been well-defined for older adults; however, these risks may be more pronounced in the geriatric population, especially those who have multiple chronic conditions. For example, cannabis causes increased heart rate, blood pressure, and respiratory rate and a quadruple increase in the risk for heart attack after the first hour of smoking it. These effects may increase the risk of cardiovascular events among older adults, particularly those who have preexisting disease. It is also important to note that THC is metabolized by CYP3A4 and CYP2C19, so inhibitors of these enzymes (e.g., macrolides, azoles, SSRIs, and PPIs) can increase THC and its active metabolite, leading to stronger intoxication, anxiety, or dissociation [13, 14]. THC itself is a weak inhibitor of both pathways and can cause small increases in levels of drugs like SSRIs, benzodiazepines, and certain antipsychotics [15]. Smoking cannabis may lead to pulmonary illness and infection, to which older adults are more vulnerable. Cannabis has been tied to cerebrovascular events, for which, again, increasing age is a risk factor. Additionally, cannabis has acute effects on cognitive function and may have residual long-term effects, which is important to consider as older adults may already have compromised cognitive function [6, 8]. THC edibles have a delayed onset of 1–3 hours as THC must undergo: gastric dissolution, intestinal absorption, and first-pass hepatic metabolism. This delay creates a window where the person may not feel anything and assume that the THC edible "isn't working", leading to a premature redose, causing "stacking"—multiple doses absorbing at once and producing a sudden intense and often overwhelming intoxication [16].

Studies show that most older adult cannabis users perceive that there is either no risk or only a slight risk associated with cannabis use. However, one particular concern related to the geriatric population is falls. Unintentional falls are common for older adults and are a major cause of morbidity and mortality, linked to functional decline and disability. A 2021 study found that in those above 50 years of age, chronic use of cannabis resulted in an increased risk of falls and a slower gait [17]. Additionally, it has been found that older adults who use cannabis are more likely to use other substances, including tobacco, alcohol, and/or illicit drugs, rendering them even more vulnerable to poor physical and mental health outcomes. Therefore, patients need to be educated about the risks of cannabis use, and more research needs to be done to study how the effects of cannabis may impact the chronic diseases, geriatric conditions, and daily functioning of older adults [8].

Substance Use and Neurocognitive Disorders

It is well-established that alcohol use disorders have neuropsychological consequences linked with permanent damage to the structure and function of the brain. However, there is debate regarding the classification of alcohol-related cognitive impairment. Currently, diagnostic systems identify two main syndromes of alcohol-associated cognitive disorders: alcohol-related dementia (ARD) and Wernicke–Korsakoff syndrome (WKS, an alcohol-induced persisting amnestic syndrome) [18].

Debate surrounding ARD and WKS involves the question of whether it is possible to have dementia directly resulting from ethanol neurotoxicity (a primary alcoholic dementia) or whether the dementia results from another underlying pathology (i.e., thiamine deficiency) or multiple factors (e.g., neurotoxicity in combination with nutritional deficiencies). Several confounding factors associated with the lifestyles of those who use alcohol have hindered the ability to clarify this distinction, including head injury, psychiatric and other substance abuse comorbidities, and a higher rate of vascular risk factors. Moreover, there has been little research into the prevalence of these comorbidities in the ARD population despite evidence that they are associated with the presence and maintenance of substance use disorders in both younger and older adults. The term "alcohol-related brain damage" is increasingly being used to encompass the heterogeneity in both etiology and clinical presentation of these disorders.

The relationship between the level of alcohol use and cognitive outcomes is complicated by varying definitions of drinking levels in the literature, which in part reflects the different definitions of a "standard drink" among different countries. Elements of drinking patterns (e.g., duration and severity of misuse, binge, and withdrawal periods) and difficulties getting an accurate self-report of past drinking also complicate attempts to establish the relationship between drinking levels and later cognitive impairment. Some studies suggest that individuals with ARD have had up to 60 years of drinking and up to 120 drinks per week at the heaviest, although the length and severity of drinking vary widely.

While heavy use increases the risk of dementia, there have been some studies that show that low to moderate drinking reduces the risk of dementia. This is certainly controversial and while low amounts may reduce the risk of dementia, it is important to note that no dose of alcohol is considered "safe" and can increase the risks of cancers, interact with medications, and worsen cognitive function in older adults among other negative effects. This is thought to be due to the inhibitory effect of ethanol on platelet aggregation, reduction of inflammatory markers, and alteration of serum lipids, which reduce the risk of coronary artery disease and ischemic stroke. On the other hand, heavier drinking may lead to adverse cerebrovascular changes (hypertension and increase triglycerides) and increased risk of arterial thrombosis, cardiac disorders, and strokes. Animal models have shown that low levels of alcohol protect cortical and hippocampal neurons against synapse damage induced by amyloid-β and α-synuclein, which may provide an explanation for the protection of alcohol against dementia syndrome.

Key characteristics differentiate alcohol-related cognitive disorders from neurodegenerative conditions, including stabilization or improvement in cognition with sobriety; cognitive deficits in executive, visuospatial, and memory domains with spared language function; and neurological symptoms such as ataxia. Neuroimaging may show atrophy in the mammillary bodies, thalamus, and cerebellum, and ventricular enlargement may be seen, though these findings vary.

Regarding potential reversibility of cognitive deficits, studies have shown individuals with alcohol use disorder had improvement on tests of nonverbal recall from short-term (working) and long-term memory, nonverbal immediate memory-attention, visuospatial abilities, and ataxia with abstinence. This may be significant for older adults as working memory is critical for many daily activities. Improved gait and balance may be particularly meaningful for physical well-being to reduce the risk of falls compounded with advancing age [19].

Treatment Considerations for the Older Adult

Opportunities to assess and refer older adults to substance use treatment are often overlooked. The geriatric population is more likely to receive referrals from non-healthcare settings (e.g., the criminal justice system, self-referral, or community social services providers) than from healthcare providers, even though many older adults in need of treatment present in healthcare settings due to other medical concerns. Older adults entering treatment for substance use disorders are more likely to be white, male, high school educated, widowed or divorced, retired, and disabled. This suggests a lack of a routine schedule associated with employment. In Sahker's analysis of individuals receiving substance use treatment in 2010–2013, up to 54% of older adults were living alone, and many widowed, suggesting a significant problem in social isolation and risk for adverse outcomes from many disorders in late life [20]. Social isolation and loneliness increased and remained worsened after the COVID19 pandemic, resulting in decreased community participation [21]. Given the recent exacerbation of an already significant problem, treatment planning should incorporate engagement with the community and improvement in social support.

Many treatment options exist for older adults, depending on the setting and severity of problems; however, access to specialized services tailored for older adults is limited. In addition to potential biases leading to the under-detection of substance use disorders in the geriatric population, other barriers that older adults face when accessing specialized treatment include stigma and shame surrounding substance-related problems, geographic isolation, financial concerns, or transportation difficulties [6].

Brief interventions include using aspects of motivational interviewing (MI) or motivational enhancement therapy; however, rigorous controlled trials of older adults and MI have yet to be conducted. Nevertheless, the limited studies that have examined MI in older adults have supported the expectation that MI is as effective with older adults as it is with younger adults [22]. Other brief interventions include providing education, focusing on alcohol and prescription medication misuse, in the primary care setting. Normative feedback, in which the older adult's drinking is compared with his or her peers, is combined with brief advice and seems to be an effective intervention for older adult drinkers.

Case and care management models, offered in primary care settings or community-based agencies, offer many advantages to the geriatric population. They provide a comprehensive approach, addressing the complexity of medical and psychiatric conditions common in the older population, and connect isolated older adults to community resources. The substance use interventions are also embedded in a broad approach addressing health, lessening stigma, and working toward a common goal among older adults: overall improved health. There is evidence that case management models are particularly effective at engaging and maintaining older at-risk drinkers in treatment.

As with younger populations, formal substance use treatment ranges from withdrawal management to outpatient treatment or aftercare. Both individual and group treatments are recommended for older adults to address their unique issues. It has been found that confrontational approaches are ill-suited for older adults, and indeed for any individual in whom the provider wishes to encourage substance use treatment. Supportive therapy models were specifically designed to focus on developing support and successful coping for older adults who misuse substances. This therapy focuses on building social support, improving self-esteem, and taking a global approach to treatment planning by addressing various biopsychosocial areas in the patient's life. There is also evidence for the effectiveness of CBT with older adults. As this therapy is highly structured and takes a didactic approach, it may be helpful to older adults with memory difficulties.

Alcoholics Anonymous and Narcotics Anonymous and their related groups can be helpful for older adults, though some experts have recommended customizing meetings for this population by slowing the pace to adapt to cognitive changes that occur in aging and devoting attention to coping with loss and extending social support.

While most FDA-approved treatments for substance use disorders appear to be safe and effective in older adults, there are some special considerations. Alcohol is the most common substance that older adults seek treatment for, and medications can be safe and effective [4]. Naltrexone is well-studied for use in older adults and has demonstrated some effectiveness with this population [23, 24]. One limitation, however, is that many older adults have chronic pain, and naltrexone blocks the effect of opiate-based pain medications. With this said, opioids are no longer recommended for treatment of chronic pain [25]. There has been previous concern that naltrexone may potentiate preexisting depressive symptoms, but this finding has not been consistent and should not prevent a trial of the medication [26]. Acamprosate is considered safe for use if the individual does not have severe kidney disease [27]. However, the impact of three times a day dosing should be considered, particularly if the individual is already taking several medications or struggles with a neurocognitive disorder. Disulfiram is likely to be last line and should only be used with significant caution as exposure to alcohol while on the medication can place extra strain on the cardiovascular system and in severe cases may cause a myocardial infarction, arrhythmia, and worsen or cause congestive heart failure [28].

The rates of opioid use disorder and misuse are on the rise in older adults, and pharmacologic treatments are effective and well tolerated. While opioids are on the Beers Criteria, methadone and buprenorphine are more specifically on the screening tool of older persons prescriptions (STOPP) criteria. Their use is not contraindicated in older adults and should be utilized for the diagnosis of opioid use disorder. In general, it is best to start low and increase slow. In older adults, buprenorphine is considered first line over methadone due to methadone's risk for QT interval prolongation and respiratory depression [29]. There should be special consideration about interactions with other medications and careful monitoring of constipation that may be more serious in the geriatric population [30].

The rate of tobacco use may be declining overtime, but this substance remains the cause of significant morbidity and mortality, and FDA-approved treatments are often underutilized. Tobacco cessation should be as aggressively addressed as it is in our younger patients. Nicotine replacement therapy should be used with caution in the presence of underlying cardiovascular disease, but the benefits should be weighed against the risks of continued exposure to tobacco smoke that poses a much higher cardiac risk. Nicotine gum should be avoided in dental disease or dentures in favor of lozenges or inhalers. Inhalers or sprays should be used with caution in those with bronchospastic disease. Varenicline appears to be safe to use with no adjustments needed specifically for older adults unless there is a history of renal impairment. If creatinine clearance is below 30 mL/minute, maintenance doses should not increase past 0.5 mg twice a day. In the case of end-stage renal disease, the maximum dose is 0.5 mg daily [31]. Lastly, bupropion sustained-release formulation appears to be well-tolerated in older adults with no special considerations that differ from younger populations [32].

As with younger populations, the off-label use of other medications for substance use disorders is common. While several medications have shown to be effective, there should be caution to avoid polypharmacy. Gabapentin is often used for cannabis withdrawal, alcohol or benzodiazepine withdrawal, and post-acute withdrawal syndrome from alcohol or benzodiazepines. In the older adult, gabapentin may contribute to an increased risk of falls or fracture and can interact with other medications (particularly opioids) to cause respiratory depression [33]. Topiramate may be effective off-label for alcohol and stimulant use disorders. It appears to be safe in an older adult who is cognitively intact. Due to its potential cognitive effects, it may be best to avoid or use with caution in an older adult diagnosed with a neurocognitive disorder [34]. Doxazosin for cocaine use disorder appears to be well-tolerated in older adults and may be additionally beneficial in addressing urinary retention if there is a co-occurring benign prostatic hyperplasia. While off-label use of these medications appears to be promising, there should be hypervigilance about potential medication interactions. It is important to keep in mind that older adults have a decreased percentage of lean body mass, decreased total body water, slower drug metabolism, and overall altered pharmacodynamics that may make them more vulnerable to the effects of substance use and our prescribed medications [35].

Chapter Review Questions

1. An 85-year-old male with a known past medical history of cardiovascular disease (past myocardial infarction, arrhythmia) presents to your office for worsening depression and anxiety. On assessment, you learn that he is drinking 8 standard drinks daily and meets criteria for alcohol use disorder. He is interested in taking medication to help reduce his use. What medication would be best to avoid in this scenario?

A. Naltrexone
B. Disulfiram
C. Acamprosate
D. Topiramate
E. Gabapentin

Answer B: Disulfiram
Explanation: In late life, disulfiram's reaction may cause significant cardiovascular effects, including heart failure and arrhythmia. It is best to first try other options or use with extreme caution, particularly if there is a cardiovascular history.

2. A 75-year-old female presents to your office for concerns about concentration and memory. During the evaluation, you ask about substance use and learn that she smokes cannabis nightly and has done so since she was in her early 20s. What other symptoms or observations may be present in older adults with a chronic history of cannabis use?

A. Reduced anxiety
B. Migraines
C. Hypotension
D. Increased risk of falls
E. Faster gait

Answer D: Increased risk of falls
Explanation: Cannabis has been associated with an increased risk of falls and a slower gait in older adults. Hypertension and not hypotension may be seen. Chronic cannabis use may worsen and not reduce anxiety. Some studies suggest cannabis may relieve migraine headaches.

3. A 71-year-old female with a history of alcohol use disorder presented to the clinic after a return to use of alcohol in the context of several psychosocial stressors. She shared that lack of support has been a precipitating factor. Which of the following has been noted after the COVID-19 pandemic?

A. Increase in community participation
B. Increased social isolation and loneliness
C. Reduction in overall substance use
D. An increase in the number of older adults receiving SUD treatment
E. A decrease in mood symptoms in the elderly

Answer B: Increased social isolation and loneliness
Explanation: After the COVID-19 pandemic there was an increase in social isolation and loneliness and a decrease in community participation. This change has appeared to persist even after lockdowns ended.

4. A 65-year-old male reports a recent increase in alcohol use after retirement. He is currently drinking more than the NIAAA recommendations and meets criteria for both binge and heavy use. What physiologic changes in late life place individuals at an increased risk for alcohol-related complications?

A. Increased total body water
B. Increased hepatic metabolism of alcohol
C. Lowered neuronal receptor sensitivity
D. Decreased lean body mass
E. Increased drug metabolism

Answer D: Decreased lean body mass

Explanation: In late life there are several physiologic changes that make one more vulnerable to adverse effects from alcohol and other substances. This includes decreased percentage of lean body mass, decreased total body water, slower drug metabolism and an increase in neuronal receptor sensitivity.

5. A 76-year-old female with a documented history of opioid use disorder reports a return to use of opioids after 20 years in recovery. She reports that she is currently using fentanyl daily and has been unable to cut down due to unbearable withdrawal symptoms. She requests treatment to manage her withdrawal and reduce her cravings. She reports that she has been diagnosed with an arrhythmia in the past and QT interval on the electrocardiogram completed in the office is 500 ms. Clinical opiate withdrawal scale (COWS) score is currently 13. What medication would be the best first choice at this time?

A. Naltrexone
B. Buprenorphine
C. Methadone
D. Clonidine
E. Lorazepam

Answer B: Buprenorphine

Explanation: Buprenorphine should be first line when there is a personal history of a prolonged QT interval. This patient is currently in moderate withdrawal and a good candidate to initiate buprenorphine at this time. While methadone is very effective in alleviating opioid withdrawal and reducing cravings, it should be used with caution in those with a prolonged QT interval. Naltrexone would not reduce withdrawal symptoms. Clonidine may be an effective symptomatic treatment to include but will not reduce cravings. Lorazepam may reduce anxiety but will not address opioid withdrawal symptoms.

References

1. Oslin DW. Evidence-based treatment of geriatric substance abuse. Psychiatr Clin North Am. 2005;28(4):897–911, ix.
2. Han B, Gfroerer JC, Colliver JD, Penne MA. Substance use disorder among older adults in the United States in 2020. Addiction. 2009;104(1):88–96.
3. Substance Abuse and Mental Health Services Administration Center for Behavioral Health Statistics and Quality. Results from the 2022 national survey on drug use and health: detailed tables [Internet]. Rockville: SAMHSA; 2022. [cited 2024 Aug 11]. Available from: https://www.samhsa.gov/data/sites/default/files/reports/rpt45341/2022-nsduh-older-adult-info.pdf.

4. Han BH, Moore AA, Sherman S, Keyes KM, Palamar JJ. Demographic trends of binge alcohol use and alcohol use disorders among older adults in the United States, 2005–2014. Drug Alcohol Depend. 2017;170:198–207.
5. Kirchner JE, Zubritsky C, Cody M, Coakley E, Chen H, Ware JH, et al. Alcohol consumption among older adults in primary care. J Gen Intern Med. 2007;22(1):92–7.
6. Kuerbis A, Sacco P, Blazer DG, Moore AA. Substance abuse among older adults. Clin Geriatr Med. 2014;30(3):629–54.
7. Brennan PL, Schutte KK, Moos RH. Pain and use of alcohol to manage pain: prevalence and 3-year outcomes among older problem and non-problem drinkers. Addiction. 2005;100(6):777–86.
8. Han BH, Sherman S, Mauro PM, Martins SS, Rotenberg J, Palamar JJ. Demographic trends among older cannabis users in the United States, 2006–13. Addiction (Abingdon, Engl). 2017;112(3):516–25. https://doi.org/10.1111/add.13670.
9. Han BH, Palamar JJ. Trends in cannabis use among older adults in the United States, 2015–2018. JAMA Intern Med. 2020;180(4):609. https://doi.org/10.1001/jamainternmed.2019.7517.
10. Simoni-Wastila L, Yang HK. Psychoactive drug abuse in older adults. Am J Geriatr Pharmacother. 2006;4(4):380–94.
11. Blow FC, Barry KL. Alcohol and substance misuse in older adults. Curr Psychiatry Rep. 2012;14(4):310–9.
12. Kuerbis AN, Hagman BT, Sacco P. Functioning of alcohol use disorders criteria among middle-aged and older adults: implications for DSM-5. Subst Use Misuse. 2013;48(4):309–22.
13. King CB, Yabut YW, Wen KT, Simon NI. CYP2C9, CYP3A and CYP2C19 metabolize Δ9-tetrahydrocannabinol to multiple metabolites but metabolism is affected by human liver fatty acid binding protein (FABP1). Biochem Pharmacol. 2024;228:116191. ISSN 0006-2952. https://doi.org/10.1016/j.bcp.2024.116191.
14. Stout SM, Cimino NM. Exogenous cannabinoids as substrates, inhibitors, and inducers of human drug-metabolizing enzymes: a systematic review. Drug Metab Rev. 2014;46(1):86–95. https://doi.org/10.3109/03602532.2013.849268.
15. Smith SA, Le GH, Teopiz KM, Kwan ATH, Rhee TG, Ho RC, Jie W, Cao B, Ceban F, McIntyre RS. Effects of cannabidiol and Δ9-tetrahydrocannabinol on cytochrome P450 enzymes: a systematic review. Drug Metab Rev. 2024;56(2):164–74.
16. Barrus DG, Capogrossi KL, Cates SC, Gourdet CK, Peiper NC, Novak SP, Lefever TW, Wiley JL. Tasty THC: promises and challenges of cannabis edibles. RTI Press Methods Report; 2016. https://doi.org/10.3768/rtipress.2016.op.0035.1611.
17. Workman CD, Fietsam AC, Sosnoff J, Rudroff T. Increased likelihood of falling in older cannabis users vs. Non-users. Brain Sci. 2021;11(2):1–12. https://doi.org/10.3390/brainsci11020134.
18. Ridley NJ, Draper B, Withall A. Alcohol-related dementia: an update of the evidence. Alzheimers Res Ther. 2013;5(1):3.
19. Sullivan EV, Rosenbloom MJ, Lim KO, Pfefferbaum A. Longitudinal changes in cognition, gait, and balance in abstinent and relapsed alcoholic men: relationships to changes in brain structure. Neuropsychology. 2000;14(2):178–88.
20. Sahker E, Schultz SK, Arndt S. Treatment of substance use disorders in older adults: implications for care delivery. J Am Geriatr Soc. 2015;63(11):2317–23.
21. Finlay J, Meltzer G, O'Shea B, Kobayashi L. Altered place engagement since COVID-19: a multi-method study of community participation and health among older Americans. Wellbeing Space Soc. 2024;6:100184. https://doi.org/10.1016/j.wss.2024.100184.
22. Serdarevic M, Lemke S. Motivational interviewing with the older adult. Int J Ment Health Promot. 2013;15(4):240–9.
23. Oslin D, Liberto JG, O'Brien J, Krois S, Norbeck J. Naltrexone as an adjunctive treatment for older patients with alcohol dependence. Am J Geriatr Psychiatr. 1997;5(4):324–32. https://doi.org/10.1097/00019442-199700540-00007.
24. Tampi RR, Chhatlani A, Ahmad H, Balaram K, Dey J, Escobar R, Lingamchetty T. Substance use disorders among older adults: a review of randomized controlled pharmacotherapy trials. World J Psychiatry. 2019;9(5):78–82. https://doi.org/10.5498/wjp.v9.i5.78.

25. Anderson TS, Wang BX, Lindenberg JH, Herzig SJ, Berens DM, Schonberg MA. Older adult and primary care practitioner perspectives on using, prescribing, and deprescribing opioids for chronic pain. JAMA Netw Open. 2024;7(3):E241342. https://doi.org/10.1001/jamanetworkopen.2024.1342.
26. Dean AJ, Saunders JB, Jones RT, Young RM, Connor JP, Lawford BR, Dean M. Does naltrexone treatment lead to depression? Findings from a randomized controlled trial in subjects with opioid dependence. J Psychiatry Neurosci. 2006;31(1):38–45.
27. Kalk NJ, Lingford-Hughes AR. The clinical pharmacology of acamprosate. Br J Clin Pharmacol. 2014;77(2):315–23. https://doi.org/10.1111/bcp.12070.
28. Huffman JC, Stern TA. Disulfiram use in an elderly man with alcoholism and heart disease: a discussion. J Clin Psychiatry. 2003;5(1):41.
29. Dufort A, Samaan Z. Problematic opioid use among older adults: epidemiology, adverse outcomes and treatment considerations. Drugs Aging. 2021;38(12):1043–53. Adis. https://doi.org/10.1007/s40266-021-00893-z.
30. Mari A, Mahamid M, Amara H, Baker FA, Yaccob A. Chronic constipation in the elderly patient: updates in evaluation and management. Korean J Family Med. 2020;41(3):139–45. https://doi.org/10.4082/kjfm.18.0182.
31. Singh D, Saadabadi A. Varenicline. [Updated 2022 Dec 14]. In: StatPearls [Internet]. Treasure Island: StatPearls Publishing; 2024. Available from: https://www.ncbi.nlm.nih.gov/books/NBK534846/.
32. Fortner M, Brown K. Bupropion SR and quality of life in the elderly depressed patients with comorbid medical disorders. J Clin Psychiatry. 1999;1(6):174.
33. Oh GY, Moga DC, Abner EL. Gabapentin utilization among older adults with different cognitive statuses enrolled in the National Alzheimer's Coordinating Center (2006–2019). Br J Clin Pharmacol. 2023;89(1):410–5. https://doi.org/10.1111/bcp.15532.
34. Sommer BR, Fenn HH. Review of topiramate for the treatment of epilepsy in elderly patients. In: Clinical interventions in aging; 2010. www.dovepress.com.
35. Yarnell S, Li L, MacGrory B, Trevisan L, Kirwin P. Substance use disorders in later life: a review and synthesis of the literature of an emerging public health concern. Am J Geriatr Psychiatry. 2020;28(2):226–36. https://doi.org/10.1016/j.jagp.2019.06.005.

Professionals 20

Jonathan C. Lee, Edwin Kim, and Penelope P. Ziegler

High-Yield Review Points

- Safety-sensitive workers with substance use disorders require intensive, multidisciplinary, multimodal treatment, often in a cohort of peers, followed by rigorous, long-term monitoring.
- Certain safety-sensitive workers have direct access to addictive substances in their work environment, increasing the risk for misuse and relapse.
- While professionals should not be stigmatized for having a health condition, impairment or potential impairment necessitates appropriate evaluation and intervention to ensure public safety.
- Specialized monitoring programs (e.g., physician health programs, lawyer assistance programs) achieve significantly higher long-term abstinence rates for professionals compared to standard treatment outcomes in the general population.
- Robust confidentiality protections (regulatory, record, application) are crucial for encouraging professionals to engage with monitoring programs as a safe, therapeutic alternative to discipline.

J. C. Lee (✉)
The Farley Center at Williamsburg Place, Williamsburg, VA, USA
e-mail: jlee@farleycenter.com

E. Kim
Federation of State Physician Health Programs, Mechanicsburg, PA, USA
e-mail: ekim@pamedsoc.org

P. P. Ziegler
Emerita Florida Professionals Resource Network, Fernandina Beach, FL, USA

C. Marienfeld, M. Soltani (eds.), *AAAP Review of Addiction Psychiatry*,
https://doi.org/10.1007/978-3-032-24174-0_20

- Effective long-term monitoring is multi-faceted, involving case management, comprehensive biological testing (e.g., urine, PEth, hair) to verify abstinence, adherence tracking, contingency management, and coordination with regulatory bodies when necessary.
- Comprehensive, multidisciplinary evaluations and specialized treatment, often utilizing cohort-specific therapy, are vital to address occupational stressors, unique psychological defenses, and profession-specific relapse risks.

Introduction

Substance use disorders (SUDs) represent a significant occupational health concern, affecting professionals across various fields. While prevalence rates among physicians, estimated at 10–12%, mirror those in the general population, relapse rates diverge dramatically based on the support systems accessed. In contrast to the general population's post-treatment relapse rates of 40–60%, physicians participating in specialized physician health programs (PHPs), which integrate treatment with long-term monitoring and continuing care, achieve remarkable long-term abstinence rates, reportedly as high as 78% over extended periods [1]. Other professions, however, may face distinct challenges; for instance, attorneys exhibit significantly higher rates of hazardous drinking, around 21%, highlighting the need for profession-specific resources like lawyer assistance programs (LAPs) [2]. The stark difference in outcomes underscores the efficacy of tailored interventions for professionals, particularly those in safety-sensitive occupation roles where impairment carries substantial risk to the public. This chapter explores the unique considerations for identifying, assessing, treating, and monitoring SUDs and other potentially impairing conditions in safety-sensitive professionals, emphasizing the specialized approaches required to facilitate recovery, ensure professional competence, and uphold public safety.

Safety Sensitive Professionals

Professionals in safety-sensitive positions have a responsibility to the public. Safety-sensitive occupations are defined by the following three factors: the size of the population that they affect, the depth of the effects from potential impairment, and the amount of public trust that is implied in that worker's occupation. Examples of safety-sensitive workers include healthcare workers, airline pilots, attorneys and judges, and public servants in the police and fire areas. Safety-sensitive workers require intensive primary treatment, typically for a minimum of 30–90 days, and continued treatment and monitoring due to potential impact on the public welfare.

Most safety-sensitive workers, with more advanced illness, do best when offered cohort-specific treatment. Certain safety-sensitive workers have direct access to addictive substances, which increases the risk of relapse [3].

Safety-sensitive workers are typically regulated by an entity to ensure safety to practice and to protect the public. Examples of regulatory agencies include licensing boards (e.g., state medical boards, boards of nursing, and state bar associations for attorneys) and the Federal Aviation Administration (FAA) for pilots. Monitoring programs, such as physician health programs (PHPs), are often available as an alternative to discipline by regulatory boards.

Physician Health Programs

PHPs provide care management to monitor adherence to continuing care and recovery activities; alcohol and drug testing to verify abstinence from intoxicating substances; advocacy and support of safety-sensitive workers in recovery; and coordination with regulatory agencies if participants fail to adhere to recommendations. Depending on the state, professional monitoring programs go beyond monitoring just substance use disorders and have the capacity to provide monitoring for psychiatric and other potentially impairing medical conditions. Some state programs also monitor healthcare professionals undergoing treatment related to unprofessional sexual behavior [4].

Many state PHPs are granted regulatory protection to aide physicians in their health concerns in a confidential manner. Appropriate legislation can further promote a safe haven for physicians by permitting PHPs the strongest opportunity to offer screening, early intervention, assessment, and connection to professional-focused treatment. These mechanisms also offer an effective therapeutic alternative to punitive approaches, thereby enabling physicians and other healthcare professionals to prioritize health and recovery [5]. Effectively providing haven relies on states codifying a Triad of Confidentiality, as set forth by the Federation of State Physician Health Programs. This triad includes:

1. Regulatory protection: Professional assistance programs are legally authorized to provide confidential assistance in lieu of a report to a disciplinary body and to receive referrals from the disciplinary body as an alternative to a disciplinary process.
2. Record protection: The records held by professional assistance programs have special legal protections against discovery in legal proceedings.
3. Application protection: Licensure and credentialing application questions related to health should focus on current impairment and not include intrusive and stigmatizing inquiry about prior mental health diagnosis and treatment. Applications should provide specific exemption to answering health-related questions (haven protections) for individuals participating in professional assistance programs.

The mere presence of a health condition—whether substance-related, psychiatric, or non-psychiatric medical—must be distinguished from evidence of actual or potential impairment resulting from that condition. A diagnosis alone does not inherently indicate work-related impairment [6]. This distinction underpins broader efforts to enhance confidentiality for healthcare professionals seeking care, while simultaneously supporting patient safety and public protection by ensuring that those with impairing or potentially impairing conditions are appropriately connected to treatment.

Identification and Assessment

If a safety-sensitive worker is identified as having a possible impairing or potentially impairing condition, they should be referred for a diagnostic evaluation. Safety-sensitive workers who are referred for substance use concerns are typically expected to refrain from practice until the PHP has sufficient information that the participant is ready to return to practice. Assessment of co-occurring psychiatric and non-psychiatric medical conditions is crucial as these conditions can exacerbate substance use disorders and impact treatment planning. Evaluations should be conducted by licensed professional(s) who specialize in assessing safety-sensitive workers; evaluators may require approval by a regulatory entity, such as the medical board. When feasible, multidisciplinary, multimodal team evaluations which include the following components are recommended: face-to-face interviews with the safety-sensitive worker; history and physical examination; mental status examination; often neurocognitive/neuropsychological testing; laboratory studies as indicated including toxicology testing; collateral contacts with referring entity, family members, supervisor(s), and others as indicated; completion of appropriate releases of information to obtain needed collateral and to allow transmission of the evaluation report to the necessary stakeholders.

Treatment

Treatment of safety-sensitive workers with moderate to severe substance use disorders may start in a residential or partial hospitalization program with full immersion into a therapeutic milieu with group and individual counseling and medication management [7]. The level of care can be adjusted based on case specifics, the ASAM criteria for safety-sensitive occupations, DSM-5 criteria, and the expectation of the regulatory and/or monitoring entity.

The treatment team should be trained in the specifics of safety-sensitive professionals' work environment that may impact their recovery. For example, access to controlled substances is common in the work environment for anesthesiologists and certified registered nurse anesthetists, and this issue affects monitoring and prognosis because of the potential for relapse on substances that are available in the work setting. Treatment team providers seek to understand and address the potential occupational stressors and traumas (e.g., first responders finding patients who are injured/dead) related to safety-sensitive positions. Staff should be aware of the psychosocial context of addiction treatment in the patient's particular cohort. For example, healthcare providers commonly struggle with accepting the role of being a patient [3]. Treatment providers should consider how licensing boards may perceive behaviors that could result from untreated addiction, such as professional boundary violations. Treatment is tailored to address common defenses and maladaptive coping skills. Staff need training to manage the dynamic defenses and coping mechanisms (e.g., intellectualization, denial, and minimization) common in safety-sensitive professionals. Clinical staff (e.g., counselors, nurses, and others providing specific treatment) may need supervision to avoid reactive judgment, which may limit self-disclosure from safety-sensitive workers.

Safety-sensitive workers benefit from profession-specific group therapy that allows for self-disclosure and discussion on boundary transgressions related to substance use disorders and professional roles. The model of cohort-specific group therapy has been studied and supported by physician health programs [7]. Peers in recovery often can confront each other on behaviors that are part of the relapse process, which may lead to using addictive substances [8]. It is important to balance the need for privacy with the involvement of professional patients' family and workplace to support their recovery.

Profession-specific mutual help groups, such as Caduceus for healthcare professionals or Birds of a Feather for pilots, can provide mentorship, sponsorship, and hope for professionals in recovery. Participation and involvement in mutual support groups (e.g., Alcoholics Anonymous, other 12-step groups, and Self-Management and Recovery Training groups) are essential parts of treatment and monitoring for professionals.

Effective treatment involves coordinating continuing care providers (for longer term recovery maintenance treatment) and monitoring entities to minimize risks for relapse during transitions in care and ensure long-term recovery support. Monitoring entities, such as physician health programs (PHPs), human intervention motivation study (HIMS) programs for commercial airline pilots, and lawyer assistance programs (LAPs), typically expect complete abstinence from alcohol and intoxicating drugs for a duration of 1–5 years or more. Signing a PHP monitoring agreement, actively participating in the PHP, and receiving formal SUD treatment are essential helpful components attributed to monitoring programs [9]. Monitoring program staff should be aware of specialty drug testing (e.g., phosphatidyl ethanol, ethyl glucuronide, and ethyl sulfate from alcohol metabolism) utilized for evaluation, treatment, and monitoring of safety-sensitive professionals. Monitoring includes case management to observe participant behaviors, compliance with the treatment plan, involvement of the worksite, adherence to recovery activities (e.g., attendance of 12-step meetings), and biological testing (e.g., urine drug screening, breathalyzer, blood testing for biomarkers of alcohol metabolites, and hair/nail drug screens).

Contingency management is a component of treatment and monitoring for safety-sensitive workers. Case managers interact with participants and provide feedback on the submission of requested data and identify emerging issues. Data collected (e.g., drug testing results, check-in reliability for drug testing, attendance at mutual support groups and therapy sessions, and tracking of appropriately prescribed medications) affect the frequency of contact with participants and frequency of drug testing. Complex drug testing may be managed by a third-party administrator with medical review officer support and carefully reviewed by the monitoring program. Participants experience positive reinforcement (convenience and decreased costs) when drug testing decreases in frequency based on adherence with check-ins and notification for lab testing, and periods of no detected substance use. When there is a concern for safety to practice, monitoring programs can utilize negative reinforcement by removing safety-sensitive workers from the workplace or fulfilling the required reporting of them to their respective regulatory agencies.

Medications for relapse prevention should be considered for safety-sensitive workers. Extended-release injectable naltrexone may be the preferred medication for opioid use disorder (MOUD) for some professionals due to return-to-work requirements enforced by a specific state medical board or monitoring programs. Alternative MOUD can be effective interventions for certain individuals seeking return to work; some programs may utilize neurocognitive examinations to assess the appropriateness of agonist treatments prior to returning to work. All evidence-based medications for alcohol use disorder (MAUD) can convey increased chances of success in a professional's recovery. It is important to understand the governing regulatory body. Due to regulations of various monitoring and licensure entities, there may be medications that are not considered appropriate due to concern for impacting the ability of the professional to practice with reasonable skill and safety.

Return-to-Work Considerations

It is important to assess cognitive and functional abilities of safety-sensitive workers. In some cases, neuropsychological testing may be required to determine safety to return-to-work recommendations. Occupational, licensing, and legal issues need to be addressed prior to the professional receiving permission to return to work—which is often in a staged and graduated manner. Work triggers or cues should be identified and be part of the relapse prevention plan. The work environment needs to make appropriate accommodations to encourage adherence to the monitoring agreement (i.e., toxicology testing, and case management) by a designated entity to provide accountability [5]. When engaged in monitoring, most healthcare professionals achieve abstinence as part of their recovery and return to and then continue to work [10]. In healthcare professionals who have responded to treatment for professional sexual misconduct, professional health programs may be beneficial in monitoring their successful return to practice without recurrent unprofessional sexual behavior [11]. Supervising personnel need to be trained in addressing profession-specific return-to-work issues for recovering safety-sensitive workers.

Conclusion

The combination of intensive, multidisciplinary, multimodal treatment in a cohort of peers followed by continuing care, long-term contingency management with monitoring and participation in mutual support groups is considered the gold standard for addiction treatment in safety-sensitive workers to sustain long-term recovery. This comprehensive model has demonstrated remarkable efficacy, particularly within established physician health programs, yielding significantly higher rates of sustained abstinence compared to standard treatment approaches. Its success stems from the integration of specialized assessments distinguishing illness from impairment, treatment tailored to address unique occupational stressors and psychological defenses, and a robust framework of extended monitoring. This long-term oversight, crucial for accountability and support, incorporates case management, biological testing to verify abstinence, adherence verification, and contingency-based strategies. Integrating profession-specific and mutual support networks further strengthens the recovery foundation. Ultimately, addressing substance use and mental health conditions in safety-sensitive professionals requires this diligent, structured approach, carefully balancing the individual's need for confidential, effective care with the overriding responsibility to protect public safety, thereby enabling professionals to achieve lasting recovery and safely continue serving their communities [7, 12, 13].

Chapter Review Questions

Bob is a 62-year-old OB/GYN physician whose medical license has been suspended due to caring for patients while intoxicated with alcohol on numerous occasions. No adverse medical outcomes were noted. He completed a residential addiction treatment program. He was recommended to continue care in an intensive outpatient program and participate in monitoring with a physician health program. Which of the following is a component of physician health programs (PHPs)?

A. Addiction treatment programs
B. Care management to monitor adherence to continuing care and recovery activities
C. Liver and metabolic panel testing
D. Diagnosis and treatment of physicians with substance use disorders
E. Exclusion of the state medical licensing board if participant fails to adhere to recommendations

Correct Answer: B
Explanation: Physician health programs (PHPs) are not addiction treatment programs, nor do they directly provide such treatment [7]. PHPs do provide care management, advocacy and support of physicians, and drug and urine test monitoring.

Okay, here are 5 board-style review questions based on the provided chapter text and our discussion:

1. A 45-year-old anesthesiologist with no prior disciplinary history is reported to the hospital's wellness committee by a colleague who suspects potential diversion of fentanyl due to observed behavioral changes and minor inventory discrepancies. The anesthesiologist denies any substance use when initially approached. According to the principles outlined for managing safety-sensitive professionals, what is the most appropriate next step?

   A. Initiate immediate termination proceedings due to the high-risk nature of the suspected behavior.
   B. Require the anesthesiologist to sign a return-to-work contract contingent on random drug screening by the hospital.
   C. Recommend participation in the hospital's general employee assistance program (EAP) for stress management.
   D. Refer the anesthesiologist for a comprehensive, multidisciplinary diagnostic evaluation coordinated through the state physician health program (PHP).
   E. Mandate weekly attendance at local Alcoholics Anonymous or Narcotics Anonymous meetings.

   Correct Answer: D
   Explanation:

   - *Why D is correct*: The text emphasizes that when a safety-sensitive worker (like an anesthesiologist with access to potent substances) is suspected of having an SUD or potentially impairing condition, referral for a specialized diagnostic evaluation is crucial. PHPs are specifically designed to facilitate such confidential, comprehensive, multidisciplinary evaluations for physicians, often as a therapeutic alternative to discipline, ensuring both physician well-being and public safety. This aligns with the need for specialized assessment before determining impairment or appropriate interventions.
   - *Why A is incorrect*: While the situation is serious, immediate termination without proper evaluation is typically not the first step, especially if a PHP pathway exists. The goal is evaluation and potential rehabilitation, balanced with public safety.
   - *Why B is incorrect*: A return-to-work contract is premature before a formal diagnosis and treatment plan are established. Monitoring without comprehensive assessment and treatment is insufficient.
   - *Why C is incorrect*: While an EAP might offer general support, it typically lacks the specialized expertise, intensive assessment capabilities, and long-term monitoring structure required for safety-sensitive professionals with potential SUDs, as outlined in the text for PHPs.
   - *Why E is incorrect*: Mandating mutual support group attendance without a diagnosis or as a standalone intervention is inappropriate. While such groups are vital components of treatment and monitoring, they follow a comprehensive evaluation and treatment plan.

2. A partner at a large law firm expresses concern about a 38-year-old associate whose work product has declined and who frequently appears disheveled and smells of alcohol after lunch. The associate dismisses concerns, attributing issues to stress. Based on the provided text regarding substance use in attorneys, which statement best reflects a key consideration in this scenario?

   A. Attorneys have SUD rates similar to physicians, suggesting standard EAP referral is sufficient.
   B. Problematic alcohol use is significantly less common among attorneys than in the general population.
   C. Lawyer assistance programs (LAPs) are primarily designed for disciplinary action rather than confidential support.
   D. Attorneys may experience higher rates of hazardous alcohol use than the general population, necessitating profession-specific support resources like LAPs.
   E. Confidentiality is not a major barrier to attorneys seeking help for substance use issues.

   Correct Answer: D
   Explanation:

- *Why D is correct*: The text explicitly states that a study of nearly 13,000 attorneys found 21% screened positive for hazardous, harmful, and potentially alcohol-dependent drinking, a rate higher than the general population. It also highlights the need for attorney-specific interventions and resources like lawyer assistance programs (LAPs), which function similarly to PHPs in providing specialized, often confidential, support.
- *Why A is incorrect*: The text contrasts attorneys' higher rates of problematic drinking with physicians' rates (which are noted as similar to the general population), implying standard EAP may be insufficient and specialized programs are needed.
- *Why B is incorrect*: The text states the opposite—attorneys in the study showed higher rates of problematic drinking than the general population.
- *Why C is incorrect*: Like PHPs, LAPs are presented as resources often available as an *alternative* to discipline, ideally providing confidential assessment, support, and connection to treatment.
- *Why E is incorrect*: While not explicitly detailed for attorneys as it was for PHPs (Triad of Confidentiality), the general principles for safety-sensitive professionals emphasize the importance of confidentiality to encourage help-seeking, making it unlikely that confidentiality is *not* a major barrier. The text supports confidential pathways (PHPs/LAPs).

3. A 52-year-old commercial airline pilot successfully completes a 90-day residential treatment program for alcohol use disorder. He is now working with the Human Intervention Motivation Study (HIMS) program and seeking reinstatement of his medical certificate from the Federal Aviation Administration (FAA). Which of the following is most critical for his long-term recovery maintenance and return to flying?

A. Attending weekly general psychotherapy sessions focused on underlying stressors.
B. Limiting mutual support group attendance to maintain privacy among colleagues.
C. Adherence to a comprehensive long-term monitoring agreement including frequent, random biological testing (e.g., PEth, urine EtG/EtS) and active participation in pilot-specific support groups.
D. Relying solely on self-monitoring and reporting any lapses directly to the FAA.
E. Taking disulfiram daily as the primary relapse prevention strategy.

Correct Answer: C
Explanation:

- *Why C is correct*: The text identifies the "gold standard" for safety-sensitive professionals as intensive treatment followed by long-term monitoring, contingency management, and mutual support. For pilots, this involves programs like HIMS coordinating with the FAA. Monitoring includes rigorous biological testing (specialty testing like PEth and EtG/EtS are mentioned) to verify complete abstinence, case management, and participation in peer/mutual support groups (like "Birds of a Feather" for pilots). This structure provides the necessary accountability and support for sustained recovery in a high-risk profession.
- *Why A is incorrect*: While therapy may be part of continuing care, it is only one component. The comprehensive monitoring and peer support structure are highlighted as essential for this population's high success rates.
- *Why B is incorrect*: The text emphasizes the *benefit* of profession-specific (cohort) groups (like Caduceus or Birds of a Feather) and mutual support participation, suggesting engagement, not privacy through avoidance, is key.
- *Why D is incorrect*: Self-monitoring alone is insufficient for safety-sensitive roles. Structured, objective, long-term monitoring by a designated entity (PHP, HIMS, LAP) is required.
- *Why E is incorrect*: While MAT like disulfiram can be part of treatment (MAUD), relying on it solely ignores the critical roles of monitoring, therapy, and peer support emphasized in the text. Furthermore, specific medication appropriateness may depend on regulatory approval.

4. A 40-year-old emergency department nurse with opioid use disorder (OUD) is enrolled in the state's nursing monitoring program following treatment. Her treatment team is considering medication for addiction treatment (MAT). Given potential regulatory and return-to-work considerations mentioned for healthcare professionals, which factor is most important when selecting MAT?

A. Choosing the medication with the lowest possible cost to the participant.
B. Prioritizing agonist therapies like methadone or buprenorphine due to highest efficacy data.

C. Selecting extended-release injectable naltrexone, as it may be preferred by some monitoring programs or boards over agonist therapies for return to work.
D. Avoiding all MAT to eliminate any risk of medication-related impairment during work hours.
E. Allowing the nurse to choose any FDA-approved MAT based solely on personal preference.

Correct Answer: C
Explanation:

- *Why C is correct*: The text specifically notes that due to regulations or return-to-work requirements imposed by monitoring programs or licensing boards, antagonist treatment (like extended-release injectable naltrexone) may be preferred over agonist treatments (methadone, buprenorphine) for some healthcare professionals with OUD. While noting agonist treatments can be effective and sometimes utilized (potentially with neurocognitive testing), it highlights naltrexone as a potentially preferred option in this specific regulatory context.
- *Why A is incorrect*: Cost is a practical factor but not the primary clinical or regulatory consideration highlighted in the text for MAT selection in this context.
- *Why B is incorrect*: While agonist therapies are highly effective, the text explicitly points out potential regulatory/monitoring program preferences or restrictions against them for return to work in safety-sensitive roles, making naltrexone a key consideration.
- *Why D is incorrect*: Avoiding all MAT is contrary to evidence-based practice for OUD and ignores potentially life-saving treatments. The text discusses *how* MAT should be considered, not avoided entirely.
- *Why E is incorrect*: While patient preference is important, the text underscores that regulatory requirements and monitoring program policies heavily influence MAT choices for safety-sensitive professionals returning to practice.

5. You are supervising a surgical resident who has become increasingly irritable, withdrawn, and whose technical skills seem slightly less precise recently. There are no definitive signs of substance use, but you are concerned about potential impairment from an underlying health issue (e.g., burnout, depression, or early substance use). Based on the chapter's distinction between illness and impairment, what is the most appropriate initial action?

   A. Immediately report the resident to the state medical board for potential impairment.
   B. Require the resident to undergo random urine drug screening supervised by the residency program director.
   C. Arrange a confidential conversation to express concern for their well-being and explore potential stressors or health issues, suggesting confidential resources like the PHP or EAP for assessment if appropriate.

D. Assume the resident is suffering from burnout and mandate a one-month leave of absence without further assessment.
E. Consult hospital legal counsel regarding the potential risks before speaking to the resident.

Correct Answer: C
Explanation:

- *Why C is correct*: The text emphasizes the crucial distinction between illness and impairment—an illness (non-psychiatric medical, mental health, or substance-related) does not automatically equate to impairment in practice. It also highlights the importance of confidentiality (safe havens like PHPs) to encourage professionals to seek help. The appropriate initial step when concern arises, short of clear evidence of acute impairment endangering patients, is a confidential conversation expressing concern and directing the individual toward appropriate, confidential assessment resources (PHP/EAP) to evaluate the situation professionally. This balances support with the need for evaluation if an impairing or potentially impairing condition exists.
- *Why A is incorrect*: Reporting to the board is a significant step, usually reserved for situations where impairment is clearly identified, the professional refuses evaluation/treatment, or poses an immediate danger. It is generally not the *initial* action based on suspicion alone, especially if confidential pathways like PHPs exist.
- *Why B is incorrect*: Mandating UDS without a broader assessment context or clear indication can be overly intrusive and may not capture underlying mental health issues. A comprehensive evaluation via PHP/EAP is preferred.
- *Why D is incorrect*: Mandating leave without assessment might provide temporary relief but does not address the underlying cause or determine fitness for duty. Assuming burnout without evaluation is insufficient.
- *Why E is incorrect*: While legal awareness is relevant in institutions, consulting legal counsel before even having a supportive, confidential conversation with the resident may escalate the situation prematurely and undermine trust. Initial supportive intervention is typically preferred.

References

1. DuPont RL, McLellan AT, Carr G, Gendel M, Skipper GE. How are addicted physicians treated? A national survey of physician health programs. J Subst Abus Treat. 2009;37:1–7.
2. Krill PR, Johnson R, Albert L. The prevalence of substance use and other mental health concerns among American attorneys. J Addict Med. 2016;10(1):46–52.
3. Baron MJ, Earley PH, Polles AG. Supporting patients working in safety sensitive occupations. In: Waller CR, Boyle MP, Daviss SR, et al., editors. The ASAM criteria: treatment criteria for addictive, substance-related, and co-occurring conditions. 4th ed. Center City: Hazelden Publishing; 2023.

4. Federation of State Physician Health Programs. State programs. https://www.fsphp.org/state-programs. Accessed 25 Sept 2024.
5. Earley PH, Bundy C. Addiction among physicians and physician health programs. In: Miller S, editor. The ASAM principles of addiction medicine. 7th ed. Philadelphia: Wolters Kluwer Health; 2024.
6. Federation of State Physician Health Programs. Public policy statement – physician illness, disability, and impairment: differentiation and responsibility. https://www.fsphp.org/fsphp-guidelines%2D%2Dpolicies%2D%2Dposition-statements. Accessed 28 Sept 2024.
7. DuPont RL, McLellan AT, White WL, Merlo LJ, Gold MS. Setting the standard for recovery: physicians' health programs. J Subst Abus Treat. 2009;32(2):159–71.
8. Angres DH, Talbott GD, Bettinardi-Angres K. Healing the healer: the addicted physician. Madison: Psychological Press; 1998.
9. Merlo LJ, Campbell MD, Shea C, et al. Essential components of physician health program monitoring for substance use disorder: a survey of participants 5 years post successful program completion. Am J Addict. 2022;31:115–22.
10. Geuijen PM, van den Broek SJM, Dijkstra BAG, Kuppens JM, de Haan HA, de Jong CAJ, Schene AH, Atsma F, Schellekens AFA. Success rates of monitoring for healthcare professionals with a substance use disorder: a meta-analysis. J Clin Med. 2021;10(2):264.
11. Polles AG, Araujo CNP, Hemphill RS, Gao H, Merlo LJ. Characterizing referrals to professional health monitoring programs for unprofessional sexual behavior. J Am Acad Psychiatry Law. 2024;52(4):1–12.
12. Body JW, Knight JR. Substance use disorders among physicians. In: Galanter M, Kleber HD, editors. Textbook of substance abuse treatment. 4th ed. Arlington: The American Psychiatric Publishing, Inc.; 2008.
13. Talbott GD, Wilson PO. Physicians and other health professionals. In: Lainson JH, Ruiz P, Millman RB, Langrod JG, editors. Substance abuse: a comprehensive textbook. 4th ed. Philadelphia: Lippincott Williams & Wilkins; 2005.

Co-occurring Medical Disorders

21

Aaron Meyer and Amutha Rajagopal

High-Yield Review Points

- Alcohol use causes a wide spectrum of liver diseases, cardiovascular complications including hypertension, arrhythmias, and dilated cardiomyopathy, myriad cancers, endocrinopathies, and neurologic diseases such as Wernicke–Korsakoff syndrome.
- Chronic benzodiazepine use has been associated with a decline in cognitive function, changes in sleep microstructure, and an increased risk of falls.
- Cocaine and amphetamine use are associated with several cardiovascular complications including hypertension, tachycardia, cardiomyopathy, aortic dissection, and acute coronary syndromes, as well as an increased risk of stroke, seizures, and pulmonary complications.
- The most recognized medical harm of opioid use is respiratory depression, which is associated with exacerbations of chronic obstructive pulmonary disease, asthma, and obstructive sleep apnea. Other common complications include opioid-induced hyperalgesia and opioid-induced hypogonadism.

A. Meyer (✉)
Department of Psychiatry, University of California San Diego, La Jolla, CA, USA
e-mail: aameyer@ucsd.edu

A. Rajagopal
Department of Medicine, Oregon Health and Science University, Portland, OR, USA
e-mail: rajagopal@ohsu.edu

C. Marienfeld, M. Soltani (eds.), *AAAP Review of Addiction Psychiatry*,
https://doi.org/10.1007/978-3-032-24174-0_21

- Heavy or chronic cannabis use has been associated with hyperemesis syndrome.
- Tobacco use remains the leading cause of preventable disease and death in the United States, leading to hypertension, stroke and coronary artery disease, respiratory diseases, and approximately one-third of all cancer deaths.
- Injection drug use increases the risks of invasive bacterial, fungal, and transmissible viral infections, including HIV, hepatitis B, and hepatitis C. Non-infectious vascular complications include phlebitis, thromboembolic disease, and venous insufficiency.

Tobacco

Cardiovascular Cigarette smoking significantly increases the risks of cardiovascular disease—heart attacks, heart failure, arrhythmias, stroke, and peripheral artery disease, and is the leading cause of preventable disease and death [1]. The United States Preventive Services Taskforce recommends one-time screening for abdominal aortic aneurysm with ultrasonography in men aged 65–75 years who have ever smoked [2]. A significantly elevated risk persists for up to 30 years following smoking cessation for peripheral arterial disease and up to 20 years for coronary heart disease or stroke. More than 40 pack-years history quadruples risk of peripheral arterial disease [3].

Respiratory Cigarette smoking is responsible for most COPD-related deaths, worsens asthma and other respiratory diseases, and increases the risks of tuberculosis and other lung infections [4]. Although e-cigarettes have been touted as a healthier alternative to cigarettes, e-cigarette use also increases blood pressure, hyperlipidemia, and other harmful cardiovascular effects via endothelial dysfunction, oxidative stress, and inflammation [5]. Electronic-cigarette, or vaping, product use-associated lung injury (EVALI) is a severe pulmonary illness associated with the presence of improperly processed vitamin E acetate [6]. Hookah use may lead to increased exposure to carcinogens compared to cigarettes [7].

Musculoskeletal Smoking is associated with low bone mineral density (BMD), an increased likelihood of fracture, delayed fracture healing, increased alveolar bone loss, increased risk of periodontitis, increased peri-implant bone loss, and implant failure [8]. Limited evidence also supports deleterious effects of smoking tobacco on muscles, cartilage, tendons, and ligaments [9]. Smoking is associated with increased rheumatoid arthritis (RA) disease activity, functional disability, and poor response to therapy [9].

Endocrine Nicotine has been associated with profound adverse effects on the hypothalamic–pituitary–gonadal axis, hypothalamic–pituitary–thyroid axis, and the hypothalamic–pituitary–adrenal axis, impacting synthesis, secretion and concentrations of gonadal steroid hormones, adrenal corticosteroid hormones, and thyroid hormones [10].

Hematological/Oncological About one out of every three cancer deaths in the United States are due to cigarette smoking; these include deaths from lung, bladder, bone marrow, cervical, gastrointestinal, hepatic, and pancreatic cancers [4]. Yearly screening for lung cancer with low-dose computed tomography has been recommended for persons 50–80 years of age with a 20-pack year history by the USPSTF and American Cancer Society [11].

Perinatal Tobacco use is recognized as one of the most important and modifiable risk factors associated with adverse perinatal outcomes. Data suggest smoking tobacco may be responsible for 15% of all preterm births, 20–30% of all infants of low birthweight, a 150% increase in overall perinatal mortality, placenta previa, abruptio placentae, premature rupture of the membranes, intrauterine growth restriction, and sudden infant death syndrome [12]. Tobacco use during pregnancy is also associated with transfers to the neonatal intensive care unit and neonatal intensive care hospitalizations longer than 7 days [13].

Alcohol

Neurologic Cognitive deficits may range from mild cognitive impairment to development of Wernicke–Korsakoff syndrome. Wernicke encephalopathy is an acute syndrome characterized by the triad of ataxia, ophthalmoplegia, and confusion, caused by thiamine deficiency. Korsakoff syndrome is a chronic amnesia caused by untreated or undertreated Wernicke encephalopathy and is often accompanied by confabulations and peripheral neuropathy [14]. Thiamine deficiency in alcohol use disorder is related to a combination of inadequate dietary intake, decreased gastrointestinal absorption, and difficulty with storage. Alcohol also damages renal epithelial cells, which leads to further thiamine excretion. Further, magnesium is a cofactor in thiamine utilization; as many with alcohol use disorder have decreased magnesium levels, thiamine is unable to be used [15]. Without thiamine, there is decreased acetylcholine formation. This deficiency can lead to microglial hyperactivity and subsequent cognitive deficits [14]. As thiamine metabolism increases with high glucose intake, clinicians must ensure that parenteral thiamine is administered prior to glucose infusion in heavy alcohol drinkers [16]. Randomized controlled clinical trials are needed to guide clinicians in the most effective duration and dose of thiamine [17]. Imaging patients with Wernicke encephalopathy has shown damage to periventricular nuclei, thalami, and mammillary bodies [15]. Imaging findings may reveal generalized cerebral atrophy and enlarged ventricles; resembling features typically seen in neurodegenerative conditions [18]. Individuals with

Korsakoff syndrome are less likely to understand socially appropriate behavior [19]. People with Korsakoff are more likely to commit crimes than those with alcohol-related dementia [20]. Korsakoff syndrome is associated with an increased risk of long-term custodial care [21].

Alcohol-induced cerebellar ataxia is due to several factors. Rodent models demonstrate that alcohol can affect cerebellar adenosine uptake, which can lead to over-activation of Purkinje cells. Alcohol can also lead to nitric oxide inhibition, which may contribute to further cerebellar damage [22]. Alcohol use has a greater effect on brain volume than any other modifiable risk factor. Higher blood pressure and body mass index increased risk for brain structure changes when co-morbid with heavy alcohol use [23].

Cardiovascular Alcohol-related cardiomyopathy contributes significantly to alcohol-attributable mortality [24]. The risk of developing cardiomyopathy increases with higher daily alcohol intake and prolonged consumption exceeding 5-years [25]. Consuming more than 100 grams of alcohol per week has been linked to an elevated risk of heart failure [26]. Notably, even moderate intake—such as one drink per day—has been associated with increased cardiovascular risk [27]. Hospitalization data further indicate that individuals who misuse alcohol face more than twice the risk of heart failure compared to non-users [28]. Cardiovascular complications with chronic use include both anatomic and electrical conduction abnormalities. Alcohol exhibits a deleterious effect on the myocardium through apoptosis and oxidative stress [29]. Additionally, cardiac MRI has demonstrated that binge drinking leads to acute inflammatory changes to the myocardium [30].

Alcohol consumption may lead to atrial fibrillation [31]. The risk is thought to arise from alcohol-induced electrophysiological, cellular, autonomic, and structural changes within the heart. Specifically, alcohol may lead to a decrease in intra- and inter-atrial conduction, elevate heart rate, alter AV-nodal conduction, and increase atrial ectopy [32]. Even after adjusting for multiple factors such as age, sex, race, chronic kidney disease, heart failure, diabetes, smoking, and obesity, individuals who misuse alcohol are approximately twice as likely to develop atrial fibrillation [25]. Notably, an increase in atrial fibrillation risk has also been observed in individuals who consume even low levels of alcohol [33, 34].

Alcohol use is correlated with increased risk of cerebrovascular accidents, primarily attributed to the impact on blood pressure [35]. Females who consume more than one drink per day and males who consume more than two drinks per day are at heightened risk of developing hypertension. The hypertensive effects of alcohol are thought to result from multiple mechanisms, including oxidative stress, heightened sympathetic nervous system activity, and activation of the renin–angiotensin–aldosterone system [36].

Respiratory Alcohol use has been associated with an increased risk of mortality from acute respiratory distress syndrome (ARDS) in individuals with COVID-19 infection [37]. Additionally, individuals who misuse alcohol are eight times more likely to develop community-acquired pneumonia [38].

Gastrointestinal Alcohol consumption can lead to increased production of acetaldehyde, a toxic metabolite that damages hepatocytes. This can lead to alcohol-associated hepatitis which may present abruptly with symptoms including fatigue, jaundice, hepatic decompensation, and coagulopathy [39, 40]. Globally, 35% of patients with alcohol use disorder will develop liver disease. Alcohol accounts for nearly 50% of all deaths globally attributed to liver disease [41].

Cirrhosis develops as a response to tissue injury [39]. A clinician should have an increased suspicion for cirrhosis in individuals with thrombocytopenia, prolonged international normalized ratio (INR), ascites, firm liver, and skin findings such as palmar erythema, or vascular spiders [42]. Countries with an average daily alcohol intake of greater than 21 grams had a higher percentage of mortality from cirrhosis [41].

Liver transplantation is indicated when medical management fails to control disease progression. Eligibility for transplantation is influenced by several factors, including the duration of abstinence from alcohol. Many transplant centers require a minimum of 6 months of abstinence prior to transplantation, though there are many new protocols that demonstrate benefit for acutely sick individuals with less time abstinent. The 6-month period is recommended both to evaluate the individual's commitment to and ability to achieve recovery and to allow time for potential improvement in liver function, which may eliminate the need for transplantation [43].

Because individuals with alcohol-related cirrhosis may not survive the required sobriety period without liver transplantation, studies have investigated the outcomes of early transplantation defined as prior to 6 months of abstinence from alcohol. Notably, the cumulative six-month survival rate was higher among persons who received early transplantation [44]. In a study of 147 persons with alcohol-associated hepatitis who underwent liver transplantation, one-year and three-year survival rates were higher than those observed for transplants performed for other indications [45]. Compared to recipients transplanted for non-alcohol-related liver disease, those with alcohol-associated liver disease tended to be younger, presented with more severe liver dysfunction, and were more likely have private insurance and higher levels of education [46].

Alcohol can lead to the development of pancreatitis through sensitization of acinar cells and release of cholecystokinin from duodenal cells [47]. Death rates from alcohol-associated pancreatitis doubled during the COVID-19 pandemic [48].

The risk of developing erosive esophagitis increases with escalating alcohol consumption [49]. Alcohol consumption can cause esophageal varices. Risks for variceal bleeding include, but are not limited to, Child-Pugh Class B/C, size of the varices, presence of ascites, and abnormal laboratory values (thrombocytopenia, high bilirubin, and low creatinine) [50]. Alcohol also increases the risk of gastritis [51].

Alcohol can also cause intestinal inflammation through a variety of mechanisms. Alcohol can disrupt the normal intestinal bacterial flora through a process called "dysbiosis." Alcohol use can also cause excess bacterial growth which can lead to toxin release and inflammation. Alcohol causes damage to intestinal epithelial cells, increasing the risk of pathogens entering the bloodstream [52].

Musculoskeletal Alcohol use carries an increased risk of gout, with the likelihood rising in parallel with greater levels of consumption [53]. Additionally, alcohol use is associated with an increased risk of falls—not only among individuals who drink moderately or excessively, but also among those with a history of alcohol use [54]. Alcohol use disorder is further associated with poorer outcomes following traumatic injuries, specifically longer intensive care and hospital stays, as well as higher mortality rates following rib fractures, compared to those without the disorder [55]. Alcohol use is associated with impaired protein synthesis, leading to skeletal muscle breakdown (wasting) [56].

Endocrine Alcohol use disrupts multiple hormone systems, contributing to an increased risk of amenorrhea in women and hypogonadism in men. It is also associated with increased prolactin levels (hyperprolactinemia) and has been linked to the development of prolactinomas [57].

Hematological/Oncological Alcohol contributes to cancer development through multiple mechanisms. It is metabolized to acetaldehyde, a known carcinogen, and promotes the formation of oxygen radicals that can damage DNA. Additionally, alcohol can increase hormones such as estradiol, which may elevate the risk of hormone-sensitive cancers [58]. The cancers associated with alcohol use are cancer of the mouth, pharynx, larynx, esophagus, liver, colorectum, and breast [59]. Alcohol consumption of more than 80 grams per day increases the risk of hepatocellular carcinoma by five times [60]. Alcohol use also increases the risk of skin cancer [61].

Women who consume less than one drink per day are at increased risk of breast cancer. Those who consume between 15- and 30-grams of alcohol daily have a 35% increased risk of breast cancer compared to non-drinkers. Lifetime cumulative alcohol intake is more strongly associated with breast cancer risk than consumption during any specific period [62]. Yet, fewer than 25% of women are aware of the link between alcohol use and breast cancer [63]. Importantly, sustained reduction in alcohol intake leads to a reduction in cancer risk [59].

Perinatal complications Alcohol use during pregnancy is associated with intrauterine growth restriction, preterm birth, and preterm premature rupture of membranes [64]. Perinatal alcohol use can cause fetal alcohol spectrum disorders, which are associated with cognitive impairment and facial dysmorphology [65].

Sedative-Hypnotics

Neurologic Benzodiazepine use is associated with cognitive impairment, particularly in the cognitive domains of attention and processing speed [66]. The association between chronic benzodiazepine use and dementia is unclear [67]. Some studies have demonstrated an association between high-dose benzodiazepine use and dementia [68, 69]. Other studies have posited that benzodiazepine use is associated with an increased risk of mild cognitive impairment but not dementia [70].

Cardiovascular In patients with heart failure, benzodiazepine use is associated with an increased risk of heart failure-related hospitalization and cardiovascular death. Individuals with heart failure who are prescribed benzodiazepines also face a higher likelihood of experiencing strokes and myocardial infarctions. These adverse outcomes are particularly pronounced in individuals with ejection fractions less than 30% [71].

Pulmonary An increased risk for obstructive sleep apnea development has been associated with benzodiazepine use as compared to Z-drug (e.g., zolpidem, zaleplon, zopiclone and eszopiclone) use. Persons who receive both benzodiazepines and Z-drugs are more likely to develop obstructive sleep apnea than those who are only prescribed benzodiazepines [72]. Benzodiazepine overdose is associated with respiratory compromise and death [73, 74].

Musculoskeletal Chronic benzodiazepine use is associated with an increase in all-cause mortality and elevated fall risk, specifically in geriatric populations. The increased fall risk is associated with a corresponding increase in fracture risk, notably hip fractures [75]. This can negatively impact mobility and lead to loss of functional independence.

Perinatal complications Benzodiazepine or Z-hypnotic use in pregnancy has been associated with small for gestational age and miscarriage [76, 77]. Chronic administration of benzodiazepines proximal to delivery is associated with neonatal toxicity and withdrawal [78].

Stimulants

Neurologic Methamphetamine use is associated with cognitive impairment across multiple domains, including executive functioning, memory, and processing speed. Methamphetamine-induced damage to central nervous system dopaminergic pathways may lead to development of parkinsonism [79]. Methamphetamine-induced hypertension is a risk factor for cerebral small vessel disease and hemorrhagic stroke [80, 81]. Methamphetamine use is also associated with seizures [82].

Cardiovascular Amphetamine use is linked to two major cardiac pathologies: pulmonary arterial hypertension (PAH) and cardiomyopathy. Despite the elevated risk of arrhythmic death, those with methamphetamine-associated cardiomyopathy were less likely to receive an implantable cardioverter-defibrillator (ICD) [83]. Additional risk factors for methamphetamine-associated cardiomyopathy include diabetes, chronic kidney disease, and chronic pulmonary disease [84]. Methamphetamine associated heart failure with reduced ejection fraction (HFrEF) improved with methamphetamine cessation. Methamphetamine-associated heart failure with preserved ejection fraction (HFpEF) did not demonstrate similar recovery [85].

Cardiovascular risks from cocaine include coronary vasospasm (from vasoconstriction), cerebrovascular accidents, and myocardial infarction. Further, a significant emergency consequence from cocaine use is aortic dissection and possible rupture [86].

Pulmonary Inhaled crack cocaine may lead to chemical pneumonitis or "crack lung" [87]. Methamphetamine use can contribute to multiple respiratory conditions, including pulmonary edema, pneumonia, pneumothorax, and pneumonitis [88].

Renal Methamphetamine-induced rhabdomyolysis can cause damage to renal tubules and has been associated with end stage renal disease. Methamphetamine use also increases the risk of disseminated intravascular coagulation, acute cortical necrosis, and vasculitis [89].

Infectious Diseases Methamphetamine use increases the risk of HIV seroconversion by intravenous drug use and high-risk sexual behaviors. There is an increased risk of HIV acquisition due to lower rates of viral suppression in populations that use methamphetamine. Methamphetamine use has also been linked to rising rates of viral hepatitis [79].

Dental A common adverse effect of smoking methamphetamine is dental decay related to combination of caries, bruxism, vasoconstriction of capillaries, and enamel exposure to chemicals [87]. Increased dental caries are also found with frequent cocaine use [88].

Hematological/oncological Cocaine exhibits a pro-thrombotic effect through multiple mechanisms [90, 91]. Cocaine-induced thrombotic microangiopathy has been proposed as a potential etiology of limb ischemia [91].

Perinatal complications Pregnancy may increase the risk of cardiovascular complications of cocaine use due to increased progesterone concentrations [92]. Chronic use of cocaine during pregnancy is associated with maternal migraines and seizures. Prenatal complications include preterm premature rupture of membranes [93].

Methamphetamine use during pregnancy is associated with gestational hypertension, placental abruption, and preterm birth [94].

Opioids

Neurologic Whether fatal or not, opioid overdose often results in hypoxic or ischemic changes with cerebral edema, ischemic neuronal damage, and ischemic neuronal loss. Differences in grey and white matter have been found in individuals with opioid use disorder (OUD) compared with healthy controls, which may explain neural network dysregulation and cognitive impairments seen in OUD because of opioids or the secondary effects from opioid use [95]. In addition to recurrent hypoxic–ischemic injury, OUD has also been associated with increased microglial activation; both factors may predispose to developing neurodegenerative disease and dementia [95, 96]. Impaired neuropsychological function, particularly with working memory, attention, and cognitive flexibility, have been associated with chronic opioid use. A sudden-onset amnestic syndrome with bilateral hippocampal damage on magnetic resonance imaging has also been associated with acute opioid use [97, 98]. Whether chronic opioid-associated memory deficits lie on a spectrum with acute opioid-associated amnestic syndrome remains unknown. Opioid-induced hyperalgesia, defined as a decrease in pain threshold or pain tolerance, may be associated with chronic opioid exposure [99].

Cardiovascular Both opioid overdose and withdrawal can trigger major adverse cardiovascular events with vascular and electrophysiological consequences [100]. Acute cardiovascular effects include hypotension, orthostasis, syncope, and bradycardia, through μ-receptor mediated vasodilation. Some opioids, including methadone, tramadol, and oxycodone, are associated with increased risk of long QT syndrome, which in turn may lead to dangerous arrhythmias including torsade de pointes [101]. The risk of long QT syndrome is significantly lower for other drugs in the opioid class, such as morphine and buprenorphine [102]. During opioid withdrawal, increased catecholaminergic tone and abrupt increases in myocardial oxygen consumption may destabilize persons, particularly those with underlying coronary artery disease, severe valvular heart disease, and ventricular systolic dysfunction [103]. Stress-induced cardiomyopathy has been described during opioid withdrawal [104]. Non-infectious vascular complications particularly from injection of drugs include phlebitis, thromboembolic disease, and venous insufficiency [105].

Infectious Diseases Opioids are among the most injected drugs [106]. Rising injection drug use, paralleling the opioid epidemic, has resulted in an increase in cases of infective endocarditis [107]. Endocarditis among persons who inject drugs often involves right-sided heart valves since peripheral veins are the portal of drug entry [101]. Injection drug use has also led to higher rates of HIV, hepatitis B, and hepatitis C transmission and hospitalizations for severe bacterial and fungal infections of the skin, soft tissue, bone, joint and central nervous system due to use of contaminated needles [108–110].

Respiratory Opioid-induced respiratory depression is characterized by slow, shallow, and irregular breathing, and in severe cases, respiratory arrest [111]. Sedation, decreased ventilation rate, decreased chemoreflexes to hypoxia and hypercapnia, decreased upper airway protective reflexes, and decreased activity of phrenic motor neurons, which innervate the diaphragm and increased rigidity of chest wall muscles, contribute to these effects [111–115]. Certain populations are at higher risk of overdose, including those who are morbidly obese, have sleep apnea, chronic obstructive pulmonary disease, chronic heart failure, certain neuromuscular diseases, or are on the age extremes [116–118]. Inhibition of upper airway patency has a range of consequences, including obstructive sleep apnea, aspiration, and difficulty swallowing [114, 119–125]. Notably, opioid agonists produce graded degrees of respiratory depression that are dose-dependent and correlate with agonist efficacy. Partial opioid receptor agonists, such as buprenorphine, which have lower intrinsic efficacy and activate receptors to a lesser extent even at maximal doses, cause reduced respiratory depression leading to a greater safety profile [126].

Gastrointestinal Due to their impact on opioid receptors in enteric neurons, opioids reduce gastrointestinal and biliary motility and may produce nausea, vomiting, constipation, intestinal pseudo-obstruction, and gastroparesis [127]. Esophageal dysmotility may present as dysphagia. Delayed gastric emptying can manifest as early satiety. Opioid-induced constipation is the most common form of opioid-induced bowel dysfunction and may increase the risk of gastrointestinal perforation [128].

Genitourinary Opioid binding receptors in the bladder and spinal cord inhibit the micturition reflex and result in urinary retention [129]. An opioid overdose can result in acute kidney injury due to dehydration, hypotension, rhabdomyolysis, and urinary retention [130].

Endocrine Endocrine complications of chronic opioid use include hypogonadism in women and in men. The consequences of opioid-induced hypogonadism include sexual dysfunction, depression, decreased quality of life, and low bone density [131]. Notably, different opioids have differing endocrine effects. For instance, the suppressive effect of methadone on the hypothalamic-pituitary-gonadal axis, resulting in hypogonadism, seems to be larger than the effect of buprenorphine in several studies comparing the two [132].

Perinatal Opioid use in pregnancy, both illicit use and prescribed, has been associated with obstetric adverse effects, including third trimester bleeding, maternal mortality, and preterm birth [133]. Adverse neonatal outcomes that have been linked with opioid use during pregnancy include small for gestational age, low birthweight, reduced head circumference, sudden infant death, respiratory complications, and neonatal opioid withdrawal syndrome (NOWS) or neonatal abstinence syndrome (NAS) [134, 135].

Cannabis

Neurologic While evidence from human studies on structural brain changes related to cannabis use remains limited, animal research has demonstrated developmental alterations associated with sustained, long-term cannabis use [136, 137]. With the long- term use of cannabis, changes in the grey matter of cortical and hippocampal regions have been reported, with impacts on motivational, emotional, and affective processing [137]. The acute administration of cannabis or THC has been shown to produce small to moderate impairments in episodic and working memory, processing speed, executive function, attention, and impulse control. These cognitive effects may persist for several days to weeks following cannabis cessation in regular users [138]. Additionally, cannabis use has been associated with increased risk of developing psychotic disorders, with early onset in vulnerable persons. Psychotic symptoms also have been observed in otherwise healthy individuals following exposure to Δ 9 -THC and synthetic cannabinoids [137, 139].

Cardiovascular Cannabis use has been associated with adverse cardiovascular outcomes, including myocardial infarction and stroke [140, 141]. The use of exogenous cannabis leads to endothelial dysfunction and increases vascular thrombosis via CB 1 receptor stimulation [142]. On the other hand, CB 2 receptors may have a beneficial anti-inflammatory response [142].

Respiratory Respiratory complications of smoking cannabis include exacerbations of asthma and chronic bronchitis, and increased susceptibility to lung infections, such as invasive pulmonary aspergillosis [143–145]. Smoking cannabis is a risk factor for the development of bullous lung disease, spontaneous pneumothorax, and hypersensitivity pneumonitis [144]. The smoke from cannabis combustion has been shown to contain many of the same toxins, irritants, and carcinogens as tobacco smoke [146], though risk for respiratory cancers is much less than for smoked tobacco.

Gastrointestinal Gastrointestinal co-morbidities associated with cannabis use include cannabinoid hyperemesis syndrome, characterized by spontaneous, recurrent episodes of nausea, vomiting, and abdominal pain. A distinctive feature of cannabis hyperemesis syndrome is symptom relief through exposure to hot water. This condition is most often associated with individuals with heavy or chronic cannabis use, and symptoms typically resolve after cessation of cannabis use [147, 148].

Perinatal Emerging data reveal that cannabis exposure during pregnancy may be associated with fetal growth restriction, respiratory distress, hypoglycemia, altered neurodevelopmental trajectories, and increased long-term risk for obesity, diabetes, and cardiovascular disease [149, 150]. Prenatal marijuana exposure has also been linked to development of psychotic symptoms [151].

Caffeine

Neurologic As a psychostimulant, caffeine exposure results in increased alertness and may be associated with tremor, insomnia, and anxiety [152].

Cardiovascular Chronic caffeine consumption at 400 mg daily has been shown to significantly impact the autonomic nervous system, raising the heart rate and blood pressure over time, while consuming moderate amounts of coffee and caffeine regularly may offer a protective effect against developing multiple cardiometabolic diseases, including type 2 diabetes, coronary heart disease, and stroke [153].

Gastrointestinal Excessive caffeine intake may be associated with short-term adverse effects including gastrointestinal upset due to stimulation of motility [154].

Perinatal One integrative review regarding perinatal outcomes of caffeine intake during pregnancy found that consumption, even below 200 mg/day (a frequently recommended level of caffeine intake during pregnancy) may be associated with pregnancy loss, low birth weight, and neurodevelopmental and neurobehavioral outcomes [155, 156].

PCP, Hallucinogens, Inhalants

Neurologic Many inhalants, like toluene, are highly lipid-soluble and can rapidly reach high concentrations in the brain, damaging the myelin sheath that insulates nerve fibers and contributing to neurocognitive and neuropsychiatric problems by activating immune-inflammatory and oxidative stress pathways [157]. Short-term effects include diplopia, memory impairment, slurred speech, and seizure. Long-term chronic effects include permanent ataxia or peripheral neuropathies, blindness, cognitive impairment, or dementia. Even a single occupational exposure leading to inhalant intoxication can produce long-term memory problems and processing speed impairments [158].

Cardiovascular Inhalants can cause fatal heart arrhythmias, potentially leading to sudden sniffing death syndrome, even after a single use. Although the exact mechanism is unknown, the inhalant is believed to sensitize the myocardium to circulating catecholamines [159].

Respiratory Asphyxiation can result from the displacement of oxygen in the lungs by prolonged or repeated inhalant use. Suffocation can occur if a plastic bag is placed over the head when inhaling the fumes and the user becomes unconscious [158].

Genitourinary Frequent ketamine use is associated with cystitis [160]. The typical presentation of ketamine cystitis is severe dysuria, urgency, frequency, and gross hematuria. Complications may include bladder wall thickening and adhesion to the peritoneum, and bladder mucosa ulceration. Cessation of ketamine is the mainstay of treatment [161].

Perinatal Data regarding perinatal outcomes with PCP, hallucinogen, and inhalant use are limited, based on few case reports and series. Case reports and series suggest a high incidence of intrauterine growth retardation, preterm delivery, and symptoms of neonatal drug withdrawal/intoxication may be associated with PCP or inhalant use during pregnancy [162, 163].

Chapter Review Questions

1. Andrew is a 70-year-old male with a 40 pack/year smoking history who currently smokes. He presents to his PCP for an annual well visit check, and he is started on atorvastatin for dyslipidemia and continued on hydrochlorothiazide for hypertension. What screening does the United States Preventive Services Task Force (USPSTF) recommend?

   A. Annual spirometry
   B. Annual non-contrast CT Chest
   C. Biannual abdominal aorta ultrasound
   D. One time biomarker screening
   E. One-time pulmonary function testing

   Correct Answer: B
   Explanation: The USPSTF recommends annual screening for lung cancer with low-dose computed tomography in adults aged 50–80 years who have a 20 pack-year smoking history and currently smoke or have quit within the past 15 years. The USPSTF recommends one-time screening for abdominal aortic aneurysm with ultrasonography in men aged 65–75 years who have ever smoked.
2. George is an 88-year-old male with generalized anxiety disorder and insomnia. He has been prescribed clonazepam 1 mg TID for the past 10 years by his primary care physician, but was referred to you, a psychiatrist, after his prescriber retired. During your discussion of the risks of benzodiazepine use, you mention which of the following?

A. Thrombocytopenia
B. Increased fall risk
C. Elevated risk of GI cancer
D. Tardive dyskinesia
E. Malnutrition

Correct Answer: B
Explanation: Long-term use of benzodiazepines has significant health consequences. Notably, the increased risk of fall has led to hip fractures in geriatric populations. There is no association with GI cancer, thrombocytopenia, tardive dyskinesia, or malnutrition. Despite these consequences, prescribers should avoid rapid discontinuation, as this can lead to seizures and potentially, withdrawal-associated psychosis or other symptoms.

3. Gina is a 28-year-old female who is currently stable in the emergency department after she experienced an overdose following intravenous fentanyl use and receiving intranasal naloxone by emergency medical services prior to her arrival in the hospital. Which of the following is most likely to require inpatient hospitalization?

A. Constipation
B. Nausea
C. Severe yawning
D. Endocarditis
E. Diarrhea

Correct Answer: D
Explanation: Intravenous fentanyl use may lead to severe bacterial infections such as endocarditis, bacteremia, or osteomyelitis. These conditions typically require intravenous antibiotics and further inpatient evaluation. While the other options may be signs of opioid withdrawal or opioid use/misuse, the other options do not require inpatient hospitalization.

4. After ingesting an unidentified substance, Elmer suddenly develops slurred speech. Which emergency condition is most important to consider in your differential diagnosis, and what was the most likely substance involved?

A. Intoxication; alcohol
B. Tardive dyskinesia; cannabis
C. Stroke; cocaine
D. Dysphagia; nicotine
E. Globus pharyngis; cannabis

Correct Answer: C
Explanation: Cocaine intoxication can cause stroke, myocardial infarction, and aortic dissection. Prompt diagnosis and treatment is crucial. Alcohol intoxication alone may not be an emergency condition. Tardive dyskinesia is not a complication of cannabis use. Sudden-onset dysphagia is not associated with nicotine use. Globus pharyngis is not an emergent consequence of cannabis use.

5. Steven is a 48-year-old male with alcohol use disorder. He has developed liver failure and requires a transplant. When should he receive a liver transplant?

   A. After 6 months of sobriety to demonstrate motivation
   B. After 6 months of sobriety to determine interval improvement and continued need for liver transplant
   C. Prior to 6 months of sobriety if clinically indicated
   D. Never; not appropriate for clinical consideration
   E. After completion of 90-day residential treatment program

   Correct Answer: C

   Explanation: Requiring an individual to wait 6 months before liver transplantation may lead to premature death. Transplantation outcomes are like other non-alcohol-associated etiologies requiring transplantation.

References

1. U.S. Department of Health and Human Services. The health consequences of smoking—50 years of progress: a report of the surgeon general. Atlanta: U.S. Department of Health and Human Services, Centers for Disease Control and Prevention, National Center for Chronic Disease Prevention and Health Promotion, Office on Smoking and Health; 2014. Accessed April 24, 2024. https://www.ncbi.nlm.nih.gov/books/NBK179276/pdf/Bookshelf_NBK179276.pdf.
2. US Preventive Services Task Force. Screening for abdominal aortic aneurysm: US Preventive Services Task Force Recommendation Statement. JAMA. 2019;322(22):2211–8. https://doi.org/10.1001/jama.2019.18928.
3. Ding N, Sang Y, Chen J, Ballew SH, Kalbaugh CA, Salameh MJ, Blaha MJ, Allison M, Heiss G, Selvin E, Coresh J, Matsushita K. Cigarette smoking, smoking cessation, and long-term risk of 3 major atherosclerotic diseases. J Am Coll Cardiol. 2019;74(4):498–507. https://doi.org/10.1016/j.jacc.2019.05.049. PMID: 31345423; PMCID: PMC6662625.
4. Centers for Disease Control and Prevention (US); National Center for Chronic Disease Prevention and Health Promotion (US); Office on Smoking and Health (US). How tobacco smoke causes disease: the biology and Behavioral basis for smoking-attributable disease: a report of the surgeon general. Atlanta: Centers for Disease Control and Prevention (US); 2010. 7, Pulmonary Diseases. Available from: https://www.ncbi.nlm.nih.gov/books/NBK53021/.
5. Espinoza-Derout J, Shao XM, Lao CJ, Hasan KM, Rivera JC, Jordan MC, Echeverria V, Roos KP, Sinha-Hikim AP, Friedman TC. Electronic cigarette use and the risk of cardiovascular diseases. Front Cardiovasc Med. 2022;9:879726. https://doi.org/10.3389/fcvm.2022.879726. PMID: 35463745; PMCID: PMC9021536.
6. Rebuli ME, Rose JJ, Noël A, Croft DP, Benowitz NL, Cohen AH, Goniewicz ML, Larsen BT, Leigh N, McGraw MD, Melzer AC, Penn AL, Rahman I, Upson D, Crotty Alexander LE, Ewart G, Jaspers I, Jordt SE, Kligerman S, Loughlin CE, McConnell R, Neptune ER, Nguyen TB, Pinkerton KE, Witek TJ Jr. The E-cigarette or vaping product use-associated lung injury epidemic: pathogenesis, management, and future directions: an Official American Thoracic Society workshop report. Ann Am Thorac Soc. 2023;20(1):1–17. https://doi.org/10.1513/AnnalsATS.202209-796ST. PMID: 36584985; PMCID: PMC9819258.
7. Jacob P 3rd, Abu Raddaha AH, Dempsey D, Havel C, Peng M, Yu L, Benowitz NL. Comparison of nicotine and carcinogen exposure with water pipe and cigarette smoking. Cancer Epidemiol Biomarkers Prev. 2013;22(5):765–72. https://doi.org/10.1158/1055-9965.EPI-12-1422. Epub 2013 Mar 5. PMID: 23462922; PMCID: PMC3650103.

8. Al-Bashaireh AM, Haddad LG, Weaver M, Kelly DL, Chengguo X, Yoon S. The effect of tobacco smoking on musculoskeletal health: a systematic review. J Environ Public Health. 2018;2018:4184190. https://doi.org/10.1155/2018/4184190. PMID: 30112011; PMCID: PMC6077562.
9. Gianfrancesco MA, Trupin L, Shiboski S, van der Laan M, Graf J, Imboden J, Yazdany J, Schmajuk G. Smoking is associated with higher disease activity in rheumatoid arthritis: a longitudinal study controlling for time-varying covariates. J Rheumatol. 2019;46(4):370–5. https://doi.org/10.3899/jrheum.180262. Epub 2018 Dec 1. PMID: 30504507; PMCID: PMC6445683.
10. Tweed JO, Hsia SH, Lutfy K, Friedman TC. The endocrine effects of nicotine and cigarette smoke. Trends Endocrinol Metab. 2012;23(7):334–42. https://doi.org/10.1016/j.tem.2012.03.006. Epub 2012 May 2. PMID: 22561025; PMCID: PMC3389568.
11. US Preventive Services Task Force. Screening for lung cancer: US Preventive Services Task Force Recommendation Statement. JAMA. 2021;325(10):962–70. https://doi.org/10.1001/jama.2021.1117.
12. Andres RL, Day MC. Perinatal complications associated with maternal tobacco use. Semin Neonatol. 2000;5(3):231–41.
13. Tarasi B, Cornuz J, Clair C, Baud D. Cigarette smoking during pregnancy and adverse perinatal outcomes: a cross-sectional study over 10 years. BMC Public Health. 2022;22(1):2403.
14. Wijnia JW. A clinician's view of Wernicke-Korsakoff syndrome. J Clin Med. 2022;11(22):6755.
15. Eva L, Brehar F-M, Florian I-A, Covache-Busuioc R-A, Costin HP, Dumitrascu D-I, et al. Neuropsychiatric and neuropsychological aspects of alcohol-related cognitive disorders: an in-depth review of Wernicke's encephalopathy and Korsakoff's syndrome. J Clin Med. 2023;12(18):6101.
16. Koguchi K, Nakatsuji Y, Abe K, Sakoda S. Wernicke's encephalopathy after glucose infusion. Neurology. 2004;62(3):512.
17. Day E, Bentham PW, Callaghan R, Kuruvilla T, George S. Thiamine for prevention and treatment of Wernicke-Korsakoff syndrome in people who abuse alcohol. Cochrane Database Syst Rev. 2013;2013(7):CD004033.
18. Malamud N, Skillicorn SA. Relationship between the Wernicke and the Korsakoff syndrome: a clinicopathologic study of seventy cases. AMA Arch Neurol Psychiatr. 1956;76(6):585–96.
19. Boere R, Oudman E, Postma A, van den Berg E. Social norms in Korsakoff's syndrome and alcohol-related dementia. J Clin Exp Neuropsychol. 2024;46(9):868–77.
20. Palm A, Talaslahti T, Vataja R, Ginters M, Kautiainen H, Elonheimo H, et al. Criminal behavior in alcohol-related dementia and Wernicke–Korsakoff syndrome: a Nationwide Register Study. Eur Arch Psychiatry Clin Neurosci. 2024;275:1–9.
21. Rasiah R, Gregoriano C, Mueller B, Kutz A, Schuetz P, editors. Hospital outcomes in medical patients with alcohol-related and non–alcohol-related Wernicke encephalopathy. Mayo Clinic proceedings. Elsevier; 2024.
22. Dar MS. Ethanol-induced cerebellar ataxia: cellular and molecular mechanisms. Cerebellum. 2015;14:447–65.
23. Topiwala A, Ebmeier KP, Maullin-Sapey T, Nichols TE. No safe level of alcohol consumption for brain health: observational cohort study of 25,378 UK Biobank participants. MedRxiv. 2021:2021.05. 10.21256931.
24. Manthey J, Rehm J. Mortality from alcoholic cardiomyopathy: exploring the gap between estimated and civil registry data. J Clin Med. 2019;8(8):1137.
25. Whitman IR, Agarwal V, Nah G, Dukes JW, Vittinghoff E, Dewland TA, et al. Alcohol abuse and cardiac disease. J Am Coll Cardiol. 2017;69(1):13–24.
26. Wood AM, Kaptoge S, Butterworth AS, Willeit P, Warnakula S, Bolton T, et al. Risk thresholds for alcohol consumption: combined analysis of individual-participant data for 599 912 current drinkers in 83 prospective studies. Lancet. 2018;391(10129):1513–23.
27. Biddinger KJ, Emdin CA, Haas ME, Wang M, Hindy G, Ellinor PT, et al. Association of habitual alcohol intake with risk of cardiovascular disease. JAMA Netw Open. 2022;5(3):e223849-e.

28. Bozkurt B, Colvin M, Cook J, Cooper LT, Deswal A, Fonarow GC, et al. Current diagnostic and treatment strategies for specific dilated cardiomyopathies: a scientific statement from the American Heart Association. Circulation. 2016;134(23):e579–646.
29. Wang S, Ren J. Role of autophagy and regulatory mechanisms in alcoholic cardiomyopathy. Biochim Biophys Acta. 2018;1864(6):2003–9.
30. Zagrosek A, Messroghli D, Schulz O, Dietz R, Schulz-Menger J. Effect of binge drinking on the heart as assessed by cardiac magnetic resonance imaging. JAMA. 2010;304(12):1328–30.
31. Beilin LJ, Puddey IB. Alcohol and hypertension: an update. Hypertension. 2006;47(6):1035–8.
32. Linz B, Hertel JN, Jespersen T, Linz D. Mechanisms and therapeutic opportunities in atrial fibrillation in relationship to alcohol use and abuse. Can J Cardiol. 2022;38(9):1352–63.
33. Csengeri D, Sprünker N-A, Di Castelnuovo A, Niiranen T, Vishram-Nielsen JK, Costanzo S, et al. Alcohol consumption, cardiac biomarkers, and risk of atrial fibrillation and adverse outcomes. Eur Heart J. 2021;42(12):1170–7.
34. Jiang H, Mei X, Jiang Y, Yao J, Shen J, Chen T, et al. Alcohol consumption and atrial fibrillation risk: an updated dose-response meta-analysis of over 10 million participants. Front Cardiovasc Med. 2022;9:979982.
35. Wood AM, Kaptoge S, Butterworth AS, Willeit P, Warnakula S, Bolton T, Paige E, Paul DS, Sweeting M, Burgess S, Bell S. Risk thresholds for alcohol consumption: combined analysis of individual-participant data for 599 912 current drinkers in 83 prospective studies. Lancet. 2018;391(10129):1513–23.
36. Middlekauff HR, Cooper ZD, Strauss SB. Drugs of misuse: focus on vascular dysfunction. Can J Cardiol. 2022;38(9):1364–77.
37. Bailey KL, Samuelson DR, Wyatt TA. Alcohol use disorder: a pre-existing condition for COVID-19? Alcohol. 2021;90:11–7.
38. Samokhvalov A, Irving H, Rehm J. Alcohol consumption as a risk factor for pneumonia: a systematic review and meta-analysis. Epidemiol Infect. 2010;138(12):1789–95.
39. Buchanan R, Sinclair JM. Alcohol use disorder and the liver. Addiction. 2021;116(5):1270–8.
40. Singal AK, Louvet A, Shah VH, Kamath PS. Grand rounds: alcoholic hepatitis. J Hepatol. 2018;69(2):534–43.
41. Stein E, Cruz-Lemini M, Altamirano J, Ndugga N, Couper D, Abraldes JG, et al. Heavy daily alcohol intake at the population level predicts the weight of alcohol in cirrhosis burden worldwide. J Hepatol. 2016;65(5):998–1005.
42. Runyon BA. A primer on detecting cirrhosis and caring for these patients without causing harm. Int J Hepatol. 2011;2011:801983.
43. Donckier V, Lucidi V, Gustot T, Moreno C. Ethical considerations regarding early liver transplantation in patients with severe alcoholic hepatitis not responding to medical therapy. J Hepatol. 2014;60(4):866–71.
44. Mathurin P, Moreno C, Samuel D, Dumortier J, Salleron J, Durand F, Castel H, Duhamel A, Pageaux GP, Leroy V, Dharancy S. Early liver transplantation for severe alcoholic hepatitis. N Engl J Med. 2011;365(19):1790–800.
45. Lee BP, Mehta N, Platt L, Gurakar A, Rice JP, Lucey MR, Im GY, Therapondos G, Han H, Victor DW, Fix OK. Outcomes of early liver transplantation for patients with severe alcoholic hepatitis. Gastroenterology. 2018;155(2):422–30.
46. Cotter TG, Sandıkçı B, Paul S, Gampa A, Wang J, Te H, Pillai A, Reddy KG, di Sabato D, Little EC, Sundaram V. Liver transplantation for alcoholic hepatitis in the United States: excellent outcomes with profound temporal and geographic variation in frequency. Am J Transplant. 2021;21(3):1039–55.
47. Lerch MM, Albrecht E, Ruthenbürger M, Mayerle J, Halangk W, Krüger B. Pathophysiology of alcohol-induced pancreatitis. Pancreas. 2003;27(4):291–6.
48. Chaudhry H, Sohal A, Sharma R, Dukovic D, Lee D, Gamboa A, et al. Increased mortality in patients with alcohol-induced pancreatitis during the COVID-19 pandemic. Ann Gastroenterol. 2022;36(1):68.
49. Sogabe M, Okahisa T, Kagawa M, Ueda H, Kagemoto K, Tanaka H, et al. Influence of alcohol consumption on the development of erosive esophagitis in both sexes: a longitudinal study. Nutrients. 2022;14(22):4760.

50. Guinazu C, Muñoz AF, Maldonado MD, De La Cruz JA, Herrera D, Arruarana VS, et al. Assessing the predictive factors for bleeding in esophageal variceal disease: a systematic review. Cureus. 2023;15(11):e48954.
51. Rugge M, Savarino E, Sbaraglia M, Bricca L, Malfertheiner P. Gastritis: the clinico-pathological spectrum. Dig Liver Dis. 2021;53(10):1237–46.
52. Bishehsari F, Magno E, Swanson G, Desai V, Voigt RM, Forsyth CB, Keshavarzian A. Alcohol and gut-derived inflammation. Alcohol Res. 2017;38(2):163.
53. Lyu J-Q, Miao M-Y, Wang J-M, Qian Y-W, Han W-W, Peng X-Z, et al. Consumption of total and specific alcoholic beverages and long-term risk of gout among men and women. JAMA Netw Open. 2024;7(8):e2430700-e.
54. Sun Y, Zhang B, Yao Q, Ma Y, Lin Y, Xu M, et al. Association between usual alcohol consumption and risk of falls in middle-aged and older Chinese adults. BMC Geriatr. 2022;22(1):750.
55. Field F, Olsson J, Hurley A. Alcohol dependence and rib fracture outcomes: a systematic review and meta-analysis. Cureus. 2023;15(7):e42639.
56. Simon L, Bourgeois BL, Molina PE. Alcohol and skeletal muscle in health and disease. Alcohol Res. 2023;43(1):04.
57. Rachdaoui N, Sarkar DK. Pathophysiology of the effects of alcohol abuse on the endocrine system. Alcohol Res. 2017;38(2):255.
58. Seitz HK, Stickel F. Molecular mechanisms of alcohol-mediated carcinogenesis. Nat Rev Cancer. 2007;7(8):599–612.
59. Yoo JE, Han K, Shin DW, Kim D, Kim BS, Chun S, Jeon KH, Jung W, Park J, Park JH, Choi KS. Association between changes in alcohol consumption and cancer risk. JAMA Netw Open. 2022;5(8):e2228544.
60. Morgan TR, Mandayam S, Jamal MM. Alcohol and hepatocellular carcinoma. Gastroenterology. 2004;127(5):S87–96.
61. Liu L, Chen J. Advances in relationship between alcohol consumption and skin diseases. Clin Cosmet Investig Dermatol. 2023;16:3785–91.
62. Terry MB, Zhang FF, Kabat G, Britton JA, Teitelbaum SL, Neugut AI, et al. Lifetime alcohol intake and breast cancer risk. Ann Epidemiol. 2006;16(3):230–40.
63. Khushalani JS, Qin J, Ekwueme DU, White A. Awareness of breast cancer risk related to a positive family history and alcohol consumption among women aged 15–44 years in United States. Prev Med Rep. 2020;17:101029.
64. Broccia M, Hansen BM, Winckler JM, Larsen T, Strandberg-Larsen K, Torp-Pedersen C, Kesmodel US. Heavy prenatal alcohol exposure and obstetric and birth outcomes: a Danish nationwide cohort study from 1996 to 2018. Lancet Public Health. 2023;8(1):e28–35.
65. Popova S, Charness ME, Burd L, Crawford A, Hoyme HE, Mukherjee RA, Riley EP, Elliott EJ. Fetal alcohol spectrum disorders. Nat Rev Dis Primers. 2023;9(1):11.
66. Zetsen SP, Schellekens AF, Paling EP, Kan CC, Kessels RP. Cognitive functioning in long-term benzodiazepine users. Eur Addict Res. 2022;28(5):377–81.
67. Wu C-C, Liao M-H, Su C-H, Poly TN, Lin M-C. Benzodiazepine use and the risk of dementia in the elderly population: an umbrella review of meta-analyses. J Personal Med. 2023;13(10):1485.
68. Chan TT, Leung WC, Li V, Wong KW, Chu WM, Leung KC, et al. Association between high cumulative dose of benzodiazepine in Chinese patients and risk of dementia: a preliminary retrospective case-control study. Psychogeriatrics. 2017;17(5):310–6.
69. Joyce G, Ferido P, Thunell J, Tysinger B, Zissimopoulos J. Benzodiazepine use and the risk of dementia. Alzheimer's Dementia Transl Res Clin Interven. 2022;8(1):e12309.
70. Teverovsky EG, Gildengers A, Ran X, Jacobsen E, Chang C-CH, Ganguli M. Benzodiazepine use and risk of incident MCI and dementia in a community sample. Int Psychogeriatr. 2024;36(2):142–8.
71. Chuang C, Hsiao F-C, Cheng Y-W, Lin C-P, Tung Y-C, Wu C-T, et al. Benzodiazepines in patients with heart failure and reduced ejection fraction. Acta Cardiologica Sinica. 2022;38(5):573.

72. Hsu T-W, Chen H-M, Chen T-Y, Chu C-S, Pan C-C. The association between use of benzodiazepine receptor agonists and the risk of obstructive sleep apnea: a nationwide population-based nested case-control study. Int J Environ Res Public Health. 2021;18(18):9720.
73. Giftson J, Hazra D, Chandy GM. A two-year retrospective observational cohort study of benzodiazepine overdose cases in the emergency department. Indian J Crit Care Med. 2025;29(3):230.
74. Kleinman RA, Weiss RD. Benzodiazepine-involved overdose deaths in the USA: 2000–2019. J Gen Intern Med. 2022;37(8):2103–9.
75. Woolcott JC, Richardson KJ, Wiens MO, Patel B, Marin J, Khan KM, Marra CA. Meta-analysis of the impact of 9 medication classes on falls in elderly persons. Arch Intern Med. 2009;169(21):1952–60.
76. Munger Clary HM. Caution: Benzodiazepines in pregnancy and risk of adverse perinatal outcomes. Epilepsy Curr. 2024;24(2):105–7.
77. Meng L, Lin C, Chuang H, Chen L, Hsiao F. Benzodiazepine use during pregnancy and risk of miscarriage. JAMA Psychiatry. 2024;81(4):366–73.
78. Ray-Griffith SL, Newport DJ, Stowe ZN. Psychopharmacology during pregnancy and lactation. In: Schatzberg AF, Nemeroff CB, editors. The American Psychiatric Association publishing textbook of psychopharmacology. 5th ed. Arlington: American Psychiatric Association Publishing; 2017. p. 1543.
79. Ciccarone D, Shoptaw S. Understanding stimulant use and use disorders in a new era. Med Clin North Am. 2022;106(1):81.
80. Zhu Z, Vanderschelden B, Lee SJ, Blackwill H, Shafie M, Soun JE, Chow D, Chang P, Stradling D, Qian T, Yu W. Methamphetamine use increases the risk of cerebral small vessel disease in young patients with acute ischemic stroke. Sci Rep. 2023;13(1):8494.
81. Hemphill K, Tierney S, Tirschwell D, Davis AP. A review of methamphetamine use and stroke in the young. Front Neurol. 2024;15:1397677.
82. Lappin JM, Sara GE. Psychostimulant use and the brain. Addiction. 2019;114(11):2065–77.
83. Zhao SX, Kwong C, Swaminathan A, Gohil A, Crawford MH. Clinical characteristics and outcome of methamphetamine-associated pulmonary arterial hypertension and dilated cardiomyopathy. JACC Heart Fail. 2018;6(3):209–18.
84. Suto DJ, Pott E, Brennan J, Jackson M, Thomas I, Coyne CJ. Risk factors and emergency department outcomes in methamphetamine-associated cardiomyopathy: a case-control study. J Emerg Med. 2024;67:e188.
85. Bhatia HS, Nishimura M, Dickson S, Adler E, Greenberg B, Thomas IC. Clinical and echocardiographic outcomes in heart failure associated with methamphetamine use and cessation. Heart. 2021;107(9):741–7.
86. Bhattacharya P, Taraman S, Shankar L, Chaturvedi S, Madhavan R. Clinical profiles, complications, and disability in cocaine-related ischemic stroke. J Stroke Cerebrovasc Dis. 2011;20(5):443–9.
87. Devlin RJ, Henry JA. Clinical review: major consequences of illicit drug consumption. Crit Care. 2008;12:1–7.
88. Tseng W, Sutter ME, Albertson TE. Stimulants and the lung: review of literature. Clin Rev Allergy Immunol. 2014;46(1):82–100.
89. Baradhi KM, Pathireddy S, Bose S, Aeddula NR. Methamphetamine (N-methylamphetamine)-induced renal disease: underevaluated cause of end-stage renal disease (ESRD). BMJ Case Rep CP. 2019;12(9):e230288.
90. Duflou J. Psychostimulant use disorder and the heart. Addiction. 2020;115(1):175–83.
91. Echevarria V, Echevarria AC, Casadesus D. Cocaine-induced four-extremity ischemia caused by a Hypercoagulable state. Cureus. 2023;15(9):e44862.
92. Smid MC, Metz TD, Gordon AJ. Stimulant use in pregnancy: an under-recognized epidemic among pregnant women. Clin Obstet Gynecol. 2019;62(1):168–84.
93. Shafai A, Landau R. Management of pregnant patients with substance use disorder. BJA Educ. 2025;25(11):455–64.

94. Pippard NS, Bandoli G, Baer RJ. Trends and adverse pregnancy and birth outcomes associated with stimulant-related disorder diagnosis. Addiction. 2024;119(11):2006–14.
95. Herlinger K, Lingford-Hughes A. Opioid use disorder and the brain: a clinical perspective. Addiction. 2022;117(2):495–505. https://doi.org/10.1111/add.15636. Epub 2021 Aug 8. PMID: 34228373.
96. Büttner A, Weis S. Neuropathological alterations in drug abusers: the involvement of neurons, glial, and vascular systems. Forensic Sci Med Pathol. 2006;2:115–26.
97. Barash JA, Somerville N, DeMaria AJ. Cluster of an unusual amnestic syndrome - Massachusetts, 2012-2016. MMWR Morb Mortal Wkly Rep. 2017;66:76–9.
98. Barash JA, Ganetsky M, Boyle KL. Acute amnestic syndrome with fentanyl overdose. N Engl J Med. 2018;378:1157–1158.
99. Trøstheim M, Eikemo M. Hyperalgesia in patients with a history of opioid use disorder: a systematic review and meta-analysis. JAMA Psychiatry. 2024;81(11):1108–17. https://doi.org/10.1001/jamapsychiatry.2024.2176.
100. Krantz M, Palmer R, Haigney M. Cardiovascular complications of opioid use: JACC state-of-the-art review. JACC. 2021;77(2):205–23. https://doi.org/10.1016/j.jacc.2020.11.002
101. Kao D, Bucker BB, Khatri V, Dart R, Mehler PS, Katz D, et al. Trends in reporting of methadone-associated cardiac arrhythmia events, 1997-2011. Ann Intern Med. 2013;158:735–40.
102. Hu J, Song Y, Huang X, Li C, Jin X, Cen L, Zhang C, Ding B, Lian J. Opioids-induced long QT syndrome: a challenge to cardiac health. Cardiovasc Toxicol. 2024;24(5):472–80. https://doi.org/10.1007/s12012-024-09853-6. Epub 2024 Apr 17. PMID: 38630336.
103. Spadotto V, Zorzi A, Elmaghawry M, et al. Heart failure due to 'stress cardiomyopathy': a severe manifestation of the opioid withdrawal syndrome. Eur Heart J Acute Cardiovasc Care. 2013;2:84–7.
104. Robertson R, Broers B, Harris M. Injecting drug use, the skin and vasculature. Addiction. 2021;116(7):1914–24. https://doi.org/10.1111/add.15283. Epub 2020 Oct 30. PMID: 33051902.
105. Colledge S, Leung J, Larney S, Peacock A, Grebely J, Hickman M, Cunningham E, Trickey A, Stone J, Vickerman P, Degenhardt L. Frequency of injecting among people who inject drugs: a systematic review and meta-analysis. Int J Drug Policy. 2020;76:102619. https://doi.org/10.1016/j.drugpo.2019.102619. Epub 2019 Dec 18. PMID: 31864107.
106. Mori M, Amabile A, Weimer MB, Geirsson A. The opioid epidemic and endocarditis: Frontiers in the management of injection drug use-related endocarditis. JTCVS Open. 2021;8:315–20. https://doi.org/10.1016/j.xjon.2021.05.021. PMID: 36004152; PMCID: PMC9390675.
107. Saldana CS, Vyas DA, Wurcel AG. Soft tissue, bone, and joint infections in people who inject drugs. Infect Dis Clin N Am. 2020;34(3):495–509. https://doi.org/10.1016/j.idc.2020.06.007. PMID: 32782098; PMCID: PMC8757538.
108. Hrycko A, Mateu-Gelabert P, Ciervo C, Linn-Walton R, Eckhardt B. Severe bacterial infections in people who inject drugs: the role of injection-related tissue damage. Harm Reduct J. 2022;19(1):41. https://doi.org/10.1186/s12954-022-00624-6. PMID: 35501854; PMCID: PMC9063270.
109. McCarthy NL, Baggs J, See I, Reddy SC, Jernigan JA, Gokhale RH, Fiore AE. Bacterial infections associated with substance use disorders, large cohort of United States hospitals, 2012–2017. Clin Infect Dis. 2020;71(7):e37–44. https://doi.org/10.1093/cid/ciaa008.
110. Marks LR, Nolan NS, Liang SY, Durkin MJ, Weimer MB. Infectious complications of injection drug use. Med Clin North Am. 2022;106(1):187–200. https://doi.org/10.1016/j.mcna.2021.08.006. PMID: 34823730.
111. Bateman JT, Saunders SE, Levitt ES. Understanding and countering opioid-induced respiratory depression. Br J Pharmacol. 2023;180(7):813–28. https://doi.org/10.1111/bph.15580. Epub 2021 Jun 26. PMID: 34089181; PMCID: PMC8997313.
112. Ferguson LM, Drummond GB. Acute effects of fentanyl on breathing pattern in anaesthetized subjects. Br J Anaesth. 2006;96:384–90. https://doi.org/10.1093/bja/ael011.

113. Hill R, Santhakumar R, Dewey W, Kelly E, Henderson G. Fentanyl depression of respiration: comparison with heroin and morphine. Br J Pharmacol. 2020;177:254–65. https://doi.org/10.1111/bph.14860.
114. Saunders SE, Levitt ES. Kölliker-Fuse/parabrachial complex mu opioid receptors contribute to fentanyl-induced apnea and respiratory rate depression. Respir Physiol Neurobiol. 2020;275:103388. https://doi.org/10.1016/j.resp.2020.103388.
115. Torralva R, Janowsky A. Noradrenergic mechanisms in fentanyl-mediated rapid death explain failure of naloxone in the opioid crisis. J Pharmacol Exp Ther. 2019;371:453–75. https://doi.org/10.1124/jpet.119.258566.
116. Dahan A, Aarts L, Smith TW. Incidence, reversal, and prevention of opioid-induced respiratory depression. Anesthesiology. 2010;112:226–38. https://doi.org/10.1097/ALN.0b013e3181c38c25.
117. Khanna AK, Bergese SD, Jungquist CR, Morimatsu H, Uezono S, Lee S, Ti LK, Urman RD, McIntyre R, Tornero C, Dahan A, Saager L, Weingarten TN, Wittmann M, Auckley D, Brazzi L, le Guen M, Soto R, Schramm F, et al. Prediction of opioid-induced respiratory depression on inpatient wards using continuous capnography and oximetry: an international prospective, observational trial. Anesth Analg. 2020;131:1012–24. https://doi.org/10.1213/ANE.0000000000004788.
118. Kinshella M-LW, Gauthier T, Lysyshyn M. Rigidity, dyskinesia and other atypical overdose presentations observed at a supervised injection site, Vancouver, Canada. Harm Reduct J. 2018;15:64. https://doi.org/10.1186/s12954-018-0271-5.
119. Christ A, Arranto CA, Schindler C, Klima T, Hunziker PR, Siegemund M, Marsch SC, Eriksson U, Mueller C. Incidence, risk factors, and outcome of aspiration pneumonitis in ICU overdose patients. Intensive Care Med. 2006;32:1423–7.
120. Walker JM, Farney RJ, Rhondeau SM, Boyle KM, Valentine K, Cloward TV, Shilling KC. Chronic opioid use is a risk factor for the development of central sleep apnea and ataxic breathing. J Clin Sleep Med. 2007;3:455–61.
121. Hajiha M, DuBord M-A, Liu H, Horner RL. Opioid receptor mechanisms at the hypoglossal motor pool and effects on tongue muscle activity in vivo. J Physiol. 2009;587:2677–92. https://doi.org/10.1113/jphysiol.2009.171678.
122. Levitt ES, Abdala AP, Paton JFR, Bissonnette JM, Williams JT. Mu opioid receptor activation hyperpolarizes respiratory-controlling Kolliker-Fuse neurons and suppresses post-inspiratory drive. J Physiol. 2015;593:4453–69. https://doi.org/10.1113/JP270822.
123. Savilampi J, Ahlstrand R, Magnuson A, Geijer H, Wattwil M. Aspiration induced by remifentanil: a double-blind, randomized, crossover study in healthy volunteers. Anesthesiology. 2014;121:52–8.
124. Tagaito Y, Isono S, Nishino T. Upper airway reflexes during a combination of propofol and fentanyl anesthesia. Anesthesiology. 1998;88:1459–66.
125. Dublin S, Walker RL, Jackson ML, Nelson JC, Weiss NS, Korff M, Jackson LA. Use of opioids or benzodiazepines and risk of pneumonia in older adults: a population-based case–control study. J Am Geriatr Soc. 2011;59:1899–907. https://doi.org/10.1111/j.1532-5415.2011.03586.x.
126. Bateman JT, Saunders SE, Levitt ES. Understanding and countering opioid-induced respiratory depression. Br J Pharmacol. 2023;180(7):813–28. https://doi.org/10.1111/bph.15580. Epub 2021 Jun 26. PMID: 34089181.
127. Camilleri M, Lembo A, Katzka DA. Opioids in gastroenterology: treating adverse effects and creating therapeutic benefits. Clin Gastroenterol Hepatol. 2017;15(9):1338–49. https://doi.org/10.1016/j.cgh.2017.05.014. Epub 2017 May 19. PMID: 28529168; PMCID: PMC5565678.
128. Mehta N, Laitman AP, Brookfield RB, Harris LA. Treatment of opioid-induced constipation: inducing laxation and understanding the risk of gastrointestinal perforation. J Clin Gastroenterol. 2025;59(6):491–6.
129. Mallappallil M, Sabu J, Friedman EA, Salifu M. What do we know about opioids and the kidney? Int J Mol Sci. 2017;18(1):223.

130. Mallappallil M, Bajracharya S, Salifu M, Yap E. Opioids and acute kidney injury. Semin Nephrol. 2021;41(1):11–8.
131. Gudin JA, Laitman A, Nalamachu S. Opioid related endocrinopathy. Pain Med. 2015;16(suppl_1):S9–S15.
132. Ortman HA, Siegel JA. The effect of methadone on the hypothalamic pituitary gonadal axis and sexual function: a systematic review. Drug Alcohol Depend. 2020;207:107823.
133. Tobon AL, Habecker E, Forray A. Opioid use in pregnancy. Curr Psychiatry Rep. 2019;21(12):118.
134. Azuine RE, Ji Y, Chang H, et al. Prenatal risk factors and perinatal and postnatal outcomes associated with maternal opioid exposure in an urban, low-income, multiethnic US population. JAMA Netw Open. 2019;2(6):e196405.
135. Grossarth S, Osmundson SS, Wiese AD, Phillips SE, Pham A, Leech AA, Patrick SW, Spieker AJ, Grijalva CG, Adgent MA. Maternal opioid use disorder and the risk of postneonatal infant mortality. JAMA Pediatr. 2023;177(7):675–83.
136. Kumar U. Cannabinoids: role in neurological diseases and psychiatric disorders. Int J Mol Sci. 2024;26(1):152. https://doi.org/10.3390/ijms26010152. PMID: 39796008; PMCID: PMC11720483.
137. Yucel M, Solowij N, Respondek C, Whittle S, Fornito A, Pantelis C, Lubman DI. Regional brain abnormalities associated with heavy long-term cannabis use. Eur Neuropsychopharmacol. 2008;18:S545–6.
138. Bourque J, Potvin S. Cannabis and cognitive functioning: from acute to residual effects, from randomized controlled trials to prospective designs. Front Psych. 2021;12:596601. https://doi.org/10.3389/fpsyt.2021.596601. PMID: 34177633; PMCID: PMC8222623.
139. Leja JA. Chronic health effects of cannabis use in childhood and adolescence. Pediatr Ann. 2025;54(6):e217–21. https://doi.org/10.3928/19382359-20250407-02. Epub 2025 Jun 1. PMID: 40489359.
140. Jeffers AM, Glantz S, Byers AL, Keyhani S. Association of Cannabis use with cardiovascular outcomes among US adults. J Am Heart Assoc. 2024;13(5):e030178. https://doi.org/10.1161/JAHA.123.030178. Epub 2024 Feb 28. PMID: 38415581; PMCID: PMC10944074.
141. Rezkalla SH, Kloner RA. A review of cardiovascular effects of Marijuana use. J Cardiopulm Rehabil Prev. 2025;45(1):2–7. https://doi.org/10.1097/HCR.0000000000000923. Epub 2024 Dec 26. PMID: 39565147.
142. Guo Y, Wei X, Pei J, Yang H, Zheng XL. Dissecting the role of cannabinoids in vascular health and disease. J Cell Physiol. 2024;239(11):e31373. https://doi.org/10.1002/jcp.31373. Epub 2024 Jul 10. PMID: 38988064.
143. National Academies of Sciences, Engineering, and Medicine; Health and Medicine Division; Board on Population Health and Public Health Practice; Committee on the Health Effects of Marijuana: An Evidence Review and Research Agenda. The health effects of cannabis and cannabinoids: the current state of evidence and recommendations for research. Washington, DC: National Academies Press (US); 2017. Respiratory Disease. Available from: https://www.ncbi.nlm.nih.gov/books/NBK425753/.
144. Khoj L, Zagà V, Amram DL, Hosein K, Pistone G, Bisconti M, Serafini A, Cammarata LM, Cattaruzza MS, Mura M. Effects of cannabis smoking on the respiratory system: a state-of-the-art review. Respir Med. 2024;221:107494. https://doi.org/10.1016/j.rmed.2023.107494. Epub 2023 Dec 5. PMID: 38056532.
145. Malvi A, Khatib MN, Balaraman AK, Roopashree R, Kaur M, Srivastava M, Barwal A, Siva Prasad GV, Rajput P, Syed R, Sharma G, Kumar S, Singh MP, Bushi G, Chilakam N, Pandey S, Brar M, Mehta R, Sah S, Gaidhane AM, Shabil M, Daniel AS. Cannabis consumption and risk of asthma: a systematic review and meta-analysis. BMC Pulm Med. 2025;25(1):48. https://doi.org/10.1186/s12890-025-03516-0. PMID: 39881272; PMCID: PMC11780798.
146. Bando JM, Tashkin DP, Barjaktarevic IZ. Impact of Marijuana use on lung health. Semin Respir Crit Care Med. 2024;45(5):548–59. https://doi.org/10.1055/s-0044-1785679. Epub 2024 Jul 5. PMID: 38968961.

147. Cue L, Chu F, Cascella M. Cannabinoid hyperemesis syndrome. [Updated 2023 Jul 3]. In: StatPearls [Internet]. Treasure Island: StatPearls Publishing; 2025. Available from: https://www.ncbi.nlm.nih.gov/books/NBK549915/.
148. Perisetti A, Gajendran M, Dasari CS, Bansal P, Aziz M, Inamdar S, Tharian B, Goyal H. Cannabis hyperemesis syndrome: an update on the pathophysiology and management. Ann Gastroenterol. 2020;33(6):571–8. https://doi.org/10.20524/aog.2020.0528. Epub 2020 Sep 16. PMID: 33162734; PMCID: PMC7599351.
149. Krishnan P, Yen E. The changing landscape of cannabis use: impact on maternal health and neonatal outcomes. Pediatr Res. 2025;99:451.
150. Prewitt KC, Hayer S, Garg B, Benson AE, Hedges MA, Caughey AB, Lo JO. Impact of prenatal cannabis use disorder on perinatal outcomes. J Addict Med. 2023;17(3):e192–8.
151. Day NL, Goldschmidt L, Day R, Larkby C, Richardson GA. Prenatal marijuana exposure, age of marijuana initiation, and the development of psychotic symptoms in young adults. Psychol Med. 2015;45(8):1779–87.
152. Planning Committee for a Workshop on Potential Health Hazards Associated with Consumption of Caffeine in Food and Dietary Supplements; Food and Nutrition Board; Board on Health Sciences Policy; Institute of Medicine. Caffeine in food and dietary supplements: examining safety: workshop summary. Washington, DC: National Academies Press (US); 2014. 6, Caffeine Effects on the Central Nervous System and Behavioral Effects Associated with Caffeine Consumption
153. New Study finds chronic high caffeine consumption may heighten risk for cardiovascular disease. American College of Cardiology, 2024, August 15. https://www.acc.org/About-ACC/Press-Releases/2024/08/15/14/46/New-Study-Finds-Chronic-High-Caffeine-Consumption-May-Heighten-Risk-for-Cardiovascular-Disease.
154. Nehlig A. Effects of coffee on the gastro-intestinal tract: a narrative review and literature update. Nutrients. 2022;14(2):399. https://doi.org/10.3390/nu14020399. PMID: 35057580; PMCID: PMC8778943.
155. Rohweder R, de Oliveira ST, Dos Santos BD, Ferreira CZ, Zanardini MK, Lopes GPTF, Barbosa CP, Moreira TD, Schuler-Faccini L, Sanseverino MTV, da Silva AA, Abeche AM, Vianna FSL, Fraga LR. Caffeine intake during pregnancy and adverse outcomes: an integrative review. Reprod Toxicol. 2024;123:108518.
156. Dube R, Kar SS, Bahutair SN, Kuruba MG, Shafi S, Zaidi H, Garg HC, Almas YM, Kidwai A, Zalat RA, Sidahmed OE. The Fetal Effect of maternal Caffeine consumption during pregnancy—a review. Biomedicine. 2025;13(2):390.
157. Howard MO, Bowen SE, Garland EL, Perron BE, Vaughn MG. Inhalant use and inhalant use disorders in the United States. Addict Sci Clin Pract. 2011;6(1):18–31. PMID: 22003419; PMCID: PMC3188822.
158. Caplan RA, Zuflacht JP, Barash JA, Fehnel CR. Neurotoxicology syndromes associated with drugs of abuse. Neurol Clin. 2020;38(4):983–96. https://doi.org/10.1016/j.ncl.2020.08.005. PMID: 33040873; PMCID: PMC7574350.
159. Samson R, Kado H, Chapman D. Huffing-induced cardiomyopathy: a case report. Cardiovasc Toxicol. 2012;12(1):90–2.
160. Shahani R, Streutker C, Dickson B, Stewart RJ. Ketamine-associated ulcerative cystitis: a new clinical entity. Urology. 2007;69(5):810–2. https://doi.org/10.1016/j.urology.2007.01.038.
161. Jhang JF, Hsu YH, Kuo HC. Possible pathophysiology of ketamine-related cystitis and associated treatment strategies. Int J Urol. 2015;22(9):816–25. https://doi.org/10.1111/iju.12841. Epub 2015 Jun 18. PMID: 26087832.
162. Kounlavong ES, Schauberger CW, Conklin JL, Jones HE. Systematic review of obstetric and child outcomes of prenatal exposure to inhalants in the context of a use disorder. J Addict Med. 2025;19(2):121–8.
163. Tabor BL, Smith-Wallace T, Yonekura ML. Perinatal outcome associated with PCP versus cocaine use. Am J Drug Alcohol Abuse. 1990;16(3–4):337–48.

Co-occurring Psychiatric Disorders

22

Sanchit Maruti

High Yield Review Points

- Co-occurring non-substance related mental health disorders (NSRMHDs) and substance use disorders (SUDs) are highly prevalent conditions and are linked to poorer outcomes for each condition individually and collectively.
- Diagnosing and treating both disorders concurrently can improve outcomes for both disorders.
- Both NSRMHDs and SUDs impact each other and are affected by each other. Thus, the diagnosis of one category of disorder can be impacted by the severity and activity of the other disorder.
- Due to the complexity of diagnosing co-occurring disorders (CODs), evaluation should be conducted through repeated, longitudinal assessments and should incorporate information from multiple sources.
- Treatment approaches for CODs should be integrated and modified based on the severity and impact of the other disorder.
- Treatment should adopt a long-term perspective and include both pharmacologic and psychosocial interventions tailored to the individual's evolving clinical needs.

S. Maruti (✉)
Department of Psychiatry, Larner College of Medicine, University of Vermont, Burlington, VT, USA
e-mail: Sanchit.maruti@uvmhealth.org

C. Marienfeld, M. Soltani (eds.), *AAAP Review of Addiction Psychiatry*,
https://doi.org/10.1007/978-3-032-24174-0_22

Introduction

The term "co-occurring disorders" (CODs) denotes the simultaneous presence of at least one non-substance related mental health disorder(s) (NSRMHD), and at least one substance use disorder(s) (SUD), all as defined in the Diagnostic and Statistical Manual of Mental Disorders, Fifth Edition Text Revision (DSM-5-TR) [1].

SUDs are part of psychiatric and mental health disorders. For the purposes of this chapter, we will reference SUDs as a distinct group within psychiatric and mental health disorders. COD refers to persons with both one or more SUD and one or more NSRMHD. This description should not be confused with the co-occurrence of multiple mental health conditions or multiple substance use conditions. Additionally, it is important to note that despite the DSM-5-TR's recognition of the frequent comorbidity of NSRMHDs and SUDs, the term "co-occurring disorder", while widely understood and used, is not a formal diagnostic classification within the manual.

Co-occurring substance use and mental disorders influence each other in a bidirectional way. The presence of a SUD can contribute to the onset or worsening of a mental disorder, while a mental disorder can increase both the likelihood and severity of a SUD. As a result, it is often difficult to determine the temporal and causal sequence between a person's SUD and NSRMHD because each condition can affect and exacerbate the other. CODs are associated with substantially more serious consequences than a single disorder, including greater functional impairment, poorer treatment outcomes, higher morbidity and mortality, increased rate of hospitalizations, elevated treatment costs, and a heightened risk of homelessness, incarceration, and suicide [2]. Consequently, current treatment guidelines recommend that people with CODs receive coordinated, concurrent treatment for both disorders [3–6].

Epidemiology and Significance

National data from the Substance Abuse and Mental Health Services Administration (SAMHSA) indicates a substantial burden of CODs across the adult population. Among adults aged 18 or older in 2024, 33.0% (or 86.6 million people) had either any mental illness (AMI) *or* a SUD in the past year [2]. In this group, 61.5 million adults had AMI and 46.3 million adults had any SUD in the past year. 8.1% of adults aged 18 or older (or 21.2 million people) had AMI *and* a SUD in the past year. The prevalence of adults in each age group who had AMI *and* a SUD in the past year have remained the same from 2021 to 2024 [2].

CODs show marked gender differences in their prevalence, presentation, and outcomes. Women entering treatment often exhibit greater overall severity of medical, behavioral, psychological, and social comorbidities, including higher rates of depression, anxiety, post-traumatic stress disorder (PTSD), and eating disorders [2]. Men with certain SUDs, such as cannabis use disorder, are more likely to exhibit co-occurring polysubstance use and antisocial personality disorder (ASPD), whereas women with comparable SUDs are more prone to developing panic and anxiety disorders. These distinct vulnerability patterns highlight the importance of nuanced, gender-informed approaches to the identification, assessment, and treatment of individuals experiencing co-occurring mental health conditions and SUDs [2].

Large epidemiologic studies have historically collected data using a gender-binary framework, limiting understanding of gender-diverse populations. Non-binary individuals bear a disproportionately high burden of co-occurring NSRMHDs and SUDs compared to cisgender people and even other transgender subgroups. Multiple large-scale studies and nationally representative studies show that non-binary people have elevated rates of depression, anxiety, psychological distress, and substance use—including hazardous drinking, problematic drug use, prescription drug misuse, and daily marijuana use—relative to both cisgender and binary transgender peers [7–17].

The elevated prevalence of co-occurring mental health conditions and SUDs among non-binary individuals is driven in part by intersecting minority stressors, including discrimination, lack of societal affirmation, housing insecurity, and limited access to affirming care. For instance, non-binary persons assigned male at birth are among the least likely to engage in behavioral health services, and non-binary identity is independently associated with higher odds of prescription drug misuse, even after accounting for psychological distress and health status [12, 17]. Structural vulnerabilities—such as unmet basic needs and discrimination in healthcare and public settings—further increase risk for both psychiatric morbidity and substance use-related harms in this population [13, 14].

Syndemic models in transgender youth, including non-binary individuals, show that the co-occurrence of substance use and depressive symptoms is strongly associated with increased suicidality, and these risks are amplified by social-structural factors such as bullying and economic deprivation. Integrated, affirming, and trauma-informed approaches to care are recommended, with attention to the unique stressors and barriers faced by non-binary individuals [9, 11].

Young adulthood also is a period of heightened vulnerability, with the highest prevalence of CODs at 14.1%, or 4.8 million individuals, observed among those aged 18–25. This elevated rate among young adults warrants attention given its potential implications for educational attainment, career development, and long-term well-being. While the prevalence decreased in subsequent age groups (10.9% or 11.3 million among adults aged 26–49, and 3.6% or 4.3 million among adults aged 50 or older) [2], significant disparities also emerged across racial and ethnic groups.

Multiracial adults had a markedly higher prevalence of either AMI or a SUD (50.0%) compared to their White (34.2%), Black (30.5%), Hispanic (30.0%), and Asian (24.3%) counterparts, underscoring possible contributions of minority stress and differential access to care [2]. These findings contribute to a growing body of literature demonstrating the substantial overlap between mental health and SUDs in the US adult population.

Significant treatment gaps persist for individuals with CODs, despite the clearly harmful nature of these conditions. The 2023 NSDUH survey revealed that a mere 30% of affected adolescents and adults received integrated mental health and SUD treatment [2].

Neurobiological Basis of Co-occurring Disorders

The neurobiological basis of CODs involves shared dysregulation involving the brain's reward, stress, and executive control circuits. A central element of this overlap is the mesolimbic dopamine system, where chronic substance use is thought to downregulate D_2 receptors and reduce dopamine signaling, producing a reward-deficient state that both resembles and worsens the anhedonia seen in major depressive disorder (MDD) and the negative symptoms of schizophrenia [18–21]. In parallel, chronic drug exposure and primary mental illness intersect on pro-inflammatory pathways, with elevated cytokines (such as IL-6 and TNF-α) promoting neuroinflammation, microglial activation, and impaired synaptic plasticity—process that may contribute to treatment-resistant presentations frequently observed in COD populations [22–26].

Beyond reward deficiency, the persistence of CODs is thought to involve recruitment of the brain's "anti-reward" or "dark side" systems. Chronic substance use can induce a state of hyperkatifeia—a heightened sensitivity to negative emotional states—driven in part by an overactive corticotropin-releasing factor (CRF) signaling pathway in the extended amygdala, paralleling the hyperarousal and emotional dysregulation characteristic of PTSD, anxiety disorders, and mood disorders [27–30]. This biological synergy is further compounded by dysfunction of the prefrontal cortex (PFC); structural and functional abnormalities in regions such as the rostral anterior cingulate cortex/ventromedial PFC and dorsolateral PFC undermine "top-down" inhibitory control and emotion regulation [31–35]. Such changes may make it biologically difficult for individuals manage cravings or regulate psychiatric symptoms, perpetuating a cycle of compulsive drug-seeking and progressive neuroadaptation [31, 34, 36–39].

Assessment of Co-occurring Disorders (CODs)

Timing of Assessment

The evaluation of individuals with suspected CODs presents unique challenges that require careful consideration of timing and methodology. A critical principle in assessment is recognizing that acute intoxication and withdrawal can significantly mask or mimic psychiatric symptoms, making accurate diagnosis difficult during these periods.

The current consensus supports early pharmacological treatment of severe substance-induced psychiatric symptoms based on symptom severity and safety concerns, rather than waiting for the traditional 4-week period of substance "clearing" for diagnostic clarification. This shift reflects recognition that untreated agitation, psychosis, and suicidality pose immediate risks that outweigh the benefits of diagnostic precision [5]. Current guidelines explicitly recommend that clinicians consider pharmacotherapy based on symptom severity and duration, even if symptoms are, for example, stimulant-induced [5]. De-escalation strategies should not delay medication use when patients are at imminent risk for severe complications. This represents a fundamental change from the traditional approach of waiting for substance clearance before initiating psychiatric treatment.

For acute agitation and psychosis, guidelines recommend immediate intervention with specific pharmacological agents. Benzodiazepines are considered first-line treatment for stimulant-induced agitation, while antipsychotic medications should be used for psychotic symptoms regardless of suspected etiology [5]. The urgency, formulation, and duration of treatment should be based on symptomatology rather than waiting to confirm whether symptoms are substance-induced or represent an independent disorder.

The rationale for early treatment rests on several key principles. Most substance-induced mental disorders improve within days to weeks of abstinence, but severe symptoms still require management even during this resolution period [1]. Suicidality may increase during waning intoxication and waxing acute withdrawal, necessitating proactive monitoring and treatment [5]. Additionally, untreated psychiatric symptoms increase risk of return to substance use [1].

Concurrent treatment of SUD and co-occurring psychiatric conditions is now standard practice. The American Academy of Addiction Psychiatry (AAAP) strongly recommends treating both conditions simultaneously using integrated behavioral and pharmacological approaches [5]. This integrated care model is more convenient and cost-effective than sequential treatment, with benefits likely outweighing risks [5]. Recent systematic reviews confirm that pharmacological treatments for dual diagnosis require personalized approaches considering the specific psychopathology, substance involved, and treatment setting.

Diagnostic uncertainty is managed through ongoing reassessment rather than delayed treatment. Clinicians should evaluate whether the clinical presentation follows the expected time course of substance-induced symptoms given the phase of use (active use, waning intoxication, acute withdrawal, post-acute withdrawal, or post-withdrawal abstinence) [5]. For stimulant-induced psychosis or mania specifically, guidelines recommend considering a gradual taper of antipsychotic medication after a period of symptom remission, allowing for diagnostic clarification over time [5].

Importantly, the DSM-5-TR notes that while symptoms of substance-induced disorders can be identical to independent mental disorders, they have different treatments and prognoses [1]. Studies requiring at least 1 week of abstinence before diagnosing depression yielded larger antidepressant effect sizes and lower placebo response, suggesting that abstinence requirements help screen out transient symptoms [40]. However, several studies observed medication effects even in actively using patients when additional diagnostic criteria were applied [40].

Comprehensive Assessment Components

Comprehensive Diagnostic Assessment

The National Institute on Alcohol Abuse and Alcoholism (NIAAA) recommends using brief validated screening tools for initial assessment [4]. Following positive screening, the AAAP recommends [5] comprehensive assessment that includes:

- Full biopsychosocial assessment evaluating trauma history, social determinants of health, biomedical and psychiatric comorbidities, and post-acute withdrawal symptoms
- Detailed substance use history including past and current use, route of administration, frequency, and age of first use
- Temporal relationship: Symptoms that preceded severe intoxication or withdrawal can indicate an independent disorder. Symptoms developed during or soon after substance intoxication, withdrawal, or medication exposure as likely to be associated with substance use.
- Persistence criterion: Disturbances persisting for at least 1 month after cessation of acute withdrawal or severe intoxication suggest an independent disorder (except for substance-induced neurocognitive disorders and hallucinogen persisting perception disorder)
- Mental status examination to identify psychosis, cognitive impairment, and risk of harm
- DSM-5-TR diagnostic criteria to classify SUD severity (mild: 2–3 criteria; moderate: 4–5 criteria; severe: 6+ criteria). Additionally, The DSM-5-TR provides specific diagnostic criteria to differentiate substance-induced from independent mental disorders [1].

Importantly, comprehensive assessment should be trauma-informed, culturally sensitive, and collaborative with patients to select an approach that best fit their goals [46]. The assessment should view the individual holistically, considering strengths, comorbidities, and social and cultural determinants rather than focusing solely on deficits.

Brief Screening Tools

Several validated screening tools and comprehensive assessment instruments are recommended for evaluating SUDs and distinguishing substance-induced from non-substance related psychiatric symptoms. For initial screening in clinical settings, see Table 22.1 for brief instruments that have demonstrated strong psychometric properties.

The US Preventive Services Task Force (USPSTF) recommends screening all adults for unhealthy drug use using validated instruments, with sensitivity for detecting drug use disorders ranging from 0.85 to 1.00 and specificity from 0.67 to 0.93 [42].

Table 22.1 Screening tools

AUDIT (Alcohol Use Disorders Identification Test)	AUDIT is the gold standard for alcohol screening, translated into many languages with decades of supporting research. The USAUDIT-C, a 3-item version, can quickly determine the presence of risky drinking and is particularly useful in busy clinical settings [41].
TAPS (Tobacco, Alcohol, Prescription medication, and other Substance use tool)	TAPS addresses both alcohol and other drugs, including illicit substances and prescription misuse [41].
ASSIST (Alcohol, Smoking and Substance Involvement Screening Test)	ASSIST is recommended by multiple guidelines and assesses frequency of drug use and associated risks. The ASSIST-2 is a modified version that can be used in specific populations [42].
DAST (Drug Abuse Screening Test)	The US Preventive Services Task Force systematic review found that the DAST-10 can detect unhealthy drug use with reasonable accuracy, with sensitivity ranging from 0.85 to 1.00 and specificity from 0.67 to 0.93 for detecting drug use disorders [42, 43]. The DAST-10 takes approximately 5 min to administer and is often used in conjunction with the AUDIT for comprehensive substance screening [44]. The tool provides severity stratification, with standard cutoffs indicating moderate-risk drug use (3–5 points) and high-risk drug use (≥6 points) [45]. The DAST is designed as a screening tool, not a diagnostic instrument. Patients with positive screening results require a diagnostic assessment to confirm SUDs [42]. The tool should be part of a comprehensive approach that includes clinical interviews and, when appropriate, referral for specialized evaluation and treatment.
Single-item screening questions	Single-item screening questions about drug frequency have shown sensitivity ranging from 0.71 to 0.94 for detecting unhealthy use of any drug [42].

Laboratory Testing

Laboratory testing must be utilized mindfully and with context in mind. It is important to understand the assays being used and their optimal utility and limitations. This includes important considerations related to the time from use to specimen collection and analysis, the presence and duration of detectable metabolites, and the potential for false-positive and false-negative results. Laboratory toxicology is never the basis of diagnosis for a SUD or a COD. Additionally, laboratory testing has limited utility in distinguishing substance-induced disorders from independent psychiatric disorder, as substance-induced symptoms may persist for up to 4 weeks after cessation of many substances used; therefore, negative toxicology results do not exclude substance-induced conditions [1].

Principles of Integrated Care

The evolution of treatment approaches for CODs has moved from sequential and parallel treatment models toward integrated care, which addresses both disorders simultaneously within a unified treatment framework.

Integrated treatment is based on the principle that CODs are interconnected conditions (see Table 22.2 for common overlapping symptoms in various non-substance related psychiatric disorders and substance related psychiatric disorders). These interconnected conditions require coordinated intervention rather than separate, specialized treatments for each disorder. Integrated treatment that addresses substance use and psychiatric disorders simultaneously represents the evidence-based standard of care for co-occurring conditions and is associated with superior outcomes compared with sequential or parallel, uncoordinated treatment approaches.

The American Society of Addiction Medicine (ASAM) strongly recommends that all SUD treatment programs be "co-occurring capable" at minimum, welcoming patients with co-occurring conditions and providing integrated services for mental health symptom management as part of routine operations [47]. The American Academy of Pediatrics (AAP) identifies three core principles: (1) young adults should receive integrated mental health and addiction care across treatment settings; (2) care should be responsive to trauma and adverse childhood experiences; and (3) programs should regularly assess and respond to evolving mental health needs, motivations, and treatment goals [48].

Table 22.2 Overlap of symptoms within substance use disorders and any mental illness

	Anxiety	Bipolar	Depression	Neurocognitive disorders	Psychosis	Sleep wake
Alcohol	x	x	x	x	x	x
Caffeine	x					x
Cannabis	x				x	x
Hallucinogens	x	x	x		x	
Inhalants	x		x	x	x	
Opioid	x		x			x
Sedative Hypnotic Anxiolytic	x	x	x	x		x
Stimulant	x	x		x	x	x
Tobacco						x
Other						

Pharmacological Management of Common Mental Health Conditions

Pharmacological treatments for CODs require personalized approaches considering the specific psychopathology, substance involved, treatment setting, and primary objective of care. A 2025 umbrella review of psychosocial interventions for SUD with co-occurring common mental health disorders found that most interventions, including treatment as usual, were associated with significant improvement in both conditions. Integrated, coordinated treatment was superior to single-condition approaches and generally outperformed parallel, uncoordinated services [49]. However, because improvement was observed across all psychosocial interventions, including active comparator conditions, the evidence did not support recommending one intervention over another.

Anxiety Disorders and Co-occurring SUDs

Selective Serotonin Reuptake Inhibitors (SSRIs) and Selective Norepinephrine Reuptake Inhibitors (SNRIs) remain first-line pharmacotherapy for anxiety disorders in general populations, with no clear superiority of any specific SSRI or SNRI compound [50]. Medication selection should be based on interactions and side-effect profile, with newer medications such as venlafaxine, escitalopram, or sertraline recommended as first-line treatment [51].

A meta-analysis of 11 randomized clinical trials found that integrated behavioral treatments for co-occurring anxiety and SUDs outperform SUD treatment alone on both substance use and anxiety outcomes, with small to moderate effect sizes favoring integrated approaches [52]. There was no significant heterogeneity across studies, suggesting consistent benefits across different integrated treatment approaches. These integrated treatments demonstrate incremental but significant and clinically meaningful improvements over SUD treatment alone [52].

See Table 22.3 for a summary of treatment recommendations for anxiety disorders when co-occurring with various substance use disorders.

Bipolar Disorders and Co-occurring SUDs

For individuals with bipolar disorders and SUDs (with consideration for child-bearing potential), valproate remains the treatment of choice, while evidence suggests lithium and quetiapine may not be effective in this population [62]. However, mood stabilization should prioritize lithium in adherent patients with bipolar disorder and AUD, as it reduces suicidality, prevents mood episode recurrence, and can be safely combined with AUD medications [63–66]. Alternative mood stabilizers include lamotrigine and atypical antipsychotics such as quetiapine, aripiprazole, and cariprazine, which are first-line agents for acute mania, bipolar depression, and maintenance treatment.

Table 22.3 Treatment of anxiety disorders and co-occurring SUDs

Alcohol Use Disorder	For co-occurring anxiety and alcohol use disorder, a Cochrane review found very low-quality evidence for pharmacotherapy efficacy. Paroxetine showed evidence for global clinical response, though there was substantial uncertainty regarding effect size [53]. There was no evidence that alcohol use was responsive to medication alone [53]. Integrated cognitive behavioral therapy (CBT) and motivational interviewing (MI) show promise for this combination. A meta-analysis found small but clinically significant decreases in depressive symptoms and alcohol consumption when combining CBT and MI compared with usual care [4].
Sedative, hypnotic, or anxiolytic use disorder	The ASAM recommends offering adjunctive psychosocial interventions to persons tapering benzodiazepines, especially those whose daily functioning has been negatively impacted by withdrawal symptoms. Clinicians should optimize evidence-based treatments for co-occurring anxiety disorders prior to initiating benzodiazepine tapering or concurrently if clinically indicated [48]. CBT combined with gradual benzodiazepine tapering demonstrates moderate-quality evidence for successful discontinuation in patients with anxiety disorders. A Cochrane review found that patients receiving CBT during tapering were more likely to successfully discontinue benzodiazepines at 1-month and 3-month post-treatment compared to tapering alone [54]. CBT combined with benzodiazepine tapering increases abstinence success rates to 70–80%, compared to only 5% for patients attempting discontinuation on their own and 25–30% with general practitioner assistance alone [55]. The effects are most robust in the short term, with less certain benefits at 6 months and beyond [55]. Note: There is limited evidence supporting the use of antipsychotic medications in sedative withdrawal, and they are generally not recommended as primary treatment. Benzodiazepines remain the gold standard for managing alcohol and sedative-hypnotic withdrawal due to superior efficacy in preventing delirium and seizures.
Cannabis Use Disorder	For cannabis use disorder with co-occurring anxiety disorders, integrated cannabis and anxiety reduction treatment (ICART) demonstrates efficacy. A pilot randomized controlled trial found that patients in the ICART condition attended significantly more treatment sessions and were more likely to be abstinent post-treatment than those receiving MET-CBT alone [56]. Treatment produced decreases in cannabis use and related problems, though therapy type did not moderate the impact on frequency of use and related problems [56]. The Department of Veterans Affairs (VA) recommends CBT, motivational enhancement therapy (MET), and combined MET-CBT for cannabis use disorder, though studies specifically examining patients with comorbid anxiety disorders are limited [57]. One study comparing MET-CBT with ICART found that the ICART group did not separate from MET-CBT in outcomes for patients with comorbid anxiety disorder, though this was a small study [57]. Psychosocial treatments such as CBT, MET, and contingency management (CM) are currently the most effective strategy for treating cannabis use disorder but are of limited benefit when comorbid with psychosis [58]. Targeted treatments for anxiety when comorbid with CUD are feasible [58].

(continued)

Table 22.3 (continued)

Opioid Use Disorder	For opioid use disorder (OUD) with co-occurring mental health symptoms including anxiety, collaborative care models show effectiveness. A 2025 cluster randomized trial found that collaborative care treating both OUD and co-occurring mental health symptoms significantly reduced opioid use more than collaborative care for mental health symptoms alone [59]. Pharmacotherapy in conjunction with psychosocial treatment should be offered to patients with OUD and co-occurring psychiatric disorders, and a patient's decision to decline psychosocial treatment should not preclude or delay pharmacological treatment of OUD [59]. A 2019 randomized clinical trial comparing extended-release naltrexone (XR-NTX) to buprenorphine-naloxone (BP-NLX) found that both treatments led to improvements in anxiety, depression, and insomnia within only a few weeks of beginning treatment [60]. The study noted that BP-NLX, as an opioid agonist, may have psychotropic effects on mood, sedation, and anxiety, and that BP-NLX is useful in the palliation of such symptoms in individuals with OUD [60]. Interestingly, XR-NTX (an opioid antagonist) showed similar improvements, suggesting that the benefits may be related to reduced illicit substance use rather than direct pharmacological effects on anxiety [60]. It is important to note that benzodiazepines and opioids both cause central nervous system depression, and benzodiazepines can potentiate opioid-induced decreases in respiratory drive. Epidemiologic studies find concurrent benzodiazepine use in some opioid-related overdose deaths. The United States Centers for Disease Control and Prevention (CDC) recommends that clinicians avoid prescribing opioid pain medication and benzodiazepines concurrently whenever possible and use extreme caution when concurrent prescribing is necessary, based on substantial evidence of increased overdose risk [111]. A 2025 randomized clinical trial examined mindfulness training versus recovery support during buprenorphine treatment, finding that mindfulness training reduced anxiety symptoms [61]. While this is a behavioral rather than pharmacological intervention, it represents an important adjunctive approach for managing anxiety during OUD treatment.
Stimulant Use Disorder	The ASAM/AAAP clinical practice guideline recommends that clinicians treat both stimulant use disorder and co-occurring anxiety disorders concurrently using an integrated behavioral treatment approach when available [5]. Clinicians should consider whether the patient's clinical presentation follows the expected time course of stimulant-induced symptoms given the phase of use (active use, waning intoxication, acute withdrawal, post-acute withdrawal, and post-withdrawal abstinence) or are present at other times [5]. Although there is no direct pharmacologic evidence supporting specific medications for the treatment of anxiety disorders in patients with stimulant use disorder, there is some consensus that or patients with cocaine use disorder and amphetamine-type stimulant (ATS) use disorder with low- to moderate-frequency (i.e., less than 18 days per month) providers can consider prescribing bupropion to promote cocaine abstinence. Additionally, clinicians can consider prescribing topiramate to reduce cocaine or ATS use [5].

Optimizing bipolar disorder treatment is the critical first step for managing concurrent SUDs. First-line pharmacologic options for bipolar disorder include:

- Lithium and valproate (in those without child-bearing potential): effective for preventing both manic and depressive episodes
- Quetiapine and olanzapine: FDA-approved for acute mania, bipolar depression, and maintenance treatment
- Lurasidone and cariprazine: FDA-approved for bipolar depression
- Lamotrigine: effective for preventing depressive episodes but not mania

See Table 22.4 for a summary of treatment recommendations for bipolar disorders when co-occurring with various substance use disorders.

Table 22.4 Treatment of bipolar disorders and co-occurring SUDs

Alcohol Use Disorder	This co-occurring combination is highly prevalent, affecting 40–70% of individuals with bipolar disorder over their lifetime, with alcohol being the most common substance of misuse [64, 65]. The comorbidity is associated with worse clinical outcomes, including earlier age of onset, more depressive episodes, rapid cycling, greater affective instability, higher suicide attempt rates, and increased mortality [64, 65]. Valproate (alone or added to lithium) and naltrexone represent the most evidence-based pharmacologic treatments for patients with bipolar disorder and comorbid alcohol use disorder, though the overall evidence base remains limited and requires individualized treatment approaches [64–66].
Sedative, hypnotic, or anxiolytic use disorder	Benzodiazepine use disorder is common in bipolar populations and poses significant clinical challenges. Chronic benzodiazepine use is associated with depression, falls, cognitive deficits, and increased mortality risk [67, 68]. The combination is particularly problematic because benzodiazepine tapering can trigger rebound psychiatric symptoms including anxiety, insomnia, and mood destabilization—potentially precipitating manic or depressive episodes in vulnerable patients [69, 70]. The ASAM and American College of Medical Toxicology recommend optimizing evidence-based treatment for psychiatric disorders prior to initiating benzodiazepine tapering or concurrently if clinically indicated [69]. Valproate and carbamazepine represent the most evidence-based pharmacologic options for patients with co-occurring bipolar disorder and benzodiazepine use disorder, as both agents treat bipolar disorder while also facilitating benzodiazepine tapering and reducing withdrawal symptoms [69]. However, the evidence base remains limited, requiring individualized, integrated treatment approaches.
Cannabis Use Disorder	Cannabis use disorder affects approximately 20% of people with bipolar disorder overall and 39% of those seeking treatment, with co-occurring cannabis use linked to worse symptom trajectory including earlier age of onset, more depressive episodes, and higher rates of suicide attempts. For bipolar disorder with cannabis use disorder specifically, evidence for valproic acid or lithium is weak. A 2025 review noted that while these mood stabilizers are used clinically, RCT evidence supporting their efficacy for cannabis use disorder in bipolar disorder is limited [64].

(continued)

Table 22.4 (continued)

Opioid Use Disorder	OUD affects approximately 6% of individuals with bipolar disorder, with higher rates in treatment-seeking populations [65]. This comorbidity is associated with worse clinical outcomes, including earlier age of onset, more depressive episodes, rapid cycling, greater inter-episodic affective instability, and higher rates of suicide attempts compared to bipolar disorder alone [65]. Co-occurring SUDs have been linked to decreased recovery time and worse psychosocial functioning [65, 71]. Buprenorphine, methadone, or naltrexone for OUD combined with mood stabilizers (lithium, valproate) or atypical antipsychotics (quetiapine, olanzapine) for bipolar disorder represent the most evidence-based pharmacologic approach, though robust randomized controlled trials specifically examining this comorbidity are lacking. Integrated treatment addressing both conditions simultaneously is essential but remains underdeveloped [65, 71, 72]. A systematic review identified valproate sodium and lamotrigine as potentially preferred pharmacological agents for co-occurring psychiatric and substance use outcomes in bipolar disorder with comorbid SUDs, though many studies were open-label designs with modest sample sizes [72]. The combination of mood stabilizers with FDA-approved medications for OUD represents a rational approach, given the potential synergistic effects observed with lithium, quetiapine, and olanzapine [73].
Stimulant Use Disorder	Stimulant use disorder affects approximately 12.5% of individuals with bipolar disorder for cocaine and 6% for amphetamines, with higher rates in treatment-seeking populations [65]. This comorbidity is associated with worse clinical outcomes, including earlier age of onset, more depressive episodes, rapid cycling, greater inter-episodic affective instability, and higher rates of suicide attempts compared to bipolar disorder alone [65]. The shared neurobiological factors include impaired cognitive control and reward processing, though evidence for the self-medication hypothesis remains scarce [65]. No FDA-approved medications exist for stimulant use disorder, and behavioral therapies remain the primary treatment modality [5]. A systematic review identified valproate sodium and lamotrigine as potentially preferred pharmacological agents for co-occurring psychiatric and substance use outcomes in bipolar disorder with comorbid SUDs [72].

Depressive Disorders and Co-occurring SUDs

Depressive disorders and SUDs co-occur at substantially higher rates than expected by chance, with bidirectional relationships and shared underlying vulnerabilities. The prevalence of any SUD in individuals with major depressive disorder (MDD) is approximately 25.0%, with illicit drug use disorder affecting 11.8% and AUD affecting 20.8% [2]. Co-occurring depressive disorders and SUDs are also associated with greater severity and worse prognosis for both disorders compared to either disorder alone [2].

See Table 22.5 for a summary of treatment recommendations for depressive disorders when co-occurring with various substance use disorders.

Table 22.5 Treatment of depressive disorders and co-occurring SUDs

Alcohol Use Disorder	Co-occurring MDD and AUD is highly prevalent, affecting approximately one-third of individuals seeking treatment for AUD [73]. This comorbidity significantly complicates diagnosis and treatment, as the bidirectional relationship between alcohol use and depression worsens outcomes for both conditions [6]. The combination is associated with reduced treatment access, poorer treatment outcomes, earlier age of onset, and increased functional impairment compared to either disorder alone [6, 73]. Differentiating primary MDD from alcohol-induced depression is essential before initiating antidepressant therapy [6, 73]. Alcohol use and withdrawal can produce mood and anxiety symptoms that mimic primary mood disorders, and psychosocial stressors associated with AUD (family issues, employment difficulties, and legal problems) can also influence mood [73]. Symptoms that appear independent of alcohol may respond better to antidepressants than substance-induced depression [73]. The American Psychiatric Association (APA) recommends against the routine use of selective serotonin reuptake inhibitors (SSRIs), including sertraline, for the pharmacological treatment of AUD, based on moderate strength of research evidence showing minimal effect or slightly detrimental effects on alcohol-related outcomes [73]. The APA's recommendation against routine use of SSRIs for AUD is based on several factors. Despite the inclusion of different antidepressants of different classes and subjects with different co-occurring conditions, the studies are consistent in showing minimal effect or a slightly detrimental effect of antidepressant medication on alcohol-related outcomes [73]. When differences were present for specific outcomes, the magnitude of the effect was small, and the effect favored placebo [73]. The overall strength of research evidence was rated as moderate, based on a number of RCTs with medium to high risk of bias and moderate sample sizes, most of which were funded by governmental agencies [73]. Thus, the evidence for antidepressants reducing substance use outcomes remains mixed, with primary benefits observed in mood symptom improvement rather than direct effects on substance use. While sertraline may be appropriate for treating co-occurring depressive or anxiety disorders in patients with AUD, it should not be prescribed with the expectation of improving alcohol-related outcomes. The evidence suggests that sertraline effectively treats PTSD symptoms in patients with co-occurring PTSD and AUD but does not provide additional benefit for reducing alcohol consumption beyond what is achieved with psychosocial interventions alone [73]. The exception is combination therapy with naltrexone, which showed superior abstinence rates and longer time to return to heavy drinking compared to either medication alone [73]. Newer FDA-approved agents such as vilazodone, vortioxetine, and levomilnacipran are also treatment options, with vortioxetine and milnacipran considered first-line in Canadian guidelines and vilazodone as second-line [78]. Naltrexone and acamprosate are first-line FDA-approved medications for AUD and can be safely combined with antidepressants [6, 73, 74]. Moderate-quality evidence shows that antidepressants as a class increase abstinence rates and reduce drinks per drinking day when used in patients with co-occurring depression [75]. Disulfiram demonstrated the highest efficacy for achieving AUD remission and increasing abstinent days in network meta-analysis, but is less commonly used due to safety concerns, particularly the risk of severe reactions that could endanger pregnancy [74, 76]. Integrated treatment addressing both disorders simultaneously yields better outcomes than sequential approaches [6]. Optimal management combines pharmacotherapy with evidence-based psychotherapies including cognitive behavioral therapy, motivational interviewing, and behavioral activation, which address both alcohol use and depressive symptoms while promoting medication adherence and prevention of return to use [6, 77]. CBTs likely reduce depressive symptoms and may slightly reduce alcohol use.

Sedative, hypnotic, or anxiolytic use disorder	Sedative, hypnotic, or anxiolytic use disorder is common in patients with MDD and poses significant clinical challenges. Chronic benzodiazepine use is associated with depression, falls, motor vehicle crashes, cognitive deficits, dementia, and increased mortality risk [68]. The comorbidity complicates treatment because benzodiazepine tapering can trigger rebound psychiatric symptoms including anxiety, insomnia, and mood destabilization—potentially worsening depressive episodes in vulnerable patients. Concurrent treatment with first-line antidepressants (SSRIs, SNRIs, bupropion, or mirtazapine) for MDD combined with gradual benzodiazepine tapering and adjunctive medications (tricyclic antidepressants, carbamazepine) to support withdrawal management represents the most evidence-based approach, as no FDA-approved medications exist for sedative, hypnotic, or anxiolytic use disorder. Importantly, bupropion is contraindicated during benzodiazepine withdrawal due to increased seizure risk (0.4% at approved doses), with specific contraindications including alcohol or benzodiazepine withdrawal, seizure disorder, bulimia, and anorexia. For insomnia during benzodiazepine tapering, recommended non-benzodiazepine medications include sedating antidepressants such as trazodone (25–150 mg/day), doxepin (10–150 mg/day), mirtazapine (7.5–30 mg/day), and trimipramine (10–150 mg/day), given 1–3 h before bedtime [69, 79]. These agents act mainly by histamine H_1 receptor antagonism and have no apparent misuse potential. Note, non-benzodiazepine sedative-hypnotics (Z-drugs) are not recommended for patients undergoing benzodiazepine taper due to similar receptor action [79].
Cannabis Use Disorder	Cannabis use disorder affects up to 30% of people who use cannabis and is highly comorbid with mental disorders, including MDD [58]. Evidence from longitudinal studies suggests a bidirectional relationship between cannabis use and depression, such that cannabis use increases the risk for depression and vice versa, with this risk possibly higher in heavy users who initiated consumption in early adolescence [58]. Clinical evidence indicates that cannabis use is associated with worse prognosis in individuals with MDD, including reduced treatment compliance and increased risk of return to use [58, 80]. No medication is FDA-approved for the treatment of cannabis use disorder [81, 82]. Note, Epidiolex (cannabidiol) is FDA-approved only for seizures associated with Lennox–Gastaut syndrome, Dravet syndrome, or tuberous sclerosis complex in patients 1 year of age and older, not for cannabis use disorder. Systematic reviews and clinical trials consistently demonstrate that SSRIs, SNRIs, bupropion, mirtazapine, and cannabinoids have not shown efficacy for cannabis use disorder. Low-strength evidence indicates that SSRIs do not reduce cannabis use or improve treatment retention [82]. A systematic review across 26 trials found that antidepressants as a class were less likely than placebo to achieve abstinence, with no difference in overall cannabis use reduction or treatment retention [57]. Individual trials of fluoxetine, nefazodone, and bupropion sustained-release failed to show primary treatment effects on cannabis use, though fluoxetine showed efficacy for depressive symptoms [81, 82]. Moderate-strength evidence shows that cannabinoids do not increase abstinence rates, with low-strength evidence that they do not reduce cannabis use or increase treatment retention [82]. Synthetic delta-9-tetrahydrocannabinol and other cannabinoids were likely ineffective for achieving abstinence [57].
Opioid Use Disorder	Depression is highly prevalent among patients with OUD. A 2022 systematic review and meta-analysis of 345 studies including 104,135 people with OUD found that current depression prevalence was 36.1% [83]. This substantially exceeds the general population prevalence of approximately 16% [84]. Among patients initiating opioid agonist therapy specifically, 14.2% had moderate/severe depression, and 34.9% had mild depression at baseline [85]. This comorbidity is associated with worse prognosis, including increased risk of suicide, unintentional overdose, treatment dropout, and all-cause mortality. In addition to front-line standard of care treatments for depression, including SSRIs, SNRIs, bupropion, and mirtazapine, buprenorphine/naloxone and methadone are first-line treatments for OUD and significantly reduce depressive symptoms and suicidal ideation [85, 86]. After 4 weeks of treatment with either medication, approximately two-thirds of participants with depression either responded (≥50% reduction in depression scores) or remitted, with no significant differences between the two medications [86]. Extended-release naltrexone shows similar effects on depression [86]. Preliminary evidence suggests that buprenorphine relieves depressed mood and suicidal behaviors in those with major depression and treatment-resistant depression [86, 87]. Given the association of OUD with suicide and the potential for medications for OUD to alleviate depressed mood and reduce suicide risk and opioid overdose, initiating these medications during psychiatric hospitalization is critical, particularly for patients admitted with suicidal ideation or suicide attempts [86, 87].

(continued)

Table 22.5 (continued)

Stimulant use disorder	The association with depression and stimulant use disorder is robust and bidirectional. A 2023 systematic review and meta-analysis examining methamphetamine exposure and depression found a significant association between any use of methamphetamine and any depression outcomes in cross-sectional studies and longitudinal estimates [88]. Individuals with a methamphetamine use disorder had significantly higher odds of depression than those without [88]. The use of amphetamines and cocaine is associated with double the odds of depression, and depressive symptoms are common in people seeking treatment for stimulant use disorder [89]. Withdrawal from heavy stimulant use can precipitate or worsen depression, and the mood-elevating effects of stimulant intoxication can lead to a vicious cycle of stimulant self-medication of depressive symptoms [89]. A 2025 study used 2021–2022 National Surveys on Drug Use and Health (NSDUH) data and found that among adults aged 18–64 years using prescription stimulants, 25% reported misuse, and 9% had prescription stimulant use disorder (PSUD) [90]. Among those with PSUD, 87% used amphetamines. Individuals using amphetamines, compared with those using methylphenidate, had higher prevalence ratios of misuse and PSUD [90]. The AAAP and ASAM strongly recommend that clinicians treat both stimulant use disorder and co-occurring psychiatric disorders (including major depressive disorder) concurrently using an integrated approach [5]. Antidepressant drug therapy reduces depression in people who use cocaine, but it does not reduce stimulant use, and some antidepressants are contraindicated for stimulant (methamphetamine) use disorder [89, 91, 92]. Bupropion shows modest efficacy for stimulant use disorder, particularly for lighter users. Two studies demonstrated that bupropion increases the likelihood of methamphetamine-free weeks among lighter users (defined as those who use half of days or less) but did not demonstrate a treatment effect for patients who used more heavily [93]. Bupropion also has some evidence of efficacy in reducing cocaine use. Topiramate shows very modest efficacy for reducing methamphetamine use and better efficacy in reducing cocaine use compared to placebo, though it requires gradual titration over several weeks to reach therapeutic dosage [5, 93]. Symptoms of depression, anxiety, insomnia, and attentional problems observed during periods of stimulant use or withdrawal should be managed with pharmacotherapy based on symptom severity and chronicity, even if symptoms are judged to be stimulant-induced [5]. Clinicians should consider whether the patient's clinical presentation follows the expected time course of stimulant-induced symptoms given the phase of use (active use, waning intoxication, acute withdrawal, post-acute withdrawal, and post-withdrawal abstinence) or are present at other times [5]. Symptoms of psychosis or mania related to or co-occurring with stimulant use disorder should be treated with indicated pharmacotherapy (antipsychotics or mood stabilizers) [5]. Acute psychoses can be treated effectively with antipsychotics, though there is only a small amount of evidence regarding the effectiveness of antipsychotics in managing acute stimulant psychosis [89]. If stimulant-induced psychosis or mania is suspected, clinicians should consider a gradual taper off antipsychotic medications after a period of symptom remission to avoid unnecessary exposure to chronic antipsychotic or mood stabilizing medications [5]. Psychological therapies such as cognitive behavioral therapy (CBT), contingency management (CM), acceptance and commitment therapy (ACT), and meditation-based therapies are evidence-based strategies to treat both depression and stimulant use disorder [5, 89].

Psychotic Disorders and Co-occurring SUDs

Epidemiology of SUDs in Psychotic Disorders

A 2018 systematic review and meta-analysis of 123 studies including 165,811 subjects found that the prevalence of any SUD in schizophrenia spectrum disorders was 41.7%, followed by illicit drugs (27.5%), cannabis (26.2%), alcohol (24.3%), and stimulant use (7.3%) [94]. Patients with SUD had an earlier age of onset of schizophrenia. Meta-regression showed prevalence increased over time for illicit drugs but not for other substances, including alcohol. The persistently high prevalence indicates that SUDs are difficult to treat in this patient population, and there is an urgent need for better prevention, detection, and treatment [94].

A 2014 study from the Genomic Psychiatry Cohort comparing 9142 individuals with severe psychotic disorders (schizophrenia, bipolar disorder with psychotic features, or schizoaffective disorder) to 10,195 population controls found dramatically elevated risks: smoking, heavy alcohol use, heavy marijuana use, and recreational drug use [95]. All races/ethnicities and both sexes had greatly elevated risks. Of specific concern, recent public health efforts that successfully decreased smoking among individuals younger than age 30 years appear to have been ineffective among individuals with severe psychotic illnesses [95].

A 2023 population-based study of 9.8 million people in Ontario, Canada, found that among individuals with an emergency department visit for substance use, 18.5% with substance-induced psychosis and 1.4% with substance use without psychosis transitioned to schizophrenia spectrum disorder within 3 years [96]. Substance-induced psychoses, particularly for cannabis use, were at high risk of transition. Given their higher prevalence, substance use without psychosis presentations were associated with 3 times the absolute number of transitions [96].

A 2025 study examining psychosis spectrum symptoms before and after adolescent cannabis use initiation noted that individuals who use cannabis are at a 2- to 4-fold increased risk of psychosis relative to those who never use cannabis [97]. This risk is further increased for individuals who initiate cannabis use in childhood and early adolescence. Cannabis initiation in early adolescence has been associated with earlier onset of psychotic disorders, more severe symptoms, and greater likelihood of return of symptoms among those who develop psychosis [97, 98].

The 2021 AAP guideline reported that one multisite study in Europe and Brazil demonstrated that daily cannabis use and use of high-potency cannabis were the strongest independent predictors of having a psychotic disorder [98]. The odds of having a psychotic disorder for individuals using cannabis daily was 3.2 times higher than for never-users, and the odds for those who used high-potency cannabis versus never-users was 1.6 times higher [98].

Treatment of Psychotic Disorders and Co-occurring SUDs

Second-generation antipsychotics represent the primary pharmacologic treatment for psychotic disorders with co-occurring SUDs, with evidence supporting their efficacy for both psychotic symptoms and, in some cases, reduction in substance use. A 2022 systematic review of 41 studies found that aripiprazole was the most frequently used drug, either orally or by long-acting formulations, followed by risperidone with oral and long-acting formulations, clozapine, olanzapine, and quetiapine. Most patients were males affected by schizophrenia, with cannabis the most misused substance, followed by alcohol [99]. Importantly, no FDA-approved pharmacologic treatments exist for hallucinogen use disorder, and the evidence base for treatment is extremely limited.

Clozapine demonstrates the strongest evidence for reducing substance use across multiple substances in patients with schizophrenia and comorbid SUD. Clozapine has been found to be superior to other antipsychotics for reduction alcohol, cocaine, and cannabis misuse among patients with schizophrenia [62, 100]. However, clozapine requires careful monitoring due to risk of agranulocytosis and other adverse effects. Alterative options include risperidone and olanzapine which have also shown efficacy, with risperidone demonstrating superiority to olanzapine for craving [62]. There is very limited direct evidence comparing third-generation antipsychotics (cariprazine and brexpiprazole) to second-generation antipsychotics in patients with psychosis and co-occurring SUDs.

Long-acting injectable (LAI) antipsychotics may provide benefits for patients with CODs due to improved adherence. A systematic review of multiple studies found significant improvements in substance use-related outcomes for schizophrenia and SUDs among patients on LAI antipsychotics [101].

Multiple psychosocial interventions have been evaluated for co-occurring psychotic disorders and SUDs, including cognitive behavioral therapy (CBT), motivational interviewing (MI), contingency management (CM), integrated models of care, skills training, and non-integrated models of care (intensive case management). Overall, no single psychosocial intervention demonstrates clear superiority. CM demonstrates the most consistent evidence for improving abstinence. MI may benefit alcohol use specifically. Overall, no single psychosocial intervention demonstrates clear superiority. However, the evidence base remains limited and heterogeneous [102–104].

Other Mental Health and Co-occurring Conditions: Hallucinogen Use Disorder

Hallucinogen use disorder is rare, with a 12-month prevalence of 0.62% in the NESARC-III study [105]. However, use is rising; 8.9% of young adults reported past-year use in 2023, up from 4.1% in 2015. While DSM-5 estimates disorder prevalence at 0.1%, rates are higher in clinical samples [1]. Use is significantly associated with other SUDs, personality disorders, PTSD, and suicide attempts [105].

Mental health outcomes vary by substance. LSD and salvia are linked to higher risks of depression and suicidality, whereas MDMA is associated with lower psychological distress [106]. Disabled adults have higher usage rates (8.37%) and report significant mental health struggles; notably, ~4% reported that hallucinogen use worsened their condition [107].

Differential Diagnosis of Hallucinogen Use Disorder

Clinicians must distinguish hallucinogen use disorder from independent psychiatric conditions, such as schizophrenia, where patients may falsely attribute symptoms to drug use [1]. Diagnosis also requires differentiating “use disorder” (characterized by impairment and loss of control) from acute intoxication or induced mental disorders [1]. If induced disorders (e.g., psychosis) are severe enough to warrant independent attention, they should be diagnosed alongside the use disorder [1].

Treatment Approaches for Co-occurring Hallucinogen Use Disorder

There are no FDA-approved medications for hallucinogen use disorder [1]. Treatment follows dual diagnosis principles, integrating care for both substance use and co-occurring psychiatric conditions [62]. Recommended psychosocial interventions include MI, CBT, and CM. While evidence varies, coordinated, multidisciplinary care remains the standard [62].

Emerging Therapeutic Uses and Safety of Hallucinogens for Co-occurring Mental Health Conditions

Research supports the efficacy of ketamine for depression and MDMA for PTSD [108]. A 2024 review identified psilocybin as the most effective psychedelic for mood disorders, with potential benefits for addiction and anxiety [109]. A 2025 review found moderate-quality evidence for MDMA in treating PTSD, but only low-grade evidence for psychedelics in treating depression [110]. Despite this therapeutic promise, concerns persist regarding adverse effects—such as psychosis—when these substances are used outside supervised clinical settings [106].

Other Mental Health and Co-occurring Conditions: Post-Traumatic Stress Disorder (PTSD)

Background

PTSD and SUDs are highly comorbid, with approximately 15–30% of individuals with alcohol use disorder (AUD) having co-occurring PTSD in the general population, and rates increasing to 50–60% among military personnel and veterans [4]. Among individuals with PTSD, up to nearly 60% also suffer from an alcohol and/or drug use disorder [112]. This comorbidity is associated with higher symptom severity, greater functional impairment, more suicide attempts, worse treatment outcomes, and increased healthcare utilization compared to either disorder alone [113, 114].

The relationship between PTSD and SUDs appears to be bidirectional and multifactorial. The self-medication hypothesis, which has the strongest empirical support, suggests that individuals use substances to manage PTSD symptoms and the resulting short-term relief reinforces ongoing substance use [115, 116]. Additional mechanisms likely play a role: heavy substance use can increase exposure to traumatic events (such as violence and assault), SUDs can erode psychological coping by disrupting arousal and cognition, and both conditions arise from shared risk factors including adverse childhood experiences, emotional dysregulation, and maladaptive coping styles [4, 117, 118].

Interpersonal and cumulative trauma exposure are especially salient risk factors for co-occurring PTSD and SUDs. Individuals who experience interpersonal trauma (for example, physical or sexual assault) have higher odds of developing both PTSD and later SUD compared to those experiencing non-interpersonal trauma, and repeated interpersonal traumas further amplify this risk [119]. PTSD is also linked to elevated craving for a range of substances, with trauma-related cues provoking intense craving that can precipitate return to use [120]. The comorbidity extends to complex PTSD, where point prevalence of AUD has been reported as high as 46%, with other SUDs showing even stronger associations [121].

Treatment of Post-Traumatic Stress Disorder (PTSD) and Co-occurring SUDs

Integrated trauma-focused psychotherapies combined with SUD treatment are the most effective evidence-based approach for co-occurring PTSD and SUDs, with specific modalities including prolonged exposure (PE), cognitive processing therapy (CPT), eye movement desensitization and reprocessing (EMDR), and imagery rescripting (ImRs) [112, 115, 124]. Notably, individuals do not need to be abstinent to initiate trauma-focused PTSD treatment, and the presence of SUD should not delay or preclude evidence-based PTSD interventions [112, 125].

Individual trauma-focused therapies demonstrate superior efficacy for reducing PTSD symptoms compared to SUD-only treatment or non-trauma-focused interventions [122, 126, 128]. Network meta-analysis shows that integrated trauma-focused therapy produces larger reductions in PTSD severity than integrated non-trauma-focused therapy or control conditions [122]. A randomized trial comparing integrated prolonged exposure (I-PE) to integrated coping skills therapy (I-CS) found significantly greater PTSD symptom reduction with I-PE, with sustained benefits at 6-month follow-up [126]. Similarly, a recent trial demonstrated that PE, EMDR, and ImRs each significantly reduced PTSD severity when added to SUD treatment, with ImRs showing the largest effect [124].

Evidence for pharmacotherapy in co-occurring PTSD and SUDs remains limited, and no medication has been definitively established specifically for this comorbidity [123]. Nonetheless, the combination of alcohol-focused pharmacotherapies with trauma-focused psychotherapies currently shows the greatest promise, yielding the largest observed improvements in both PTSD symptom severity and alcohol use outcomes by end of treatment [122]. For PTSD symptom reduction, SSRIs (paroxetine and sertraline) remain first-line pharmacotherapy based on moderate-certainty evidence from PTSD-only trials, and the 2023 VA/DoD guidelines recommend that comorbid SUDs should not preclude their use [125, 131].

The most comprehensive recent pharmacology evidence comes from the 2023 Project Harmony meta-analysis [130]. This study analyzed 36 trials with 4046 participants and found that combining trauma-focused therapy with pharmacotherapy for SUDs showed the largest comparative effect sizes for both PTSD severity and alcohol use severity at end of treatment.

A 2024 network meta-analysis systematically reviewed psychotherapy and pharmacologic trials from 1995–2019, including 24 randomized controlled trials in the network analysis [122]. This study confirmed that alcohol-targeted medications combined with trauma-focused psychotherapy were more effective than either approach alone for reducing both PTSD and alcohol use severity.

The 2022 Cochrane systematic review on pharmacotherapy for PTSD offers the most rigorous evidence synthesis on PTSD medications generally, finding moderate-certainty evidence for SSRIs (paroxetine, sertraline) and low-certainty evidence for mirtazapine and amitriptyline, though it does not specifically focus on comorbid SUD populations [131].

Pharmacotherapy with SSRIs or SNRIs represents an alternative first-line option, particularly when psychotherapy is unavailable, declined, or when patients have co-occurring MDD [132]. The 2023 VA/DoD guidelines continue to recommend paroxetine and sertraline (both FDA-approved for PTSD) along with venlafaxine as first-line pharmacologic options, all of which maintain robust individual trial evidence supporting their efficacy. Note, fluoxetine also has evidence for efficacy, though it was removed from the 2023 VA/DoD first-line recommendations due to lack of benefit in recent trials [125].

The 2023 VA/DoD Clinical Practice Guidelines recommend against benzodiazepines for PTSD treatment due to lack of evidence of benefits and the presence of known harms. Evidence demonstrates that benzodiazepines are associated with misuse, decreased effectiveness of recommended PTSD treatments, and adverse cognitive changes, especially in the elderly [125]. This recommendation is particularly important in patients with active SUDs given the high risk of misuse and potential for worsening addiction. The guidelines also recommend against cannabis or cannabis derivatives for PTSD treatment because of the lack of well-designed RCTs and potentially serious side effects associated with cannabis use [125]. This is especially relevant for patients with SUDs, as cannabis use may complicate recovery.

Personality Disorders and SUDs

Co-occurring personality disorders and SUDs are highly prevalent, with approximately 60% of patients with SUDs having a personality disorder, and among patients with borderline personality disorder (BPD), the lifetime prevalence of

SUDs reaches 78%. This comorbidity is associated with significant clinical consequences including greater functional impairment, higher all-cause mortality, more complex treatment presentations, poorer treatment outcomes, and lower treatment retention rates compared to either disorder alone [135–138].

Prevalence estimates vary by specific personality disorder and substance. Among patients with substance use disorders, 12-month prevalence shows significant associations with antisocial personality disorder (ASPD), BPD, and schizotypal personality disorder [139]. For AUD specifically, a 2018 meta-analysis found lifetime prevalence of 77% in people with ASPD, 52% in people with BPD, and 39% in people with other personality disorders [140]. The National Epidemiologic Survey on Alcohol and Related Conditions demonstrated that individuals with severe lifetime AUD had odds ratios of 2.4 for ASPD and 2.5 for BPD, respectively [140].

BPD and ASPD show the strongest associations with SUDs. These two disorders are consistently identified as the most robust predictors of both alcohol and drug use disorders across multiple large epidemiological studies [135, 141, 142]. A population-based twin study found that BPD and ASPD criteria were the strongest predictors of phenotypic and genotypic liability to alcohol use and AUD. Genetic variation associated with these personality disorder criteria accounted for an estimated 5–10% of the variance in AUD criteria at baseline, increasing to approximately 17–33% at follow-up [142].

The clinical impact of this comorbidity is profound. Patients with co-occurring SUD and BPD tend to be younger, more functionally impaired, less satisfied with their social relationships, and exhibit higher levels of impulsivity, emotion regulation difficulties, and alexithymia than those with SUD alone [143]. They also show higher rates of cannabis use disorder, polysubstance use, and comorbid anxiety, obsessive-compulsive, and post-traumatic stress disorder [143]. The comorbidity markedly complicates care, contributing to lower retention rates in SUD treatment programs among individuals with co-occurring personality disorders [140].

Proposed mechanisms underlying this co-occurrence include shared etiology and behavioral disinhibition. The behavioral disinhibition hypothesis posits that individuals with antisocial and impulsive traits have lower thresholds for deviant behaviors, which combined with low constraint, low harm avoidance, and lack of social conformity, and favors early alcohol use and development of SUDs [140]. Personality traits in childhood, particularly low harm avoidance and high novelty seeking at age 11, exponentially increase risk for alcohol misuse in adulthood [140]. Additional mechanisms include emotional dysregulation, shared genetic factors, and certain neurotransmitter pathways [136].

Treatment utilization remains critically low despite high prevalence. Among respondents with 12-month drug use disorder, only 13.5% received treatment, and among those with lifetime drug use disorder, only 24.6% received treatment [139]. This treatment gap, combined with the complexity of dual diagnosis presentations, underscores the urgent need to destigmatize these conditions and educate clinicians and policy makers about evidence-based treatment approaches [139].

Substantial evidence supports dialectical behavior therapy (DBT) for treating co-occurring BPD and SUDs. A 2021 review noted beneficial effects despite elevated dropout risks, finding that treatment completers respond similarly to those without personality disorders [144]. A 2023 review confirmed that DBT reduces symptom severity more effectively than usual care (medium effect sizes), which is crucial given the high rate (78%) of co-occurring SUD in this population [145].

Multiple reviews confirm DBT's impact on key metrics [149, 150]. A 2022 meta-analysis found that standalone DBT significantly reduced self-harm and improved psychosocial functioning, while adjunctive skills training specifically reduced BPD severity [146]. These findings were echoed in a 2022 practice guideline, which noted improvements in severity, self-harm incidence, and functioning compared to usual treatment [148]. Additionally, intensive 28-day DBT programs have been shown to significantly reduce depression and improve coping skills in dual-diagnosis patients [147].

Eating Disorders and SUDs

Approximately one in seven males and one in five females will experience any eating disorder by age 40, with 95% of first-time cases occurring by age 25 [178]. Women are affected 2–3 times more frequently than men (lifetime: 1.25%–3.5% in women vs. 0.42%–2.0% in men) [1]. Prevalence appears comparable across ethnoracial groups in the United States, though Mexican Americans show higher rates than their counterparts in Mexico. Co-occurring eating disorders and SUDs are common, with a pooled lifetime prevalence of 21.9% for any comorbid SUD among individuals with eating disorders, though prevalence varies substantially by eating disorder subtype, with binge-purge presentations showing higher rates than restrictive presentations. The most prevalent substance use (not necessarily disorders) comorbidities are tobacco (36.1%), caffeine (23.8%), and alcohol (20.6%) [127]. Among specific eating disorder subtypes, the lifetime prevalence of major depression is highest in bulimia nervosa (76.3%), followed by binge-eating disorder (65.5%) and anorexia nervosa (49.5%) [173]. SUDs are particularly common in binge-purge-type eating disorders, with AUD and stimulant use disorder being frequently comorbid conditions [1, 173].

Individuals with eating disorders often use substances in ways that directly server their eating-related goals or emotional needs. Cigarette smoking (including vaping) may be used to suppress appetite; stimulants or over-the-counter medications such as laxatives or diuretics may be used to promote weight loss and/or boost energy; and alcohol or other psychoactive substances may be used for emotional regulation or as part of a pattern of impulsive behavior [174, 175]. This functional relationship between eating disorders and substance use varies within and across eating disorder subtypes and depends on the specific substance involved [174].

The co-occurrence of eating disorders and substance use substantially worsens prognosis. Individuals with eating disorders who misuse substances exhibit more severe core eating disorder symptoms and broader psychopathology, more frequent general medical complications, longer recovery trajectories, poorer functional outcomes, and higher rates of substance use relapse than those with eating disorders alone [174]. Outcomes are further compromised, and mortality risk increases when an additional psychiatric disorder is present [175].

The APA recommends that all patients undergoing initial psychiatric evaluation should be assessed for use of caffeine, tobacco, alcohol, cannabinoids, and other substances, as well as any misuse of prescribed or over-the-counter medications or supplements [175]. A comprehensive substance use history is essential in patients with potential eating disorders given the high comorbidity rates [175]. Specific inquiry should be made about the use or misuse of prescribed or non-prescribed medications that suppress appetite (e.g., OTC weight loss products, stimulants) or enhance muscularity (e.g., supplements, androgens) [175]. The functional relationship between an eating disorder and substance use should be evaluated individually for each patient to determine whether substances are being used to facilitate weight loss, increase energy, regulate emotions, or reflect broader patterns of impulsive behavior [174].

In terms of treatment recommendations, the eating disorder and SUD should be addressed simultaneously using a multidisciplinary approach [174]. The need for medical stabilization, hospitalization, or inpatient treatment should be assessed based on general medical and psychiatric considerations [179, 180]. Individuals with eating disorders should be regularly screened and offered treatment for SUDs concurrently during treatment for the eating disorder [127].

Common elements across therapeutic interventions include psychoeducation about the shared etiology, risks, and consequences of concurrent eating disorder behaviors and substance misuse, dietary education and planning, cognitive restructuring of disordered eating beliefs and attitudes; skills training and development of adaptive coping strategies; targeted work on barriers to change; and structured relapse-prevention focused on both eating disorder symptoms and substance use [174, 180].

CBT has been frequently used in the treatment of comorbid eating disorders and SUDs, though there are no randomized controlled trials. More recently, evidence has been found for the efficacy of DBT in reducing both eating disorder and substance use behaviors [174]. Emphasis should be placed on building a collaborative therapeutic relationship and avoiding power struggles [174].

Emerging pharmacological approaches show promise for co-occurring conditions. Olanzapine and ketamine may improve compulsive behaviors and mood in anorexia nervosa and SUDs, while GLP-1 receptor agonists may reduce binge episodes and cravings in binge-eating disorder and SUDs [176]. However, currently only lisdexamfetamine (for binge-eating disorder) and fluoxetine (for bulimia nervosa) have regulatory approval for eating disorders [177, 181].

Acute Management of Co-occurring Disorders

Alcohol and Sedative Withdrawal

Clinical management guidelines for alcohol and sedative withdrawal in patients with co-occurring psychiatric disorders emphasize integrated treatment, careful medication selection, and higher levels of monitoring compared to patients with SUDs alone.

The presence of co-occurring psychiatric disorders fundamentally alters both assessment and treatment planning. Comprehensive evaluation must include withdrawal severity (using tools like CIWA-Ar), psychiatric comorbidity, and risk factors for complicated withdrawal [133, 134]. Patients with dual diagnosis often need a higher level of care with inpatient treatment indicated not only for standard reasons such as severe withdrawal or a history of delirium tremens, but also for active psychosis, marked cognitive impairment, or an inability to safely or effectively participate in outpatient programs [151].

Pharmacologic management requires careful consideration of psychiatric comorbidity. For alcohol withdrawal, benzodiazepines remain first-line, but when patients have co-occurring sedative use disorder or psychiatric conditions, alternatives including gabapentin, carbamazepine, and valproic acid may be preferred to avoid reinforcing sedative use disorder [133, 151, 152]. For sedative withdrawal with psychiatric comorbidity, clinicians should optimize evidence-based psychiatric treatment prior to or concurrent with benzodiazepine tapering [153]. The taper may need to proceed more slowly, and monitoring sleep is critical—particularly in bipolar disorder where sleep disturbance can trigger manic episodes [153]. If significant psychiatric symptoms emerge during tapering, the taper should be paused until symptoms resolve [153, 154].

Integrated treatment addressing both conditions simultaneously produces superior outcomes compared to fragmented approaches [4]. This includes combining medications and behavioral therapies such as CBT and MI, with skills to manage both disorders increasingly offered in the same session [4]. For patients with more severe psychiatric comorbidities, care teams should include specialists with appropriate expertise to design personalized, multimodal treatment plans [4].

When managing concurrent withdrawal from multiple substances, patients should be placed in the level of care appropriate to their most acute problem, which may be sedative withdrawal rather than alcohol withdrawal [79]. Patients with physiological benzodiazepine use disorder should not receive standard alcohol withdrawal protocols but instead require slow, individualized tapering [79]. For patients with co-occurring OUD, the medications for opioid use disorder (MOUD) should typically be initiated and stabilized before beginning benzodiazepine tapering, with the opioid medication dose kept stable throughout [151].

Stimulant Intoxication

Clinical management guidelines for stimulant intoxication in patients with co-occurring psychiatric disorders emphasize concurrent treatment of both conditions using integrated approaches, whereas management in patients with stimulant use disorder alone focuses primarily on acute symptom control without the need for ongoing psychiatric medication coordination [5]. The ASAM and AAAP recommend that clinicians treat both stimulant use disorder and co-occurring psychiatric disorders concurrently using integrated behavioral treatment approaches whenever possible [5].

Pharmacologic management of agitation and psychosis during stimulant intoxication follows similar protocols regardless of CODs. Benzodiazepines are considered first-line treatment for stimulant-induced agitation and confusion, while antipsychotic medications should be used for psychotic symptoms [5]. However, chlorpromazine and clozapine should be avoided due to increased seizure risk [5]. The urgency, formulation, and duration of antipsychotic therapy should be based on etiology and symptomatology [5].

A key distinction in dual diagnosis management is the approach to psychiatric symptoms. In patients with CODs, clinicians should consider pharmacotherapy for depression, anxiety, insomnia, and attentional problems based on symptom severity and duration, even if symptoms are stimulant-induced [5]. The clinical presentation should be evaluated to determine whether symptoms follow the expected time course of stimulant-induced symptoms (active use, waning intoxication, acute withdrawal, post-acute withdrawal, or post-withdrawal abstinence) or represent preexisting psychiatric conditions [5].

For patients with dual diagnosis, behavioral therapies should be tailored to address interactions between stimulant use disorder and co-occurring psychiatric conditions [5]. Clinicians should be aware that adherence to and effectiveness of psychiatric medications may be reduced during ongoing stimulant use, and unknown adverse interactions between medications and stimulants could occur [5].

In contrast, management of stimulant intoxication in patients without co-occurring psychiatric disorders focuses on acute symptom control through de-escalation strategies and pharmacotherapy as needed, without requiring integration with ongoing psychiatric treatment plans [5]. Mild stimulant intoxication can typically be managed with behavioral and environmental interventions to help patients feel calm and safe [5].

The evidence base for dual diagnosis management remains limited, with very few mental health interventions evaluated specifically in people with stimulant use disorders [89]. Recent systematic reviews indicate mixed findings regarding optimal pharmacological strategies, with effectiveness varying according to specific psychopathology, the particular substance involved, treatment setting, and primary care objectives [63]. Further research is needed to develop individualized treatment plans and understand the biological underpinnings of dual diagnosis to create more targeted interventions [63].

Psychosocial Interventions for Co-occurring Disorders

Motivational Interviewing and Motivational Enhancement Therapy

Motivational interviewing (MI) and motivational enhancement therapy (MET) show promise for treating co-occurring mental illness and SUDs, with the strongest evidence supporting their use in combination with cognitive-behavioral therapy (CBT) and for increasing treatment engagement, though the overall quality of evidence remains limited.

A 2009 systematic review of 54 studies found that MI had the most quality evidence for reducing substance use over the short term in psychiatric settings [155]. When combined with CBT, improvements in mental state were also apparent, suggesting synergistic effects when addressing both conditions simultaneously.

For patients with AUD and co-occurring anxiety or depressive disorders, the combination of CBT plus MI appears more effective than comparison conditions [151]. A meta-analysis demonstrated small but clinically significant decreases in both depressive symptoms and alcohol consumption when combining CBT and MI to treat depression and AUD, compared with usual care [4].

Recent evidence from a 2022 randomized trial showed that MI resulted in greater likelihood of abstaining from unhealthy alcohol use (70.0% vs. 60.2%, $p < 0.01$) and cannabis use (74.6% vs. 63.9%, $p < 0.01$) at 6 months among patients with depression, though outcomes did not differ at 12 months [156]. A 2024 review confirmed that MI techniques can be administered both in-person and online to decrease substance misuse and anxiety among patients with elevated anxiety and substance misuse [157].

For patients with severe mental illness and substance misuse, individual studies within a 2019 Cochrane review found specific benefits: one study ($n = 28$) showed MI improved alcohol abstinence at 6 months compared to treatment as usual [102, 158]. However, the overall review of 41 trials found no high-quality evidence supporting any one psychosocial treatment over standard care for remaining in treatment, reduction in substance use, or improving mental or global state [102].

MET is delivered as a more structured intervention over four 60-min sessions, using systematic assessment with personalized feedback and MI principles to elicit commitment to change [151]. As a stand-alone treatment, MET provided over 3–4 sessions yielded comparable benefits to more intensive manualized interventions (CBT or TSF) involving 8–12 sessions [151]. The ASAM recommends that MI and MET are highly effective evidence-based practices for increasing patients' internal motivation for change, which can increase engagement and retention in care [159]. MI principles can be integrated into program procedures at various points, from first contact through clinical services, and research has demonstrated it can be feasibly and effectively implemented in community-based settings when clinicians are provided with training and supervision [159].

Despite all this evidence, certain limitations and caveats need to be borne in mind. A 2023 Cochrane review of MI for substance use reduction found only low to very low-certainty evidence across most comparisons, with substantial heterogeneity between studies [160]. The review emphasized the importance of counselor adherence to, and transparent reporting of, intervention fidelity and quality conditions to ensure that only studies in which MI was truly implemented are included in evidence synthesis [160].

For patients with first-episode psychosis and schizophrenia with co-occurring substance use, a 2023 VA/DoD guideline review found very low-quality evidence with no overall difference in outcomes when comparing various psychosocial interventions including MI to treatment as usual, though individual studies showed some benefits [158].

Overall, the evidence suggests MI/MET is most valuable as part of integrated treatment approaches, particularly when combined with CBT, and for enhancing engagement and short-term outcomes in dual diagnosis populations, though longer-term benefits and superiority over other active treatments remain uncertain.

Cognitive Behavioral Therapy

CBT shows modest efficacy for treating co-occurring mental illness and substance use disorders, with the strongest evidence supporting integrated CBT approaches that simultaneously address both conditions, though effect sizes are generally small and evidence quality remains limited.

A 2025 meta-analysis of 47 randomized trials found that CBT-based interventions targeting CODs provided benefit over usual care for substance use consumption outcomes, but not psychosocial outcomes [161]. Conversely, when CBT was added to usual care and compared to usual care alone, benefits emerged for psychosocial outcomes but not consumption [161]. An earlier 2021 meta-analysis of 15 trials showed small effect sizes for both substance use and mental health outcomes, with only mental health outcomes reaching statistical significance [162].

The NIAAA recommends that integrated treatment plans might include CBT for both AUD and co-occurring conditions (depression, anxiety, PTSD, or sleep disorders), with skills to manage both disorders increasingly offered in the same session rather than alternating sessions [4]. A meta-analysis found small but clinically significant decreases in depressive symptoms and alcohol consumption when combining CBT and MI to treat depression and AUD, compared with usual care [4].

For depression and SUDs, a 2019 Cochrane review found insufficient high-quality evidence to support any specific psychological intervention over standard care [163]. Two studies comparing integrated cognitive behavioral therapy (ICBT) with twelve-step facilitation (TSF) showed that while TSF produced lower depression scores at post-treatment, there was no difference at 6–12-month follow-up. However, ICBT resulted in greater proportion of days abstinent at follow-up [163].

For severe mental illness and substance misuse, a 2019 Cochrane review of 41 trials found no high-quality evidence supporting any one psychosocial treatment over standard care for remaining in treatment, reduction in substance use, or improving mental or global state [102].

For stimulant use disorder with co-occurring conditions, some evidence supports CBT as superior to usual treatment options on stimulant use and abstinence outcomes during treatment and at follow-up, as well as for treatment retention [5]. However, CBT has not been found superior for longest duration of continuous stimulant abstinence or stimulant use at study endpoint [5].

When CBT was compared directly to other specific therapies, treatment effects were consistently nonsignificant across outcomes and follow-up time points [164]. A 2019 meta-analysis of 30 trials found that CBT showed moderate and significant effects compared to minimal treatment, and significant effects for consumption frequency and quantity at early (but not late) follow-up when compared to nonspecific therapy, but no superior efficacy compared to other specific treatment modalities [164].

Importantly, CBT requires trained clinicians for proper delivery and can be delivered in individual or group sessions [5, 151]. The ASAM and AAAP recommend using evidence-based CBT manuals such as Project MATCH's Cognitive-Behavioral Coping Skills Therapy Manual or NIDA's Therapy Manual for Drug Addiction [5]. Combined pharmacotherapy and CBT may enhance outcomes. An early review found effect sizes were roughly 5 times higher when CBT was combined with pharmacotherapy than when delivered as a stand-alone intervention, though this was based on only 4 studies [165].

The evidence base on CBT is limited by methodological challenges including small sample sizes, high attrition rates, heterogeneous interventions and outcome measures, and high risk of bias in most studies [102, 161–163]. Most studies were conducted in the United States with predominantly Caucasian samples, limiting generalizability [163]. The 2021 meta-analysis noted that the most promising effect sizes were observed for integrated CBT compared with single disorder interventions for follow-up outcomes and for interventions targeting alcohol use and/or PTSD [162].

Trauma Informed Care

There is substantial evidence supporting trauma-informed care (TIC) in treating patients with co-occurring PTSD and SUDs, with the strongest evidence favoring integrated trauma-focused psychotherapies that simultaneously address both conditions.

The SAMHSA model of trauma-informed care recognizes the role of prior traumatic experiences in illness and recovery, emphasizing evidence-informed healthcare interactions to reduce revictimization risk and improve trust in the healthcare system [166]. Key domains include patient and provider safety, transparency and trust-building, shared decision-making, involvement of peers or navigators, and personalization of care with attention to cultural context [166]. Both clients and staff in residential SUD treatment facilities perceive TIC as essential, viewing it as a multi-faceted and consistent approach to service delivery that creates a safe and supportive environment [167].

Individual trauma-focused psychological therapy delivered alongside SUD intervention is more effective than treatment as usual for reducing PTSD severity post-treatment and at 3–4- and 5–7-months follow-up [129]. A 2024 network meta-analysis found that integrated trauma-focused therapy for PTSD and substance use was more effective at reducing PTSD symptoms than integrated non-trauma-focused therapy, substance-focused psychotherapy alone, and control psychotherapies [122].

Prolonged exposure (PE), concurrent treatment of PTSD and SUDs using PE (COPE), and cognitive processing therapy (CPT) show promise as trauma-focused treatments [115]. A 2025 randomized trial of integrated treatment (COPE) in women with PTSD and AUD demonstrated significant reductions in both PTSD symptom severity and alcohol use. The combination of trauma-focused therapy and pharmacotherapy for SUDs showed the largest comparative effect sizes for PTSD severity and alcohol use severity at end of treatment [114, 130].

An important clinical consideration is that patients do not need to be abstinent to initiate or benefit from evidence-based PTSD treatment [112]. The VA/DoD guidelines suggest that the presence of comorbid SUD should not prevent delivery of trauma-focused psychotherapies like PE and CPT, as evidence shows persons with comorbid conditions can tolerate and benefit from these treatments [123]. The presence of comorbid conditions does not alter treatment effectiveness and should not delay PTSD treatment [123].

However, fewer participants complete trauma-focused therapy than treatment as usual, raising tolerability concerns [129]. Treatment effects, while consistent, are generally small, and individuals with more severe presentations (serious mental illness, cognitive impairment, and suicidal ideation) were excluded from most studies, limiting generalizability [129].

Various explanations for the link between SUDs and PTSD include the self-medication hypothesis—that individuals with PTSD seek symptom relief through drug use. Psychological interventions are expected to elicit change through facilitating effective coping skills, processing trauma memories, promoting attitudinal changes, and increasing understanding of cognitive and situational factors associated with substance use, particularly those related to past trauma [117].

Family and Social Support Interventions

There is substantial evidence supporting family and social support interventions in treating patients with co-occurring mental illness and SUDs, with the strongest evidence favoring integrated family interventions that combine education with communication and problem-solving skills training.

A randomized controlled trial of 108 clients (77% with schizophrenia-spectrum disorders) and their relatives compared brief Family Education (2–3 months) with longer-term Family Intervention for Dual Disorders (FIDD, 9–18 months) that combined education with communication and problem-solving skills training. Clients in FIDD had significantly less severe overall psychiatric symptoms and psychotic symptoms and tended to improve more in functioning, while relatives in FIDD improved more in mental health functioning and knowledge of CODs [168]. Both programs showed improvements in psychiatric, substance misuse, and functional outcomes, though there were no consistent differences in substance misuse severity or family burden between programs.

A 2023 systematic review of family therapy for SUDs found that incorporation of family members in treatment produces benefits by diminishing consumption and improving family functioning [169]. The review noted that family therapy influences not only personal variables but also promotes changes in family dynamics. Research on recovery homes demonstrates the importance of abstinence-specific social support. A study of 368 individuals living in Oxford Houses found that abstinence social support had a full mediating effect on the relationship between stress and length of stay for residents with psychiatric comorbidity, whereas general social support showed only partial mediating effects [170]. This suggests that specific components of social support optimize outcomes for those with psychiatric comorbidity. Peer support interventions in criminal justice settings have been shown to reduce risk behaviors and improve mental health, SUDs, and health service engagement [171].

A 2025 umbrella review found that integrated (coordinated) treatment for co-occurring diagnosis patients was better than treating one condition alone, and usually better than parallel uncoordinated services [49]. This supports the importance of coordinating family and social support interventions with other treatment modalities. However, retention of families in treatment programs remains a challenge. The FIDD trial noted that rates of retention of families in both programs were moderate, suggesting the need to modify these programs to retain more families in treatment to provide them with the information and skills they need [168].

In summary, while family and social support interventions show promise in improving outcomes, the evidence base has limitations including small sample sizes, high attrition rates, heterogeneous interventions, and short follow-up periods [172].

Technology-Enhanced Interventions

Technology-based interventions—including web-based, smartphone-based, artificial intelligence (AI) platform and computer-delivered approaches—show promise for treating co-occurring mental health and SUDs, with the strongest evidence supporting their use as supplements to in-person care rather than replacements.

When remote interventions supplement in-person care, there is 39% lower odds of return to use and a reduction in mean days of substance use compared with in-person care alone [182]. The VA/DoD guidelines suggest using technology-based interventions such as automated text or voice messaging and smartphone apps in addition to usual care for AUD, though evidence for other SUDs is insufficient [183].

Web-based CBT interventions show promise. Computer-Based training for CBT (CBT4CBT) has demonstrated significant reductions in substance use and improved retention in treatment relative to in-person CBT [5]. The therapeutic education system (TES), an interactive web-based program based on community reinforcement approach with a CBT component, showed that patients experienced more days of abstinence and remained in treatment longer than those in treatment as usual [151]. However, these effects are not always durable [5].

Smartphone applications can be effective for continuing care. A systematic review found that out of four studies using control groups, three showed significant differences favoring smartphone interventions over control conditions [184]. The FDA cleared the ReSET application, which delivers community reinforcement approach via smartphone [151]. VA-developed apps including VetChange for AUD and Stay Quit Coach for tobacco relapse prevention have shown reductions in problematic substance use [185].

For patients with co-occurring depression and problematic alcohol use, digital interventions show small but significant effects on depressive symptoms at 3-month follow-up and on alcohol use at 6-month follow-up, though the latter finding was sensitive to statistical estimator choice [186]. A 2019 systematic review found medium to large short-term improvements in both depression severity and substance use symptoms, plus global improvement in functioning, though longer-term effectiveness could not be established [187]. However, another systematic review found limited evidence for the superiority of combined digital interventions over therapist-delivered approaches, single condition interventions, or assessment-only controls for comorbid heavy drinking and depression [188].

When remote interventions replace or partially replace in-person care, there is a 49% lower odds of return to use compared with in-person care, but evidence for reduction in days of use is less conclusive [182]. The VA/DoD guidelines found insufficient evidence to recommend computer-delivered behavioral treatments either for or against as replacements for in-person care, noting that most studies were not designed as non-inferiority studies [151].

Telemedicine-delivered treatment appears generally as effective as in-person care for substance use reduction and treatment retention, though most studies lack rigorous designs and follow-up durations are brief (≤3 months) [189]. The VA/DoD guidelines note that despite considerable interest in telemedicine-delivered SUD treatment, no published major studies have compared telemedicine with clinic-based care [183].

Technology-based interventions allow for standardized implementation, reduced staff burden, and increased access to care [5]. They appear particularly beneficial for patients who prefer digital interventions or lack access to in-person care. High client satisfaction, therapeutic alliance, and engagement have been reported [187]. However, access and utilization may vary by platform. Telephone-based platforms (versus video) are positively associated with older age, lower education, and no prior overdose [189]. External validity of existing studies is generally low, limiting generalizability [187].

The evidence base has substantial limitations. Over 70% of outcomes in one meta-analysis were judged to be at high risk of bias [182]. Most systematic reviews conclude that evidence for mental health apps is weak, inconclusive, and hampered by substantial heterogeneity in study designs [190]. Quality of evidence ranges from moderate to very low across most comparisons [151, 186].

Generally, effect sizes for Internet-based interventions treating eating disorders and SUDs are lower compared with interventions for depression and anxiety. The literature reveals less evidence of efficacy for amphetamine-type stimulants and methamphetamine use compared to cocaine use [5].

Summary: Co-occurring Non-substance Related Psychiatric Disorders and SUDs

CODs consist of the simultaneous presence of a SUD and a NSRMHD. Approximately 8.1% of adults in the United States, or roughly 21.2 million people, can be characterized as having CODs. These disorders share a complex, bidirectional relationship where each condition can exacerbate the severity and prognosis of the other. Individuals with CODs face significantly poorer outcomes compared to those with a single disorder, including higher rates of homelessness, incarceration, suicide, and mortality. Epidemiological data indicates that young adulthood (ages 18–25) is a period of peak vulnerability, with prevalence rates reaching 14.1%. Significant disparities exist across demographic groups; multiracial adults exhibit the highest prevalence of combined mental illness or SUD, and non-binary individuals face disproportionately high risks due to minority stress. Furthermore, gender differences influence clinical presentation, with women more likely to present with mood and anxiety comorbidities, while men are more prone to antisocial personality traits and polysubstance use.

The neurobiological underpinnings of CODs involve shared dysregulation in brain circuitry governing reward, stress, and executive control. Chronic substance use often precipitates a "reward deficiency" state—characterized by downregulated dopamine transmission—that mirrors the anhedonia found in depression. Simultaneously, the recruitment of stress systems in the extended amygdala leads to "hyperkatifeia," a hypersensitivity to negative emotional states that perpetuates the cycle of addiction to escape distress. Assessment of these conditions has evolved; current guidelines reject the traditional practice of delaying psychiatric treatment until abstinence is achieved. Instead, clinicians are urged to treat severe symptoms such as agitation or psychosis immediately. Distinguishing between substance-induced and independent disorders remains critical, with symptoms persisting for more than 1 month after the cessation of acute withdrawal generally indicating an independent psychiatric condition.

Integrated care, where both conditions are treated concurrently within a unified framework, is now the gold standard of treatment. For anxiety and SUDs, selective serotonin reuptake inhibitors (SSRIs) are the first-line pharmacotherapy, while benzodiazepines are generally contraindicated due to misuse risk. In the context of bipolar disorder, which has a 40–70% comorbidity rate with AUD, mood stabilization with valproate or lithium is prioritized to reduce suicidality and reduce return to use. Depression is also highly comorbid with SUDs; while antidepressants effectively treat mood symptoms, they rarely reduce substance use on their own, often necessitating combination therapies like naltrexone. For psychotic disorders, particularly schizophrenia, cannabis use is a significant risk factor, increasing the likelihood of psychosis two- to four-fold. Clozapine and long-acting injectable antipsychotics have demonstrated the strongest evidence for reducing substance use in this population.

Trauma is a central theme in CODs, particularly regarding PTSD. The "self-medication" hypothesis suggests that individuals use substances to cope with hyperarousal and intrusive memories. Treatment guidelines emphasize that patients need not be abstinent to benefit from trauma-focused therapies such as prolonged exposure or cognitive processing therapy; delaying trauma work often hinders recovery. Similarly, personality disorders—specifically BPD and ASPD—are robust predictors of SUDs. DBT has emerged as the most effective intervention for these co-occurring presentations, improving both emotional regulation and retention in treatment.

Psychosocial interventions remain a cornerstone of management. MI is effective for enhancing engagement, while CBT aids in skill-building, though effect sizes are modest. Family and social support interventions that address family dynamics show promise in improving functioning. Finally, technology-enhanced interventions, such as smartphone applications and web-based CBT, serve as effective adjuncts to in-person care—reducing the odds of return to use—but are not recommended as standalone replacements for clinical treatment.

Chapter Review Questions

1. Treatment Approaches for CODs

   A 42-year-old man with a history of schizophrenia and severe AUD presents to the emergency department after being found intoxicated and with altered mental status. He has been hospitalized three times in the past year for psychotic exacerbations, each precipitated by a return to alcohol use. He has previously attended a residential treatment program but stopped taking his antipsychotic medication while there because "they didn't understand my mental health." Conversely, when treated in acute inpatient psychiatry setting, he often returns to use of alcohol shortly after discharge due to a lack of substance use support. Which of the following treatment models is most likely to improve this patient's long-term prognosis?

   A. Sequential treatment of psychiatric disorder followed by substance use disorder
   B. Treatment focusing primarily on substance use disorder with psychiatric consultation as needed
   C. Parallel treatment in separate programs with coordinated care plans

D. Integrated treatment addressing both disorders concurrently
E. Treatment of the more severe disorder with monitoring of the secondary condition

Correct Answer: D

Explanation: Integrated treatment—where both the mental health and substance use disorders are addressed simultaneously within a unified framework—has been shown to result in superior outcomes, including reduced psychiatric symptoms and decreased substance use. Sequential, parallel, or hierarchical treatment models are less effective because they fail to address the complex interactions between psychiatric and substance use symptoms.

References: American Academy of Addiction Psychiatry [93], Bahji et al. [6], Murthy et al. [62], Wolitzky-Taylor [52].

2. Alcohol Use Screening in the Primary Care Setting

A 35-year-old man presents to his primary care physician for an annual wellness visit. He has no significant past medical history. As part of the routine intake, the physician intends to screen for unhealthy alcohol use using the brief, single-item screening tool recommended by the U.S. Preventive Services Task Force (USPSTF) for its balance of sensitivity and specificity in primary care settings. Which of the following questions should the physician ask?

A. "How many times in the past year have you had 5 (for men) or 4 (for women) or more drinks in a day?"
B. "How many days per week do you typically consume alcohol?"
C. "How many drinks containing alcohol do you have on a typical day when drinking?"
D. "How many times in the past month have you felt you needed to cut down on drinking?"
E. "How many drinks do you consume in a typical week?"

Correct Answer: A

Explanation: This Single Alcohol Screening Question (SASQ) is endorsed by the USPSTF due to its brevity, validated sensitivity and specificity, and clinical utility for detecting unhealthy alcohol use in adults. The question specifically identifies binge drinking episodes, which is a strong indicator of unhealthy alcohol use. A response of one or more times indicates a positive screen.

References: US Preventive Services Task Force et al. [42], Patnode et al. [43].

3. Pharmacological Treatment of Anxiety in CODs

A 45-year-old woman with severe alcohol use disorder in early remission and generalized anxiety disorder presents for follow-up. She has been abstinent from alcohol for 6 months and is actively engaged in outpatient therapy and mutual support groups. Despite psychosocial interventions, she reports persistent, impairing anxiety symptoms and requests medication. Which of the following is the most appropriate initial pharmacological treatment?

A. Sertraline 25–50 mg daily with plan to increase dose in the future
B. Alprazolam 0.5 mg three times daily

C. Buspirone 10 mg twice daily
D. Clonazepam 0.5 mg twice daily
E. Lorazepam 1 mg as needed for anxiety

Correct Answer: A

Explanation: SSRIs, particularly sertraline, have demonstrated effectiveness in treating anxiety disorders (including generalized anxiety disorder and panic disorder) in patients with co-occurring alcohol use disorder. Non-benzodiazepine anxiolytics and antidepressants are preferred first-line treatments for anxiety disorders in patients with co-occurring SUDs due to their favorable safety profile and while avoiding benzodiazepine-associated risks of developing a benzodiazepine use disorder, cognitive impairment, and return to substance use,

References: Department of Veterans Affairs, Department of Defense [57] (Guidelines typically recommend against the use of benzodiazepines in patients with active or remitted SUDs due to misuse liability), Ipser et al. [53] (This is the most direct evidence, reviewing medication efficacy specifically for this dual diagnosis and supporting the use of antidepressants), Szuhany and Simon [50] (Establish SSRIs, such as sertraline, as the first-line pharmacotherapy for generalized anxiety disorder).

4. Comprehensive Substance Screening

A 32-year-old man presents to primary care for an annual physical examination. The physician selects a validated screening instrument designed explicitly for primary care that assesses tobacco, alcohol, illicit drugs, and nonmedical use of prescription medications to generate a risk-level stratification. Which of the following tools has the physician selected?

A. AUDIT (Alcohol Use Disorders Identification Test)
B. TAPS (Tobacco, Alcohol, Prescription medications, and other Substances) Tool
C. DAST-10 (Drug Abuse Screening Test)
D. CAGE-AID (Cut down, Annoyed, Guilty, Eye-opener—Adapted to Include Drugs)
E. NIDA Quick Screen

Correct Answer: B.

Explanation: The TAPS tool was specifically designed and validated for primary care use to assess a broad range of substance use, offering a comprehensive but brief screening method. While CAGE-AID and NIDA Quick Screen can assess multiple substances, the TAPS tool provides the most systematic approach to screening across tobacco, alcohol, prescription medications, and illicit substances with validated scoring thresholds. The AUDIT screens for alcohol only, and the DAST-10 screens for drug use only.

References: McNeely et al. [45], Kowalchuk et al. [44].

5. Benzodiazepine Management in Panic Disorder with Alcohol Use Disorder

A 52-year-old woman with panic disorder and severe alcohol use disorder in early remission presents to an outpatient clinic. She successfully completed residential treatment for alcohol use 45 days ago and remains abstinent. She has been taking alprazolam 1 mg four times daily for 8 years. Despite adherence, she reports having 2–3 panic attacks weekly and admits to requesting early refills twice in the past month. She consumes 6–8 cups of coffee daily. Which of the following is the most appropriate management strategy?

A. Continue alprazolam at the current dose to support sobriety and prevent withdrawal
B. Abruptly discontinue alprazolam and initiate sertraline 50 mg daily
C. Switch to an equivalent dose of clonazepam, initiate sertraline, and begin a slow taper of clonazepam with caffeine reduction counseling
D. Initiate a slow taper of alprazolam over 8–12 weeks while simultaneously starting sertraline and counseling on caffeine reduction
E. Increase alprazolam to 1.5 mg four times daily to control breakthrough panic symptoms

Correct Answer: C—Convert to equivalent-dose clonazepam, initiate sertraline, and then taper clonazepam over 8–12 weeks with caffeine reduction counseling

Explanation: Why C is correct:

Switching to a long-acting benzodiazepine (clonazepam) minimizes inter-dose withdrawal and facilitates a smoother taper compared to short-acting agents like alprazolam. The conversion typically uses a 2:1 ratio (alprazolam 4 mg daily = clonazepam 2 mg daily), often divided into twice-daily dosing. After conversion and stabilization (typically 1–2 weeks), a gradual taper can be initiated, reducing the dose by 10–25% every 1–2 weeks over 8–12 weeks or longer given her 8-year history of use. Concurrent initiation of an SSRI (sertraline) ensures therapeutic coverage for panic disorder as the benzodiazepine is withdrawn. Addressing the patient's excessive caffeine intake eliminates a significant physiological precipitant of anxiety. This comprehensive strategy safely manages physiological dependence while mitigating the high risks of misuse and return to alcohol—evidenced here by her early refill requests—associated with benzodiazepine use in patients with alcohol use disorder.

References: American College of Medical Toxicology; American Society of Addiction Medicine [69], Ipser et al. [53] (Supports the transition to antidepressants), Szuhany and Simon [50].

References

1. American Psychiatric Association. Diagnostic and statistical manual of mental disorders. 5th ed., text rev. ed. Washington, DC: American Psychiatric Association; 2022.
2. Substance Abuse and Mental Health Services Administration. Key substance use and mental health indicators in the United States: results from the 2024 National Survey on Drug Use and Health. Rockville: Center for Behavioral Health Statistics and Quality, Substance Abuse and Mental Health Services Administration; 2025. Publication No.: PEP25-07-007.
3. Boyle MP, Gibson E, Lien J, et al. Clinical considerations for engagement and retention of nonabstinent patients in care. J Addict Med. 2025;19(5):504–6.

4. De Aquino JP, Petrakis IL. Alcohol use disorder and common co-occurring conditions. Alcohol Res. 2025;45(1):e1.
5. Batki S, Ciccarone D, Hadland SE. Clinical Guideline Committee. The ASAM/AAAP clinical practice guideline on the management of stimulant use disorder. J Addict Med. 2024;18(1):1–56.
6. Bahji A, Tang V, Danilewitz M. Integrated management of co-occurring alcohol use disorder and depression: clinical approaches for concurrent disorders. Can J Psychiatr. 2025;3:7067437251374564. [Epub ahead of print].
7. Aguayo-Romero R, Beccia A, Trinh MH, Reisner SL. Psychological distress and substance use among transgender and gender diverse adults in the United States: an intersectional multilevel analysis of individual heterogeneity and discriminatory accuracy. Ann Behav Med. 2025;59(1):kaaf022.
8. Bailey S, Newton N, Perry Y, et al. Prevalence, distribution, and inequitable co-occurrence of mental ill-health and substance use among gender and sexuality diverse young people in Australia: epidemiological findings from a population-based cohort study. Soc Psychiatry Psychiatr Epidemiol. 2024;59(12):2323–37.
9. Bailey S, Lin A, Cook A, et al. Contextualising experiences of co-occurring mental ill-health and substance use among trans, non-binary, and gender diverse young people: implications for tailored harm reduction approaches. Community Ment Health J. 2025;61(1):181–92.
10. Eccles H, Abramovich A, Patte KA, et al. Mental disorders and suicidality in transgender and gender-diverse people. JAMA Netw Open. 2024;7(10):e2436883.
11. Felner JK, Wisdom JP, Williams T et al. Stress, coping, and context: examining substance use among LGBTQ young adults with probable substance use disorders. Psychiatr Serv. 2020;71(2):112–20.
12. Kidd JD, Goetz TG, Shea EA, Bockting WO. Prevalence and minority-stress correlates of past 12-month prescription drug misuse in a national sample of transgender and gender nonbinary adults: results from the U.S. Transgender Survey. Drug Alcohol Depend. 2021;219:108474.
13. Kidd JD, Tettamanti NA, Kaczmarkiewicz R, et al. Prevalence of substance use and mental health problems among transgender and cisgender U.S. adults: results from a national probability sample. Psychiatry Res. 2023;326:115339.
14. King WM, Gamarel KE, Iwamoto M et al. Structural needs, substance use, and mental health among transgender and nonbinary young adults in the San Francisco Bay Area: findings from the Phoenix Study. J Urban Health. 2023;100(1):190–203
15. Lett E, Abrams MP, Moberg E, et al. Syndemic relationship of depressive symptoms, substance use, and suicidality in transgender youth: a cross-sectional study using the U.S. Youth Risk Behavior Surveillance System. Soc Psychiatry Psychiatr Epidemiol. 2022;57(11):2293–304
16. Ruppert R, Kattari SK, Sussman S. Review: prevalence of addictions among transgender and gender diverse subgroups. Int J Environ Res Public Health. 2021;18(16):8843.
17. Stanton AM, Batchelder AW, Kirakosian N, et al. Differences in mental health symptom severity and care engagement among transgender and gender diverse individuals: findings from a large community health center. PLoS One. 2021;16(1):e0245872.
18. Dobbs LK, Lemos JC, Alvarez VA. Restructuring of basal ganglia circuitry and associated behaviors triggered by low striatal D2 receptor expression: implications for substance use disorders. Genes Brain Behav. 2016;15(2):227–39.
19. Tanabe J, Regner M, Sakai J, et al. Neuroimaging reward, craving, learning, and cognitive control in substance use disorders: review and implications for treatment. Br J Radiol. 2019;92(1101):20180541.
20. Chen W, Nong Z, Li Y, et al. Role of dopamine signaling in drug addiction. Curr Top Med Chem. 2017;17(21):2412–24.
21. Luijten M, Schellekens AF, Kühn S, et al. Disruption of reward processing in addiction: an image-based metaanalysis of functional magnetic resonance imaging studies. JAMA Psychiatry. 2017;74(4):387–95.
22. Smiley CE, Wood SK. Stress- and drug-induced neuroimmune signaling as a therapeutic target for comorbid anxiety and substance use disorders. Pharmacol Ther. 2022;231:107971.

23. Agarwal K, Manza P, Chapman M, et al. Inflammatory markers in substance use and mood disorders: a neuroimaging perspective. Front Psych. 2022;13:832321.
24. Li H, Watkins LR, Wang X. Microglia in neuroimmunopharmacology and drug addiction. Mol Psychiatry. 2024;29(1):15–28.
25. Namba MD, Leyrer-Jackson JM, Nagy EK et al. Neuroimmune mechanisms as novel treatment targets for substance use disorders and associated comorbidities. Front Neurosci. 2021;15:713439.
26. Sharma P, Sawaya MF, Dumitrescu AM, et al. Novel neurotherapeutic targets for substance use disorders: neuroplasticity, neuroinflammation, gasotransmitters and non-canonical organ systems. Neurotherapeutics. 2025;22(1):152–68.
27. Koob GF. Drug addiction: hyperkatifeia/negative reinforcement as a framework for medications development. Pharmacol Rev. 2021;73(1):163–201.
28. Koob GF. Neurobiology of opioid addiction: opponent process, hyperkatifeia, and negative reinforcement. Biol Psychiatry. 2020;87(1):44–53.
29. Simpson S, Shankar K, Kimbrough A, George O. Role of corticotropin-releasing factor in alcohol and nicotine addiction. Brain Res. 2020;1728:146554.
30. Zorrilla EP, Logrip ML, Koob GF. Corticotropin releasing factor: a key role in the neurobiology of addiction. Front Neuroendocrinol. 2014;35(2):234–44.
31. Ceceli AO, Bradberry CW, Goldstein RZ. The neurobiology of drug addiction: cross-species insights into the dysfunction and recovery of the prefrontal cortex. Neuropsychopharmacology. 2022;47(1):126–41.
32. Yan H, Xiao S, Fu S, et al. Functional and structural brain abnormalities in substance use disorder: a multimodal meta-analysis of neuroimaging studies. Acta Psychiatr Scand. 2023;147(3):234–48.
33. Wilcox CE, Pommy JM, Adinoff B. Neural circuitry of impaired emotion regulation in substance use disorders. Am J Psychiatry. 2016;173(4):344–61.
34. Goldstein RZ, Volkow ND. Dysfunction of the prefrontal cortex in addiction: neuroimaging findings and clinical implications. Nat Rev Neurosci. 2011;12(11):652–69.
35. Le TM, Potvin S, Zhornitsky S, Li CR. Distinct patterns of prefrontal cortical disengagement during inhibitory control in addiction: a meta-analysis based on population characteristics. Neurosci Biobehav Rev. 2021;127:255–69.
36. Bart CP, Titone MK, Ng TH et al. Neural reward circuit dysfunction as a risk factor for bipolar spectrum disorders and substance use disorders: a review and integration. Clin Psychol Rev. 2021;87:102043.
37. Gómez-Coronado N, Sethi R, Bortolasci CC, et al. A review of the neurobiological underpinning of comorbid substance use and mood disorders. J Affect Disord. 2018;235:277–84.
38. Jang SK, Saunders G, Liu M, et al. Genetic correlation, pleiotropy, and causal associations between substance use and psychiatric disorder. Psychol Med. 2022;52(10):1872–81.
39. Gerring ZF, Thorp JG, Gamazon ER, Derks EM. A local genetic correlation analysis provides biological insights into the shared genetic architecture of psychiatric and substance use phenotypes. Biol Psychiatry. 2022;92(12):951–60.
40. Nunes EV, Levin FR. Treatment of depression in patients with alcohol or other drug dependence: a meta-analysis. JAMA. 2004;291(15):1887–96.
41. American College of Surgeons Committee on Trauma. Best practices guidelines: screening and intervention for mental health disorders and substance use and misuse in the acute trauma patient. Chicago: American College of Surgeons; 2022.
42. US Preventive Services Task Force, Krist AH, Davidson KW, Mangione CM, et al. Screening for unhealthy drug use: US Preventive Services Task Force recommendation statement. JAMA. 2020;323(22):2301–9.
43. Patnode CD, Perdue LA, Rushkin M, et al. Screening for unhealthy drug use: updated evidence report and systematic review for the US Preventive Services Task Force. JAMA. 2020;323(22):2310–28.
44. Kowalchuk A, Gonzalez SJ, Zoorob RJ. Substance misuse in adults: a primary care approach. Am Fam Physician. 2024;109(5):430–40.

45. McNeely J, Adam A, Rotrosen J, et al. Comparison of methods for alcohol and drug screening in primary care clinics. JAMA Netw Open. 2021;4(5):e2110721.
46. Boness CL, Carlos Gonzalez J, Sleep C, et al. Evidence-based assessment of substance use disorder. Assessment.2024;31(1):168–90.
47. American Society of Addiction Medicine. Engagement and retention of nonabstinent patients in substance use treatment: clinical consideration for addiction treatment providers. Rockville: American Society of Addiction Medicine; 2024.
48. Spencer AE, Valentine SE, Sikov J, et al. Principles of care for young adults with co-occurring psychiatric and substance use disorders. Pediatrics. 2021;147(Suppl 2):229–39.
49. Simpson EL, Essat M, Wong R, et al. Effectiveness of psychosocial interventions for adults with substance use disorder that have a co-occurring common mental health disorder: an umbrella review. Drug Alcohol Rev. 2026;45(1):e70066.
50. Szuhany KL, Simon NM. Anxiety disorders: a review. JAMA. 2022;328(24):2431–45.
51. Penninx BW, Pine DS, Holmes EA, Reif A. Anxiety disorders. Lancet. 2021;397(10277):914–27.
52. Wolitzky-Taylor K. Integrated behavioral treatments for comorbid anxiety and substance use disorders: a model for understanding integrated treatment approaches and meta-analysis to evaluate their efficacy. Drug Alcohol Depend. 2023;253:110990.
53. Ipser JC, Wilson D, Akindipe TO, et al. Pharmacotherapy for anxiety and comorbid alcohol use disorders. Cochrane Database Syst Rev. 2015;1(1):CD007505.
54. Takeshima M, Otsubo T, Funada D, et al. Does cognitive behavioral therapy for anxiety disorders assist the discontinuation of benzodiazepines among patients with anxiety disorders? A systematic review and metaanalysis. Psychiatry Clin Neurosci. 2021;75(4):119–27.
55. Chapoutot M, Peter-Derex L, Bastuji H, et al. Cognitive behavioral therapy and acceptance and commitment therapy for the discontinuation of long-term benzodiazepine use in insomnia and anxiety disorders. Int J Environ Res Public Health. 2021;18(19):10222.
56. Buckner JD, Zvolensky MJ, Ecker AH, et al. Integrated cognitive behavioral therapy for comorbid cannabis use and anxiety disorders: a pilot randomized controlled trial. Behav Res Ther. 2019;115:38–45.
57. Department of Veterans Affairs, Department of Defense. VA/DoD clinical practice guideline for the management of substance use disorders. Washington, DC: Department of Veterans Affairs; 2021.
58. Lees R, Hines LA, D'Souza DC, et al. Psychosocial and pharmacological treatments for cannabis use disorder and mental health comorbidities: a narrative review. Psychol Med. 2021;51(3):353–64.
59. Fortney JC, Ratzliff AD, Blanchard BE, et al. Collaborative care for opioid use disorder in primary care: a hybrid type 2 cluster randomized clinical trial. JAMA Psychiatry. 2025;82(10):956–66.
60. Latif Z, Šaltytė Benth J, Solli KK, et al. Anxiety, depression, and insomnia among adults with opioid dependence treated with extended-release naltrexone vs buprenorphine-naloxone: a randomized clinical trial and follow-up study. JAMA Psychiatry. 2019;76(2):127–34.
61. Schuman-Olivier Z, Goodman H, Rosansky J, et al. Mindfulness training vs recovery support for opioid use, craving, and anxiety during buprenorphine treatment: a randomized clinical trial. JAMA Netw Open. 2025;8(1):e2454950.
62. Murthy P, Mahadevan J, Chand PK. Treatment of substance use disorders with co-occurring severe mental health disorders. Curr Opin Psychiatry. 2019;32(4):293–9.
63. Chiappini S, Mosca A, Semeraro F, et al. Navigating the challenges of substance use and psychopathology in depression, bipolar disorder, and schizophrenia. Compr Psychiatry. 2025;136:152532.
64. Singh B, Swartz HA, Cuellar-Barboza AB, et al. Bipolar disorder. Lancet. 2025;406(10506):963–78.
65. Grunze H, Soyka M. The pharmacotherapeutic management of comorbid bipolar disorder and alcohol use disorder. Expert Opin Pharmacother. 2022;23(10):1181–93.

66. Naglich A, Adinoff B, Brown ES. Pharmacological treatment of bipolar disorder with comorbid alcohol use disorder. CNS Drugs. 2017;31(8):665–74.
67. Department of Veterans Affairs, Department of Defense. VA/DoD clinical practice guideline for the management of bipolar disorder. Washington, DC: Department of Veterans Affairs; 2023.
68. Robertson S, Peacock EE, Scott R. Benzodiazepine use disorder: common questions and answers. Am Fam Physician. 2023;108(3):260–6.
69. American College of Medical Toxicology; American Society of Addiction Medicine. The joint clinical practice guideline on benzodiazepine tapering: considerations when benzodiazepine risks outweigh benefits. Phoenix: American College of Medical Toxicology; 2024.
70. Salloum IM, Brown ES. Management of comorbid bipolar disorder and substance use disorders. Am J Drug Alcohol Abuse. 2017;43(4):366–76.
71. Coles AS, Sasiadek J, George TP. Pharmacotherapies for co-occurring substance use and bipolar disorders: a systematic review. Bipolar Disord. 2019;21(7):595–610.
72. Patel K, Waldron D, Graziane N. Re-purposing FDA-approved drugs for opioid use disorder. Subst Use Misuse. 2023;58(13):1751–60.
73. Reus VI, Fochtmann LJ, Bukstein O, et al. The American Psychiatric Association practice guideline for the pharmacological treatment of patients with alcohol use disorder. Washington, DC: American Psychiatric Association; 2018.
74. Poorman E, McQuade BM, Messmer S. Medications for alcohol use disorder. Am Fam Physician. 2024;109(1):71–8.
75. Agabio R, Trogu E, Pani PP. Antidepressants for the treatment of people with co-occurring depression and alcohol dependence. Cochrane Database Syst Rev. 2018;4(4):CD008581.
76. Li J, Wang H, Li M, et al. Efficacy of pharmacotherapeutics for patients comorbid with alcohol use disorders and depressive symptoms - a Bayesian network meta-analysis. CNS Neurosci Ther. 2020;26(11):1185–97.
77. Grant S, Azhar G, Han E, et al. Clinical interventions for adults with comorbid alcohol use and depressive disorders: a systematic review and network meta-analysis. PLoS Med. 2021;18(10):e1003822.
78. Park LT, Zarate CA Jr. Depression in the primary care setting. N Engl J Med. 2019;380(6):559–68.
79. Soyka M. Treatment of benzodiazepine dependence. N Engl J Med. 2017;376(12):1147–57.
80. Langlois C, Potvin S, Khullar A, Tourjman SV. Down and high: reflections regarding depression and cannabis. Front Psych. 2021;12:625158.
81. Gorelick DA. Cannabis-related disorders and toxic effects. N Engl J Med. 2023;389(24):2267–75.
82. Kondo KK, Morasco BJ, Nugent SM, Ayers CK, O'Neil ME, Freeman M, Kansagara D. Pharmacotherapy for the treatment of cannabis use disorder: a systematic review. Ann Intern Med. 2020;172(6):398–412.
83. Santo T Jr, Campbell G, Gisev N, et al. Prevalence of mental disorders among people with opioid use disorder: a systematic review and meta-analysis. Drug Alcohol Depend. 2022;238:109551
84. Rosoff DB, Davey Smith G, Lohoff FW. Prescription opioid use and risk for major depressive disorder and anxiety and stress-related disorders: a multivariable Mendelian randomization analysis. JAMA Psychiatry. 2021;78(2):151–60.
85. Na PJ, Scodes J, Fishman M, et al. Co-occurring depression and suicidal ideation in opioid use disorder: prevalence and response during treatment with buprenorphine-naloxone and injection naltrexone. J Clin Psychiatry. 2022;83(3):21m14140.
86. Funk MC, Nash S, Smith A, et al. Treatment of opioid use disorder in the general hospital. Washington, DC: American Psychiatric Association; 2022.
87. Serafini G, Adavastro G, Canepa G, et al. The efficacy of buprenorphine in major depression, treatmentresistant depression and suicidal behavior: a systematic review. Int J Mol Sci. 2018;19(8):2410.

88. Leung J, Mekonen T, Wang X, et al. Methamphetamine exposure and depression - a systematic review and meta-analysis. Drug Alcohol Rev. 2023;42(6):1438–49.
89. Farrell M, Martin NK, Stockings E, et al. Responding to global stimulant use: challenges and opportunities. Lancet. 2019;394(10209):1652–67.
90. Han B, Jones CM, Volkow ND, et al. Prescription stimulant use, misuse, and use disorder among US adults aged 18 to 64 years. JAMA Psychiatry. 2025;82(6):572–81.
91. Hartikainen M, Taipale H, Tanskanen A, et al. Association of pharmacological treatments and hospitalization and death in individuals with amphetamine use disorders in a Swedish nationwide cohort of 13 965 patients. JAMA Psychiatry. 2023;80(1):31–9.
92. Siefried KJ, Acheson LS, Lintzeris N, Ezard N. Pharmacological treatment of methamphetamine/amphetamine dependence: a systematic review. CNS Drugs. 2020;34(4):337–65.
93. American Academy of Addiction Psychiatry. Core competencies for use of collaborative care in the treatment of substance use disorders (guidance). East Providence: American Academy of Addiction Psychiatry; 2024.
94. Hunt GE, Large MM, Cleary M, et al. Prevalence of comorbid substance use in schizophrenia spectrum disorders in community and clinical settings, 1990-2017: systematic review and meta-analysis. Drug Alcohol Depend. 2018;191:234–58.
95. Hartz SM, Pato CN, Medeiros H, et al. Comorbidity of severe psychotic disorders with measures of substance use. JAMA Psychiatry. 2014;71(3):248–54.
96. Myran DT, Harrison LD, Pugliese M, et al. Transition to schizophrenia spectrum disorder following emergency department visits due to substance use with and without psychosis. JAMA Psychiatry. 2023;80(11):1169–74.
97. Chiappini S, Mosca A, Miuli A, et al. Exploring dual diagnoses: psychopathological characteristics in the co-occurrence of schizophrenia and addiction - a scoping review. Psychopathology. 2025;22:1–55. https://doi.org/10.1159/000547322. Epub ahead of print. PMID: 40982399.
98. Osborne KJ, Barch DM, Jackson JJ, Karcher NR. Psychosis spectrum symptoms before and after adolescent cannabis use initiation. JAMA Psychiatry. 2025;82(2):181–90.
99. Martinotti G, Chiappini S, Mosca A, et al. Atypical antipsychotic drugs in dual disorders: current evidence for clinical practice. Curr Pharm Des. 2022;28(27):2259.
100. Krause M, Huhn M, Schneider-Thoma J, et al. Efficacy, acceptability and tolerability of antipsychotics inpatients with schizophrenia and comorbid substance use. A systematic review and meta-analysis. Eur Neuropsychopharmacol. 2019;29(1):32–45.
101. Coles AS, Knezevic D, George TP, et al. Long-acting injectable antipsychotic treatment in schizophrenia and co-occurring substance use disorders: a systematic review. Front Psych. 2021;12:808002.
102. Hunt GE, Siegfried N, Morley K, et al. Psychosocial interventions for people with both severe mental illness and substance misuse. Cochrane Database Syst Rev. 2019;12(12):CD001088.
103. Department of Veterans Affairs, Department of Defense. VA/DoD clinical practice guideline for the management of first-episode psychosis and schizophrenia. Washington, DC: U.S. Government Printing Office; 2023.
104. Siddiqui S, Mehta D, Coles A. Psychosocial interventions for individuals with comorbid psychosis and substance use disorders: systematic review and meta-analysis of randomized studies. Schizophr Bull. 2024;28:sbae101.
105. Shalit N, Rehm J, Lev-Ran S. Epidemiology of hallucinogen use in the U.S.: results from the National Epidemiologic Survey on Alcohol and Related Conditions III. Addict Behav. 2019;89:35–44.
106. Yang KH, Han BH, Palamar JJ. Past-year hallucinogen use in relation to psychological distress, depression, and suicidality among US adults. Addict Behav. 2022;135:107446.
107. Ross-Cypcar SM, Haegele JA, Garcia JM. Hallucinogenic drug use and depression, psychological distress and suicidality among disabled adults in the US. Addict Behav. 2025;160:108170.

108. De Gregorio D, Aguilar-Valles A, Preller KH et al. Hallucinogens in mental health: preclinical and clinical studies on LSD, psilocybin, MDMA, and ketamine. J Neurosci. 2021;41(5):891–900.
109. Yao Y, Guo D, Lu TS, et al. Efficacy and safety of psychedelics for the treatment of mental disorders: a systematic review and meta-analysis. Psychiatry Res. 2024;336:115918.
110. Højlund M, Kafali HY, Kırmızı B, et al. Efficacy, all-cause discontinuation, and safety of serotonergic psychedelics and MDMA to treat mental disorders: a living systematic review with meta-analysis. Eur Neuropsychopharmacol. 2025;90:22–38.
111. Xu KY, Hartz SM, Borodovsky JT, et al. Association between benzodiazepine use with or without opioid use and all-cause mortality in the United States, 1999-2015. JAMA Netw Open. 2020;3(12):e2028557.
112. Back SE, Jarnecke AM, Norman SB, et al. State of the science: treatment of comorbid posttraumatic stress disorder and substance use disorders. J Trauma Stress. 2024;37(6):803–13.
113. Sartor Z, Kelley L, Laschober R. Posttraumatic stress disorder: evaluation and treatment. Am Fam Physician. 2023;107(3):273–81. PMID: 36920821.
114. Persson A, Axén Å, Johansson Capusan A, et al. Concurrent treatment of posttraumatic stress disorder and alcohol use disorder in women: a randomized clinical trial. JAMA Netw Open. 2025;8(7):e2521087.
115. Patton SC, Watkins LE, Killeen TK, Hien DA. Posttraumatic stress disorder and substance use disorder screening, assessment, and treatment. Curr Psychiatry Rep. 2024;26(12):843–51.
116. Danielson CK, Adams Z, McCart MR, et al. Safety and efficacy of exposure-based risk reduction through family therapy for co-occurring substance use problems and posttraumatic stress disorder symptoms among adolescents: a randomized clinical trial. JAMA Psychiatry. 2020;77(6):574–86.
117. Upadhyay J, Verrico CD, Cay M, et al. Neurocircuitry basis of the opioid use disorder-post-traumatic stress disorder comorbid state: conceptual analyses using a dimensional framework. Lancet Psychiatry. 2022;9(1):84–96. https://doi.org/10.1016/S2215-0366(21)00008-0. Epub 2021 Nov 11. Erratum in: Lancet Psychiatry. 2022 Jun;9(6):e23.
118. María-Ríos CE, Morrow JD. Mechanisms of shared vulnerability to post-traumatic stress disorder and substance use disorders. Front Behav Neurosci. 2020;14:6.
119. Dell'Aquila A, Berle D. Predictors of alcohol and substance use among people with post-traumatic stress disorder (PTSD): findings from the NESARC-III study. Soc Psychiatry Psychiatr Epidemiol. 2023;58(10):1509–22.
120. Renaud F, Jakubiec L, Swendsen J, Fatseas M. The impact of co-occurring post-traumatic stress disorder and substance use disorders on craving: a systematic review of the literature. Front Psych. 2021;12:786664.
121. Maercker A, Cloitre M, Bachem R, et al. Complex post-traumatic stress disorder. Lancet.2022;400(10345):60–72.
122. Hien DA, Papini S, Saavedra LM, et al. Project harmony: a systematic review and network meta-analysis of psychotherapy and pharmacologic trials for comorbid posttraumatic stress, alcohol, and other drug use disorders. Psychol Bull. 2024;150(3):319–53.
123. Schnurr PP, Hamblen JL, Wolf J et al. The management of posttraumatic stress disorder and acute stress disorder: synopsis of the 2023 U.S. Department of Veterans Affairs and U.S. Department of Defense clinical practice guideline. Ann Intern Med. 2024;177(3):363–74.
124. Lortye S, Will JP, Marquenie LA, et al. Effectiveness of treating post-traumatic stress disorder in patients with co-occurring substance use disorder with prolonged exposure, eye movement desensitization and reprocessing or imagery rescripting: a randomized controlled trial. Addiction. 2025;120(11):2231–44.
125. Schnurr PP, Hamblen JL, Wolf J, et al. The management of posttraumatic stress disorder and acute stress disorder: synopsis of the 2023 U.S. Department of Veterans Affairs and U.S. Department of Defense clinical practice guideline. Ann Intern Med. 2024;177(3):363–74.
126. Norman SB, Trim R, Haller M, et al. Efficacy of integrated exposure therapy vs integrated coping skills therapy for comorbid posttraumatic stress disorder and alcohol use disorder: a randomized clinical trial. JAMA Psychiatry. 2019;76(8):791–9.

127. Bahji A, Mazhar MN, Hudson CC, et al. Prevalence of substance use disorder comorbidity among individuals with eating disorders: A systematic review and meta-analysis. Psychiatry Res. 2019;273:58–66.
128. Roberts NP, Roberts PA, Jones N, Bisson JI. Psychological interventions for post-traumatic stress disorder and comorbid substance use disorder: a systematic review and meta-analysis. Clin Psychol Rev. 2015;38:25–38.
129. Roberts NP, Roberts PA, Jones N, Bisson JI. Psychological therapies for post-traumatic stress disorder and comorbid substance use disorder. Cochrane Database Syst Rev. 2016;4(4):CD010204.
130. Hien DA, Morgan-López AA, Saavedra LM, et al. Project harmony: a meta-analysis with individual patient data on behavioral and pharmacologic trials for comorbid posttraumatic stress and alcohol or other drug use disorders. Am J Psychiatry. 2023;180(2):155–66.
131. Williams T, Phillips NJ, Stein DJ, Ipser JC. Pharmacotherapy for post traumatic stress disorder (PTSD). Cochrane Database Syst Rev. 2022;3(3):CD002795.
132. Merz J, Schwarzer G, Gerger H. Comparative efficacy and acceptability of pharmacological, psychotherapeutic, and combination treatments in adults with posttraumatic stress disorder: a network meta-analysis. JAMA Psychiatry. 2019;76(9):904–13.
133. Connors NJ, Alsakha A, Larocque A, et al. Antipsychotics for the treatment of sympathomimetic toxicity: a systematic review. Am J Emerg Med. 2019;37(10):1880–90.
134. Haber PS. Identification and treatment of alcohol use disorder. N Engl J Med. 2025;392(3):258–66.
135. Stetsiv K, McNamara IA, Nance M, Carpenter RW. The co-occurrence of personality disorders and substance use disorders. Curr Psychiatry Rep. 2023;25(11):625–36.
136. Smith NDL, Cottler LB. What's old is new again: updated findings on personality disorders and substance use disorders. Curr Opin Psychiatry. 2019;32(6):532–9.
137. Sharp C, Wall K. Personality disorders. N Engl J Med. 2022;387(10):916–23.
138. Skodol AE, Oldham JM, Gallaher PE. Axis II comorbidity of substance use disorders among patients referred for treatment of personality disorders. Am J Psychiatry. 1999;156(5):733–8.
139. Grant BF, Saha TD, Ruan WJ, et al. Epidemiology of DSM-5 drug use disorder: results from the National Epidemiologic Survey on alcohol and related conditions–III. JAMA Psychiatry. 2016;73(1):39–47.
140. Castillo-Carniglia A, Keyes KM, Hasin DS, Cerdá M. Psychiatric comorbidities in alcohol use disorder. Lancet Psychiatry. 2019;6(12):1068–80.
141. Helle AC, Watts AL, Trull TJ, Sher KJ. Alcohol use disorder and antisocial and borderline personality disorders. Alcohol Res. 2019;40(1):arcr.v40.1.05.
142. Long EC, Aggen SH, Neale MC, et al. The association between personality disorders with alcohol use and misuse: a population-based twin study. Drug Alcohol Depend. 2017;174:174–80.
143. Blay M, Verne M, Durpoix A, et al. Clinical specificities of patients with substance use disorder and comorbid borderline personality disorder compared to patients with substance use disorder only: a retrospective study. J Addict Dis. 2025;43(3):225–31.
144. Bohus M, Stoffers-Winterling J, Sharp C, et al. Borderline personality disorder. Lancet. 2021;398(10310):1528–40.
145. Stoffers-Winterling JM, Storebø OJ, Kongerslev MT, et al. Psychotherapies for borderline personality disorder: a focused systematic review and meta-analysis. Br J Psychiatry. 2022;221(6):728–41.
146. Leichsenring F, Heim N, Leweke F, et al. Borderline personality disorder: a review. JAMA. 2023;329(8):670–9.
147. Buono FD, Larkin K, Rowe D, et al. Intensive Dialectical Behavior Treatment for Individuals With Borderline Personality Disorder With and Without Substance Use Disorders. Front Psychol. 2021 Aug 23;12:629842.
148. Cohen D, Lau K, Lau S. Effect of psychotherapy on patients with borderline personality disorder. Am Fam Physician. 2022;106(6):715–6.
149. Warner N, Murphy M. Dialectical behaviour therapy skills training for individuals with substance use disorder: a systematic review. Drug Alcohol Rev. 2022;41(4):711–28.

150. Lee NK, Cameron J, Jenner L. A systematic review of interventions for co-occurring substance use and borderline personality disorders. Drug Alcohol Rev. 2015;34(6):663–72.
151. Atkinson T, Baldridge C, Burden J, et al. Management of substance use disorder. Washington, DC: Department of Veterans Affairs(US); 2021:1–36.
152. Tiglao SM, Meisenheimer ES, Oh RC. Alcohol withdrawal syndrome: outpatient management. Am Fam Physician. 2021;104(3):253–62.
153. Brunner E, Chen CA, Klein T, et al. Clinical Guideline Committee (CGC) Members; ASAM Staff and Contractors. Joint Clinical Practice Guideline on Benzodiazepine Tapering: Considerations When Risks Outweigh Benefits. J Gen Intern Med. 2025;40(12):2814–59.
154. Shuey B, Anderson TS, Park TW. Implementing benzodiazepine deprescribing in the primary care clinic. JAMA Intern Med. 2026;186(1):120–1.
155. Cleary M, Hunt GE, Matheson S, Walter G. Psychosocial treatments for people with co-occurring severe mental illness and substance misuse: systematic review. J Adv Nurs. 2009;65(2):238–58.
156. Satre DD, Parthasarathy S, Young-Wolff KC et al. Cost-effectiveness of motivational interviewing to reduce alcohol and cannabis use among patients with depression. J Stud Alcohol Drugs. 2022;83(5):662–71.
157. Buckner JD. Motivational interviewing-based interventions with patients with comorbid anxiety and substance use disorders. Curr Opin Psychol. 2024;60:101934.
158. Arias-Reynoso M, Bell JL, Blueford P, et al. Management of first-episode psychosis and schizophrenia (SCZ). Washington, DC: Department of Veterans Affairs (US); 2023.
159. Gibson E, Lien J, Manages S, et al. Engagement and retention of nonabstinent patients in substance use treatment: clinical consideration for addiction treatment providers. Rockville: American Society of Addiction Medicine; 2024.
160. Schwenker R, Dietrich CE, Hirpa S, et al. Motivational interviewing for substance use reduction. Cochrane Database Syst Rev. 2023;12(12):CD008063.
161. Magill M, Helminen EC, Lynch-Gadaleta B, et al. Cognitive-behavioral interventions for co-occurring substance use and mental health disorders. Drug Alcohol Depend. 2025.
162. Mehta K, Hoadley A, Ray LA, et al. Cognitive-behavioral interventions targeting alcohol or other drug use and co-occurring mental health disorders: a meta-analysis. Alcohol Alcohol. 2021;56(5):535–44.
163. Hides L, Quinn C, Stoyanov S, et al. Psychological interventions for co-occurring depression and substance use disorders. Cochrane Database Syst Rev. 2019;2019(11).
164. Magill M, Ray L, Kiluk B, et al. A meta-analysis of cognitive-behavioral therapy for alcohol or other drug use disorders: treatment efficacy by contrast condition. J Consult Clin Psychol. 2019;87(12):1093–105.
165. Ray LA, Meredith LR, Kiluk BD, et al. Combined pharmacotherapy and cognitive behavioral therapy for adults with alcohol or substance use disorders: a systematic review and meta-analysis. JAMA Netw Open. 2020.
166. Brasel KJ, deRoon-Cassini TA, Bernard A, et al. Best practices guidelines screening and intervention for mental health disorders and substance use and misuse in the acute trauma patient. Chicago: American College of Surgeons; 2022.
167. Mefodeva V, Carlyle M, Walter Z, Hides L. Client and staff perceptions of the integration of trauma informed care and specialist posttraumatic stress disorder treatment in residential treatment facilities for substance use: A qualitative study. Drug Alcohol Rev. 2023;42(1):181–92.
168. Mueser KT, Glynn SM, Cather C, et al. A randomized controlled trial of family intervention for co-occurring substance use and severe psychiatric disorders. Schizophr Bull. 2013;39(3):658–72.
169. Esteban J, Suárez-Relinque C, Jiménez TI. Effects of family therapy for substance abuse: a systematic review of recent research. Fam Process. 2023;62(1):49–73.
170. Majer JM, Jason LA, Bobak TJ. An examination of abstinence social support among recovery home residents with psychiatric comorbidity. Drug Alcohol Depend. 2021;228:108971.
171. Luchenski S, Maguire N, Aldridge RW, et al. What works in inclusion health: overview of effective interventions for marginalised and excluded populations. Lancet. 2018;391(10117):266–80.

172. Horsfall J, Cleary M, Hunt GE, Walter G. Psychosocial treatments for people with co-occurring severe mental illnesses and substance use disorders (dual diagnosis): a review of empirical evidence. Harv Rev Psychiatry. 2009;17(1):24–34.
173. Attia E, Walsh BT. Eating disorders: a review. JAMA. 2025;333(14):1242–52.
174. Gregorowski C, Seedat S, Jordaan GP. A clinical approach to the assessment and management of co-morbid eating disorders and substance use disorders. BMC Psychiatry. 2013;13:289.
175. American Psychiatric Association. American Psychiatric Association practice guideline for the treatment of patients with eating disorders. Washington, DC: American Psychiatric Association; 2023.
176. Xi ZX, Galaj E. Novel potential pharmacological approaches in treating eating disorders comorbid with substance use disorders. Biomed Pharmacother. 2025;189:118327.
177. Rodan SC, Maguire S, Meez N, et al. Prescription and nonprescription drug use among people with eating disorders. JAMA Netw Open. 2025;8(7):e2522406.
178. Ward ZJ, Rodriguez P, Wright DR, Austin SB, Long MW. Estimation of eating disorders prevalence by age and associations with mortality in a simulated nationally representative US cohort. JAMA Netw Open. 2019;2(10):e1912925.
179. Grilo CM. Treatment of eating disorders: current status, challenges, and future directions. Annu Rev Clin Psychol. 2024;20:97–123.
180. Grilo CM. Interventions for weight management in binge-eating disorder: current findings and issues. Curr Psychiatry Rep. 2025;27:572–83.
181. Grilo CM, Ivezaj V, Yurkow S, Tek C, Gueorguieva R. Cognitive-behavioral therapy and lisdexamfetamine, alone and combined, for binge-eating disorder: secondary outcomes of a randomized controlled trial. Int J Eat Disord. 2025;58:1970–8.
182. Kwan I, Burchett HED, Macdowall W, D'Souza P, Stansfield C, Kneale D, Sutcliffe K. How effective are remote and/or digital interventions as part of alcohol and drug treatment and recovery support? A systematic review and meta-analysis. Addiction. 2025.
183. Perry C, Liberto J, Milliken C, et al. The management of substance use disorders: synopsis of the 2021 U.S. Department of Veterans Affairs and U.S. Department of Defense clinical practice guideline. Ann Intern Med. 2022;175(2):ITC33–48.
184. Ramadas E, de Lima MP, Caetano T, Lopes J, Dixe MDACR. Effectiveness of smartphone interventions as continuing care for substance use disorders: A systematic review. Acta Psychol (Amst). 2023;240:104046.
185. Schouten MJE, Christ C, Dekker JJM, Riper H, Goudriaan AE, Blankers M. Digital interventions for people with co-occurring depression and problematic alcohol use: a systematic review and meta-analysis. Alcohol Alcohol. 2022;57(4):423–32.
186. Holmes NA, van Agteren JE, Dorstyn DS. A systematic review of technology-assisted interventions for co-morbid depression and substance use. J Telemed Telecare. 2019;25(3):131–46.
187. O'Donnell A, Schmidt CS, Beyer F, et al. Effectiveness of digital interventions for people with comorbid heavy drinking and depression: a systematic review and narrative synthesis. J Affect Disord. 2022;298(Pt A):315–26.
188. Pham H, Lin C, Zhu Y, et al. Telemedicine-delivered treatment for substance use disorder: a scoping review. J Telemed Telecare. 2025.
189. Manning V, Whelan D, Piercy H. The current evidence for substance use disorder apps. Curr Opin Psychiatry. 2022;35(4):325–32.
190. Taylor CB, Graham AK, Flatt RE, et al. Current state of scientific evidence on internet-based interventions for the treatment of depression, anxiety, eating disorders and substance abuse: an overview of systematic reviews and meta-analyses. Eur J Public Health. 2021;31(Suppl 1):i3-i10. https://doi.org/10.1093/eurpub/ckz208. Erratum in: Eur J Public Health. 2021;7;31(Supplement_1):i94. https://doi.org/10.1093/eurpub/ckab104. PMID: 32918448; PMCID: PMC8495688.

Part IV

Other Topics

Prevention, Public Health, and Public Policy

23

María Luisa Zúñiga, Sarah A. Rojas, Victor Manuel Magaña, and Nafisa Ferdous

High-Yield Review Points

- Prevention of substance use disorders (SUDs) applies research-driven interventions and policies that target individual-level and community-level factors that can be modified to decrease risky substance use behavior that may lead to a substance use disorder.
- There are three general types of prevention in public health: Primary prevention, which seeks to stop problems before they start; secondary prevention, which focuses on early detection and intervention; and tertiary prevention, which manages existing conditions to minimize harm.

M. L. Zúñiga (✉) · V. M. Magaña
San Diego State University, School of Social Work, Joint Doctoral Program in Interdisciplinary Research on Substance Use, San Diego, CA, USA
e-mail: mlzuniga@sdsu.edu

S. A. Rojas
San Ysidro Health San Diego, San Diego, CA, USA
e-mail: sarah.rojas@syhealth.org

N. Ferdous
San Diego State University, School of Social Work, Joint Doctoral Program in Interdisciplinary Research on Substance Use, San Diego, CA, USA

Thirdhand Smoke Resource Center, San Diego State University, San Diego, CA, USA
e-mail: nferdous@sdsu.edu

C. Marienfeld, M. Soltani (eds.), *AAAP Review of Addiction Psychiatry*,
https://doi.org/10.1007/978-3-032-24174-0_23

- Public health allows us to identify, understand, and reduce high-risk drug-using behaviors, promote SUD screening and treatment, and address underlying factors that may contribute to the societal burden of addiction, including poverty, stigma and discrimination, health inequities, and inadequate access to medication treatment.
- Public policy involves regulations, rules, and laws designed to achieve a public benefit through shaping or controlling drug availability, access, and use, and environmental factors that shape access and use.

Introduction

The addiction psychiatrist is well positioned to advocate for and influence prevention addiction-related public health efforts and policies to prevent substance use disorders and improve treatment outcomes at community and population levels. In this chapter, we describe approaches that clinicians can use to leverage their power to impact community health through prevention, public health, and policy. We frame prevention, public health, and public policy as interrelated approaches to reduce the societal impact and burden of substance use disorders.

Prevention

Prevention is a core health principle and clinical approach to avert or decrease the likelihood of a poor health outcome. Prevention traditionally has been conceptualized into three categories: primary, secondary, and tertiary. Primary prevention involves interventions to prevent substance use disorders, while secondary prevention focuses on screening, managing comorbidities, and reducing complications in individuals who may not be ready for medication-assisted treatment. Tertiary prevention includes efforts aimed at improving quality of life, reducing disease progression, and aiding symptom management. In this chapter, we will consider these avenues of prevention and clinical and nonclinical approaches to reducing the burden of substance use disorders at individual, community, and population levels.

Public Health

Public health refers to the discipline of promoting health and well-being within a population through efforts that target individual, community, societal, environmental, and policy levels. Public health is founded on research to understand and reduce factors that undermine health and promote factors that favor good health. Public health operates at local, regional, national, and global scales that require integrated approaches and transdisciplinary collaboration. Prevention is a key tenet of public health. Public health promotes the best health of a community or population through scaling up and disseminating evidence-based interventions such as medication treatment for opioid use disorder. Public health also involves interventions designed to address root causes of disease and poor health, including *social determinants of health*, which are factors such as poverty and inadequate access to health care. Public health and clinical research together develop, evaluate, and disseminate effective interventions to reduce the burden of SUDs and to promote best health and recovery in a manner that is best suited for the needs of individuals and their communities.

Public Policy

Public policy refers to principles that form the basis for organizational or governmental rules, regulations, and laws that shape and guide individual and organizational behavior. Its primary purpose is to encourage actions that benefit the public. This chapter focuses on public policy within the context of public health for SUDs, specifically policies designed to influence substance use behavior, treatment, and drug availability (commonly referred to as drug policies). The development of public policies is a complex process shaped by societal expectations, perceptions, economic goals, and political interest. Addiction psychiatrists play a vital role in shaping substance use treatment policies by ensuring they are grounded in scientific research and evidence. Policies informed by scientific evidence tend to lead to better health outcomes and are often referred to as "evidence-based" policies [1]. This evidence-based approach parallels clinical treatments and interventions, which are evaluated for their efficacy (short-term impact) and effectiveness (long-term impact) to ensure positive health outcomes.

Prevention, public health, and public policy are interrelated and complementary approaches to reduce the burden of substance use and misuse and addiction rather than discrete, independent topics. Because stigma and discrimination against persons who use drugs are common and undermine prevention and public health treatment and recovery efforts, this chapter will also include brief discussion of stigma in healthcare settings. We also describe opportunities for clinician leadership in prevention, public health, and policy to reduce stigmatizing attitudes and policies that pose serious risk to effective treatment and recovery of persons suffering from SUDs.

Prevention

In public health, prevention is broadly defined as activities aimed at reducing or eliminating the risk of negative or worsening health outcomes. These efforts can target different levels, including individuals, families, communities, and societies, where behaviors and environmental or contextual and factors influence substance use risk and the potential for dependence. Prevention activities may include a variety of approaches, such as educational programs (e.g., classroom instruction, peer-led initiatives, and parenting education), the development and enforcement of effective public health policies, and evidence-based interventions (e.g., school programs designed to reduce adolescent depression or substance use). Additionally, behavioral and medical treatments can support prevention by promoting health and reducing likelihood of misuse or progression to substance use disorders. Prevention efforts can be initiated by individuals to improve their own health or by professionals, such as clinicians and organizations, to address broader public health concerns. These activities take place in diverse settings, including clinical practices, schools, and community environments. The public health model categorizes prevention into three types: primary prevention, which seeks to stop problems before they start; secondary prevention, which focuses on early detection and intervention; and tertiary prevention, which manages existing conditions to minimize harm. Many prevention efforts, however, combine elements from these categories, creating an integrated approach rather than treating them as separate stages.

Primary Prevention

Primary prevention involves activities that promote health and reduce the risk of individuals or groups engaging in harmful substance use or progressing from experimentation to a substance use disorder. Primary prevention efforts frequently target youth to support early adoption of healthy behaviors for lifelong positive health outcomes.

Examples of primary prevention activities help illustrate how prevention works at the individual level. These may include clinical interventions, such as a clinician offering anticipatory guidance to an adolescent or parent about the risks of youth experimenting with marijuana. For an adolescent who has not experimented with marijuana or reports minimal experimentation, a prevention approach may involve the clinician using motivational interviewing techniques to encourage the adolescent to identify personal reasons for abstaining from use and strategies for resisting peer pressure that support their decision. Interventions like *Project Chill* offer the primary care specialist the utility of a computer-based program that has been shown effective at lowering marijuana use among adolescents in urban health centers. Another example of primary prevention is clinician efforts to adopt opioid prescribing guidelines and pain management strategies that reduce the risk of a person developing an opioid use disorder.

Primary prevention also includes group- or societal-level efforts, such as public health policies effective in reducing risky substance use behavior. For instance, one well-studied policy shown to reduce alcohol-related harms among adolescents is the enforcement of age restriction laws that limit youth access to alcohol.

Secondary Prevention

Secondary prevention involves timely screening, diagnosis, and treatment of a disease or disorder. The objective in secondary prevention in addiction is diagnosis and treatment before progression to the life-threatening events [2]. Approaches to secondary prevention may include screening, brief intervention, and referral to treatment (SBIRT) with populations who may be at heightened risk for substance use disorders, including those served at HIV care clinics. Expansion of access to treatment for substance use disorders (e.g., continuing medical education in clinical management of substance use and addiction and expanded third-party payer coverage) will also support secondary prevention efforts to screen and treat persons with substance use disorders [2].

Tertiary Prevention

Tertiary prevention involves managing and reducing the symptoms of chronic disease and co-occurring problems, including prevention of life-threatening adverse outcomes. An example of tertiary prevention includes harm reduction approaches, defined below, such as providing naloxone to prevent death from opioid overdose to individuals who may or may not be receiving treatment for their substance use disorder [2, 6]. Provision of naloxone to others with whom individuals at risk for overdose live or spend time with is also an important part of supporting persons who are living with or in recovery from opioid use disorders. This can be expanded further by providing naloxone and appropriate training to law officers and emergency response personnel. Within tertiary prevention we may also consider relapse prevention and recovery support activities that can improve an individual's ability to manage their substance use disorder symptoms and related problems to achieve and maintain optimal health and well-being.

Prevention Through Harm Reduction

Harm reduction refers to a set of strategies and approaches designed to reduce negative consequences of drug use, especially for persons who are not ready to seek or interested in treatment. One example of harm reduction is the evidence-based public health practice of making sterile syringes available to persons who inject drugs [12]. The significance of this single intervention is that it (a) reduces the likelihood that the person who injects drugs will transmit or acquire a virus such as Hepatitis C or HIV, (b) respects the person's autonomy by leaving them in control of their use while offering treatment options and safer means to use, and (c) can meaningfully reduce stigma associated with injection drug use by providing a nonjudgmental environment where persons who are not yet ready to quit can more safely manage their use [12]. Sterile syringe exchange programs are an example of *primary prevention*, as they help stop the spread of infectious diseases by reducing syringe-sharing. Since the person may already have a substance use disorder, then we could also consider a sterile syringe program as a *secondary prevention* approach when, for example, HIV or Hepatitis C testing and treatment are also provided. This same intervention could be considered *tertiary prevention* when the availability of sterile syringes is also reducing the likelihood that the individual's chronic condition (e.g., SUD or Hepatitis C) will be exacerbated by acquisition of yet another condition, such as HIV [12]. Harm reduction strategies, like sterile syringes programs, demonstrate how primary, secondary, and tertiary prevention efforts often overlap and work together to improve public health outcomes.

Public Health

Public health is a multidisciplinary and interdisciplinary field that uses research, practice and policy approaches, strategies, methodologies, and interventions to promote best health and well-being at a population level. Public health is also devoted to understanding and addressing societal, contextual, and environmental factors that undermine health and those factors that favor resilience, good health outcomes, and well-being. The Centers for Disease Control (CDC) and World Health Organization (WHO) characterize ten essential public health services that comprise the overarching roles and activities of the field of public health (https://www.cdc.gov/publichealthgateway/publichealthservices/pdf/ten_essential_services_and_sdoh.pdf). The following section outlines the ten essential public health services, highlighting their relevance to substance use, misuse, and addiction. Additionally, we present an overview of a public health strategy implemented to reduce Hepatitis C in New York City [5].

Ten Essential Services of Public Health

On a global and national scale, there is general concordance in what constitutes public health services and corresponding activities. In each service category we provide an example of what this service would look like in a substance use or addiction context.

1. *Surveillance*: Monitor health indicators to identify and address community health problems.
2. *Identify and Investigate*: Identify and investigate population-level health problems, address their root causes, and propose actions to eliminate them.
3. *Health Promotion*: Empower individuals to improve their health, protect public health through services like free or low-cost Hepatitis A vaccinations, and to provide timely, accurate information to educate the public about health issues affecting them, their families, and their communities.
4. *Disease Prevention*: This includes
   (a) *Primary prevention*: strategies to prevent poor health outcomes, such as cannabis laws that reduce youth access.

   (b) *Secondary prevention*: strategies to promote screening and treatment. This may include expanded access to medication for opioid use disorder.
   (c) *Tertiary prevention*: providing services to manage chronic conditions and prevent further harms to health, such as sterile syringes for people who inject drugs to prevent Hepatitis C or HIV, or using fentanyl test strips as a strategy to avoid opioid overdose where individuals who use substances may be made aware of whether their substance may contain fentanyl.
5. *Community Mobilization and Engagement*: Build partnerships between public health organizations and communities to increase responsiveness and involvement in solving public health problems.
6. *Policy Development*: Create polices based on research and program evaluation to protect public health, such as protocols to prevent needle-stick injury among healthcare professionals and Hepatitis A vaccination guidelines.
7. *Policy Enforcement*: Ensure compliance with national or state public health recommendations and laws, like mandatory registration in state Prescription Drug Monitoring Programs (PDMP) for prescribers and/or pharmacists.
8. *Linking the Public to Health Services*: Increase public awareness of available health services and ensure equitable access.
9. *Public Health Infrastructure*: Develop and maintain robust organizational structures and a well-trained public health workforce to meet public health needs.
10. *Research*: Conduct studies to understand health outcomes, identify trends (e.g., changes in types of drugs that contribute to overdose deaths in the United States over time), develop interventions (e.g., scaling up naloxone availability to prevent overdose deaths), and evaluate the effectiveness of current public health initiatives, like PDMP in reducing new cases of opioid use disorder.

Case Example: Public Health Strategy to Reduce Transmission of Hepatitis C in New York City [5]

Given that Hepatitis C virus (HCV) transmission in the United States is driven largely by lack of access to and low use of clean syringes and injection equipment among persons who inject drugs, public health efforts are well positioned to reduce and eliminate HCV transmission. Let us consider a public health approach using the ten-principle public health services to consider how HCV transmission can be reduced and stopped.

Public health *Surveillance* of new HCV cases (i.e., incidence) allows local, state, and national bodies to monitor changes in new cases over time as well as changes in HCV genotypes that may warrant changes in treatment protocols. By *identifying and investigating* HCV transmission, we can determine which populations are most affected (e.g., persons who inject drugs, homeless individuals), uncover factors contributing to transmission (e.g., limited access to sterile injection equipment), and address barriers to reducing HCV such as the lack of sterile syringe programs (SSP), inadequate political or social support, and stigma toward people who inject drugs. Effective *Health Promotion* efforts to reduce transmission include timely and accurate information about HCV prevention and treatment to educate key populations as well as efforts to reduce stigmatizing attitudes among clinicians and the public. In a systematic review of studies investigating stigmatizing attitudes among healthcare professionals, study authors found that some providers hold negative attitudes toward patients with SUD including perceptions that persons who use illicit substances may be violent, manipulative, or unmotivated to change the behavior [13]. The study also found that perceived discrimination from healthcare professionals has led to discontinuation of treatment among individuals with SUD [13]. *Disease prevention* strategies and activities to prevent behaviors or conditions that lead to transmission could include increased availability of SSP (i.e., primary prevention) and expanded testing and treatment for HCV among key populations (secondary prevention). Treatment of substance use disorder among key populations is also a form of secondary prevention and may include medications such as buprenorphine and methadone for treatment of opioid use disorder. *Community mobilization and engagement* to reduce HCV transmission include involvement of substance-using communities to provide recommendations on reducing their barriers to HCV treatment and related clinical care and services. Local, state, and national *policy development and enforcement* is needed to reduce barriers to availability of SSP and other effective public health measures (e.g., safe injection facilities) that could further reduce transmission and increase access to treatment. Activities that could increase access to treatment, *linking the public to health services*, could include, for example, outreach workers who can work with key populations in settings where they can be more effectively reached (e.g., street-based settings). Efforts to increase *public health infrastructure and workforce capacity* could include educational efforts to reduce stigmatizing attitudes among clinicians and staff that may undermine treatment efficacy or adherence. *Research* can serve to inform the types of interventions that may be needed for specific subpopulations at risk for HCV, including efforts to promote optimal adherence to treatment for increasing successful HCV cure rate.

Public Health Conclusions

Public health approaches play a crucial role in reducing the societal burden of substance misuse and substance use disorders through integrated, multidisciplinary, and comprehensive approaches to substance use problems and, importantly, the root factors that may contribute to development of problematic use and addiction. Clinicians are well positioned to play an important role in wider public health efforts through many avenues, including advocacy for policy changes and increased access to medication treatment.

Public Policy

Public policy refers to agency and governmental guidelines, regulations, and laws that are designed to influence behavior of individuals and groups to reduce negative health outcomes, societal problems, and costs to society. Policies can be regional, state, or federal, can change considerably over time, and span a broad spectrum of influences and contexts. For example, US clinical drug access and availability, access and availability of treatment for disorders, and laws that govern availability of substances or criminalize the possession or use of substances have changed substantially over time. In this section, we will focus on recent health policies that impact substance use treatment access and availability.

Substance Use Treatment Access and Expansion Policies

There are several federal laws that have influenced access to substance use disorder treatment. For example, the *Affordable Care Act 2010* [10] is an example of movement toward reforming health care as well as access to treatment for substance use disorders. In 2010, the Affordable Care Act was enacted by the US government to increase health insurance coverage for individuals, families, and small business owners. The Affordable Care Act also includes a provision on prevention, early intervention, and treatment of substance use disorders and mental health problems as an "essential health benefit" [10]. Another federal law designed to target substance use treatment is the *Mental Health Parity and Addiction Equity Act of* 2008 that requires insurance groups that provide health coverage to make benefits for substance use and/or mental health disorders no more restrictive than benefits offered for other medical care [10]. To address the concern around underage drinking, the *Sober Truth on Preventing Underage Drinking Act (STOP Act)* of 2006 was authorized by the US federal government. Nationwide, the STOP Act provides additional funds to grantees under the Drug Free Communities Act of 1997 to prevent and reduce alcohol use among youth ages 12–20 years [10].

In the face of longstanding opioid misuse in the United States, federal legislation, regulation, and guidelines for Opioid Treatment Program (OTP) and Medication Treatment (MT) (formerly Medication-Assisted Treatment [MAT]) have been developed. SAMSHA's Division of Pharmacologic Therapies (DPT), which is a part of SAMHSA Center for Substance Abuse Treatment (CSAT), together with the Drug Enforcement Administration (DEA) supervise the standards and certification process for OTPs and regulate certain medications used in MT. The *Controlled Substance Act* governs medication used in MT and includes drug policy on regulation of manufacture, importation, possession, use, and distribution of controlled substances [9] OTPs provide MT for individuals diagnosed with an opioid use disorder (OUD) with the goal of reducing, preventing, or eliminating use of illicit opioids (such as heroin or fentanyl) and provide a safe and controlled level of medications like methadone, buprenorphine, and naltrexone to stop or reduce the use of non-therapeutic opioids.

The *Drug Addiction Treatment Act of* 2000 *(DATA* 2000*)* allows clinical practitioners to treat OUD with Schedule III, IV, and V medications or combinations of such medications that have received FDA approval for those conditions. Currently the only approved medication for this is the Schedule III drug buprenorphine. This Act also allowed physicians to obtain a waiver from the separate registration requirements of the *Narcotic Addict Treatment ACT* 1974 [9].

Since DATA 2000 act, new policies that eliminate the need for a waiver to treat persons with a substance use disorder have been enacted through the Consolidated Appropriations Act of 2023, signed into law on December 29, 2022 [14]. The key provisions that dismantled the waiver system are found within two specific sections of the omnibus spending bill:

The Mainstreaming Addiction Treatment (MAT) Act: Section 1262 of the Consolidated Appropriations Act, 2023, officially repealed the section of the Controlled Substances Act that mandated the waiver. This means that any practitioner with a standard Drug Enforcement Administration (DEA) registration to prescribe schedule III-controlled substances can now prescribe buprenorphine for OUD, subject to state laws [15].

The Medication Access and Training Expansion (MATE) Act: While the MAT Act eliminated the waiver, Section 1263 of the same appropriations bill introduced a new, one-time training requirement for all DEA-registered practitioners (except veterinarians) who prescribe any controlled substances. This provision mandates that prescribers complete 8 hours of training on identifying and managing patients with substance use disorders, including opioid use disorder, before obtaining or renewing their DEA registration. This training requirement went into effect on June 27, 2023 [15].

Opioid Treatment Program (OTP) regulations such as *Certification of Opioid Treatment Programs* and the 42 *Code of Federal Regulations (CFR) Part* 8 are behind the accreditation and certification of services for OTPs, with supervision from SAMSHA. It regulates use of narcotic drugs to treat opioid dependency [9]. 42 *CFR Part* 2 of the regulation protects patient confidentiality via restrictions in use and disclosure of patient information related to substance use treatment [9].

In 2015, *Federal Guidelines for Opioid Treatment Programs* were established. These guidelines help accrediting programs prepare for and meet accreditation standards for opioid treatment and provide guidance and information on how programs can meet federal regulations and maintain compliance. The 2015 guidelines were an update from 2007 *Guidelines for the Accreditation of Opioid Treatment Programs* [9].

Methadone Policy Updates

Recent policy changes, driven by lessons from the COVID-19 pandemic, have significantly altered methadone prescribing regulations to increase access and flexibility. In February 2024, the Department of Health and Human Services and SAMHSA issued a final rule that permanently codified and expanded many of the pandemic-era methadone take-home flexibilities. This new rule, the first major update to

Opioid Treatment Program (OTP) regulations (42 CFR Part 8) in over two decades, allows for greater clinical discretion in providing multiple take-home doses of methadone earlier in treatment, authorizes the use of telehealth for patient evaluations, and removes the requirement for a one-year history of addiction prior to admission, all aiming to reduce treatment barriers and promote patient-centered care [16, 17].

Public Health Success Story: Naloxone Access and Expansion Policies

Naloxone is an opioid agonist medication that reverses the effect of opioid overdose and reduces the likelihood of death [4]. It is a harm reduction approach and form of *tertiary prevention* since it is given to reduce fatalities among individuals who have overdosed from an opioid such as fentanyl. Naloxone and policies that expand naloxone access are hailed as key components of a public health success story because of their role in reducing deaths from opioid overdose, especially when coupled with overdose education, increased access to medication for opioid use disorder and recovery supports [18, 19].

In 2024, the United States saw its first decrease in opioid overdose deaths since 2019; this represents a 27% reduction in deaths in 2023 [20]. Policy changes to improve naloxone access and availability in the United States have played an important role in reducing overdose deaths and have received growing recognition from policymakers, substance use researchers, clinicians, public health advocates, and impacted communities alike. Below we examine changes in naloxone prescribing and access policies that have allowed this life-saving medication to reach more individuals at risk for an opioid overdose.

Naloxone access laws vary from state to state and by jurisdiction. As of January 2023, all 50 states, the District of Columbia and all U.S. territories have naloxone access laws and related immunity protections, with some states having enacted laws since the early 2000s [4, 18]. Policy research on factors that reduce opioid overdose deaths that variations in naloxone access policies, including state-level variations in Medicaid policy, play a role in reducing barriers to naloxone [18]. The following examples are key to reduce barriers and improve access to naloxone: co-prescription of naloxone with an opioid prescription, not needing to show an identification to obtain naloxone, policies that expand access through pharmacies and community-based agencies, federal funding to purchase naloxone, and expanded naloxone distribution infrastructure [18].

Currently 33 states have a statewide standing order for naloxone [4] meaning that naloxone can be made available, under a pre-approved prescription, to anyone who is at risk for an opioid overdose or may know someone at risk, which forgoes the need for clinicians to prescribe naloxone directly to patients [21]. The *Naloxone Access: Summary of State Laws* report, developed and updated by the Legislative Analysis and Public Policy Association (LAPPA), provides a summary of naloxone access laws by state, including who is able to prescribe, dispense, or administer naloxone; types of immunity granted to them (e.g., immunity for prescribes or Good Samaritan laws that protect someone who administers naloxone in good faith); co-prescription requirements (e.g., prescribing naloxone to a patient who is also prescribed opioid therapy); insurer requirements and school-based naloxone availability [4]. In March 2023, the Food and Drug Administration approved naloxone nasal spray for over the counter, nonprescription, use, which further increased access to naloxone across the United States [22].

In summary, expanded naloxone access is an evidence-based intervention, that when coupled with overdose education, improved treatment engagement in MOUD, and treatment retention, contribute to short and long-term major reductions in opioid overdose deaths [19]. As of this writing, proposed U.S. federal government budget cuts that may drastically reduce funding for critical public health efforts such naloxone distribution and access to life-saving treatment for OUD will undermine progress. Realized and proposed cuts include defunding the Substance Abuse and Mental Health Services Administration, substantial funding reduction for NIH, and other federal agencies, and cuts to Medicaid programs. Additional proposed cuts will result in reduced access to naloxone and treatment for opioid use disorder and undermine evidence-based public health efforts that led to a 27% reduction of opioid overdose deaths observed in the United States in 2024 [20, 23].

Public Policy Conclusions

Substance-use-related public policies are broad in scope, and some will directly influence clinician prescribing behavior and patient access to evidence-based harm reduction strategies and treatment. Physicians and professional organizations play a critical role in advocating for acceleration and adoption of public policies, as well as actively participating in the research process and public health efforts to reduce the burden of substance use disorders at individual, community, and societal levels.

Conclusion

This chapter was designed to expand the clinician's concept of substance use prevention and policy by introducing a public health perspective on substance use and related diseases. The chapter highlighted the various levels at which prevention efforts can take place (i.e., individual, community, and policy) and the various points of intervention within each level. The public health perspective highlights how the integration and harmonization of epidemiological and health behavior findings can identify and leverage actions that can be taken by the clinician to reduce the societal burden of addiction. Finally, we present policy-level efforts at controlling use of and access to substances, harm reduction, and treatment, and how these efforts influence community- and individual-level factors and population-level health. With this knowledge, we understand that substance use interventions require complementary and transdisciplinary approaches. A public health perspective highlights the complex landscape of substance use and comorbidities where clinicians, researchers, and policymakers can play significant roles to prevent, address, and reduce the burden of substance use, misuse, and addiction and intervene at key points throughout the course of addiction.

Chapter Review Questions

1. Naloxone, an effective medication for reversal of opioid overdose, is more widely available to the public. Universities are providing it at no cost in vending machines. A 20-year-old student whose roommate uses opioids obtained naloxone from the university vending machine. They also participated in the university's naloxone training. Wider availability of and training individuals in the administration of Naloxone are examples of _______ prevention.

   A. Primary
   B. Primary AND secondary
   C. Secondary
   D. Secondary AND tertiary
   E. Tertiary

   Answer: E

   Explanation: For substance use disorders and addiction, expanding harm reduction services to prevent life-threatening adverse outcomes among persons who use opioids is tertiary prevention. Primary prevention is reducing the need to use substances, controlling access to substances, and promoting protective factors. Secondary prevention is diagnosing and treating substance use disorders.

   Reference: Butler et al. [2]

2. As part of fellowship training, you provide opioid overdose prevention patient education in a community clinic. This prevention education, coupled with which of the following, comprise comprehensive, evidence-based approaches that form the foundation for reducing opioid overdose deaths?

   A. Naloxone access through harm reduction organizations and pharmacies, reduced insurance co-payment for medication for opioid use disorder (MOUD), and family support
   B. Naloxone standing orders, MOUD treatment, and recovery support
   C. Expanded naloxone access policies, MOUD treatment engagement and retention, and recovery support
   D. Medicaid expansion of naloxone access, MOUD treatment engagement, and recovery support
   E. Naloxone standing orders and co-prescription of naloxone with opioid prescriptions, MOUD treatment engagement, and family support

   Answer: C

   Explanation: Overdose prevention education and expanded naloxone access policies broadly, including further expansion through an FDA approval in March

2023 for over-the-counter purchase, are short-term ways to reduce overdose deaths; coupled with improved MOUD treatment access and retention and recovery supports provide the foundation for long-term reduction in death due to opioid overdose [19].

Reference: Nataraj [19] and Legislative Analysis and Public Policy Association [4]

3. Public health strategies to reduce Hepatitis C virus (HCV) transmission among persons who inject drugs should prioritize which of the following?

   A. Identify which populations are most affected by HCV; dissemination information about HCV prevention to practitioners, and address community stigma towards persons who inject drugs
   B. Identify which populations are most affected by HCV; provide timely and accurate information about HCV prevention and treatment to key populations; and address community and practitioner stigmatizing attitudes towards persons who inject drugs
   C. Provide timely and accurate information about HCV prevention and treatment to key populations; address community stigmatizing attitudes towards persons who inject drugs; and engage community clinics in identifying new cases of HCV
   D. Expand syringe exchange programs across clinic and hospital settings; provide timely and accurate information about HCV prevention and treatment to key populations; and reduce stigmatizing attitudes among practitioners
   E. Identify which populations are most affected by HCV; work with community clinics to increase access to HCV treatment; and address stigmatizing attitudes towards persons who inject drugs

   Answer: B

   Explanation: Public health efforts to reduce HCV transmission include epidemiological surveillance to identify key populations who are most affected; increase access to sterile syringe programs and promoting treatment engagement; providing timely HCV prevention and treatment information to the public and practitioners; and continuous efforts to reduce stigma relating to persons who inject drugs among clinicians, law enforcement, and the public.

   Reference: van Boekel LC [13]

4. Expansion of public health efforts in the city in which you are working includes implementing a series of opioid overdose prevention policies. In addition to naloxone access, which of the following *tertiary* prevention efforts could contribute to reducing harms among persons who inject drugs?

   A. Syringe exchange programs, availability of fentanyl test strips and wound care to treat abscesses
   B. Syringe exchange programs, access to medication for opioid use disorder, and engagement in recovery programs

C. Syringe exchange programs, availability of fentanyl test strips, and access to medication for opioid use disorder
D. Availability of fentanyl test strips, access to naloxone, and access to medication for opioid use disorder
E. Syringe exchange programs, access to naloxone, and recovery programs

Answer: A

Explanation: Opioid overdose prevention policies that focus on *tertiary prevention* are the hallmark harm reduction efforts to further reduce the health impacts on persons with an opioid use disorder, including persons who are in treatment and persons who have relapsed or are not currently in treatment.

Reference: Chapter 5: Recovery: the many paths to wellness [12]

5. New policies that eliminate the need for a waiver to treat persons with a substance use disorder have led to expanded access to treatment. This expansion was enacted through the Consolidated Appropriations Act of 2023. One of the significant changes in this Act expanded treatment access through:

A. Rescheduling buprenorphine so it is no longer on the list of Schedule III controlled substances
B. Repealing the Controlled Substances Act that expanded practitioner ability to prescribe buprenorphine for OUD
C. Repeal of the Controlled Substances Act that expanded state naloxone access laws
D. Aligning state laws and policies for prescribing buprenorphine
E. Increased DEA training hours required for practitioners who prescribe any controlled substances

Answer: B

Explanation: The Consolidated Appropriations Act (2023) included the Mainstreaming Addiction Treatment Act that any practitioner with a standard Drug Enforcement Administration (DEA) registration to prescribe schedule III-controlled substances could now prescribe buprenorphine for OUD, subject to state laws [15].

Reference: Pub. L. No. 117-238. *Consolidated Appropriations Act*, 2023 https://www.congress.gov/117/plaws/publ328/PLAW-117publ328.pdf

References

1. Brownson RC, Chriqui JF, Stamatakis KA. Understanding evidence-based public health policy. Am J Public Health. 2009;99(9):1576–83.
2. Butler JC. 2017 ASTHO president's challenge: public health approaches to preventing substance misuse and addiction. J Public Health Manag Pract. 2017;23(5):531–6.
3. DeSimone EM, Tilleman JA, Kaku KA, Erickson CT. Expanding access to naloxone. US Pharm. 2018;43(3):16–20.

4. Legislative Analysis and Public Policy Association. Naloxone access: summary of state laws. 2023. [cited 2025 Jun 21]. Available from: https://legislativeanalysis.org/wp-content/uploads/2023/02/Naloxone-Access-Summary-of-State-Laws.pdf.
5. Laraque F, Varma JK. A public health approach to hepatitis C in an urban setting. Am J Public Health. 2017;107(6):922–6.
6. Peglow SL, Binswanger IA. Preventing opioid overdose in the clinic and hospital: analgesia and opioid antagonists. Med Clin North Am. 2018;102(4):621–34.
7. Pitt AL, Humphreys K, Brandeau ML. Modeling health benefits and harms of public policy responses to the US opioid epidemic. Am J Public Health. 2018;108(10):1394–400.
8. Ryan SA, Ammerman SD, Committee on Substance Use and Prevention. Counseling parents and teens about marijuana use in the era of legalization of marijuana. Pediatrics. 2017;139(3):e20164069.
9. SAMHSA. MAT statutes, regulations, and guidelines [Internet]. 2019 [cited 2019 May 17]. Available from: https://www.samhsa.gov/medication-assisted-treatment/statutes-regulations-guidelines.
10. SAMHSA. Laws and regulations [Internet]. 2019 [cited 2019 May 17]. Available from: https://www.samhsa.gov/about-us/who-we-are/laws-regulations.
11. SAMHSA. Medication and counseling treatment [Internet]. 2019 [cited 2019 May 17]. Available from: https://www.samhsa.gov/medication-assisted-treatment/treatment.
12. Chapter 5: Recovery: the many paths to wellness. In: Facing addiction in America: the surgeon general's report on alcohol, drugs, and health [Internet]. US Department of Health and Human Services; 2016 [cited 2018 Nov 16]. Available from: https://www.ncbi.nlm.nih.gov/books/NBK424846/.
13. van Boekel LC, Brouwers EPM, van Weeghel J, Garretsen HFL. Stigma among health professionals towards patients with substance use disorders and its consequences for healthcare delivery: systematic review. Drug Alcohol Depend. 2013;131(1):23–35.
14. Consolidated Appropriations Act, 2023, Pub. L. No. 117-328, 136 Stat. 4459 (2022).
15. Substance Abuse and Mental Health Services Administration. Waiver elimination (MAT Act) [Internet]. Washington, DC: U.S. Department of Health & Human Services. [cited 2025 Jun 11]. Available from: https://www.samhsa.gov/substance-use/treatment/statutes-regulations-guidelines/mat-acthttps://www.samhsa.gov/substance-use/treatment/statutes-regulations-guidelines/mat-act.
16. U.S. Department of Health and Human Services, Substance Abuse and Mental Health Services Administration. Medications for the treatment of opioid use disorder. Fed Regist [Internet]. 2024 [cited 2025 Jun 11];89(23):7528–63. Available from: https://www.federalregister.gov/documents/2024/02/02/2024-01693/medications-for-the-treatment-of-opioid-use-disorderhttps://www.federalregister.gov/documents/2024/02/02/2024-01693/medications-for-the-treatment-of-opioid-use-disorder.
17. Substance Abuse and Mental Health Services Administration. The 42 CFR Part 8 final rule table of changes [Internet]. Washington, DC: U.S. Department of Health & Human Services. [updated 2024 Jan 31; cited 2025 Jun 11]. Available from: https://www.samhsa.gov/substance-use/treatment/opioid-treatment-program/42-cfr-part-8/changeshttps://www.samhsa.gov/substance-use/treatment/opioid-treatment-program/42-cfr-part-8/changes.
18. Bohler RM, Freeman PR, Villani J, Hunt T, Linas BS, Walley AY, Green TC, Lofwall MR, Bridden C, Frazier LA, Fanucchi LC, Talbert JC, Chandler R. The policy landscape for naloxone distribution in four states highly impacted by fatal opioid overdoses. Drug Alcohol Depend Rep. 2023;6:100126. https://doi.org/10.1016/j.dadr.2022.100126. Epub 2022 Dec 5. PMID: 36643788; PMCID: PMC9838196.
19. Nataraj N, Rikard SM, Zhang K, Jiang X, Guy GP Jr, Rice K, Mattson CL, Gladden RM, Mustaquim DM, Illg ZN, Seth P, Noonan RK, Losby JL. Public health interventions and overdose-related outcomes among persons with opioid use disorder. JAMA Netw Open. 2024;7(4):e244617. https://doi.org/10.1001/jamanetworkopen.2024.4617. PMID: 38568691; PMCID: PMC10993074.

20. Ahmad FB, Cisewski JA, Rossen LM, Sutton P. Provisional drug overdose death counts. National Center for Health Statistics; 2025. https://doi.org/10.15620/cdc/20250305008.
21. Gravlee E, Ramachandran S, Cafer A, Holmes E, McGregor J, Jordan T, Rosenthal M. Naloxone accessibility under the state standing order across Mississippi. JAMA Netw Open. 2023;6(7):e2321939. https://doi.org/10.1001/jamanetworkopen.2023.21939. PMID: 37410464; PMCID: PMC10326645.
22. U.S. Food and Drug Administration. FDA approves first over-the-counter naloxone nasal spray. [Press release]. 2023. https://www.fda.gov/news-events/press-announcements/fda-approves-first-over-counter-naloxone-nasal-spray. Accessed on 23 June 2025.
23. Frederique K. Trump's funding cuts jeopardize fentanyl overdose prevention and recovery. Drug Policy Alliance; 2025. https://drugpolicy.org/news/trumps-funding-cuts-jeopardize-fentanyl-overdose-prevention-and-recovery/. Accessed on 22 June 2025.

Ethical and Legal Considerations

24

María Luisa Mittal, Leo Beletsky, and Peter J. Davidson

High-Yield Review Points

- The key ethical principles of beneficence, non-maleficence, respect for autonomy, and justice should guide the practice of addiction psychiatry.
- Everyday stigma faced by persons with substance use disorder can be magnified by stigma of medication-assisted treatment for opioid use disorders, and this can influence treatment access and retention.
- Current legal interventions to reduce overdose mortality in the United States include laws expanding access and availability to naloxone to help bystanders and/or first responders to reverse opioid overdoses.
- Regulatory frameworks under which opioid treatments have been delivered in the United States were marked by a period of limited regulation followed by a period marked by extreme regulation.
- Coordination and integration of primary care and substance use treatment must protect patient privacy using the general rule established by CFR 42 Part 2 and the HIPAA Privacy Rule.

M. L. Mittal · P. J. Davidson (✉)
Department of Medicine, University of California San Diego, La Jolla, CA, USA
e-mail: pdavidson@health.ucsd.edu

L. Beletsky
Department of Medicine, University of California San Diego, La Jolla, CA, USA

School of Law & Bouvé College of Health Sciences, Northeastern University, Boston, MA, USA
e-mail: l.beletsky@neu.edu

C. Marienfeld, M. Soltani (eds.), *AAAP Review of Addiction Psychiatry*,
https://doi.org/10.1007/978-3-032-24174-0_24

Introduction

Addiction psychiatry is a medical practice that manages substance use disorders with evidence-based clinical interventions. Ethics, stigma and discrimination, and legal discussions are presented using several examples from persons with opioid use disorders (OUDs) seeking medication for addiction treatment (MAT) as illustration. The approach to screening, assessment, and clinical care for persons with SUDs is based within the four principles of biomedical ethics. Any stigma or discrimination the patient has experienced due to their diagnosis should be addressed. Additionally, the practitioner should be informed of current regulatory frameworks that may guide implementation and utilization of treatment options. With this information in hand, the addiction psychiatrist will offer the best approach and information to address the person's needs at the time.

Medical Ethics

Addiction psychiatry, like all clinical practices, often encounters difficult healthcare decisions. Beauchamp and Childress' principles of biomedical ethics allow us to question patient care and improve clinical decision-making for patients and their families [1]. The four basic principles of biomedical ethics are: (1) beneficence, (2) non-maleficence, (3) respect for autonomy, and (4) justice. Many readers may be familiar with these principles in the clinical research context, particularly as they discuss informed consent when enrolling or referring patients into trials. Additionally, physicians must build trust with their patients and have a fiduciary duty to protect information [2]. These principles should also guide daily patient care.

The principle of beneficence requires the physician's intent of doing good for the patient (i.e., tailoring care to avoid additional burdens for the patient). Non-maleficence explicitly requires the physician do no harm to the patient. Respect for autonomy ensures the patient's decision-making process in enrolling in or denying substance use treatment is free of coercion. To help respect a patient's autonomy, it is important to fully explain the risks and benefits of all treatment options so they can make an informed decision. The principle of justice requires that treatment options be fair to all patient populations and that they remain in compliance with federal and state regulations. Finally, physicians are also responsible for social and political advocacy to improve substance use treatment resources to improve patient health.

Clinical settings with substance use disorders can rely upon ethical principles to ensure patients understand the physical and legal implications of their diagnosis and treatment options. It is challenging to apply the non-maleficence principle when the treatment itself will allow a person with an opioid use disorder to experience opioid withdrawal; however, one can rely on the principle of beneficence to explain the net benefit of medication for addiction treatment (MAT) for this person. Together, the patient and the addiction psychiatrist can use ethical principles to discuss the physical (e.g., side effects) and psychosocial risks (e.g., stigma and discrimination), as well as the benefits, when they tailor treatment plans. By doing so, the patient will be fully informed and know the implications of agreeing to start a treatment regimen. Physicians must uphold the principle of respect for autonomy when physician and patient goals differ. For example, a physician may insist on methadone as the optimal treatment to reduce the risks associated with a patient's opioid use disorder, including overdose and death. However, if the patient's competing priorities place more value on their quality of life and is expressing concern over methadone clinics, the physician can respect the patient's autonomy and offer pros and cons on alternative treatments such as buprenorphine, naltrexone, or non-pharmacologic treatments.

Using the principle of justice, the addiction psychiatrist can help ensure fair distribution of treatment resources among patient populations with substance use disorders. For example, one should ensure that if medication options like buprenorphine and methadone are equally available in their clinical setting, they should be equally available to all patients with opioid use disorder regardless of gender, race, or ethnicity. This principle must be used with the principle of non-maleficence to ensure the optimal dosing for each treatment option. This is particularly important since methadone under-dosing is more common among programs and clinical trials serving high proportions of African American patients, raising critical concerns in care delivery to reduce racial disparities [3, 4]. Please refer to Part III, Chap. 18, for additional information on treatment disparities among underserved populations.

Informed consent includes a discussion with the patient to address concerns and confirm the knowledge guiding their decision to participate or not participate in substance use treatment. To protect the patient and others from harm, the addiction psychiatrist should be aware that they may need to balance the respect for autonomy of a person with impaired judgment, alongside obligations of beneficence, non-maleficence, and justice. One should be prepared to revisit informed consent discussions and document them as part of the medical record as the patient's clinical presentation and decisions change. Using the principle of respect for autonomy, one should recognize that a signed consent to treatment is not equivalent to an informed consent. Given the complexities of multifaceted MAT programs, patient consent to start a treatment plan requires a carefully documented patient orientation on treatment options and requirements [5]. To give an informed consent, the patient must know and understand the benefits and consequences of enrolling in MAT. A transparent approach to consenting to treatment will include full disclosure of all procedures involved in MAT, recordkeeping of personal data and confidentiality (i.e., networks with access to that data, divulging information without additional consent), involuntary discharge procedures, and facility safety instructions [5].

Stigma and Discrimination

Stigmatized persons are often labeled by an individual trait or characteristic that culturally devalues them [6]. Link and Phelan describe status loss and discrimination as the consequences of stigma when a person is labeled with an undesirable characteristic [6]. Consequently, discrimination of persons with substance use disorders may lead to unequal treatment outcomes [7, 8]. Patients may be facing double stigma related to seeking MAT and to the underlying substance use disorder, which may produce exclusion from social and economic life [9, 10]. Discrimination and stigma related to substance use may be a complex barrier to accessing and receiving treatment [11–13] and is associated with poorer physical and mental health [14]. Stigma can be enacted by different people, including healthcare providers, and experienced differently by different types of patients, but it can be modifiable [10, 15]. To minimize stigma and discrimination for persons with substance use disorders, it is important to treat patients with compassion, respect, and dignity regardless of substance use career, race, age, gender, disabilities, or sexual orientation [16].

MAT-related stigma can be driven by different attributes in the substance use patient. Stigma can also affect the internal operation of MAT programs when healthcare staff absorb society's MAT-related stigma and deliver services with punitive behavior. For example, some factors associated with increased stigma among methadone patients have been previously described as concurrent drug use, co-occurring psychiatric disorders (e.g., anxiety and depression), self-reported positive HIV status, current pain or discomfort, a previous history of substance use treatment, and higher education (i.e., attended college) [17–19]. When addressing patient questions related to starting treatment, it would be helpful to probe for MAT-related stigma concerns (e.g., job discrimination, worries about swapping one drug for another) and take the time to address any negative thoughts or feelings that could diminish the patient's self-image resulting from starting MAT. Leadership, supervision, and educational efforts can help improve attitudes toward persons in MAT [5, 16].

Addictions and the Law

Internationally, drug policies vary widely based on the nation's approach to reduce drug production, trafficking, and consumption. The United States maintains a criminal justice oriented approach to drug use rather than a health-oriented approach. Drug control efforts in the United States have traditionally focused on international eradication of product, trafficking suppression, and criminalizing consumers. Despite this drug policy approach, overdose deaths in the United States, driven by synthetic opioids (other than methadone), continue to increase significantly [20, 21]. In response, in 2017 the United States declared a national public health emergency to address the national opioid overdose crisis to improve "prevention, treatment, and recovery support services" and improve opioid prescribing practices, among other strategies to reduce opioid use [22]. Other countries have moved toward a more public health-oriented approach, regulating drug consumption while improving access to substance use treatment. For example, in 2001, Portugal introduced Law 30/2000 to decriminalize personal drug use, ending penal sanctions for possession, and rapidly expanded the provision of evidence-based treatment, which led to significant reductions in drug-related deaths [23].

A history of tough sentencing rules for drug violations has exacerbated racial disparities in the criminal justice system in the United States. For example, the Rockefeller Drug Laws in New York State in 1973 raised criminal penalties for the sale and possession of drugs, primarily heroin. But an ambiguity in the law permitted discretionary exceptions that would allow for those being arrested to come primarily from black and Latino neighborhoods [24]. More than 5.4 million persons are currently under the supervision of US adult correctional systems and have been shown to have unmet healthcare needs and high rates of substance use disorders [25]. Different models for linking persons with substance use disorders at several stages of the criminal justice system process into detoxification management and substance use treatment for alcohol and opioids can be found in Chap. 18.

Other legal interventions that can help expand access to substance use treatment are the expansion of Medicaid to provide coverage for previously uninsured Americans. Following the Affordable Care Act (ACA) in 2008 and the 2012 Supreme Court's decision on Medicaid expansion, US states decided whether to adopt the Medicaid expansion for most low-income adults to 138% of the federal poverty level. As of 2024, 41 states including the District of Columbia had approved Medicaid expansion [26]. However, there is a need to repeal the Medicaid Inmate Exclusion Policy and reform reimbursement for substance use treatment inside correctional systems [27]. The Section 1115 waivers are an opportunity for Medicaid programs to improve the continuum of care for opioid use disorders among the incarcerated prior to their release but are vulnerable to inconsistencies in coverage [28, 29].

Using the principle of justice, many leaders have called for drug policy reforms to prevent the harms associated with substance use. The criminalization of consumers in US drug policy has evolved to public health efforts aimed at reducing overdose and blood-borne infections driven by substance use. Resistance to needle-exchange programs persists in most states, and the Department of Justice is threatening criminal prosecution for those involved in supervised injection facilities [30]. Current legal interventions to reduce overdose mortality in the United States include expanding naloxone access to help bystanders and/or first responders to reverse opioid overdoses. All 50 states and the District of Columbia have modified their laws to increase access to naloxone, which aids in reducing liability fears for those prescribing or dispensing naloxone [31]. Additionally, as of 2023, 48 states and the District of Columbia had passed overdose Good Samaritan laws to protect bystanders from arrest or prosecution when they report an overdose in good faith [31].

Medical Licensure and Credentialing in Addiction Psychiatry

Addiction psychiatrists should be aware of the regulatory frameworks under which opioid agonist treatments have been delivered in the United States. Before the Harrison Narcotic Tax Act of 1914, there was a period of limited regulation favoring the clinical independence of individual providers, which was followed by a period marked by extreme regulation. The Harrison Narcotics Tax Act, introduced to implement a treaty obligation to regulate the manufacture and trade of opioids, contained a clause relating to the medical use of narcotics that the Supreme Court interpreted as prohibiting the prescription of narcotics to habitual users on the grounds that addiction was not a disease [32, 33]. Later cases, particularly *Linder v. United States* in 1925, reestablished the right of a physician to prescribe opioids to a patient in her direct care on the basis that such behavior amounted to the exercise of "professional conduct with which Congress never intended to interfere" [34]. However, by this time opioid agonist treatment was limited to a very small number of specialized clinics.

In 1958, a joint committee of the American Bar Association and the American Medical Association recommended trials of opioid agonist treatment in outpatient settings [5]. Later, the Controlled Substances Act of 1970 required registration with the Drug Enforcement Administration (DEA) for prescribing, dispensing, and administering controlled substances. As support for treatment options continued to grow, Congress amended the Controlled Substances Act with the Narcotic Addict Treatment Act of 1974. This Act brought several changes and improved coordination between the US Department of Health and Human Services (DHHS) and the DEA. It established the National Institute on Drug Abuse (NIDA) independently from the National Institute on Mental Health and split opioid treatment regulation between NIDA (responsible for treatment standards) and the Food and Drug Administration (FDA; responsible for safety, effectiveness, and approval of new drugs for treatment). The Narcotic Addict Treatment Act defined maintenance treatment in federal law and required separate DEA registration for dispensing opioids for opioid use disorder treatment. Therefore, a physician would no longer be able to prescribe methadone for OUD without additional registration. Once the DHHS determined a medical practitioner was qualified based on treatment standards established by NIDA, they could apply for and obtain registration from the DEA [5]. Outpatient methadone treatment can only be provided by opioid treatment programs (OTPs), which are registered by the DEA and certified at the federal level by Substance Abuse and Mental Health Services Administration (SAMHSA) [5, 35]. OTPs can include outpatient, intensive outpatient, residential, and hospital settings, which are in conformance with Title 42 of the Code of Federal Regulations Part 8 (CFR Part 8) [5, 36, 37].

The Drug Addiction Treatment Act (DATA 2000) amended the Narcotic Addict Treatment Act by allowing physicians to obtain a waiver from separate registration requirements for Schedule III, IV, and V medications approved by the FDA to treat opioid use disorder. However, physicians (MD or DO; and later nurse practitioners and physicians' assistants) had to meet certain qualifications under DATA provisions that include state license, DEA registration, certification/training for treatment and management of opioid use disorders, treat a maximum of 30 patients within the first year, and have the capacity to refer patients to counseling and ancillary services [5, 38]. Given that DATA 2000 does not disqualify practitioners in residency programs, SAMHSA granted waivers to those with unrestricted licenses and DEA registration [38]. In 2002, the FDA-approved buprenorphine for opioid use disorder treatment and for supervised withdrawal, which allowed physicians with the waiver in non-opioid treatment program settings to prescribe to patients. In 2013, modifications to 42 CFR Part 8 allowed buprenorphine products to be dispensed without adhering to a time in treatment [36, 37], and in 2023 Section 1262 of the Consolidated Appropriations Act removed the need for practitioners to have a waiver and allowing any practitioner who has a current DEA registration with Schedule III authority to prescribe buprenorphine for OUD [39].

Privacy Laws in the Context of Addiction Psychiatry

Guided by the principles of beneficence and non-maleficence, the addiction psychiatrist may need to disclose patient information about substance use treatment to improve coordination and integration of primary care and substance use treatment. The Health Insurance Portability and Accountability Act of 1996 (HIPAA) Privacy Rule (45 CFR Parts 160 and 164) sets limits and conditions on the uses of personal health information and patient medical records without patient consent [40]. If a substance use treatment program (including individual providers and provider organizations) transmits health information in an electronic form (e.g., inquiry of eligibility to health plans, submission of claims) it is considered a covered entity, and they must comply with the Privacy Rule. Under the Privacy Rule, a program may not use or disclose protected health information, which includes information that may identify a patient such as medical record numbers and employment information [40].

As previously mentioned, stigma related to substance use disorders may act as a barrier to seek or stay in treatment. Therefore, Congress moved to improve confidentiality laws and extend legal protection to substance use treatment records in the 1970s. This set of healthcare regulations are known as Title 42 of the Code of Federal Regulations Part 2 (42 CFR Part 2) [40], or Part 2. Part 2 ensures that a patient does not face adverse consequences related to criminal and domestic proceedings because they are receiving substance use treatment. Part 2 prohibits disclosing any information that could identify a patient as having a history of substance use without written consent. Part 2 and the HIPAA Privacy Rule have different general rules regarding the use of patient health information. Substance use programs will not disclose information without consent or identify an exception to the rule in Part 2 that allows disclosure and ensure that it is permitted by the Privacy Rule [40]. For example, Part 2 allows programs to report limited information to law enforcement on crimes that occur on program premises, including patient name and address [40]. Part 2 will also allow programs to release information in response to a subpoena if the patient provides written consent, which will also comply with the Privacy Rule qualified protective order [40]. Providers are also required by law to report child abuse and neglect to local authorities [5]. It is important to identify if the type of setting the provider is in, and if Part 2, HIPAA Privacy Rule, or both apply. The Office of the National Coordinator (ONC) for Health Information

Technology and the SAMHSA offer technical guidance to help stakeholders understand how Part 2 applies in complex healthcare settings.

Chapter Review Questions

1. A 23-year-old African American man engaged in commercial sex work and a 42-year-old Latinx woman homemaker with a history of back problems both present to an opioid treatment program seeking maintenance treatment for opioid use disorder. Which of the following principles of biomedical ethics is most likely to be used when offering treatment options equally among patients with substance use disorders?

   A. Beneficence
   B. Justice
   C. Non-maleficence
   D. Insurance
   E. Fiduciary

   Correct Answer: B. Justice. Justice is the medical ethical principle that requires that treatment options are fair to all patient populations and that they remain in compliance with federal and state regulations. Beneficence and non-maleficence are other medical ethical principles unrelated to equity of treatment. Insurance is a distracting answer and not a medical ethical principle.
2. A 35-year-old female construction worker residing in a suburban area is unable to commute to the methadone opioid treatment program (OTP) for her opioid use disorder. She found a general medicine practitioner at a local community clinic who prescribes buprenorphine. Which of the following legislations allowed healthcare providers with a current DEA registration that includes Schedule III authority to prescribe buprenorphine for opioid use disorders?

   A. Narcotic Addict Treatment Act of 1974
   B. Harrison Narcotics Tax Act of 1914
   C. Drug Addiction Treatment Act of 2000
   D. Affordable Care Act of 2010
   E. Section 1262 of the Consolidated Appropriations Act, 2023

   Correct Answer: E. Section 1262 of the Consolidated Appropriations Act, 2023 removed the original Drug Addiction Treatment Act (DATA 2000) requirement that providers first apply for and receive a waiver from separate registration requirements. DATA 200 amended the Narcotic Addict Treatment Act by allowing physicians (MD or DO; and later nurse practitioners and physicians' assistants) to obtain a waiver from separate registration requirements for Schedule III, IV, and V medications approved by the FDA to treat opioid use disorder. The Harrison Narcotics Tax Act of 1914 does not regulate the clinical independence of individual providers. The Affordable Care Act of 2010 is a distracting answer.

3. A 34-year-old female jewellery sales associate with a history of opioid use disorder recently completed a residential treatment program. After a stressful week back at work, she used her regular oxycodone dose and experienced an overdose. Fortunately, her sister called 911 and first responders arrived in time to reverse the overdose. Which of the following legal interventions have helped reduce opioid overdoses in the United States?

   A. Law 30/2000
   B. Rockefeller Drug Laws in New York State in 1973
   C. Title 42 of the Code of Federal Regulations Part 2
   D. Expansion of naloxone access
   E. NATA (Narcotic Addict Treatment Act) of 1970

   Correct Answer: A. The expansion of naloxone access has directly reduced opioid overdoses by increasing the availability of an overdose reversal drug in the community. Law 30/2000 has helped reduce opioid overdoses in Portugal. Rockefeller Drug Laws raised criminal penalties for the sale and possession of drugs, primarily heroin. Part 2 is a distracting answer and is related to privacy laws.

4. A 48-year-old male park maintenance worker is concerned he may not make his shift on time if he starts methadone maintenance treatment for his opioid use disorder. He fears he may be fired from his job and questions would arise if he requests a later start time. Which of the following consequences of stigma should be addressed when probing for patient concerns regarding treatment?

   A. Positive stereotypes
   B. Status loss and discrimination
   C. Impartial treatment
   D. Improved self-image
   E. Acceptance

   Correct Answer: B. If the patient's employer finds out he needs a later start time to start treatment for an opioid use disorder, they will know he is using opioids. Link and Phelan describe status loss and discrimination as the consequences of stigma when a person is labeled with an undesirable characteristic. Positive stereotypes, improved self-image, acceptance, and impartial treatment are the opposite of experiences related to stigma.

5. A 22-year-old male with 3 years of methadone maintenance treatment recently changed jobs and lost insurance coverage. If a substance use treatment program is subject to both 42 CFR Part 2 and HIPPA Privacy Rule, can they disclose a medical record number to obtain authorization for referring an individual to another healthcare provider?

   A. Yes, the medical record number can be used to identify the patient by sources external to the program.

B. Yes, even though the medical record number can identify the patient, it is important to not delay the referral while waiting for patient consent.
C. No, a medical record number is considered protected health information.
D. No, since only the HIPPA Privacy Rule applies to the referring provider.
E. No, one must contact legal counsel for assistance before reaching a decision.

Correct Answer: C. Under the Privacy Rule, a program may not use or disclose protected health information, which includes information that may identify a patient such as the medical record number. The other options are distracting answers.

References

1. Beauchamp TL, Childress JF. Principles of biomedical ethics. 7th ed. New York: Oxford University Press; 2012.
2. Dickens BM, Cook RJ. Law and ethics in conflict over confidentiality? Int J Gynecol Obstet. 2000;70(3):385–91.
3. D'Aunno T, Park S, Pollack HA. Evidence-based treatment for opioid use disorders: a national study of T methadone dose levels, 2011–2017. J Subst Abus Treat. 2019;96:18–22.
4. Ross RK, Inose S, Shulman M. Variation in opioid agonist dosing in clinical trials by race and ethnicity. JAMA Netw Open. 2024;7(10):e2436612.
5. U.S. Department of Health and Human Services. Medication for opioid use disorder (Treatment Improvement Protocol Series, No. 63). DHHS publication No. PEP21-02-01-002. Rockville: Substance Abuse and Mental Health Services Administration; 2021.
6. Link BG, Phelan JC. Conceptualizing stigma. Annu Rev Sociol. 2001;27(1):363–85.
7. Bommersbach TJ, Jegede O, Na PJ, Stefanovics EA, Rhee TG, Rosenheck RA. Treatment of substance use disorders among black and white adults: ratees, correlates, and racial discrimination. J Addict Dis. 2022;40(3):345–56.
8. Crapanzano KA, Hammarlund R, Ahmad B, Hunsinger N, Kullar R. The association between perceived stigma and substance use disorder treatment outcomes: a review. Subst Abus Rehabil. 2019:1–12.
9. Parker R, Aggleton P. HIV and AIDS-related stigma and discrimination: a conceptual framework and implications for action. Soc Sci Med. 2003;57(1):13–24.
10. Smith LR, Earnshaw VA, Copenhaver MM, Cunningham CO. Substance use stigma: reliability and validity of a theory-based scale for substance-using populations. Drug Alcohol Depend. 2016;162:34–43.
11. American Association for the Treatment of Opioid Dependence (AATOD). Canon of ethics [Internet]. AATOD; 2025. [cited 2025 Oct10]. Available from: https://www.aatod.org/apply/canon-of-ethics/.
12. Skinner N, Feather NT, Freeman T, Roche A. Stigma and discrimination in health-care provision to drug users: the role of values, affect, and deservingness judgments. J Appl Soc Psych. 2007;37(1):163–86.
13. Deering DE, Sheridan J, Sellman JD, Adamson SJ, Pooley S, Robertson R, Henderson C. Consumer and treatment provider perspectives on reducing barriers to opioid substitution treatment and improving treatment attractiveness. Addict Behav. 2011;36(6):636–42.
14. Lago RR, Peter E, Bógus CM. Harm reduction and tensions in trust and distrust in a mental health service: a qualitative approach. Subst Abuse Treat Prev Policy. 2017;12(1):12.
15. Ahern J, Stuber J, Galea S. Stigma, discrimination and the health of illicit drug users. Drug Alcohol Depend. 2007;88(2):188–96.

16. Kulesza M, Larimer ME, Rao D. Substance use related stigma: what we know and the way forward. J Addict Behav Ther Rehabil. 2013;2(2):2–6.
17. Tran BX, Vu PB, Nguyen LH, et al. Drug addiction stigma in relation to methadone maintenance treatment by different service delivery models in Vietnam. BMC Public Health. 2016;16(1):238.
18. Luoma JB, Twohig MP, Waltz T, et al. An investigation of stigma in individuals receiving treatment for substance abuse. Addict Behav. 2007;32(7):1331–46.
19. Carl A, Pasman E, Broman MJ, Lister JJ, Agius E, Resko SM. Experiences of healthcare and substance use treatment provider-based stigma among patients receiving methadone. Drug Alcohol Depend Rep. 2023;6:100138.
20. Scholl L, Seth P, Kariisa M, Wilson N, Baldwin G. Drug and opioid-involved overdose deaths – United States, 2013–2017. Morb Mortal Wkly Rep. 2019;67(5152):1419–27.
21. Tanz LJ. Routes of drug use among drug overdose deaths – United States, 2020–2022. Morb Mortal Wkly Rep. 2024;73:124–30.
22. U.S. Department of Health and Human Services. Determination that a public health emergency exists. 2017. [cited 2025 Oct 23]. Available from: https://aspr.hhs.gov/legal/PHE/Pages/opioids.aspx.
23. Hughes CE, Stevens A. What can we learn from the Portuguese decriminalization of illicit drugs? Br J Criminol. 2010;50(6):999–1022.
24. National Institute of Law Enforcement and Criminal Justice. The nation's toughest drug law: evaluating the New York experience – final report of the Joint Committee on New York Drug Law Evaluation. New York: The Association of the Bar of the City of New York; 1978.
25. Gann S, Kaeble D. Correctional populations in the United States, 2023. U.S. Department of Justice, Office of Justice Programs, Bureau of Justice Statistics, NCJ 310413; 2025. p. 1–25. [cited 2025 Oct 23]. Available from: https://bjs.ojp.gov/document/cpus23st.pdf.
26. Kaiser Family Foundation. Status of state Medicaid expansion decisions [Internet]. KFF State Health Facts; 2025. [cited 2025 Oct 23]. Available from: https://www.kff.org/affordable-care-act/issue-brief/status-of-state-medicaid-expansion-decisions-interactive-map/.
27. Fiscella K, Beletsky L, Wakeman SE. The inmate exception and reform of correctional health care. Am J Public Health. 2017;107(3):384.
28. Saunders S, Panchal N. Addressing the opioid crisis: a look at the evolving landscape of federal OUD treatment policies [Internet]. Kaiser Family Foundation; 2025. [cited 2025 Oct 23]. Available from: https://www.kff.org/mental-health/addressing-the-opioid-crisis-a-look-at-the-evolving-landscape-of-federal-oud-treatment-policies/.
29. RTI International. Medicaid Section 1115 Substance Use Disorder (SUD) demonstrations: features of state approaches to improve Medicaid SUD treatment delivery systems. Baltimore: Centers for Medicare & Medicaid Services; 2022. [cited 2025 Oct 22]. Available from: https://www.medicaid.gov/medicaid/section-1115-demonstrations/downloads/sud-1115-rcr-features.pdf.
30. Gostin LO, Hodge JG, Noe SA. Reframing the opioid epidemic as a national emergency. JAMA. 2017;318(16):1539–40.
31. Lieberman A, Davis C. Legal interventions to reduce overdose mortality: overdose good Samaritan Laws. Network for Public Health Law (USA); 2024 [cited Oct 7, 2025]. Available from: https://www.networkforphl.org/wp-content/uploads/2024/11/Legal-Interventions-to-Reduce-Overdose-Mortality_Overdose-Good-Samaritan-Laws.pdf.
32. Harrison Narcotics Tax Act. Public law # 63–223. 1914.
33. Webb v. United States, 249 U.S. 96, 39 S. Ct. 217, 63 L. Ed. 497. 1919.
34. Linder v. United States, 268 U.S. 5, 45 S. Ct. 446, 69 L. Ed. 819. 1925.
35. U.S. Food and Drug Administration. Methadone oral concentrate (methadone hydrochloride oral concentrate USP) and methadone sugar- free oral concentrate (methadone hydrochloride oral concentrate USP) dye-free, sugar-free, unflavored. [cited 2025 Oct 10]. Available from https://www.accessdata.fda.gov/drugsatfda_docs/label/2018/017116s032lbl.pdf.

36. Opioid drugs in maintenance and detoxification treatment of opiate addiction; proposed modification of dispensing restrictions for buprenorphine and buprenorphine combination as used in approved opioid treatment medications; correction. 42 C.F.R. § 8.12 (2015) [regulation on the Internet]. [cited 2025 Oct 23]. Available from: https://www.federalregister.gov/documents/2015/06/18/2015-14421/opioid-drugs-in-maintenance-and-detoxification-treatment-of-opiate-addiction-proposed-modification.
37. Medication Assisted Treatment for Opioid Use Disorders. 42 C.F.R. § 8 (2016) [regulation on the Internet]. [cited 2025 Oct 23]. Available from: https://www.federalregister.gov/documents/2016/07/08/2016-16120/medication-assisted-treatment-for-opioid-use-disorders.
38. U.S. Department of Health and Human Services. Qualify for a practitioner waiver [Internet]. Substance Abuse and Mental Health Services Administration; 2019. Available from: https://www.samhsa.gov/medication-assisted-treatment/buprenorphine-waiver-management/qualify-for-practitioner-waiver.
39. U.S. Department of Health and Human Services. Waiver elimination (MAT Act). Rockville: Substance Abuse and Mental Health Services Administration; 2024. [cited 2025 Oct 23]. Available from: https://www.samhsa.gov/substance-use/treatment/statutes-regulations-guidelines/mat-act.
40. CSAT (Center for Substance Abuse Treatment). The confidentiality of alcohol and drug abuse patient records regulation and the HIPAA privacy rule: implications for alcohol and substance abuse programs. DHHS publication no. (SMA) 04-3947. Rockville: Substance Abuse and Mental Health Services Administration; 2004. [cited 2025 Oct 23]. Available from: https://www.samhsa.gov/sites/default/files/part2-hipaa-comparison2004.pdf.

Index

C. Marienfeld, M. Soltani (eds.), *AAAP Review of Addiction Psychiatry*,
https://doi.org/10.1007/978-3-032-24174-0

C

T

MIX
Papier aus verantwortungsvollen Quellen
Paper from responsible sources
FSC® C105338
FSC
www.fsc.org

If you have any concerns about our products,
you can contact us on
ProductSafety@springernature.com

In case Publisher is established outside the EU,
the EU authorized representative is:
Springer Nature Customer Service Center GmbH
Europaplatz 3, 69115 Heidelberg, Germany

Printed by Libri Plureos GmbH
in Hamburg, Germany